# BROUGHTON ISLANDS
## CRUISING GUIDE

**FORMERLY TITLED
NORTH OF DESOLATION SOUND**

## Stuart Island to the Broughton Archipelago, Blackfish Sound to Port Hardy, Seymour Inlet and Cape Caution to the Discovery Coast

### Destinations, Passages, Marinas, Marine Parks and Anchorages

Other books by the same author

Cruising Handbooks:
Docks and Destinations
Anchorages and Marine Parks

Mariner Cruising Guides:
Gulf Islands Cruising Guide
Cruising to Desolation Sound

Others:
Mariner Artist John M. Horton

Antiques Afloat
From the Golden Age of boating in British Columbia

## PETER VASSILOPOULOS

# www.marineguides.com

Contents copyright © 2011 Peter Vassilopoulos.
Pacific Marine Publishing, Canada.
Prepress design and production Pacific Marine Publishing.
Printed in Canada.
Photographs and illustrations by author unless indicated otherwise.

All information and illustrations in this book are provided without guarantee and it is up to the boat operator to ensure the proper use of navigational charts and other aids to navigation. Use of charts, depth sounders, BC Sailing Directions, Small Craft Guide and other sources is recommended. Hydrographic Charts and tide and current tables should be used at all times when navigating waterways, bays, coves, harbours and marinas.
The publisher and author is not liable for marine operations leading to accident, damage or injury in any way connected with reference to this book.

Waypoints included were taken by the author at the point of reading, using a marine GPS unit. Every effort has been made to ensure accuracy but this is subject to transposition and final information cannot be guaranteed.

All rights reserved. No part of this book may be reproduced or transmitted in any form by any means without the permission of the publisher, except by a reviewer, who may show any two page sections in a review unless otherwise arranged with the publisher.
First edition–October 2003. Second printing June 2005.
New edition–Broughton Islands Cruising Guide–2011.

**Library and Archives Canada Cataloguing in Publication**

Vassilopoulos, Peter, 1940-
Broughton Islands cruising guide : a mariner's guide to the popular Broughton Islands / Peter Vassilopoulos.

Prev. ed. published with title: North of Desolation Sound.
Includes bibliographical references and index.

ISBN 978-0-919317-46-8

1. Boats and boating--British Columbia--Broughton Island Region.
2. Broughton Island Region (B.C.)--Guidebooks. I. Title.
GV776.15.B7V362 2011      797.109711'1      C2011-906108-2

Copies available from marine stores, marinas and book stores. Distribution and acquisition enquiries to Pacific Marine Publishing. Phone (604) 943-4618.
*boating@dccnet.com   www.marineguides.com*
The author welcomes emails from readers.

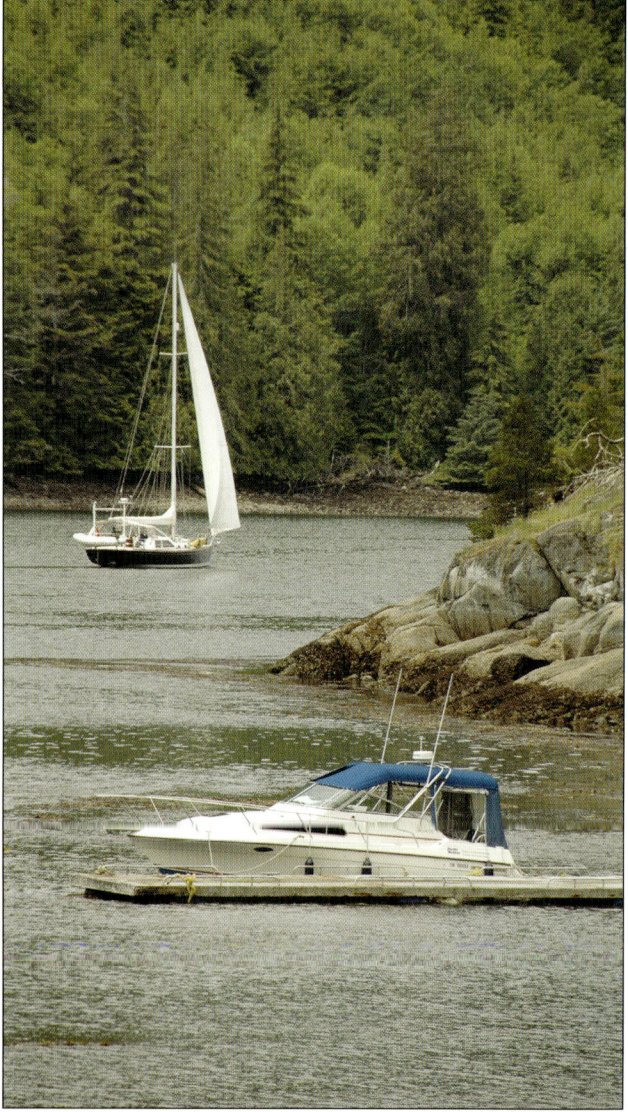

*The author's Monaro 27 used for acquiring information for this book. It is shown docked at Chatham Channel Post Office float near Minstrel Island in 2011.*

Peter Vassilopoulos is a veteran boater of over 35 years in the Pacific Northwest and British Columbia waters. He and his wife, Carla, in their boat, above, are well-known in western waters where they spend their time maintaining their marine guides that include:
**Docks and Destinations** and **Anchorages and Marine Parks.**
This book is dedicated to the memory of John Chappel who provided first hand information and direction to the author and his wife on their early voyages beyond Desolation Sound.

*Cover: A private pleasure boat with its canoes at the ready for exploring, cruises peacefully through the backwaters of the Broughton Archipelago Marine Provincial Park.*

PETER VASSILOPOULOS

# BROUGHTON ISLANDS
## CRUISING GUIDE

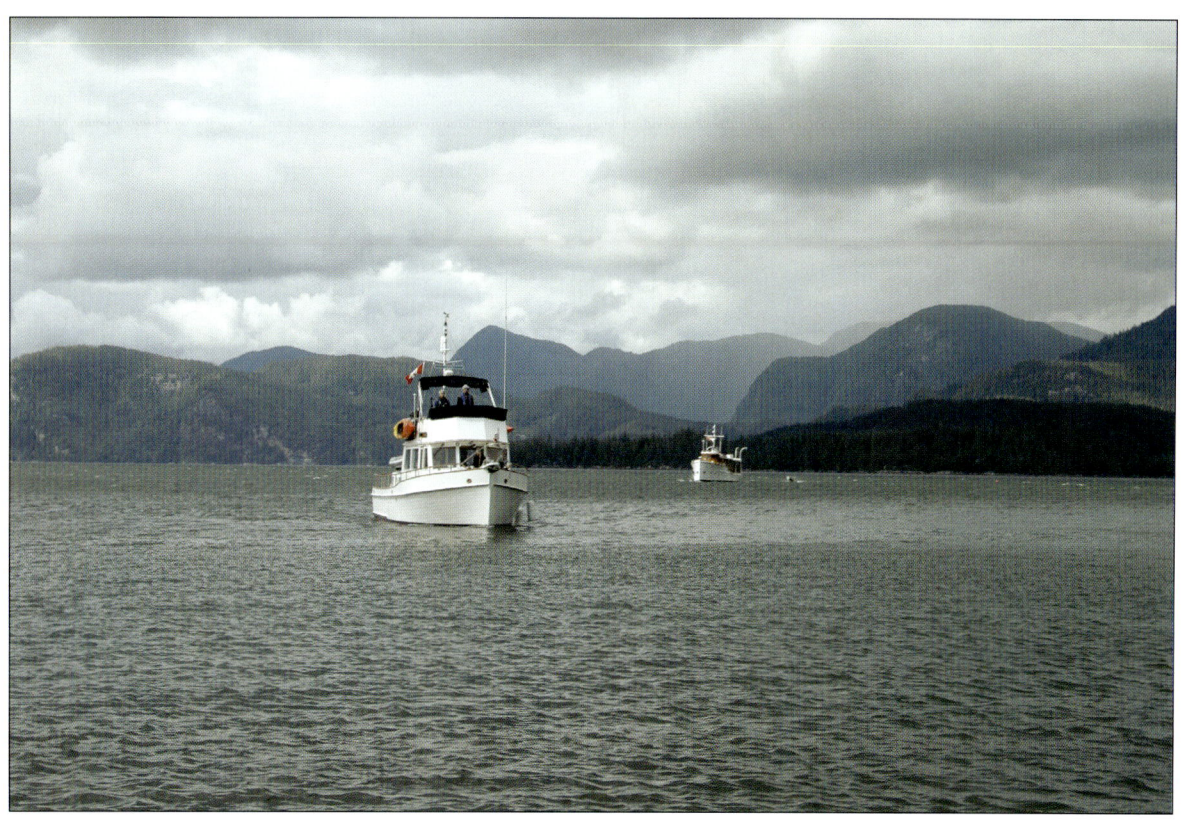

### FEATURING
ROUTES THROUGH THE TIDAL WATERS BEYOND DESOLATION SOUND,
TO THE HISTORIC NATIVE VILLAGES OF THE BROUGHTON ISLANDS, TO
SEYMOUR INLET AND AROUND CAPE CAUTION TO RIVERS INLET

WITH
### SEYMOUR INLET
BY DAVID HOAR AND NOREEN RUDD

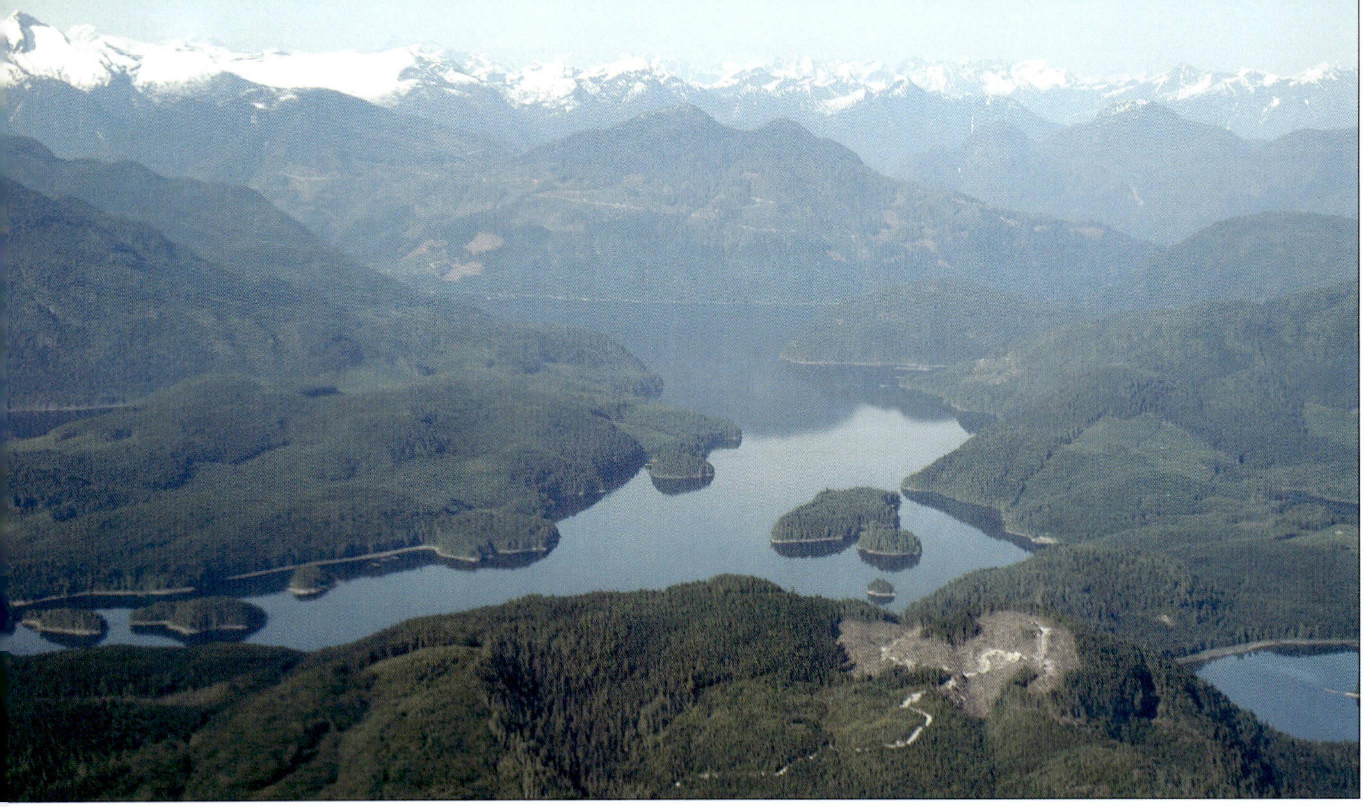

*Above: Looking east over Cordero Channel from above West Thurlow Island. Greene Point Rapids is off to the left. Mayne Channel is centre, to the right of Mink and Erasmus Islands at Crawford Anchorage. Below: Entering Drury Inlet near Sullivan Bay.*

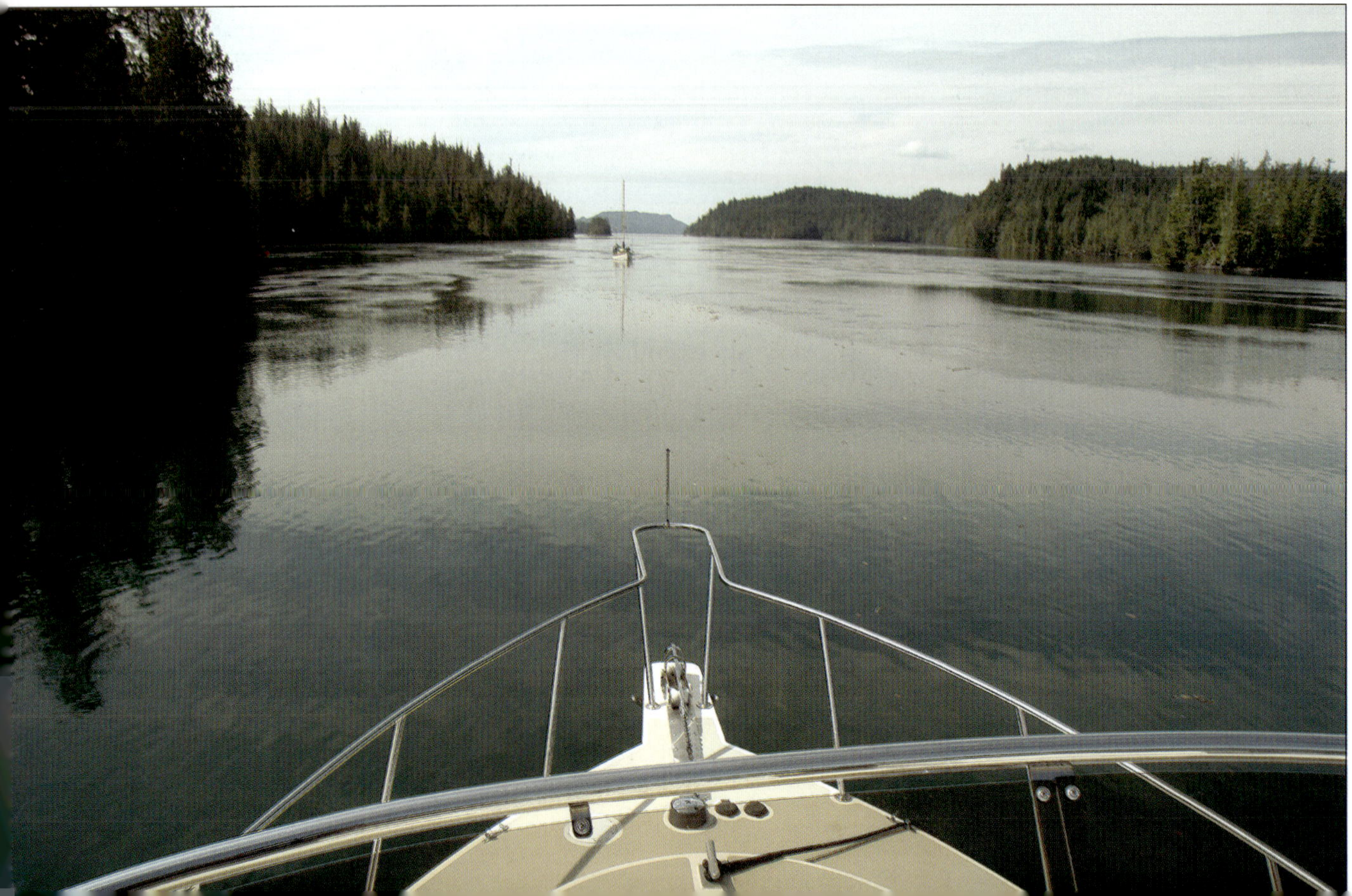

# BROUGHTON ISLANDS CRUISING GUIDE

## Marina and public dock locations

| | |
|---|---|
| Stuart Island | 27 |
| Shoal Bay | 34 |
| Cordero Channel | 37 |
| *Blind Channel | 38 |
| Kelsey Bay | 54 |
| Port Neville | 58 |
| Port Harvey | 62 |
| Minstrel Island | 68 |
| *Lagoon Cove | 71 |
| Kwatsi Bay | 79 |
| New Vancouver | 103 |
| *Echo Bay | 128 |
| Shawl Bay | 143 |
| *Sullivan Bay | 159 |
| Jennis Bay | 180 |
| **Telegraph Cove | 206 |
| Alert Bay | 207 |
| *Port McNeill | 218 |
| Sointula | 223 |
| *Port Hardy | 232 |
| *Duncanby | 246 |
| *Dawsons Landing | 249 |

*Fuel available.* ** *Gas only*

The author wishes to express gratitude to those who assisted in the acquisition of material in this book. Special thanks to Bruce Jackman, Craig Houston and pilot Krista Houston of Grizzly Helicopters and to Peter Barrett and Terry Eisfeldt of West Coast Helicopters and pilot Catherine Wykes. Thanks also to Heinz Bold and Henry Karcz for their flights. A special thanks to my wife Carla, and to Chris Fraser and Janice Graham-Andrews for their input and assistance in editing and proof reading the entire work. Many thanks go to others who have assisted in providing and correcting some of the material in this book. These include Sharon Allman, Iz Goto, David Hoar and Noreen Rudd, Norm Elliott, Carl Tenning and David Castimore. My appreciation and many thanks to Peter Schlieck of Canadian Flight Centre and to Bruce and Steve Jackman of Port McNeill Fuel Dock for assistance with boat and air trasportation into and over the Broughton Islands and to Pierre and Tove Landry and Jerome and Lucy Rose for their overnight hospitality at Echo Bay during the updating of this book.

–Peter Vassilopoulos

## CONTENTS

| | |
|---|---|
| Preface | 6 |
| Foreword | 8 |
| Pretrip Planning | 10 |
| Heading North | 13 |
| GPS References | 15 |
| Introduction | 16 |
| First Nations Villages | 18 |
| Tides and Currents | 20 |

### Sections

| | |
|---|---|
| Big Bay to Forward Harbour | 22 |
| Discovery Pass to Knight Inlet | 49 |
| Tribune Channel | 77 |
| Havannah Channel to the Broughtons | 87 |
| Knight Inlet to Fife Sound | 113 |
| The Mainland | 125 |
| Grappler, McKenzie Sounds | 164 |
| Drury Inlet, Actaeon Sound | 173 |
| Wells Pass to Allison Harbour | 184 |
| Seymour Inlet | 194 |
| Broughton Strait to Port Hardy | 202 |
| Cape Caution to Hakai Pass | 237 |
| Index | 260 |
| Bibliography | 263 |

Pacific Marine Publishing • Canada

# Preface

In the 1980s a well-known local mariner and cruise guide author, John Chappel and I met several times and discussed the Broughton Islands. His *Beyond Desolation Sound* cruising guide was not long off the press and I told him of my experience using it on a trip to the north island area. The account is related in the foreword of this book. We discussed my trip and the many passages that he had included in his book, some of which I had missed on that first journey. That discussion was to inspire me to visit them or most of them on future cruises. This I did, on numerous trips into the area since that meeting with John.

Although I have been to all areas discussed, except deep inside Seymour Inlet, I have not stopped at every single anchorage mentioned in this book. But if I have not stopped at them I have at least cruised by or into them and out again, checking depths and acknowledging as much as possible what I have heard from others who have stopped there. With my wife Carla, our years of boating have taken us to practically every channel, bay and cove on the west coast of British Columbia and in Puget Sound. In this book I follow my own passages, stopping in at all the marinas and favoured anchorages where mariners can find shelter, company, moorage and enjoyment of the nature and history of the still unspoiled coast. The area covered consists of routes from Stuart Island and Discovery Passage to Rivers Inlet with reference to some places up to Hakai Pass. The emphasis, however, is on the Broughton Archipelago Marine Park and its neighbouring waterways, inlets and passages.

In the references to the various anchorages in the following pages I have included information about the bays and coves, passages and islands, with details regarding currents, winds and their effect on anchoring, rocks, reefs and hazards and recommended routes. This information comes from my own notes and observations and from discussions with other mariners and reference to the BC Sailing Directions. Books such as this latter one were referenced to ensure I had not overlooked any important details. However I do not believe a book such as this can be absolutely complete. There is always something that will be missed, overlooked or different. Different because of changes that have come about, even recently, since my last visit. Every attempt has been made to provide current, correct information. However it is up to the individual mariner to verify for him- or herself the current status of any area into which they might voyage. And also to check on local weather conditions, to correctly read charts and current and tide tables and to ensure their own safety and that of their crew and guests.

The diagrams in this book have been done entirely by free hand, not attempting to use any scale or precision. Always use the correct large scale navigational charts produced by the Canadian Hydrographical Services for details. In this guide waterways are depicted in blue with light blue used to denote approximate shallows and hazards. Land areas are depicted in tan. The drawings of marinas are intended as computer-graphic artistic renditions of the facilities, showing approximate dock layout, and are not accurate in detail.

It is my hope that this guide will serve as a teaser to prompt you to explore farther afield, to discover the area that has provided so much joy for others and to discover things that writers and other adventurers may have missed.

I thank those who have assisted me with the material in this book: Tom Taylor of Greenway Sound was particularly helpful and encouraging; Kevin Monahan, Ken Burton and the late Henry Karcz for assisting me with GPS waypoints and other information. Thanks to Jodi Brochno for her introduction to tides and currents and to Dr Phil Nuytten for his notes on the First Nations inhabitants of Alert Bay and nearby islands; Rick Bradley, who owns and operates the *Black Tie* in Vancouver Harbour and has done many trips into the Broughton Islands area. I thank him for confirming important facts on navigating through some waterways.

---

In the Broughton Islands and beyond there are many tiny nooks and coves in which to anchor, or places of interest to visit that are the personal findings or choices of some mariners who have visited the area or who will do so in the future. While every one of these places cannot be included in this guide, the author welcomes suggestions from mariners for future editions. Correspondence by email: boating@dccnet.com

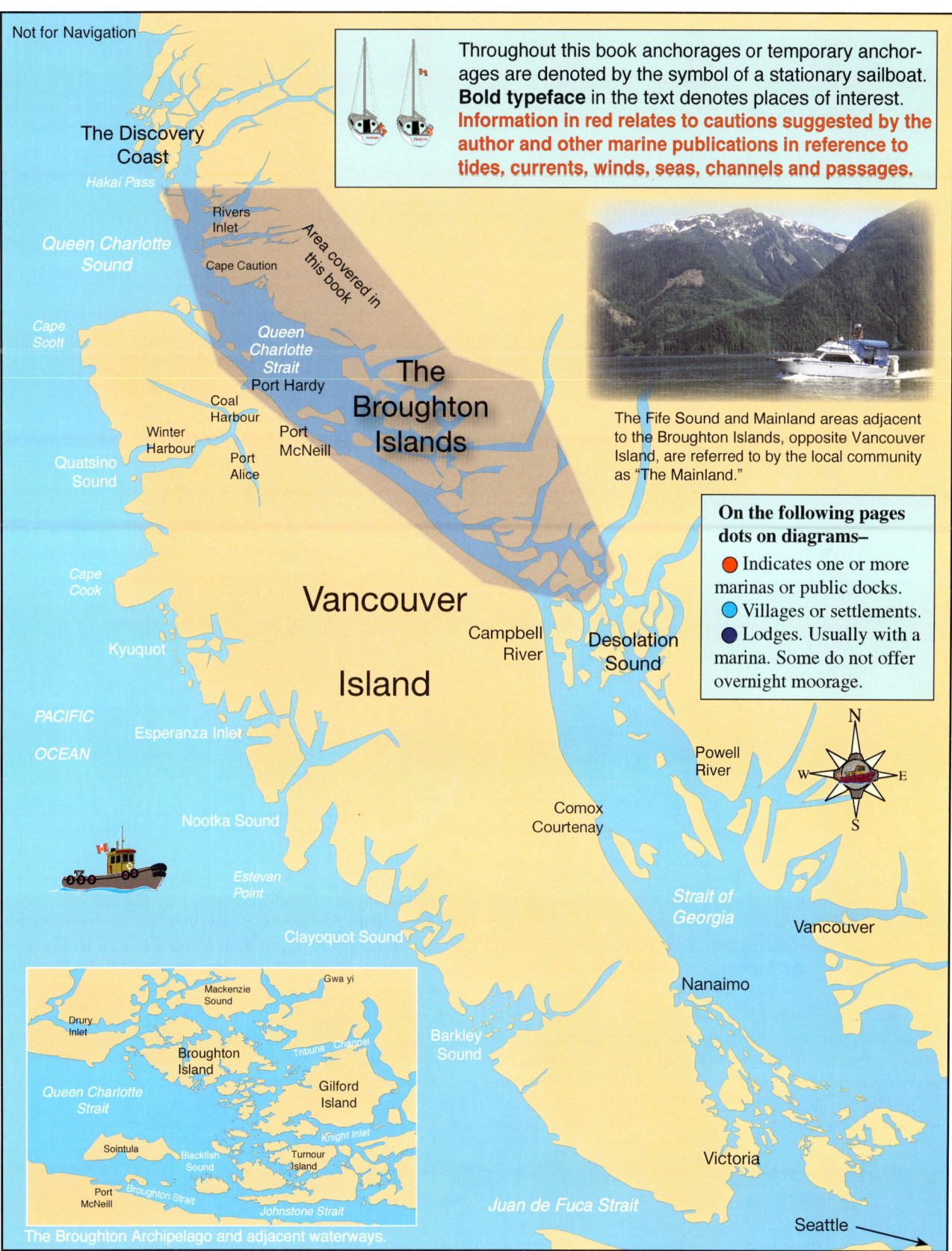

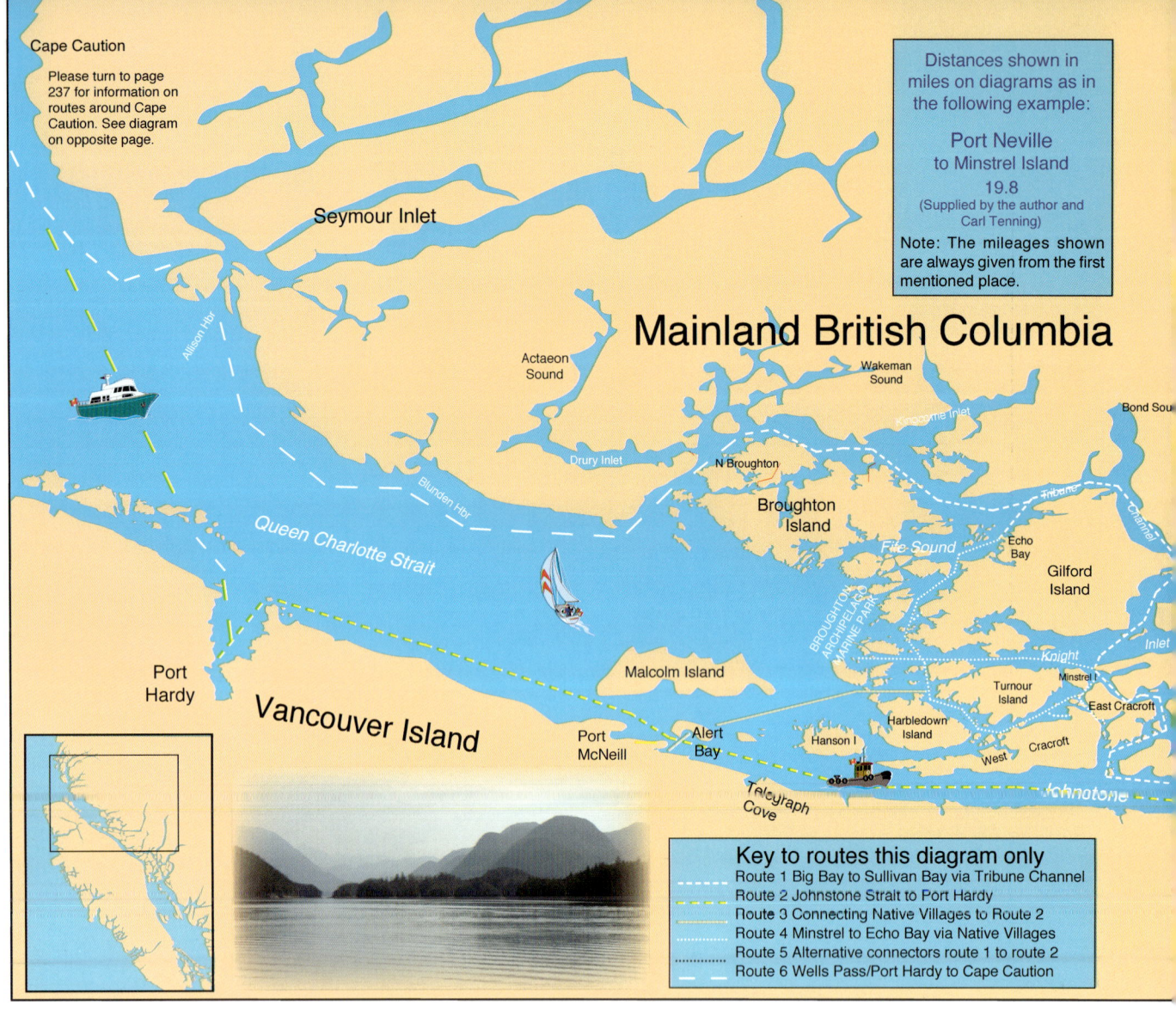

# Foreword

The first time I navigated my own boat through the rapids north of Desolation Sound I was lucky. Carla and I had set off with some apprehension about navigating through the reputedly treacherous waters of the Yucultas, Gillard, Dent, Greene Point and Whirlpool rapids. We were armed with all the necessary navigational charts and a copy of John Chappel's newly published *Cruising Beyond Desolation Sound* guide. It was 1979. We were cruising northward through Desolation Sound *en route* to the waters of Blackfish Sound and Minstrel Island. Our expected time of entering the first set of rapids, the Yucultas, was at about 1 pm on the 8th of July. In his book, Chappel provided an example for calculating the time of slack at these and two other sets of rapids. In the example he cited the expected slack at the Yucultas for July the 8th. He had done my first calculations for me. At least I had his calculations as a reference and backup for my own. John was a professor at UBC and I felt as though my teacher had seen and corrected my homework.

Needless to say we passed through the rapids with ease, although travelling slowly we began to experience the force of the swiftly flowing streams as we motored on to the farther rapids of the route. By the time we reached the approaches to Greene Point rapids we thankfully turned in to Blind Channel and spent the night, waiting for the tide and currents to be in our favour for the following day's run through Whirlpool Rapids in Wellbore Channel.

This was actually my second time through the rapids. The previous trip had been easier. I had accompanied a friend to

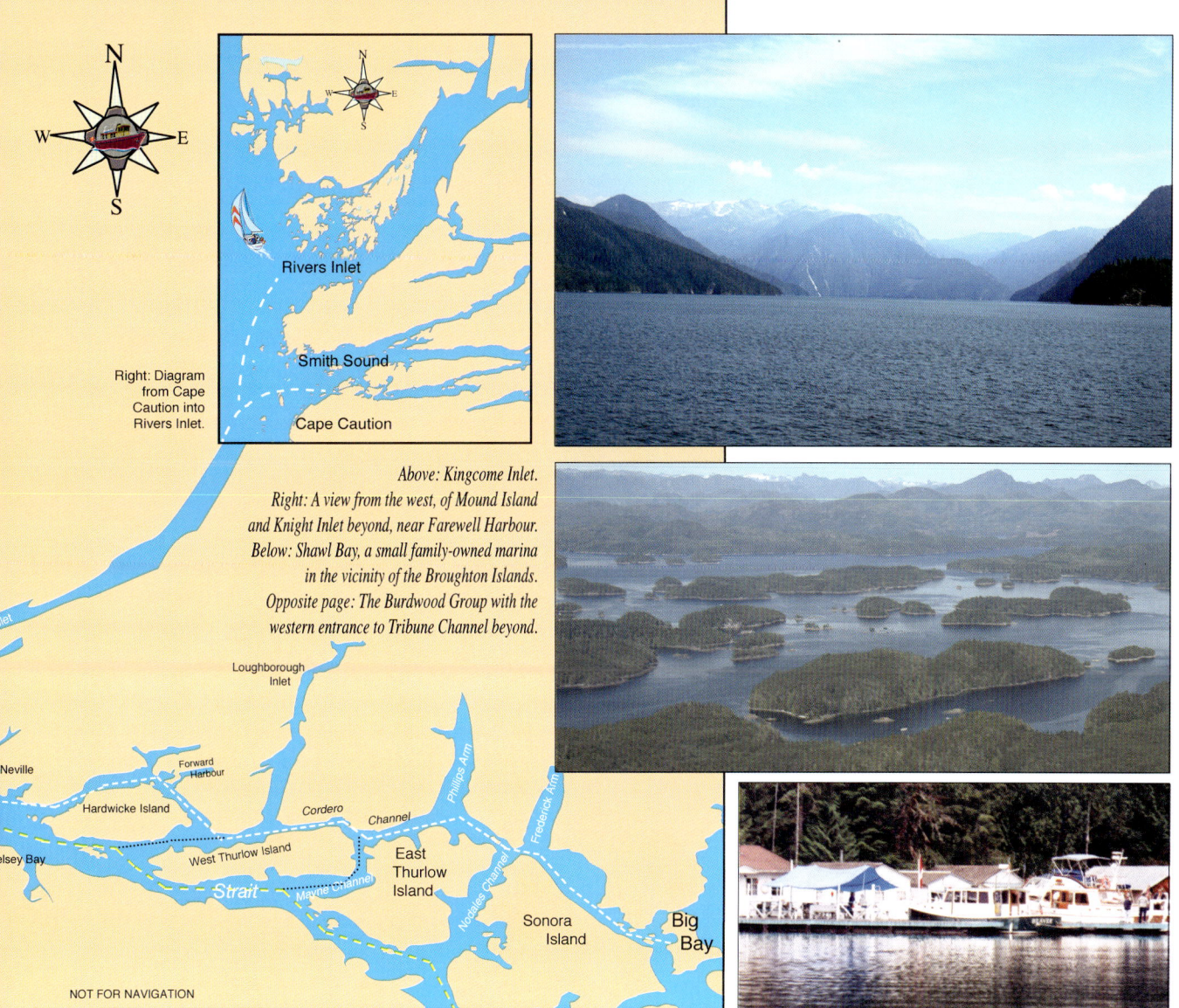

*Above: Kingcome Inlet.*
*Right: A view from the west, of Mound Island and Knight Inlet beyond, near Farewell Harbour.*
*Below: Shawl Bay, a small family-owned marina in the vicinity of the Broughton Islands.*
*Opposite page: The Burdwood Group with the western entrance to Tribune Channel beyond.*

Desolation Sound—via the west coast of Vancouver Island, clockwise, around Cape Scott and down the inside passage. Easier, because he had done all the calculations.

Having travelled extensively and often, through the waters covered in this book, I now feel qualified to produce this reference to the area and recommend that anyone travelling into the Broughtons first read as much as possible about the history and geography of the area and study its weather and currents. To assist you in a selection of reading material I have provided, at the end of this book, a short bibliography as well as reference to several books on the Broughtons.

This book follows the coast from south to north, beginning at Stuart Island, through the Dent Rapids out of Big Bay, then beyond through Cordero Channel and the Greene Point Rapids, Chancellor, Wellbore (Whirlpool Rapids) and Sunderland Channels into Johnstone Strait. Alternatively from Seymour Narrows just north of Campbell River, it takes the route north via Johnstone Strait, from Discovery Passage up Johnstone Strait via Kelsey Bay to Port Neville, Port Harvey and Minstrel Island. Then Tribune Channel to Echo Bay.

On either route you can reach Minstrel Island and detour through Clio Passage and Beware Passage visiting some of the anchorages and islands in the area. Visit the native villages at New Vancouver, Mamalilaculla and Karlukwees then travel through the Broughton Archipelago to Echo Bay, Shawl Bay and Sullivan Bay with more anchorages, marinas and beautiful channels along the way. Poke around Blackfish Sound, Telegraph Cove, Alert Bay and Port McNeil and then on to the northern reaches of Queen Charlotte Strait Port Hardy or Allison Harbour. The area covered in this book continues around Cape Caution to Rivers Inlet and on to Hakai Pass.

The diagram above shows the various routes taken to the Broughton Islands. Sections are repeated throughout the book in conjunction with information on the areas traversed.

# Pretrip Planning

Refer to the *Canadian Tide and Current Tables* or to *Ports and Passes,* a respected tide and current guidebook.

Numerous boat owners spend most of their summers in familiar waters, even though it is their intention to travel farther afield. One of the areas on the short list is the area north of Desolation Sound. This area has a character and charm that is unique on the coast. It lies beyond a series of tidal rapids that are intimidating to not only novices but also to some seasoned skippers.

While Desolation Sound and farther south are basking in balmy days of mid summer, the climate north of the rapids is mostly mild or cool. However, on cloudless days hot conditions can prevail, sometimes accompanied by fog and usually afternoon wind. These conditions, or cloudy skies and rain, could drive you back to Desolation Sound in search of the summer sun you just spent a long winter awaiting.

**Access to facilities**

It is essential that you travel beyond Desolation Sound prepared for a possibly cooler climate. There are facilities to provide shelter from the weather, accommodations, meals, moorage, service and repairs. There are establishments providing excursions such as dive charters and whale and bear watching trips. Many of these places are serviced by water taxis or float plane transportation. They are the means for many to reach outlying marinas, villages and commercial or residential installations. Some of these services are beneficial to those travelling up Vancouver Island by road, and also to mariners looking for a variety of options in accessing coastal areas where they may choose to travel other than in their private vessels. For example some guests fly or drive to marinas or embarkation points to join up with cruising yachtsmen for part of a trip.

We have sometimes moored our boat at a marina and taken a ferry to one of the serviced islands that was out of our way. This way we have been able to walk local roads and visit some of the attractions, just for a day, returning to the boat later to stay the night before continuing our travels.

When venturing into less populated marine areas it is wise to carry suitable tools and spares for minor eventualities requiring such inventory. It is also wise to carry medical supplies and equipment, although help is not too far away if it is needed.

There are hospitals and clinics at major centres such as Alert Bay, Port Hardy, Port McNeill and Campbell River and these can be reached within relatively short time by boat or in emergency by float plane or water taxi and ground transportation.

Whale watching is very popular and successful in Johnstone Strait and Blackfish Sound. If you stop at Telegraph Cove you would do well to join a whale watching boat trip. In your own craft you are cautioned about approaching whales if you see them. The law is very strict about harassing whales, and mariners must not pursue them in any way.

Tourism is alive and well in British Columbia. However, the province has many natural features that have been overlooked. Few people realize, for example, that Alert Bay has a wondrous phenomenon in its Ecological Reserve (formerly known as Gator Gardens) that sits atop the hill above the town. The people of Alert Bay have discovered the importance of tourism and are conducting guided visits to their ancient villages, but there are other areas that could be doing the same.

**Tides and currents**

The tide enters Queen Charlotte Strait and Johnstone Strait every day by curling around Cape Scott at the north end of Vancouver Island. Just as it does to the south, where it flows into Juan de Fuca Strait. The tides and currents tables are an essential part of a mariner's equipment. From them we are able to determine when it is safest to navigate the sometimes furious waters of the rapidly flowing passages and high speed narrows on the coast.

To reach the waters north of Desolation Sound requires an understanding of the flow of water from low to high tide and back again. It is essential to understand the effect of currents and other weather elements on the tides. Basically, and most

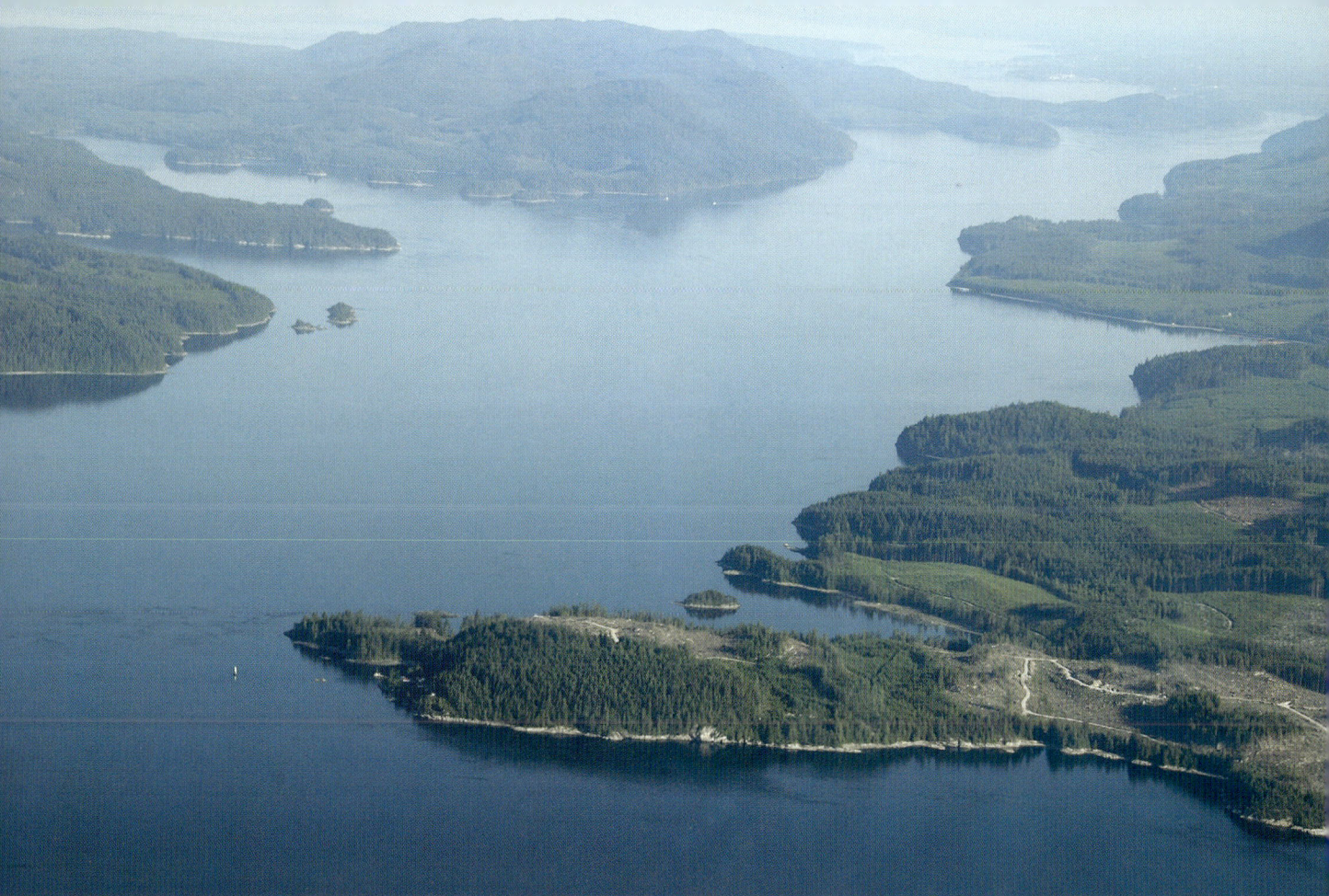

*Discovery Passage with Seymour Narrows in the distance and Chatham Point in the foreground. Otter Cove is just beyond the point and Kanish Bay is on the opposite side of the passage (upper left in photo).*

boat owners come to know this fairly soon in their involvement with boats, it is the influence of the pull of the moon, and to a much lesser extent the sun and local barometric pressure, that dictates the tides. What most people don't realize is that the effect of this pull affects not only the waters of the oceans but also the precession of the earth, not that this latter action is really of significant consequence to the mariner.

In the Pacific Northwest, with its labyrinth of islands and waterways there are blockages in the form of narrow passages that cause a build-up of water resulting in higher and lower tidal heights than in most other parts of the world. These heights range to about four metres, and at some places more. Frobisher Bay in the Arctic has ranges to over 10 metres and the Bay of Fundy on Canada's east coast sees tides of about 16 metres. It is not only the narrows and channels that are affected by tide. Mariners are surprised when running along the open west coast to find some severe currents and turbulence caused by the tidal changes.

The times for high tide and low tide vary throughout the coastal waterways (as they do worldwide). But in the Pacific Northwest it can be difficult to understand all of the variations during these tidal changes. In some constricted waterways, because of the bottleneck effect, tidal changes can be quite a bit later or earlier than those just outside. In Seymour Inlet, for example, while the tidal range outside the entrance can be in excess of four metres, it is only a little over one metre inside. Mariners familiar with the area can attest to the short duration of slack at the narrow mouth where Nakwakto Rapids can run at a quivering 24 knots during the exchange at major tides.

Mariners are advised to be cautious when navigating swift-flowing, current-swept waterways. But do not be intimidated by navigable passages. Rather, use the tide and current tables to plan your travels and thereby enjoy the scenic nature of the coastal features of the area.

**Wind and weather**

The prevailing winds in Johnstone Strait and Queen Charlotte Strait are westerly in summer and easterly in winter. Richard E. Thompson's *Oceanography of the British Columbia Coast* explains: "In general, strong winds along the main channels are associated with the passage of frontal systems. During summer there is a distinct sea-breeze effect in Johnstone and Queen Charlotte Straits as rising air over the heated mainland coast draws cooler marine air inland. On clear sunny days these westerly winds build in strength beginning in the late morning and, combined with the prevailing air flow, can lead to wind speeds of 30 knots by late afternoon. The western portion of Johnstone Strait appears to be particularly susceptible to these winds, the eastern portion less so. The sea breeze dies out before dusk and is replaced by a considerably weaker land breeze from the east, whose influence is most confined to the more exposed waters of Queen Charlotte Strait."

The geography of Johnstone Strait prevents long rolling seas from occurring, although a choppy buildup can be experienced in most areas depending on wind and tidal activity. We have found the best time to travel is early in the morning or late in the day. This is particularly true in a slower boat. We have travelled the area in a 10 knot trawler type boat as well as in faster boats (to 30 knots plus) and find a fast boat will get you from one sheltered point to the next, in many instances, before there is a major wind or weather change. While mariners are reminded that cruising into this area is pleasurable and generally easy and safe, it is important that forecasts are taken very seriously in any type of boat.

Johnstone Strait requires some planning and weather watching. Slow moving boats must be operated according to weather predictions along with the tides and currents. When there is a southeasterly wind blowing against a large flood of three or four knots the short wavelength can prove overwhelming. Equally, westerlies against an ebb can be devastating. We have stopped at Port Neville in calm, clear weather with just a light breeze blowing up the strait and left for places north believing we were in for a mostly calm passage. But, as the wind picked up and the tide changed we found ourselves scurrying for shelter in Port Harvey rather than continuing on to Telegraph Cove or Port McNeill. Of course, such changes in plans usually lead to discovering new and alternative destinations, so all is not lost. Just make sure to keep out of serious sea conditions by monitoring weather reports and observing telltale weather signs.

Fast moving clouds indicate wind and approaching system changes. If you want to be informed about clouds and weather patterns study some of the publications on the subject including Thompson's *Oceanography*.

### Navigational considerations

Johnstone Strait is a major route for commercial marine traffic. It was charted by Captain George Vancouver in the summer of 1792. Today it is the passage for numerous cruise ships on the way to and from Alaska, as well as tugs, freighters, bulk carriers, barges and pleasure craft. For the pleasure boat operator, it is not only weather that dictates great caution while navigating but also these numerous vessels that require a wide berth in many cases. They generally operate along the deeper, less convoluted south side of Johnstone Strait more than the north side where most of the smaller pleasure craft tend to travel.

One area that dictates extreme caution is Race Passage off Kelsey Bay. Back in 1850, John Sebastian Helmcken, a medical officer aboard the Hudson's Bay company steamer *Beaver* asked the captain the name of the island they were passing off Kelsey Bay. Typically there was a strong current of six knots kicking up high seas against a flood tide at that point and the slow, uncomfortable progress had the good doctor on edge. The captain named the island then and there, in honour of Helmcken.

While greater depths can be found in Knight Inlet and Bute Inlet, the depth of Johnstone Strait reaches about 500 metres. The maximum in the Strait of Georgia is about 420 and in the Strait of Juan de Fuca 275 metres. It follows that the depths and the high, steep slopes of the south shoreline of Johnstone Strait allow few safe, shallow anchorages. This is why pleasure craft will be found running along the opposite shore of Johnstone Strait where access to anchorages and shelter is more readily available in the event of contrary weather. Because of the depth of the water combined with its constant, swift ebb and flow, water temperatures remain lower than those in the Strait of Georgia where temperatures can exceed 20° Celsius.

There is less opportunity in summer to find suitable waters in the Johnstone Strait area in which to bathe, other than some of the lakes easily accessible from shore. Temperatures seldom reach 10° C in mid summer and are more like 7° C in spring and winter. Surface water temperatures in Queen Charlotte Strait are actually warmer than in Johnstone Strait and its adjacent waterways.

### Options

If you plan a trip to the Broughton Islands and have enough time to include a period in Desolation Sound consider your options: You may stay in Desolation Sound for the first part of your trip or you may end up there as the balance of a trip north of the Sound. Let the weather predictions determine your decision.

We have always gone directly through the rapids and on to Knight Inlet and beyond if the weather forecast favours doing so. If not we dally in Desolation Sound or stop at Big Bay until we get a weather break.

When we are in the Broughton Islands we begin our weather watch days before we have to return. If a system is moving in that threatens a lengthy duration we may scoot back into Desolation Sound for the remainder of our vacation. Our return south to Vancouver is determined by the same set of rules. The same goes for continuing past Cape Caution.

> NOTE: *Reference to anchorages for small boats usually means under 50 feet. When discussing shallow, drying passages small boats refers to runabouts, dinghies, kayaks and canoes.*

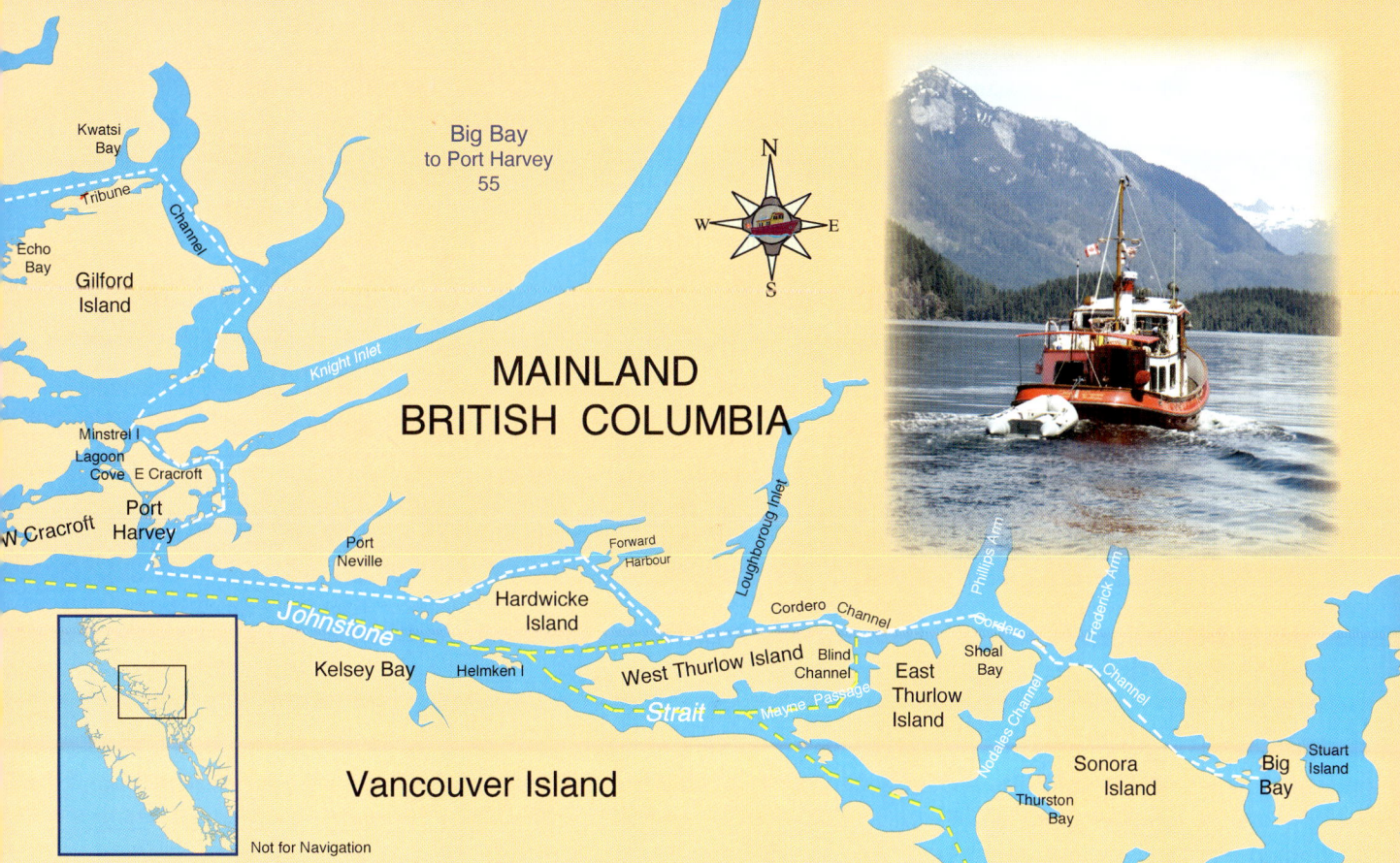

# Heading North–First Impressions

Along the waterways of Queen Charlotte Strait, Kingcome Inlet and Tribune Channel, I felt as though I had travelled uphill and could look down over the world of Vancouver Island and Desolation Sound far below. There the sets of turbulent rapids free the upper waters from their mountainous reservoir channels to flow and surge into the valleys of Desolation Sound and over the northern tip of Vancouver Island into the open Pacific. In Desolation Sound they mingle with the northward flood from the Strait of Georgia and Juan de Fuca Strait. Swiftly running currents tug at kelp beds lining the shore. They ripple and eddy, carry flotsam rapidly through narrow passages and sometimes form fascinating whirlpools.

First time voyagers to the waters beyond Desolation Sound set out initially in fear of the awesome rapids: the Yucultas, Dent and Greene Point and Whirlpool Rapids. Sailboating writers with their inevitably slower boats, made me fearful of the rapids until the first time I navigated them. Many boat owners never even plan to take in those waters during their years of cruising—perhaps because of a subconscious dread of the rapids and the swirling waters sometimes conjured up unintentionally in the works of some experienced writers. But there is no need to fear the rapids north of Desolation Sound–just respect them. Respect them and work closely in conjunction with the tide and currents tables. Be cautious. Don't try to rush through them. Learn how to use them to your advantage.

With a slow, hull-speed boat, following the advice of sail boaters makes sense, but when you would otherwise sit and wait in a slower boat, a fast powerboat will often carry you through easily. However, caution must be observed no matter what boat you have. Rapids and tide rips can be dangerous and navigating fast flowing channels at maximum or near maximum currents is foolish and can be disastrous. My log-book entry for July 1979 reads:

*We passed through one set of rapids in the Yucultas area, stopped at Stuart Island, smack in between the Yucultas and Dent, and waited for the following slack before continuing and passing through the second set. In between we hiked along an island trail (that is no longer accessible) to Arran Rapids to watch them run at full flood.*

13

The Arran Rapids, one of the most respected in the area, pours through a narrow channel and on a full ebb creates a massive whirlpool at the southwestern end.

I wrote: *It was a moderate flood that we saw, and no problem–boats large and small passed through in either direction. However, they were mostly high speed power boats ranging from 13 foot fishing tenders to 28 or 30 foot sportsfishermen. One 12 knot fish boat ran through with the flood with no apparent concern.*

The channels, straits and sounds beyond the Yucultas are a cruising yachtsman's paradise. They are relatively desolate, environmentally clean, aesthetically unspoiled and naturally quite undisturbed. There are whales, fish, river otters, mink and eagles. We saw many, many bald eagles and one gigantic golden eagle. There are dolphins, orcas, bear and deer and sightings of such wildlife can be quite frequent.

Journal entry: *Cruising out of Johnstone Strait at Alert Bay, it was convenient to transit Blackfish Sound, pass around Swanson Island into the entrance of Knight Inlet and around Midsummer Island off to port, up Retreat Passage. Then to the most isolated, beautiful cove in the world at the north end of Bonwick Island. It was Waddington Bay. We anchored and set off in the dinghy to drop traps in the hopes of crab for dinner. Success. We went ashore and dug clams for chowder. And this prompted an urge to get on with some fishing. Spring salmon were running and in no time at all we hooked a couple of small ones–but eight pounds apiece is plenty. We had prawns too–fished out of 45 fathoms off Minstrel Island.*

We had intended to conclude our northward passage with a run up to the head of Kingcome Inlet of Margaret Craven's *I Heard the Owl Call My Name* fame, but heavy, inclement weather kept us in Cypress Harbour opposite its mouth until time simply ran out and we had to begin the 'downhill' run back towards Vancouver. On a future trip we went up the Kingcome River in an inflatable as far as the First Nations village of Gwa'yi. Then, later sitting out the weather in Cypress Harbour time was not wasted. We went out to look for salmon. The thrill of catching a big one is hard to equal.

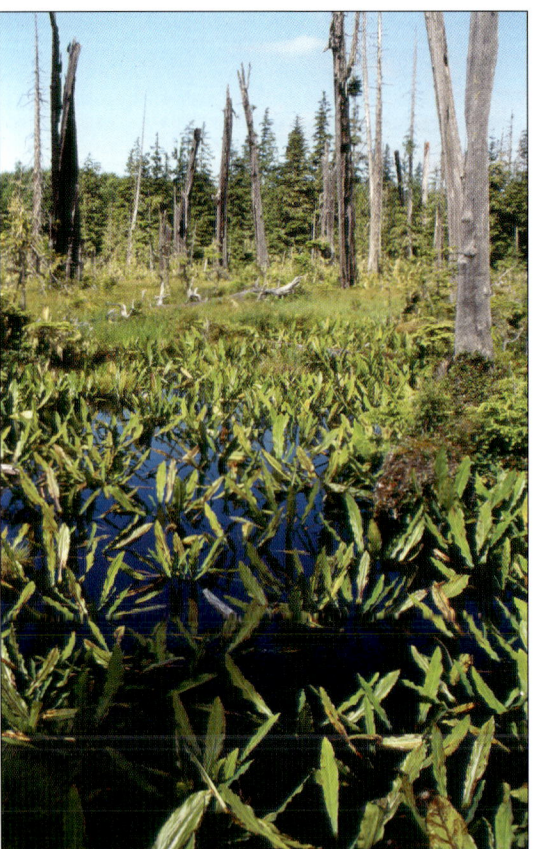

*Ecological Park at Alert Bay–see page 214.*

First Nations villages are as exciting as the very names of the islands on which they are located or the channels that serve them. Arrow, Indian and Village Channels, Village, Owl and Midsummer Islands all conjure up romantic notions. The now deserted villages of Karlukwees and Mamililaculla have about them an air of pressing history. In the past few years some members of the Kwakwaka'wakw people have cleaned up some of their villages and welcome visitors each summer for a fee towards the maintenance and upkeep of the property. We made our way into Mamililaculla after anchoring near its ramshackle jetty (since gone) and clambering along the rocky shore to the beach in front of the deserted village. The path from the landing had been cleared and could be used to reach the historic site.

I wrote on my first visit to Mamaliliculla: *Sitting on a low ledge overlooking Native Anchorage, grey, weathered houses sit forlornly looking across the water. Long grass and weeds grow up around woodwork, porch steps and ancient longhouse frames. Totems and house posts, horizontal and fallen, slowly yield to the decay of time and the elements. A gentle breeze flaps ragged cloth in window frames, or torn plastic used for temporary coverage since the village's abandonment—there are signs of recent overnight visitors.*

Pathways, homes, community and the school were fast succumbing to the encroaching foliage–a sad confirmation of the prophetic accounts of Ms Wiley Blanchet in her *Curve of Time*. We have since learned that, while the crumbling of an old village is a sad loss, this is the traditional way of the Kwakwaka'wakw. It is their belief that when a totem falls to the ground it must be left for mother nature to reclaim. This is why, we discovered, some of the fine totems and the twin whale arch at the Alert Bay cemetery have disappeared and not been re-erected.

We visited Village Island during trips through the Broughtons in recent years and found the village all but gone and overgrown with salal, trees and grass.

# GPS References

Published by FineEdge.com
Anacortes, WA

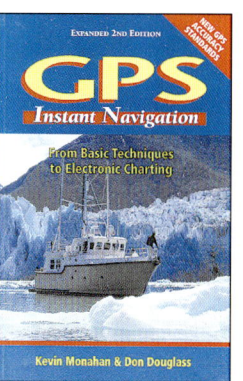

*Kevin Monahan of Shipwrite Productions and author of the book,* **GPS–Instant Navigation**, *has kindly written the following about the use of the GPS coordinates in this guide:*

### Latitude and Longitude—It's not quite that simple

Boaters using a modern GPS receiver can probably determine their position more accurately than was possible even for map makers until just a few years ago. An unassisted GPS can now resolve a position to within 10 to 15 metres, 95% of the time. As a result, your GPS may be more accurate than your chart. As if this wasn't enough, the chart may also be drawn to a different horizontal datum than is used in your GPS, resulting in errors of up to metres in northern BC.

A datum is simply a reference point from which latitude and longitude are measured. In 1927, map-makers in North America established the first truly continental datum at Meade's Ranch in Kansas, This datum was known as North American Datum 1927 (NAD27).

By 1983, using satellite telemetry data scientists had learned enough about the shape of the earth, that they were able to accurately model the surface of the earth. This allowed a new horizontal datum to be developed in North America—(NAD83)—a datum that did not rely on any single reference point.

When charts were drawn to the new datum, cartographers discovered that the positions of geographic features on older charts could not be reconciled with their positions on new charts—the lines of latitude and longitude on the older charts were in the wrong places. In many areas of the continent these differences are minimal—just a few metres—but in northern BC and Alaska, the difference between NAD27 and NAD83 is over 200 metres.

Now that world-wide satellite positioning is available, GPS uses a truly universal chart datum—World Geodetic Survey 1984 (WGS84). In North Amcrica, WGS84 is equivalent to NAD83.

So much for the idea that latitude and longitude are absolute. Any one location can be represented by different lat/long coordinates, depending on the datum that is used. So in order to accurately identify a position on a chart, you must reconcile not only the latitude and longitude, but the horizontal datum used as well.

The positions of the various docks etc. in this guide have been taken directly from a Garmin GPS set to the WGS84 Horizontal Datum. In general, it is best to match the datum your GPS reads out to the datum of the chart you are using. Boaters using electronic navigation systems with electronic charts will find that all their electronic charts have been compensated to read out in NAD83, and should simply ensure that their GPS is set to NAD83 at all times.

However, if you are using an older style GPS without a chart display and plotting your position on a paper chart—and if those charts are drawn to NAD27—the latitudes and longitudes of positions on the chart will not match the same positions given in this guide or as indicated by the GPS. If you set your GPS to read out in NAD27, your GPS and paper chart will agree, but will not match the positions given in this guide.

The only way to resolve these discrepancies is to convert the latitudes and longitudes, using the conversion factors set out on the paper chart. Every chart should incorporate a Horizontal Datum Note describing the datum used in that particular chart and the corrections to be applied to convert to NAD83 (or NAD27 as the case may be). Once you have converted the latitude and longitude given by the GPS you can plot it on the chart. To input positions taken from the paper chart simply apply the conversion factors in reverse.

Canada still publishes charts that are drawn to NAD27. Each year some of these charts are updated and replaced. But until they have all been replaced—especially in out-of-the-way places—you should check the horizontal datum of your chart to ensure that you are aware of any discrepancies that may exist.

—*Kevin Monahan*

For more information on GPS and Horizontal Datums, visit www.shipwrite.bc.ca

---

## Use of weights and measures in this guide

**Temperatures:**
A Fahrenheit is smaller than a Centigrade (Celsius) degree. It is 5/9 of a Celsius degree.

**Conversion method**
To convert Celsius to Fahrenheit multiply by 9, divide by 5 and add 32.
To convert Fahrenheit to Celsius, subtract 32, multiply by 5 and divide by 9.

Throughout this guide chart distance references have been made in nautical miles and depths in metres. Tides affect depths and therefore all suggested anchoring depths are approximate. More precise measurements, if needed, can be calculated with the use of your nautical charts or taken from official publications such as the *BC Sailing Directions*. The above suggested method of conversion is intended as a quick way for the mariner to convert measures and distances to their preferred standard.

**Measures:**
1 US gallon ................0.833 Imperial gallon
1 US gallon ................3.785 litres
1 Imperial gallon ........1.201 US gallons
1 Imperial gallon ........4.546 litres
1 litre .........................0.264 US gallon
2 pints........................1 quart
4 quarts......................1 gallon
1 litre .........................1.0567 quarts
1 quart .......................0.9463 litre

**Mariners' Measures:**
6 feet..........................1 fathom
1 metre ......................39.37 inches (1.0936 yards)
120 fathoms...............1 cable (length)
5,280 feet...................1 statute mile
6,067.11 feet..............1 nautical mile

**Linear Measure:**
1 metre ......................39.37 inches (1.0936 yards)
1 kilometre ................0.621 mile
1 mile ........................1.609 kilometres

# Introduction
# Boating Beyond Desolation Sound

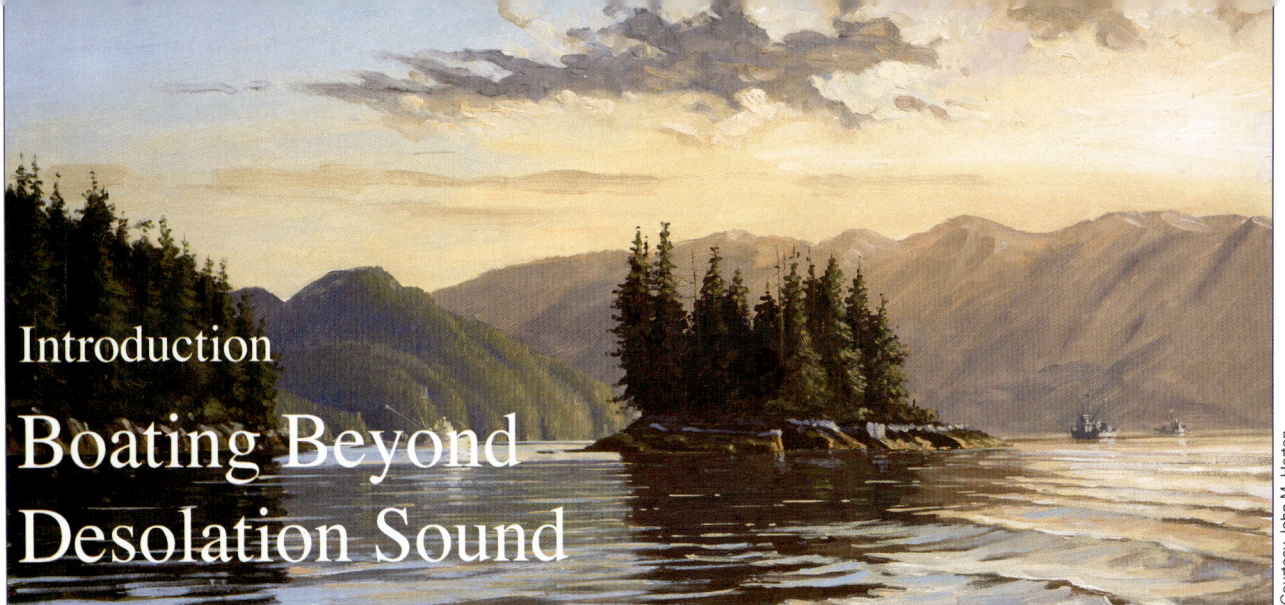

The coast between Desolation Sound and the Broughton Islands is steeped in history of settlement and abandonment. Many villages, logging camps and other communities existed for a while in places today visited only briefly by passing mariners or used as destinations to sit at docks and enjoy the peace and tranquility of being away from it all.

In the early 1900s people tired of eking out a meagre living in the cities, or those arriving in British Columbia from abroad with no job potential or just wanting to try to make a living off the coast, moved into sheltered coves and bays where they set up home, some to log the forests, some to fish and hunt. For them, of course, home at first was a crude shelter by today's standards. Some were improved upon while others yielded to the unrelenting growth of vegetation under the rainy skies of the west coast.

A number of settlers opened their new found residences as lodges, stores and post offices and today there remains a sparse albeit significant scattering of these settlements. At one time the stores on the coast thrived even more than they do today on the many loggers and settlers in nearby and neighbouring coves and inlets who would row in for supplies and news.

The islands and inlets that we visit in these pages are mostly with minimal population if any. Native villages that once thrived are all but gone, some remnants being carefully guarded by descendants of the last residents, others simply abandoned to the ravages of time. Visit Stuart Island where local history begins. Take in the facilities now provided for a short but intense summer tourist season. Venture on beyond the famous Yuculta Rapids and Johnstone Strait to Knight Inlet, Lagoon Cove and the Broughton Archipelago area with the adjacent communities at Echo Bay, Shawl Bay, Sullivan Bay and on to Rivers Inlet beyond Cape Caution. Enjoy the ambience of remote waterways, narrow channels, the presence of bears, cougars, eagles, whales and wolves.

Indulge yourself in the pleasure of meeting the people of the coast who have made the area home and who are sustaining it for the future, just as the people of the past sustained it. Poignantly, many settlements have declined and all but disappeared. Hopefully the businesses that remain will find economic success and be there or leave behind facilities for the next generation of mariners to enjoy. Theirs is a very short season in which to conduct business, and to survive economically they need all the traffic possible, and that in a period of barely more than two months.

Mariners going to Alaska for the summer begin trickling through this area in early spring. The months of March, April and May see the flow increasing steadily until summer begins with the main flow of holiday makers cruising beyond Desolation Sound commencing in July. Then as the school break comes to an end the tide of traffic turns and ebbs back southbound.

At one time the stream of Alaska- or Hakai Pass and Rivers Inlet-bound boats made the marinas between Minstrel Island and Sullivan Bay their main stops on the way north. Today, with improved facilities at Port McNeill they have tended to follow that route rather than delay reaching Alaska by stopping in the Broughton islands. This has been an economic blow to the marinas in the area. Yet they survive, partly because it is the proprietors' life-style to be where they are. Some, however, are very dependant on the all-too-short season of tourist traffic to survive through the years. This is true, of course, of all marinas on the coast, but nowhere is the short season as critical as it is north of Desolation Sound.

For some mariners, getting to the Broughton Islands is a matter of just going. Leave your departure point and make it your intention to get there, stopping along the way only for an overnight rest as needed. Once there, the choice of anchorages is vast, with several extremely safe, sheltered coves and bays and many temporary havens to escape the winds that prevail throughout summer.

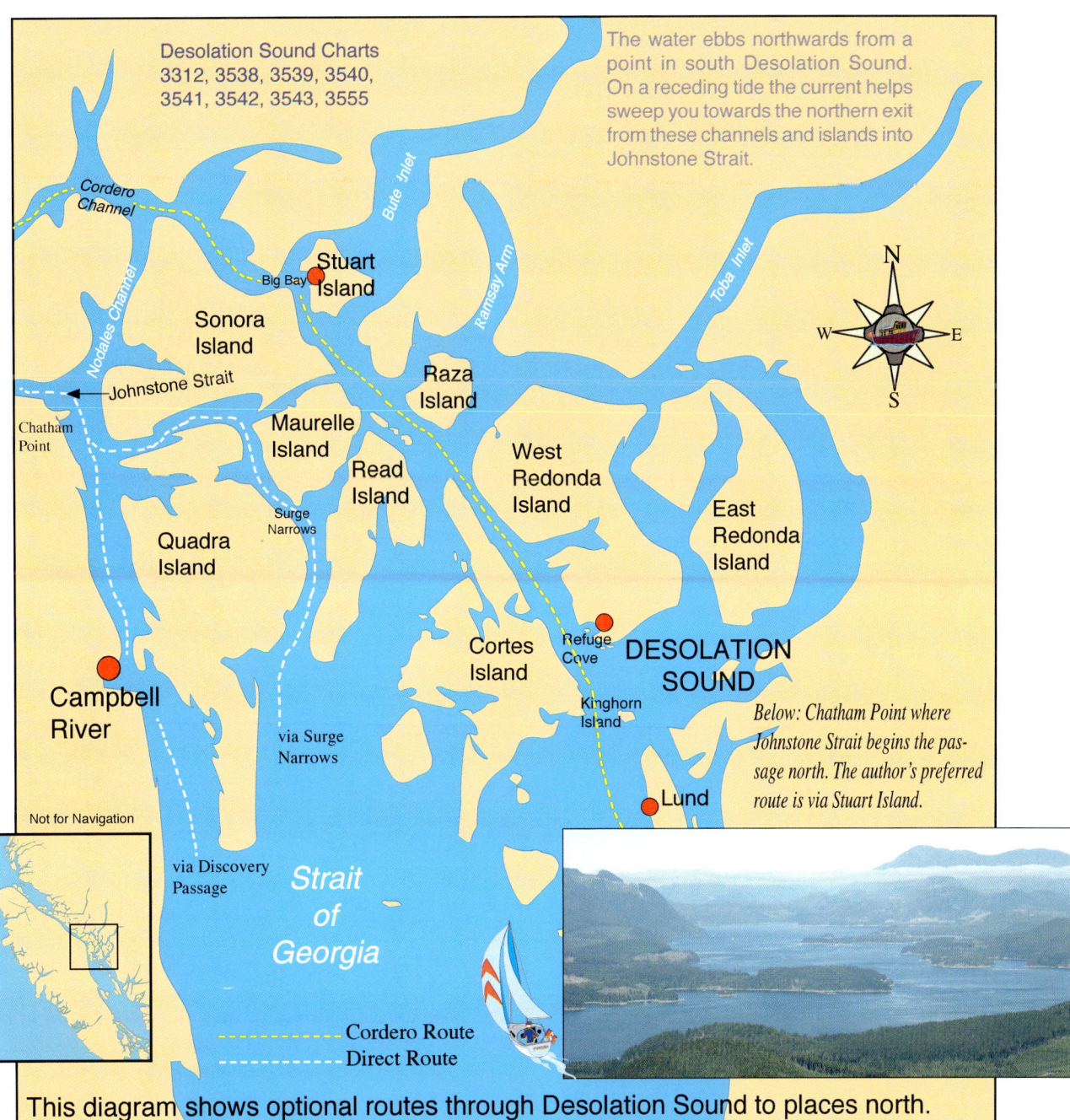

This diagram shows optional routes through Desolation Sound to places north.

Some concern has been expressed in recent years about the presence of fish farms and the effects on wild salmon that fish farming is having. You may encounter numerous fish farms throughout the area, some where they are stated to be and others unexpectedly located in what has been recommended a good anchorage.

Fish farms may have appeared, been moved or removed since the gathering of material for this book. The best policy is to expect them when and where you see them and plan your anchoring or cruising routes accordingly.

This book's focus of concern is with helping recreational mariners find their way safely and make new discoveries in the pursuit of the pleasure of being in one of British Columbia's prime boating wilderness locations.

An increase in traffic to the Broughton Archipelago area will boost the economy of the marinas and tourism industry of the region. The publication of this book is intended to prompt mariners to travel to the area more frequently, stay longer and treat the historical sites with respect. It is our responsibility to ensure the Broughton area remains a pristine wilderness.

# First Nations Villages

Notes on the pre-contact origin of some B.C. coastal place-names.

### By Dr Phil Nuytten
Author of *The Totem Carvers*

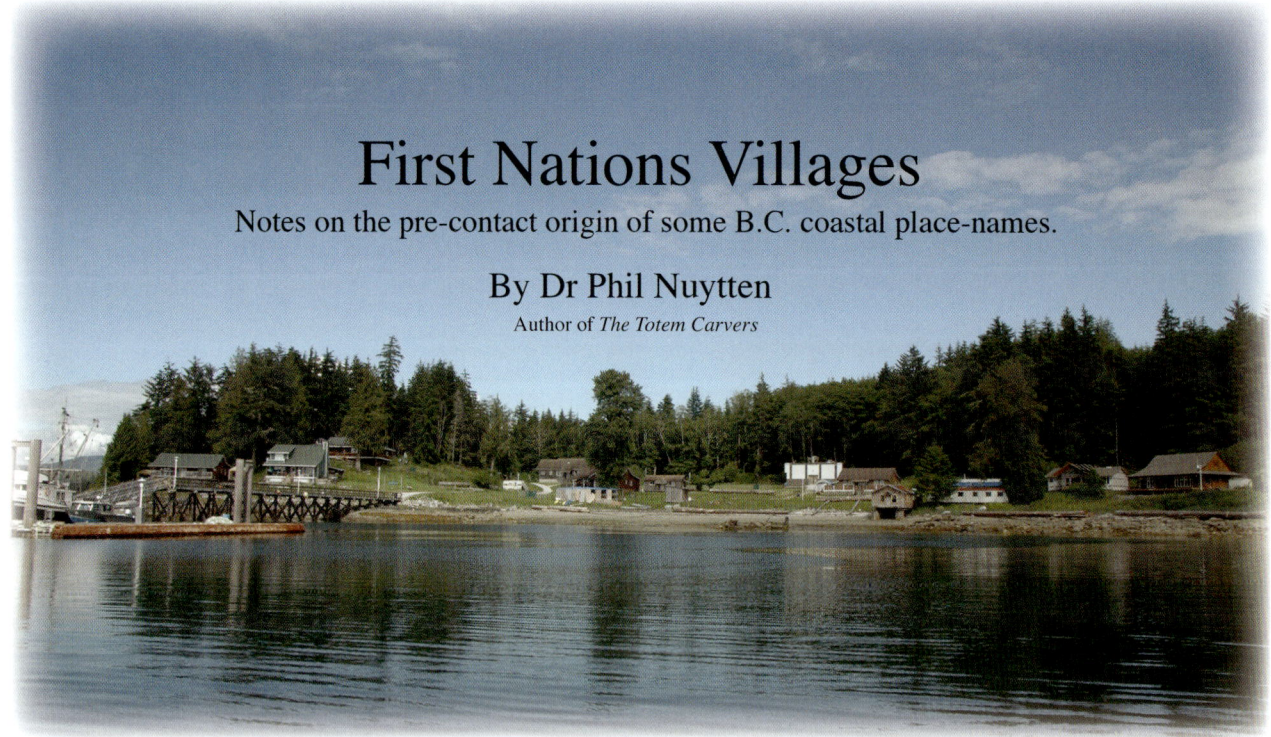

*The village of New Vancouver on Harbledown Island is a place where the First Nations culture can be experienced. Opposite: Young dancer at Alert Bay.*

Marine travellers in the Strait of Georgia, Johnstone Strait, and heading up Queen Charlotte Strait often remark on the abundance of First Nations place names. Northward of Comox, on the east coast of Vancouver Island, and northward of Bute Inlet on the mainland side, almost all the native names derive from a tribal group now called the *Kwakwaka'wakw*. This jawbreaker replaces the former 'Kwakiutl', (which really isn't much better in terms of how to pronounce it with an english-speaking mouth!) *Kwakwaka'wakw* is said as *Kwok-wuhk-kyuh-wuhk* and add a very softly said *wuh* on the end, (for the last "w"), and you have it, or, at least, fairly close to it! Many old people don't care for the new tribal designation, preferring the former *Kwa-gyulth*, the approximate native pronunciation of the anglicized *Kwakiutl*. The native place-names south of Bute Inlet and south of Brooks peninsula (on the west coast of Vancouver Island) are typically either from Salish or Nu-chahl-nath people, respectively.

The language of the *Kwakwaka'wakw* people is called *Kwak'wala* (*Kwok-wuh-luh*) and that's what *Kwakwaka'wakw* means; *those who speak Kwak'wala*. The dialects of individual villages can be different, the cadences can be quite differ-

> Dr Phil Nuytten is of First Nations descent through the Metis people of the Red River Valley, Manitoba. He is an adopted member of the Village Island band (Mamalilicula) of the Kwakwaka'wakw nation. He explains in this introduction what the various villages represent to the native peoples of the coast, their place in their culture and in the history of BC.

ent (The people from Rivers Inlet sound, to many others, like they are 'singing' their language), even many words are different–but all *Kwak'wala* speaking people understand one another.

The *Kwa-gyulth* were true sea-people and they spent far more time in their canoes, paddling and sailing this enormous inland sea, than they did in the forest. It's no wonder, then, that most of the native place names describe how the island or bay or reef looks from a near water-level perspective. If you are looking for *the island that looks like a sleeping seal* just past *stinking river beach*, you don't need GPS to know when you've arrived!

Many of the names are rather humorous, some even risque. 'Ya-lees' (or Yalis) is the native name for the town of Alert Bay, on tiny Cormorant Island. When approaching Alert Bay, the two hills on either side of the bay resemble the bent knees of a person lying on his or her back...and *Yal-lees* is right in the centre! Some of the names are repeated in different areas–*Numas* ('Old person'–but, usually 'Old Man') is very often used to describe any small island or large rock; the ever-present bird-lime resembles white hair and the rock, itself, is like the craggy features of an elderly man. *Numas* is also a rock that overhangs the water or a rock that is at the

18

end of a peninsula at low tide–and by itself at high tide. "So, which *Numas* is it? The one by stinking river beach, of course!" Actually, it gets even more complicated since there is a legend about an old man named *Numas* who was ultimately turned into a sea-rock and most kids know it as the rock by their village. They really get bent out of shape when their cousins claim it's the rock by *their* village!

Sometimes the villages are named after the chief who founded them. Mamalilakula (sic), for example, is the name of the native village shown on your charts as being located on Village Island. Mamaliliculla is spelled many different ways, all usually acceptable. Other than in this introduction, it is spelled Mamaliliculla throughout this book. Mamalilakula is just the plural for Mamlilakula the chief who caused this village to be built, and it means *all those of Mamlilikula*.

Pretty simple...except it's not really the native name of the village–it's the name of the island! The village is called *Mem-kumlees* only it cannot be found on the chart. A kwak'wala speaker would shrug and say "Hey, we didn't name it 'Village Island.'–You guys did!"

That is another amusing, and somewhat confusing, thing about north island native place names. Very often, the locals (white and native) only know the local spots by their original names. Someone says "Good fishing at Tlak'wa'gila Bay." So you look on the chart and guess what, there's no such place. You say, " It's not on the chart."

"Oh, no," he says, "It's an Indian name."–"Well, what is it in English?– "Lets see, Coppermaker Bay, I guess". You look it up again. Still not on the chart. Bring the chart over. "Where?" Finger goes on to chart. "Right here". "Wait a minute," you say, "That says 'Thompson Bay.'" He shrugs and says, "Yeah, I dunno why they put that name on the chart... everybody knows it's Tlak'wa'gila".

Very often the Kwa'yulth names have meanings within meanings. Negei Island, for example, shown on your chart as just north of Port Hardy is an easy one to figure out once you see it! *Nug-eh* means mountain and that's exactly what the whole island looks like–a mountain. Simple–but, actually it was named for a famous chief called *Nage'dzi*–which you would pronounce 'Nuh-ged-zee'–and that means 'Great Mountain'. Well, a big mountain, then. No, the 'mountain' doesn't refer to the actual mountain on the island, but to "An overhanging mountain of wealth threatening to slide down and bury the chief's rivals (during the enormous wealth-giving feasts known as 'potlatches')". Now that's a pretty long name even for a great potlatch chief, so he was just known as 'Great Mountain' in Kwak'wala and just 'Mountain' in English. They named the island after him. "But it looks like a mountain" you say. Another shrug. "Coincidence".

When you near the top end of Vancouver Island, on the inside passage, one of the best areas for poking around is called the 'Indian Group". It is surrounded by Midsummer Island, Village Island, Turnour Island, West Cracroft Island, Gilford Island, and a bunch of smaller ones. All of these cluster together with the appropriately-named 'Indian Group' in the centre. It is easy to find: Just follow the directions in this book: Up Johnstone Strait, veer right at Blackfish Sound, turn up 'Indian Channel', and you're there! This is the heart of Kwa'gulth country. Alert Bay (*Ya-lees*) is close-by, to the northwest, with Port Hardy and Fort Rupert (*Sa-hees*) to the north, and ancient village sites all around you.

In the quiet anchorages in front of long-abandoned villages, some mariners say they have heard the plaintive cries of the Giantess called *Dsu-no-kwa*, the 'wild-woman-of-the-woods', echo across the still night waters. Others claim to have caught sight of the shy, diminutive, *Buk-wis*, the 'man-of- the-forest' on the beaches at dawn. Still others say it's only the wind and the shifting morning shadows. But I've been there, and I can tell you that the goose-bump readings are of a high order!

A good way to become immersed in the local culture, when travelling in the Kwa'gulth Nation, is to select a couple of books that explain some of the origins of common place-names. It's interesting how often the place you pass looks exactly as you would expect it to, by its name. And it's gratifying how often you can elicit a smile of surprise and delight when you call a place by the name that goes back to its earliest beginnings.

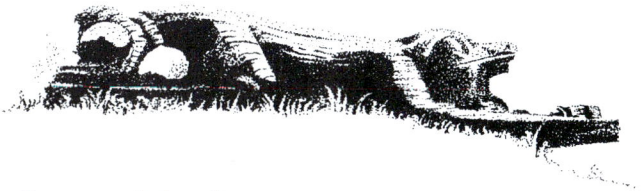

**Recommended reading:**
*Raincoast Place Names*. Andrew Scott. Harbour Publishing.
*Sailing Directions–British Columbia Coast*. Canadian Hydrographic Service– Department of the Environment, Ottawa, Ontario, Canada K1A 0E6.

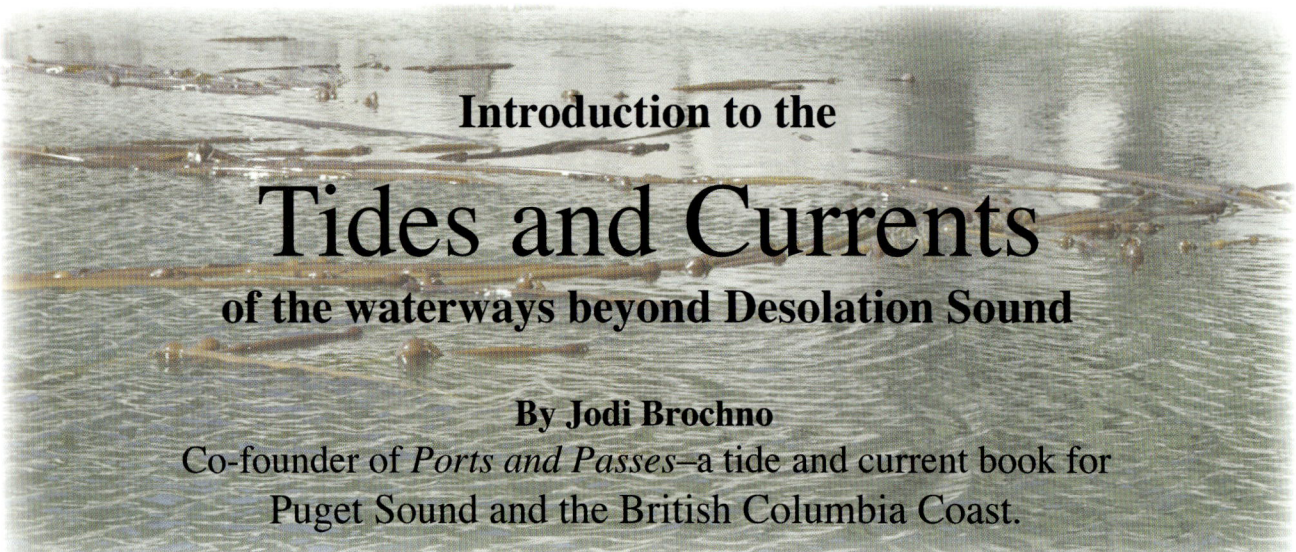

# Introduction to the
# Tides and Currents
### of the waterways beyond Desolation Sound

**By Jodi Brochno**
Co-founder of *Ports and Passes*–a tide and current book for Puget Sound and the British Columbia Coast.

Cruising the waters of British Columbia demands some knowledge of tidal currents. When one understands what causes whirlpools and backeddies, it is that much easier to avoid them. Some of the most beautiful cruising areas are only accessible by travelling though areas where the rapids and turbulence require caution. As noted earlier, one should always plan to navigate through rapids only during slack current.

The optimum situation is to arrive at the narrows just before the current turns to the direction you want to travel. This will give a small favourable push. If you enter the same channel on the opposite tide, with the flow turning against, you will see an uncomfortable situation turn progressively worse as the current strengthens. When the current starts moving, backeddies begin to form. If these backeddies become strong enough, whirlpools appear near the centre of the channel. Whirlpools also form behind points and outcroppings, where the backeddies force water around against the shore. If the boat enters a whirlpool where the water is moving in the same direction, it is easier to control and the boat will usually ride out with the water.

Johnstone Strait is the highway to the North. A residual westerly current at the surface gives a gentle push towards Alert Bay and many days can pass before there is any appreciable flood current. The strongest currents are on the mainland side of the channel. This surface current makes it impossible to guess the times of slack based on the tide predictions. The effects of this current weaken as one approaches Seymour Narrows where a large flood is reflected in an eastward movement of water from Race Pass to Chatham Point. Winter's prevailing southeast winds tend to increase the ebb and reduce the duration of the flood current; in summer, the northwest winds have the opposite effect. At Chatham Point, the junction of Discovery Passage and Johnstone Strait, the maximum flood occurs 30 minutes later than at Johnstone Strait (Central) and the maximum ebb is 50 minutes later. The times of slack water are very close to those at Seymour Narrows.

On the northeast side of Sonora Island, lie Yuculta Rapids, Dent Rapids, Gillard Passage and Barber Passage. Collectively known as the Yucultas, they are the gateway to a serene and unspoiled region. Slack water here is very brief. Effects of the weather and river runoff can make this short period seem non-existent. The Yuculta Rapids can be dangerous with strong east winds. The turbulence caused by wind against the current can produce much rougher waters than would be expected in open areas. With a flood current, the strong wind causes the east side of the channel to race south while the west side tumbles northwards. In calm weather, one can anticipate small whirlpools in Big Bay, larger whirlpools south of Whirlpool Point along the east side of the channel and white water in the centre of the channel off Kelsey Point. The worst rapids in the Yucultas are found at Dent Island, with dangerous overfalls and violent eddies. The CHS Sailing Directions and local knowledge all suggest staying close to the shore of Sonora Island.

It is extremely important to carry the latest edition of the Tide and Current Tables for the region, and know how to use them. Calculations to determine slack water must be made when travelling through many of the passes north of Desolation Sound. The mathematical procedure is quite simple and can often be performed quickly without a calculator. Yuculta and Dent Rapids are both referenced to Gillard Passage. One would think, by looking at the chart that the times of slack

## Secondary Current Stations, British Columbia

| Current Station | Dir of flood | Position Lat N | Position Long W | Time Difference Turn to flood | Time Difference Max Flood | Time Difference Turn to Ebb | Time Difference Max Ebb | Max Rate FLd | Max Rate Ebb | % Ref Rate Fld | % Ref Rate Ebb |
|---|---|---|---|---|---|---|---|---|---|---|---|
| | °True | 0 / | 0 / | h min | h min | h min | h min | knts | knts | % | % |
| **British Columbia - North** Based on Gillard Passage | | | | | | | | | | | |
| Yuculta Rapids 3/4 mile S of Gillard Light | 180 | 50 23 | 125 09 | +0 25 | - | +0 05 | - | 10.0 | 8.0 | - | - |
| Dent Rapids | 140 | 20 25 | 125 13 | -0 15 | - | -0 25 | - | 11.0 | 9.5 | - | - |

water should be very close to each other. In reality, the Turn to Flood in Yuculta Rapids, only 3/4 mile south of Gillard Light is 25 minutes after the same turn at Gillard. The table above outlines the time differences calculated by years of observation by the Canadian Hydrographic Service.

To apply the time differences and calculate the predicted time of slack water, one must add the appropriate time difference to the corresponding turn of tide at the reference station. For example, if the turn to flood at Gillard Passage occurs at 1:00 pm and the turn to ebb is at 7:00 pm, we know that Yuculta Rapids will turn at 1:25 pm (to flood) and 7:05 pm (to ebb). Dent Rapids turns will take place at 12:45 pm (to flood) and 6:35 pm (to ebb).

### Duration of weak current near time of slack water

The prudent mariner knows the safest time to negotiate any narrows is during the turn of the tide. The most critical areas are those with the strongest maximum currents and they have the shortest period of slack water. There is a period on each side of the predicted time of slack water, during which the current is very weak and safely navigable.

The accompanying table helps approximate the length of time during which these weak currents can be expected. The duration given refers to the entire period of time encompassing the turn; half of the interval will be before and half after the time of slack water.

Occasionally, in areas of extremely swift currents, a time of "slack water" does not occur. In these areas, the tide will change direction or "turn" without ever reaching slack water.

**NOTE:**
When there is a large difference between the speed of the maximum flood and ebb before and after the slack for which the duration is desired, find the duration for each maximum separately and average the two.
—Excerpt from Ports and Passes.

*GPS users will generally find handy tide and current information in the programme that came with their equipment. This is an easy method of finding tide and current information. But, as with nautical charts, this should not be relied on absolutely to replace a working knowledge and understanding of navigation.*

| Maximum Current | Period with a speed not more than: | | | | |
|---|---|---|---|---|---|
| | 0.1 knot | 0.2 knot | 0.3 knot | 0.4 knot | 0.5 knot |
| Knots | Minutes | Minutes | Minutes | Minutes | Minutes |
| 1 | 23 | 46 | 70 | 97 | 120 |
| 1.5 | 15 | 31 | 46 | 62 | 78 |
| 2 | 11 | 23 | 35 | 46 | 58 |
| 3 | 8 | 15 | 23 | 31 | 35 |
| 4 | 6 | 11 | 17 | 23 | 29 |
| 5 | 5 | 9 | 1 | 18 | 23 |
| 6 | 4 | 8 | 11 | 15 | 19 |
| 7 | 3 | 7 | 10 | 13 | 16 |
| 8 | 3 | 6 | 9 | 11 | 14 |
| 9 | 3 | 5 | 8 | 10 | 13 |
| 10 | 2 | 5 | 7 | 9 | 11 |

# Big Bay to Forward Harbour

## Entrance to the passages of flowing waters

Charts 3312, 3541, 3542, 3543, 3544

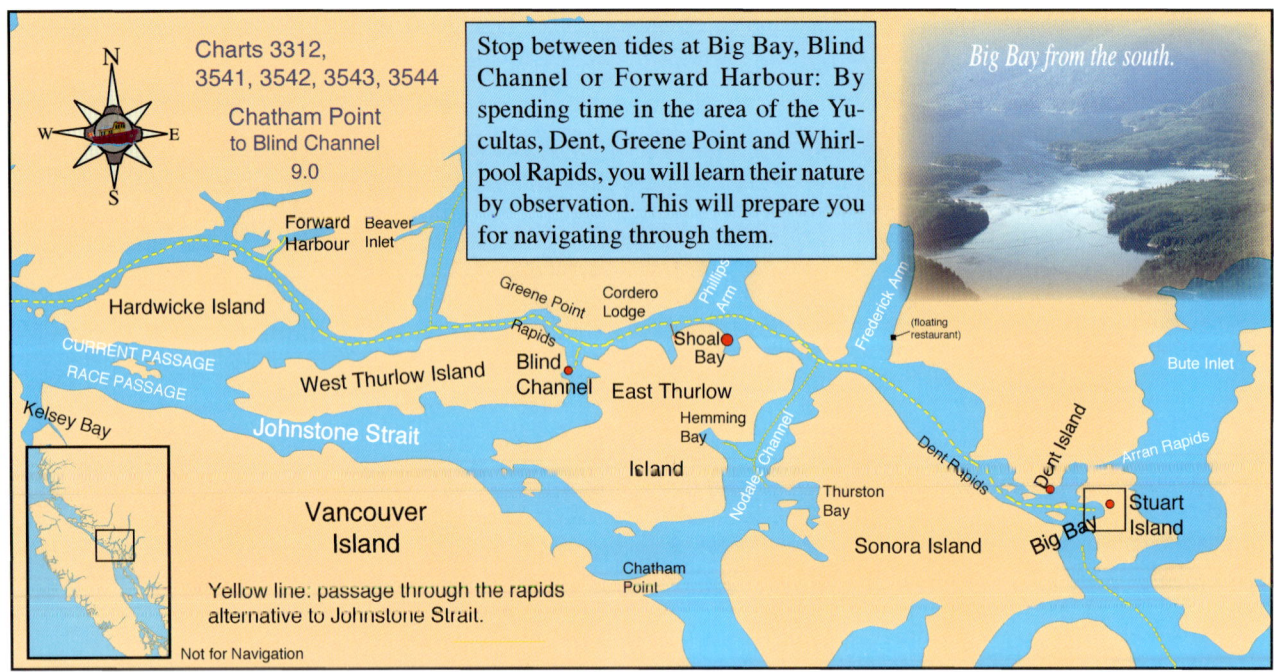

### Yucultas, Dent Rapids  charts 3312, 3541, 3543

The water ebbs northwards from near Kinghorn Island in Desolation Sound. On a receding tide the current helps sweep you past Stuart Island towards the northern exit from these channels and islands into Johnstone Strait.

From Stuart Island the route north leads through Gillard Passage between Gillard Island and Jimmy Judd Island into Cordero Channel. This goes past Dent Island and through the rapids. In the middle of these rapids, between Sonora and Dent Islands there is an area known as Devil's Hole, a swirling whirlpool with violent eddies that erupts into a dish-like depression through which you will pass if the tide and currents are strong. Watch for tugs with barges in tow. They have very limited control of their charges and cannot be expected to avoid small pleasure craft that move into a dangerous course with them.

Running a fast boat through this 'dent' in the water can be like driving a car through a depression in the road causing you to lift off as you clear the ridge and emerge back onto level ground. I have done this and concluded that this phenomenon must have been what gave the Dent Rapids their (appropriate) name.

Don't be mistaken into believing that a fast boat is immune from the power of the tidal currents. Surfacing logs and debris could put a fast boat out of action. Exercise great caution and good judgement before attempting any fast moving waters. You need to use the Canadian Tide and Current Tables Volume 6 and plan to stay put somewhere safe until slack water.

### Big Bay, Stuart Island  charts 3312, 3543

When we stopped at Big Bay for the first time, in the 1970s, Big Bay Marina was in its infancy. It comprised a number of old, small buildings including the home of the owners, Bruce and Kay Knierim and their daughters. The house was the primary structure on the property. At that time they were

## Twenty miles of rapids

Options are to travel via Seymour Narrows north of Campbell River or go through the Yucultas. We take you through the northern route first, as this is the passage of choice to avoid commercial traffic and strong currents with almost no relief off Kelsey Bay.

A slow moving boat of perhaps 6 to 12 knots may not be able to pass through the Yucultas, Gillard Passage, Dent Rapids, Greene Point Rapids and Whirlpool Rapids all in one leg. Break it with selected stops such as in Big Bay, Thurston Marine Park, Shoal Bay, Blind Channel and Forward Harbour and possibly others.

Through the Dent Rapids and up Cordero Channel to where Nodales Channel and Frederick Arm intersect, the water is very deep. Not to suggest doing it, but a boat can run very close to shore, practically sweeping the branches of overhanging trees as it passes by.

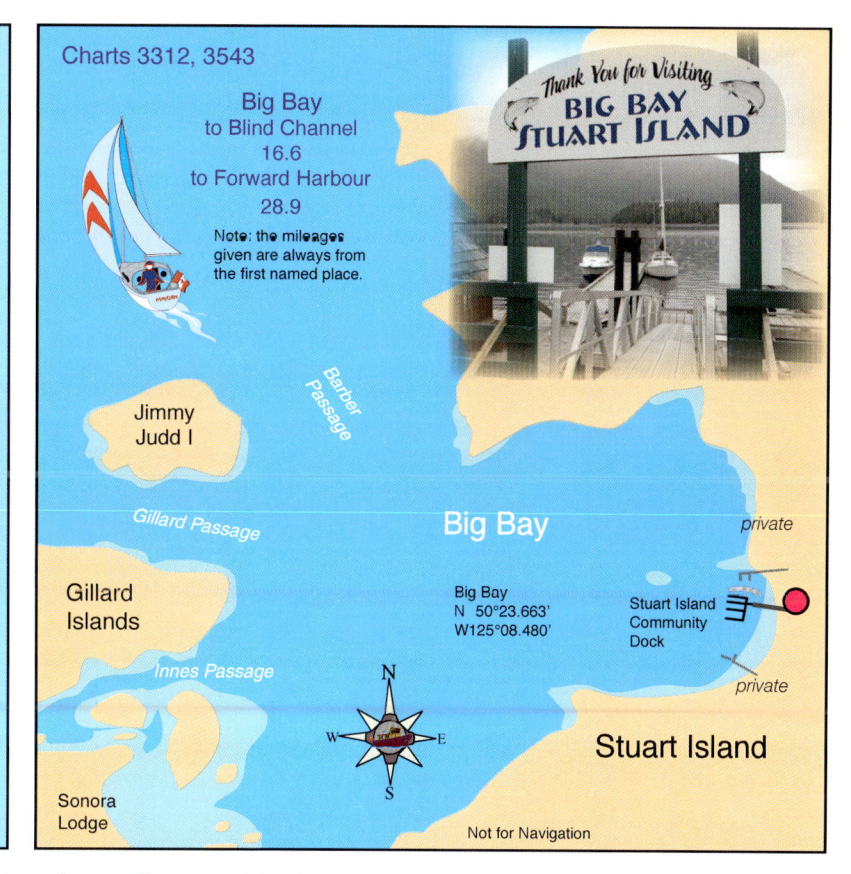

Charts 3312, 3543

Big Bay
to Blind Channel
16.6
to Forward Harbour
28.9

Note: the mileages given are always from the first named place.

Jimmy Judd I

Barber Passage

Gillard Passage

Big Bay

Gillard Islands

Big Bay
N 50°23.663'
W125°08.480'

private

Stuart Island Community Dock

private

Innes Passage

Sonora Lodge

Stuart Island

Thank You for Visiting
BIG BAY
STUART ISLAND

Not for Navigation

---

talking about the fishing, catering to tourists and expanding their moorage for the benefit of overnight visitors. They even talked of the good scuba diving in the clear waters of the bay and nearby Arran Rapids–during slack tides, of course.

We had stopped at the public dock, not even aware that there was a marina in the making nearby. A short walk through the scrub and towering trees along a well-worn path took us through a small school yard and alongside the local residents' cottages with their quaintly fenced-off, colourful gardens invaded by indigenous growths of salal and such, before reaching the home of the Knierims.

In later years when we returned to the bay we discovered a developed marina and eventual construction and opening of their large, spacious restaurant and later their new store. We also discovered the pub and its overnight moorage nearby. We walked to Arran Rapids to watch the fast flowing water, from the safety of land. Now Big Bay Marina is gone. However, the community has rallied and developed the public dock and built adjacent facilities for visiting mariners. Once again there is a store and amenities.

On one occasion we sat at the public dock and marvelled at the ebb and flow of the waters during the changing of tides, and at how crystal clear the waters were, despite the fact it was summer when most waters in BC darken and become cloudy with the bloom of plankton in the sunlight.

The fishermen were out. Guides from the resorts ran back and forth in their small boatss. They steered their boats with their sports fishermen charges to and from the swirling tide rips and streams in the outer bay, invariably returning with big spring salmon and even bigger smiles. We tried our luck. It would be too dangerous to attempt fishing out there ourselves, not understanding yet the peculiarities of the rushing waters and not having the right equipment to handle it.

We employed a guide and spent several hours mooching in the rapids. Carla is a lucky fisherman. She had nibbles. Then bites, then landed her first fish. I had nothing. She had more strikes and then landed a second. I had nothing. So we traded sides of the boat. I still caught nothing. She caught fish. We traded rods. She caught. I had nothing.

The guide was aghast when I asked him to cut the catch into fillets. Guests usually want to take the salmon away whole. I wanted them to fit into the small freezer we had on our boat, so that we could continue our trip north to the Broughtons without having to worry about what to do with several large fish.

We learned a lot about fishing from that short interlude. We also learned a lot about British Columbia's tidal rapids. A small fast boat can handle the swift running water. But it is still wise to keep out of the worst of the flow. Use the backeddies to work around the current. Most of all stay put and wait for conditions to change to those that your boat can more readily handle.

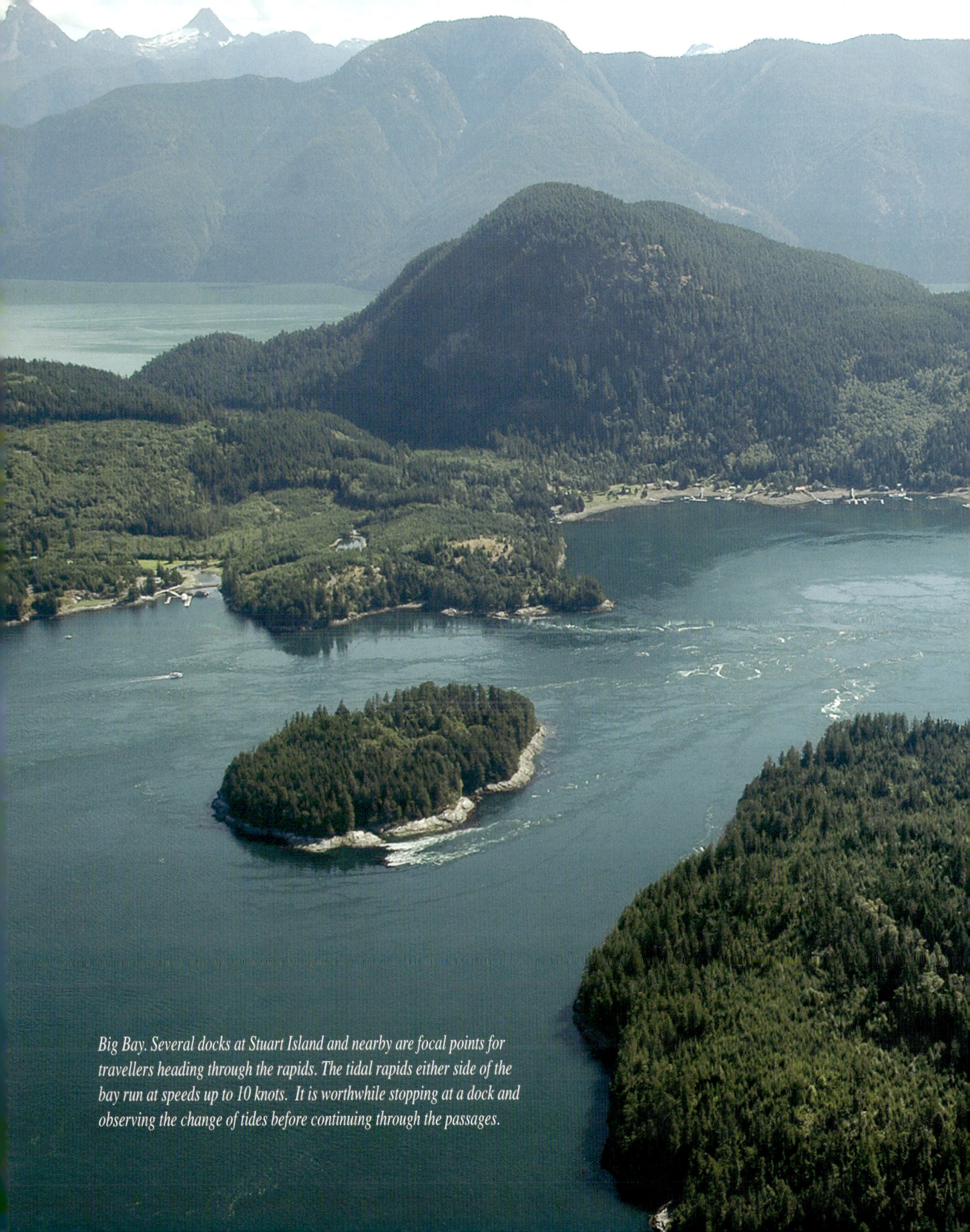

*Big Bay. Several docks at Stuart Island and nearby are focal points for travellers heading through the rapids. The tidal rapids either side of the bay run at speeds up to 10 knots. It is worthwhile stopping at a dock and observing the change of tides before continuing through the passages.*

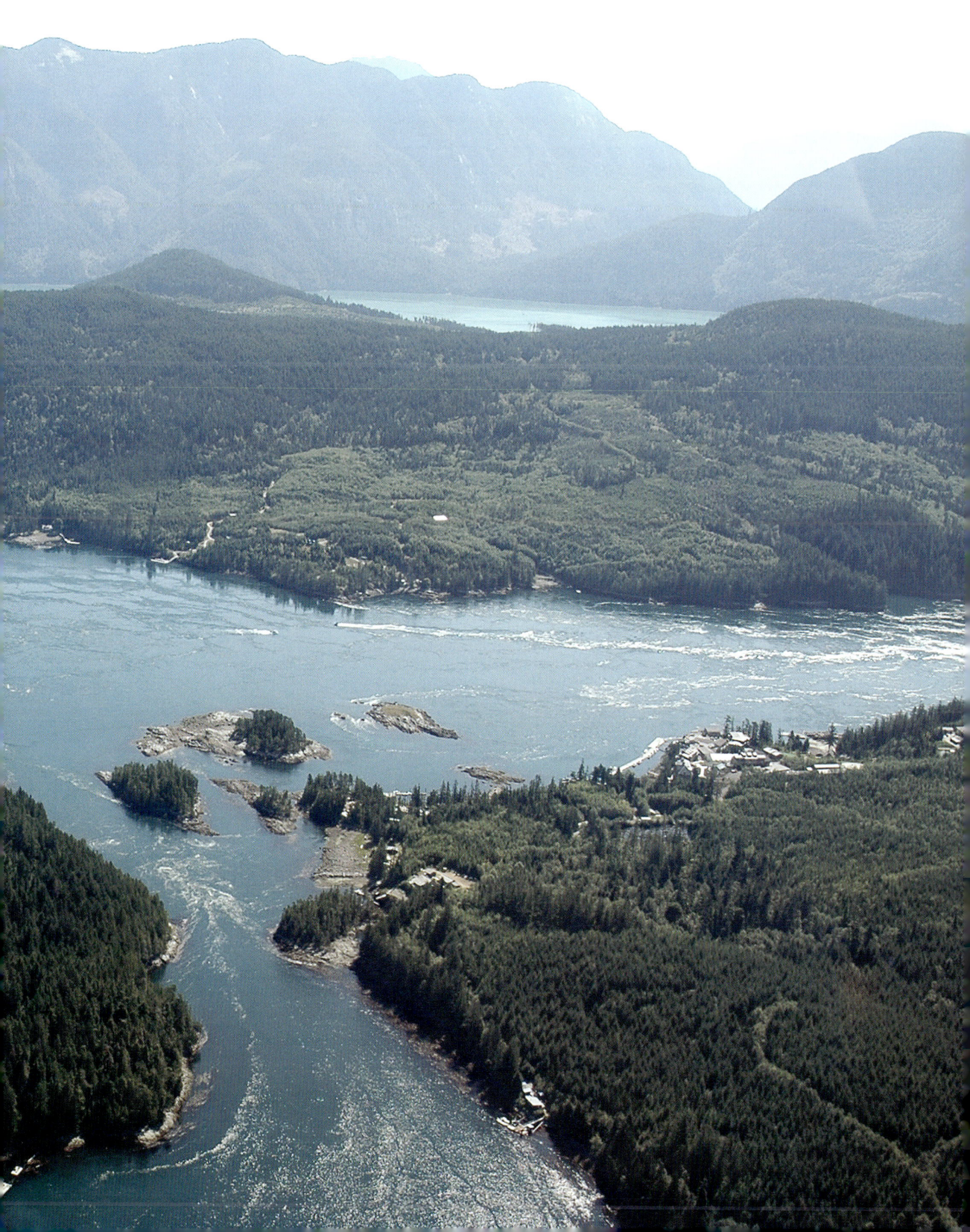

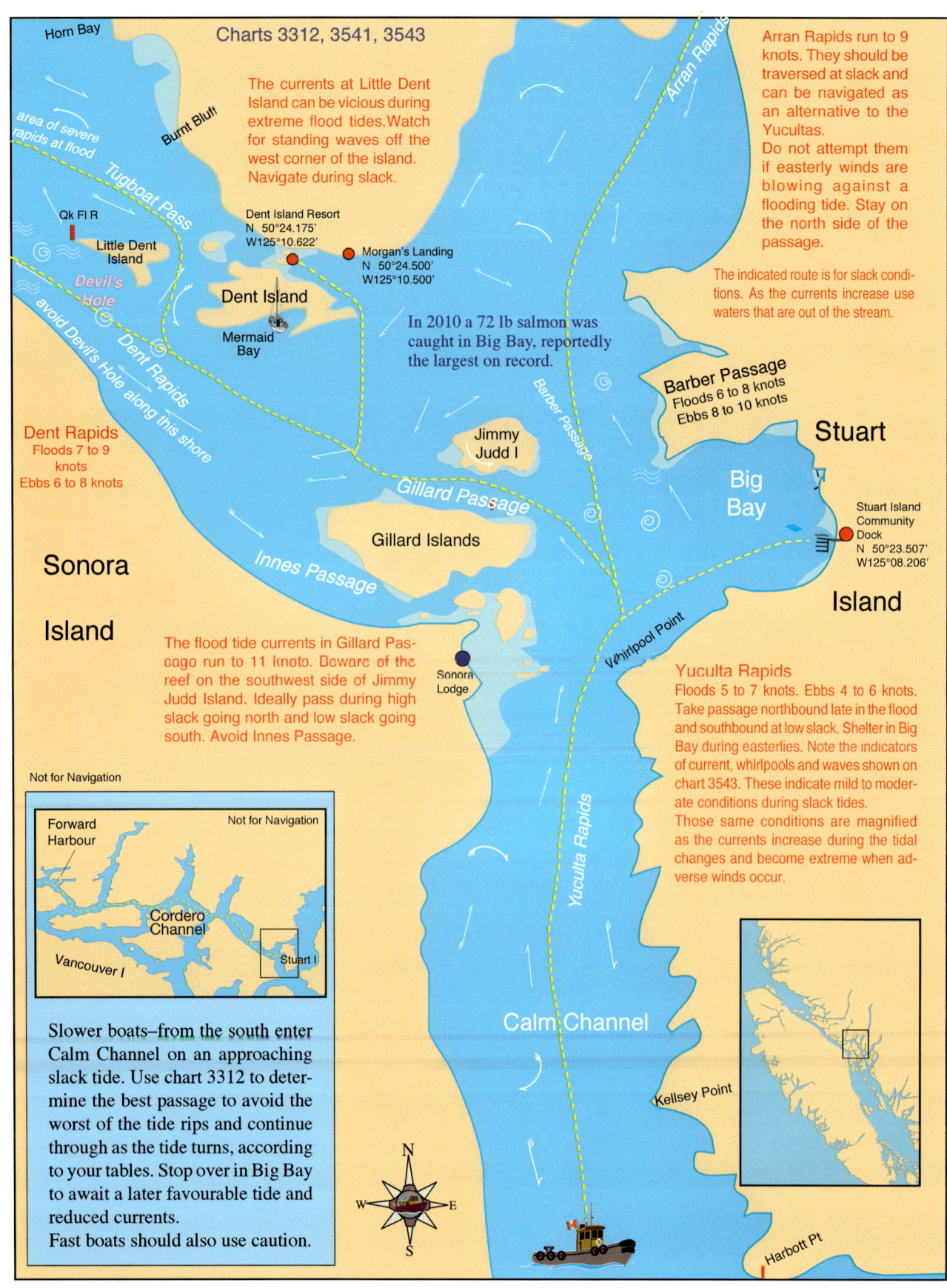

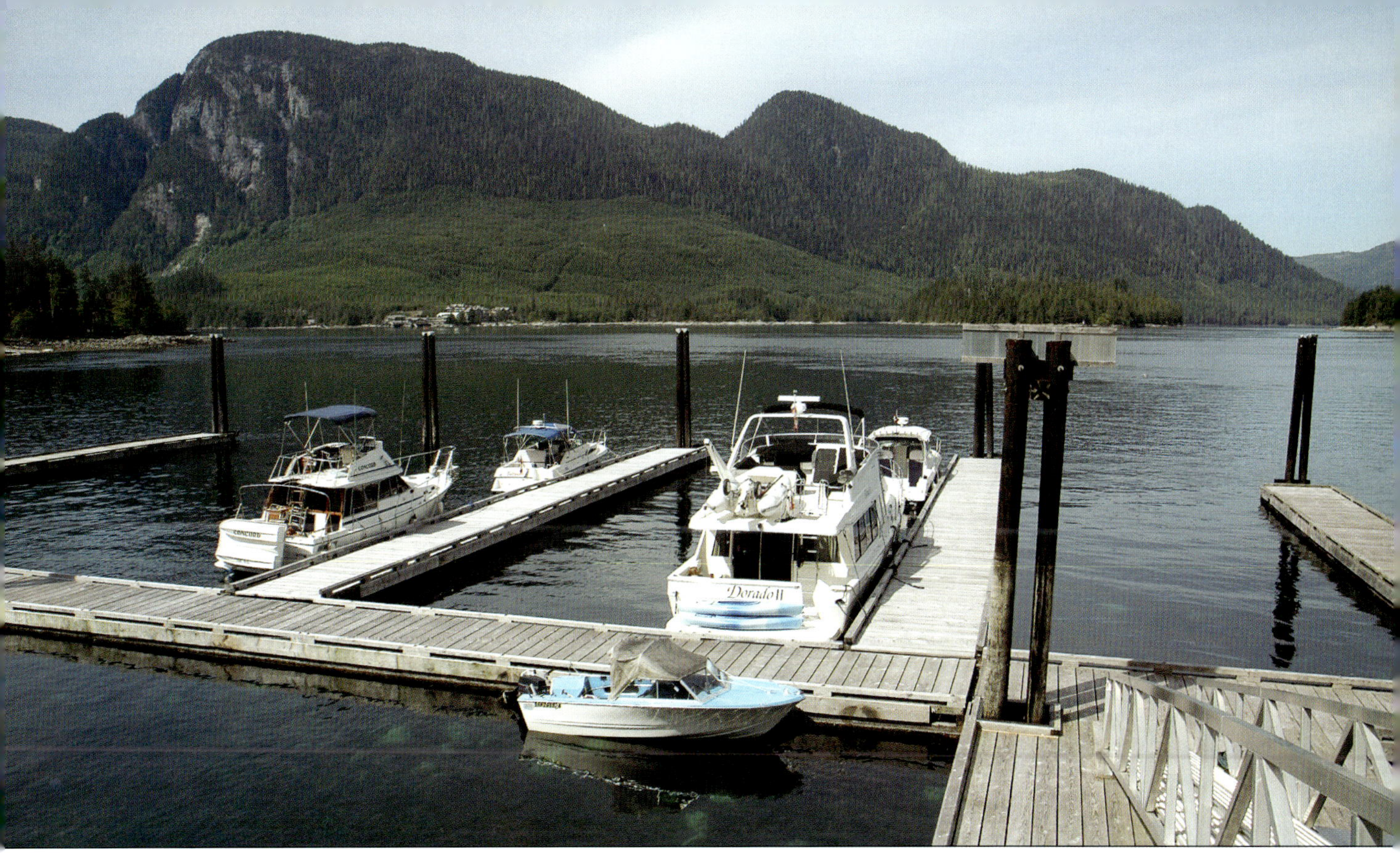

## Stuart Island Community Dock
PO Stuart Island BC V0P 1V0
Phone 250-202-3625    VHF 66A
*email: stuartislandca@aol.com*
*www.stuartislanddock.com*

Boats to 150' can be accommodated at the public floats. There is water but no power at the dock. Showers, washrooms and laundry are available ashore. The community has a coffee shop, grocery store with local crafts and fresh produce, liquor agency and post office. The store has fishing supplies to equip you for the very good fishing in local waters. A Saturday event on the August long weekend supports local salmon enhancement. There are picnic tables on a sheltered deck and facilities for group events. Those looking for exercise can walk to Eagle Lake. Big Bay has good cell phone reception. Float plane and water taxi service is available.

**Navigate with caution in Big Bay. Watch for kelp over the charted reef near shore as you approach the marina and public dock. Currents swirl around the bay at all tides.**

*Right and above: The public dock dominates the waterfront in Big Bay. Note Sonora Lodge in the photo at top of page.*

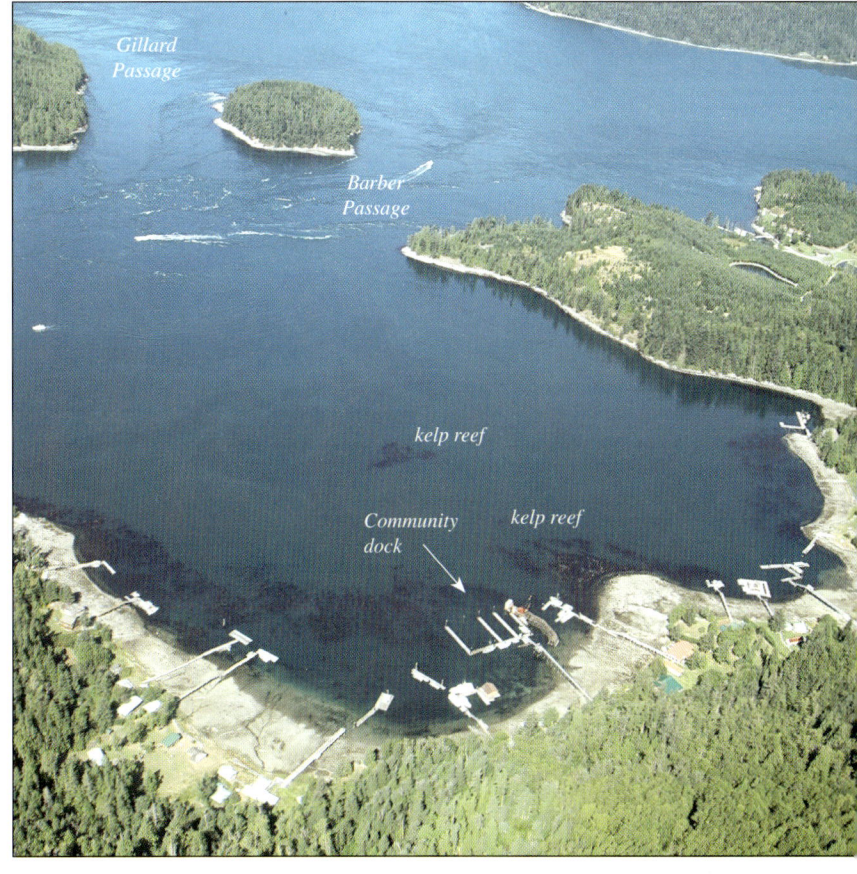

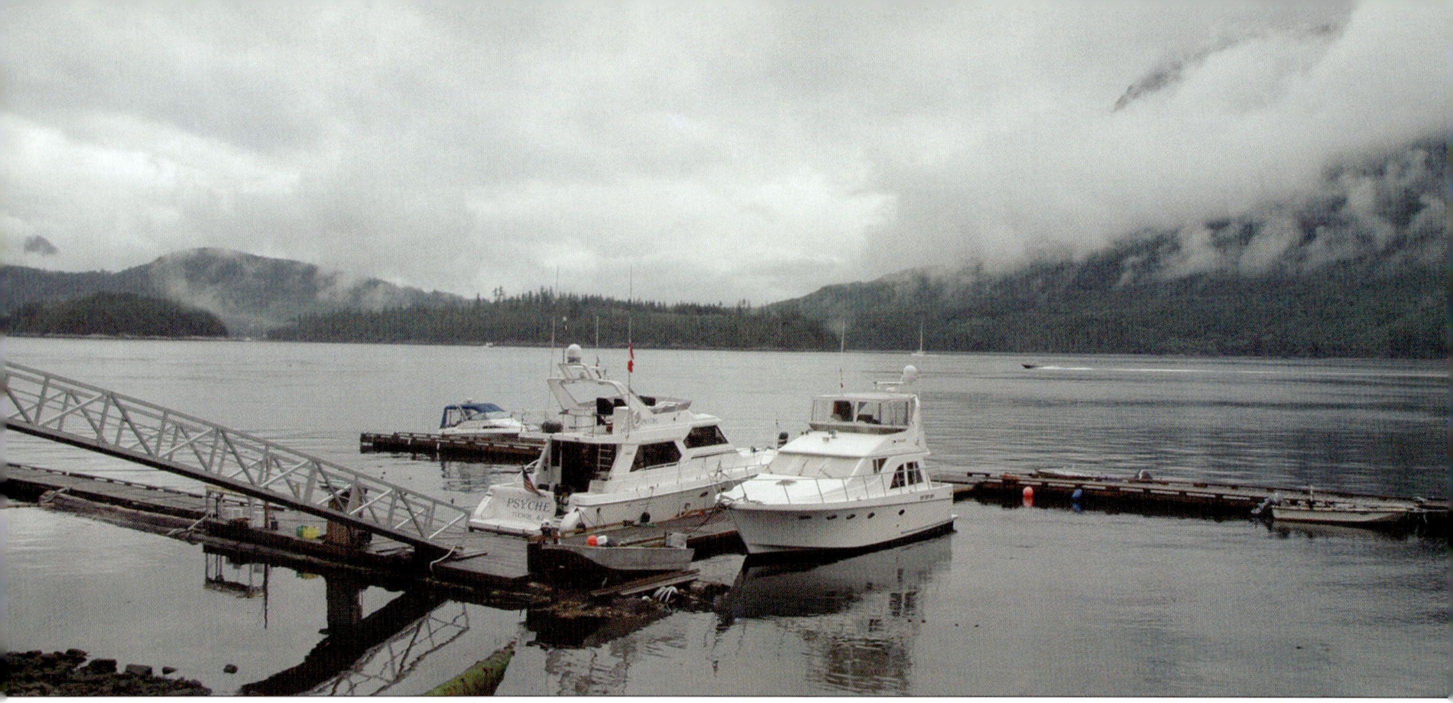

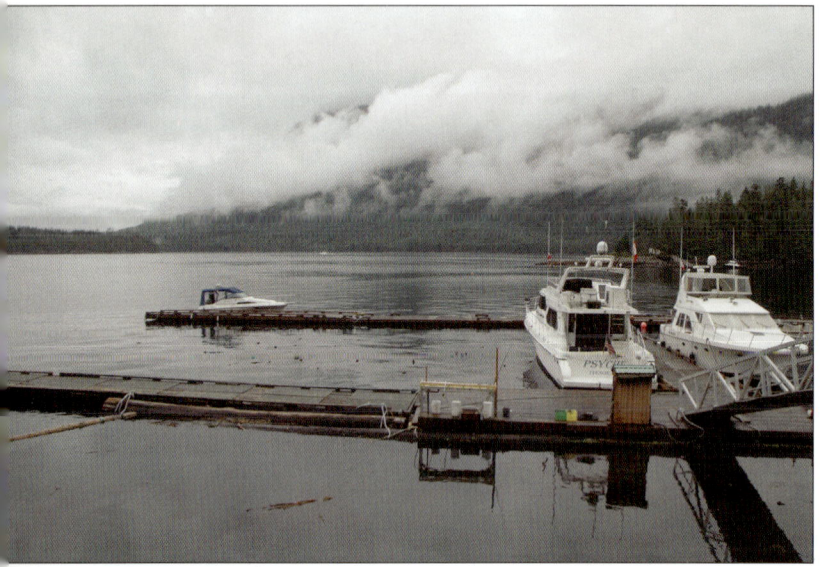

## Morgan's Landing Wilderness Retreat
General Delivery Stuart Island BC V0P 1V0
Phone 250-287-0237
email: jodemorgan@hotmail.com
www.facebook.com/pages/Morgans-Landing

The docks at this resort have been expanded to accommodate additional visiting boats. It has some 375 feet of dock. Bait, ice and fishing licences are available. There is water and power at the docks. At weekends the restaurant is open to visitors as well as guests at the resort. Rental rooms are available and there are guided bear and wildlife watching tours in season.

*Top and left: Moorage at Morgan's Landing. The view is across Big Bay with Gillard Islands in the background.*
*Bottom: The luxurious Sonora Lodge, left, and the Arran Rapids.*
*Opposite page: The dock at Dent Island.*

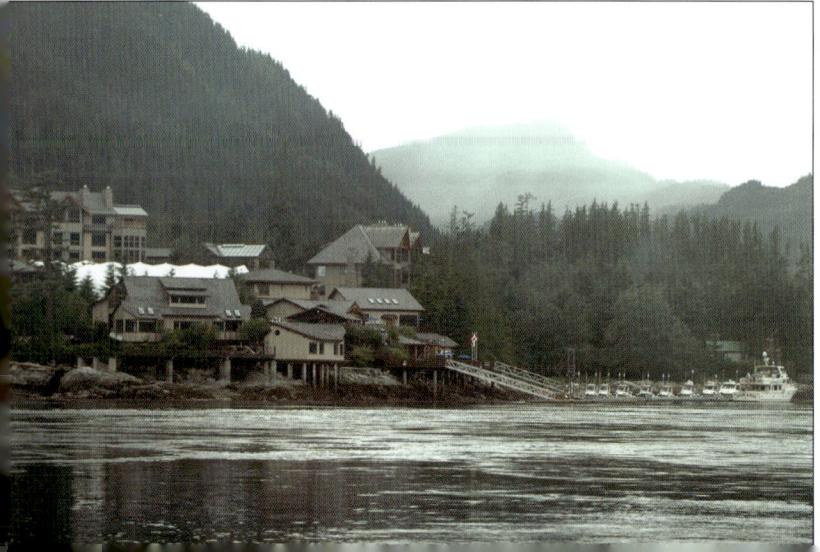

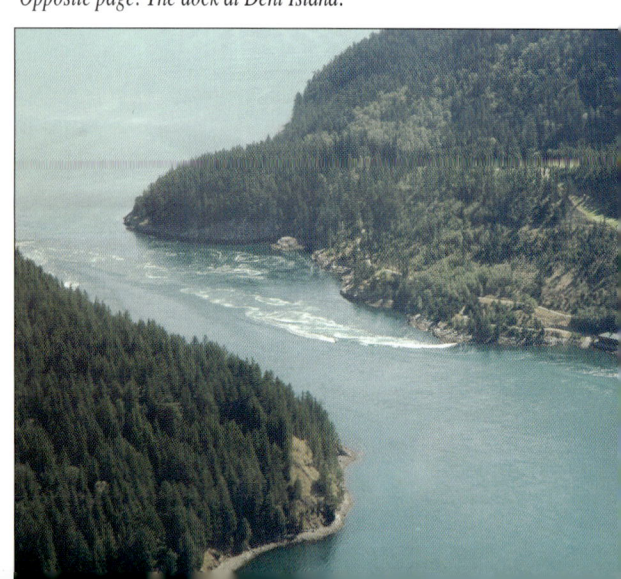

## Dent and Sonora Islands

Although the swirling waters of the adjacent rapids run strong around Dent Island, the docks at Dent Island Resort are somewhat protected from the turbulence. In summer it is a busy place and when you can find space, or have reserved a slip, you will be able to enjoy the ambience and hospitality of a luxurious yet easygoing facility. The lodge is built on the small islands between Dent Island and the mainland with patios and a hot tub extended over narrow Canoe Pass at what has come to be termed Hot Tub Point. The water in this passage runs fairly swiftly at most times. The narrow boat passage is used by fast, small boats and is not suitable for general navigation. The marina is located beyond the fast movement of tidal waters on the islets that separate Dent Island from the mainland. Tidal water passes alongside the resort's west patio, like a mountain stream, with the occasional small fishing boat slipping through between its shores at high tide. The lodge has a gym with large picture windows overlooking the lower reaches of Cordero Channel. Guest cabins are on the second island. Tie up at the floats and stay a while or find anchorage in **Mermaid Bay** at the south end of Dent Island. This anchorage is considered a temporary stop. If you wish to remain in the area longer make sure you have reservations at the lodge docks. On nearby Sonora Island, Sonora Lodge is a luxurious and exclusive fishing destination that caters to fly-in guests. Moorage is available to guests of the lodge only.

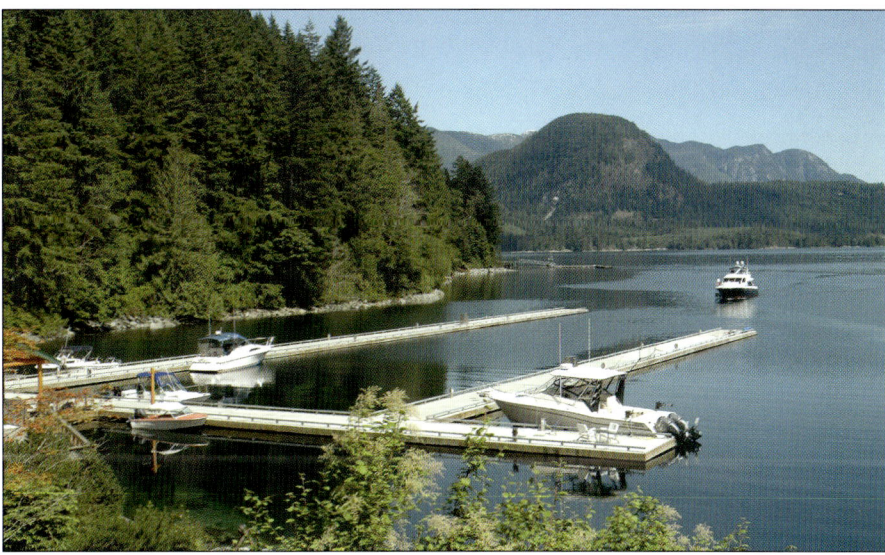

### Dent Island Resort charts 3312, 3543
Stuart Island BC V0P 1V0
Phone 250-203-2553 Fax 250-203-1041
email: info@dentisland.com   www.dentisland.com
There are more than 300 metres of dock space for visitors. The Dent Island Lodge has become renowned for its outstanding location, its atmosphere, gourmet meals and fine accommodations. Shore power is 30, 50 and 100 amps and there is wireless internet available. The resort offers showers, hot tub and sauna, gym, restaurant, fishing guides and accommodations.

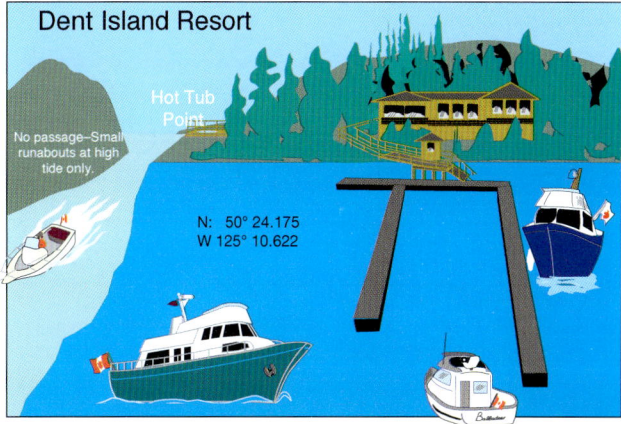

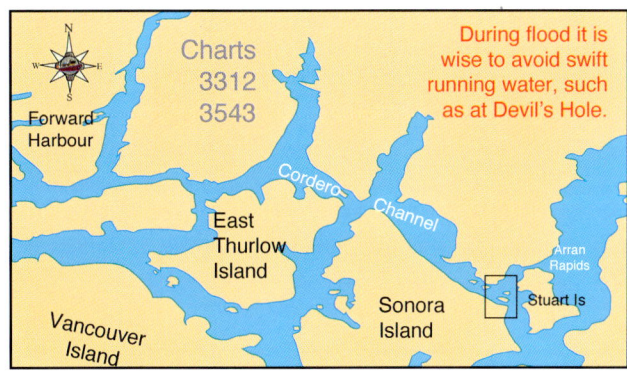

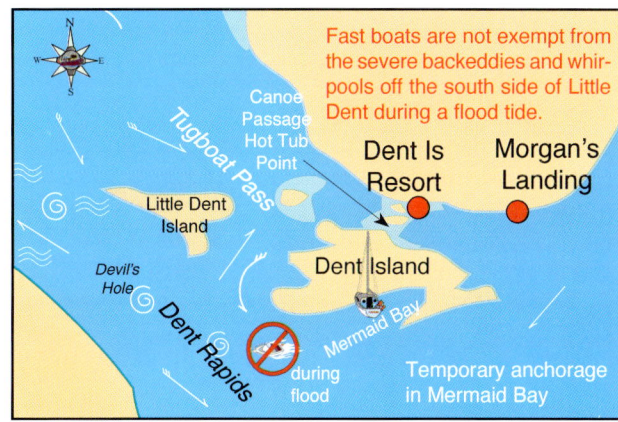

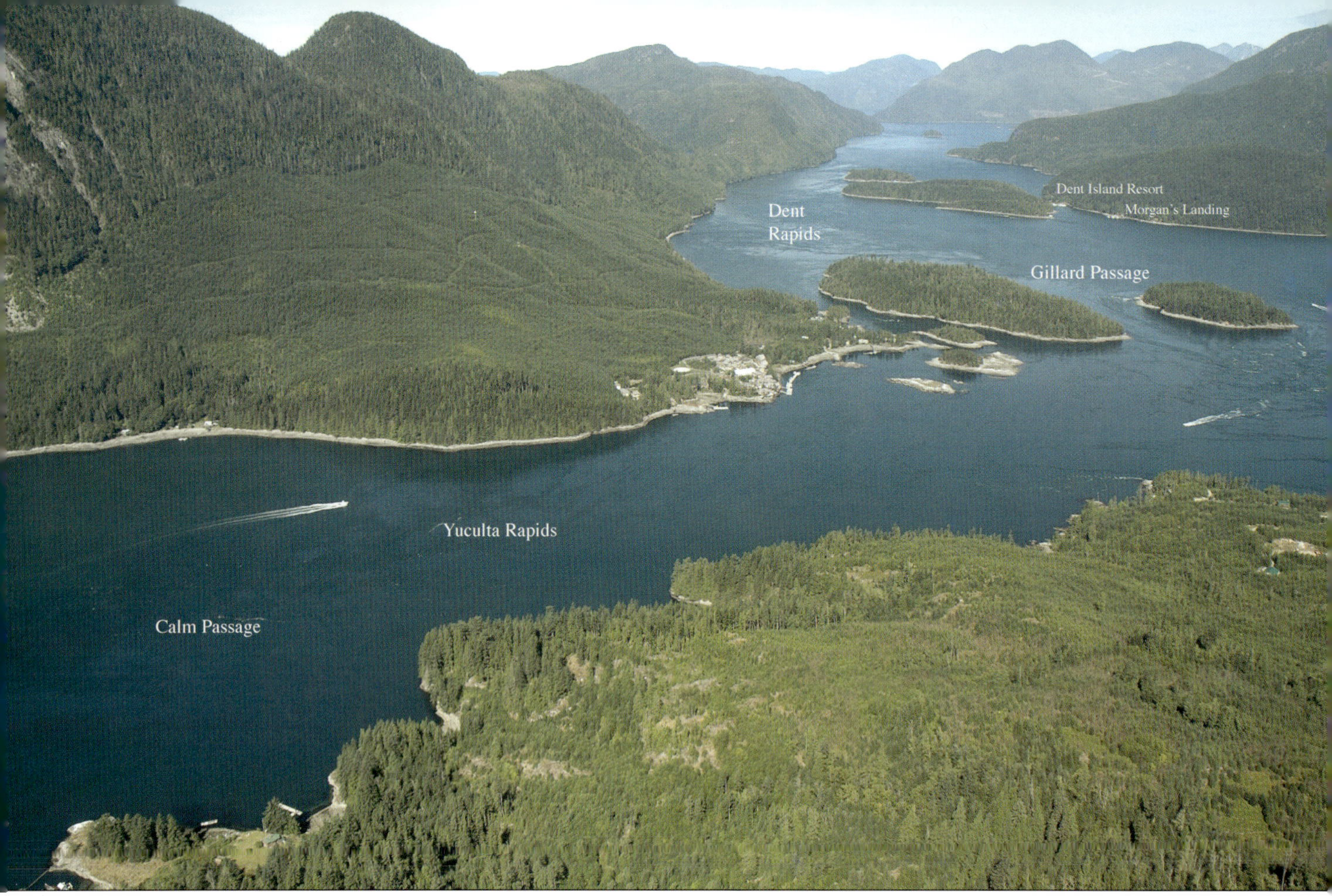

*Looking up Cordero Channel from above Stuart Island. Sonora Lodge can be seen on the shore of Sonora Island. Dent Rapids lies beyond Gillard Passage.*

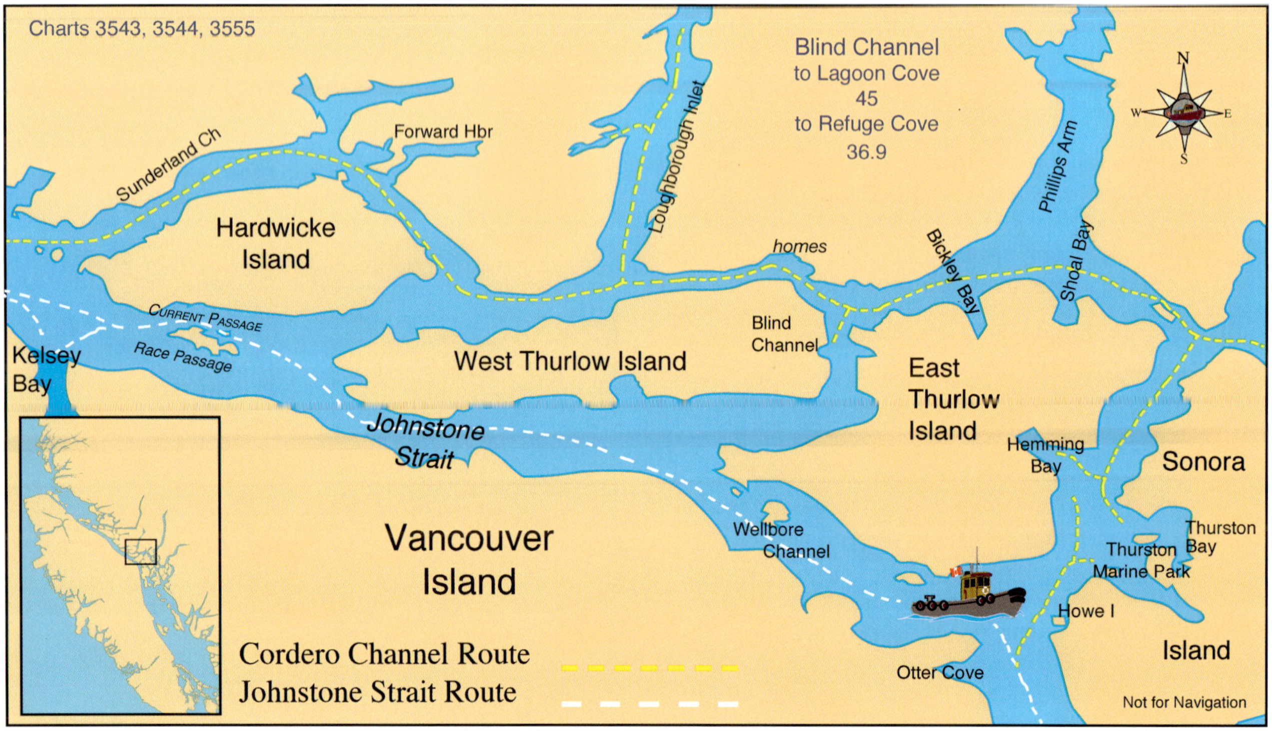

30

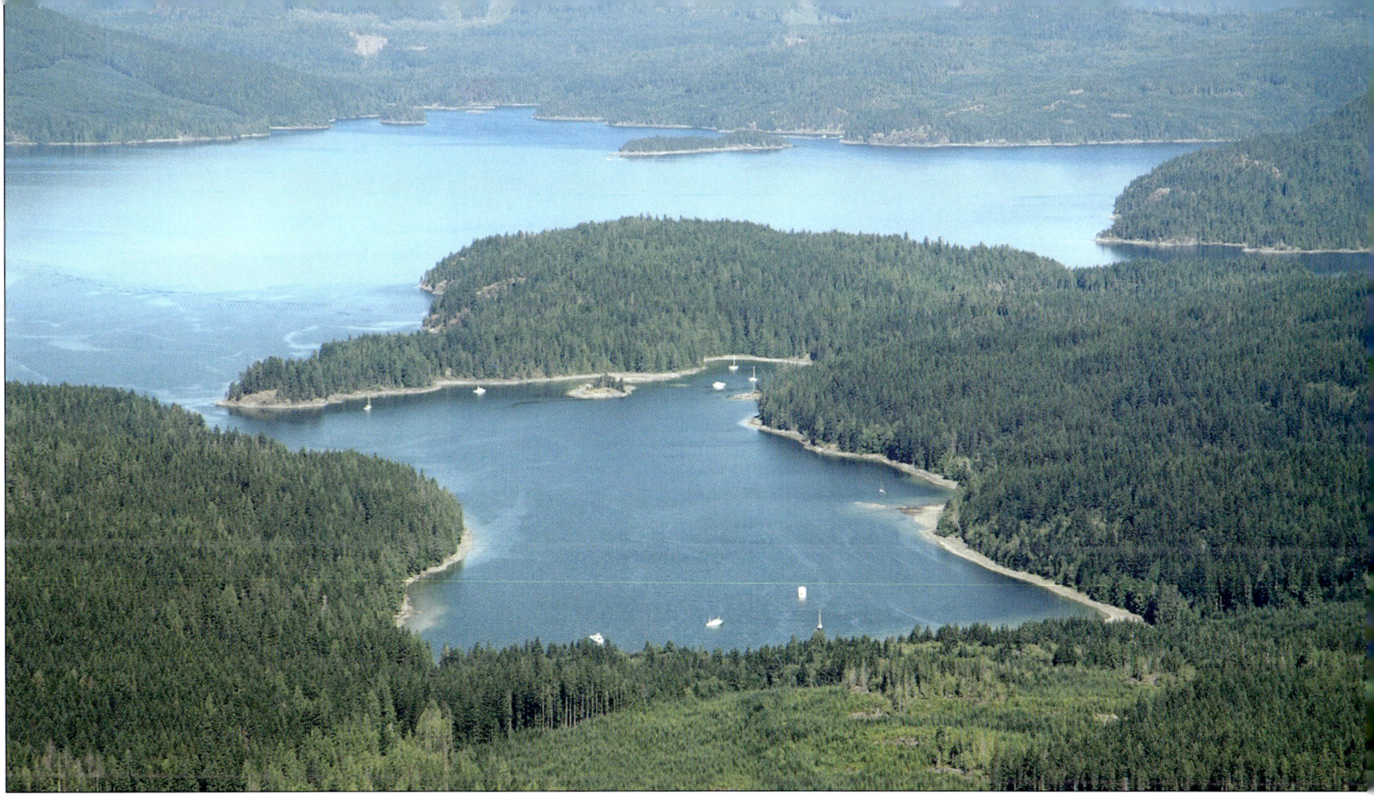

*Thurston Bay Marine Park with Piddell Bay in Cameleon Harbour in the foreground and Handfield Bay opening to the right. Thurston Bay is off to the right (see diagram below). Anchorage is popular in both locations and many mariners make these pristine bays a destination. Beware Maycock Rock, Entry Ledge and Douglas Rock as you approach or leave Handfield Bay. The lagoon cannot be seen in the photo. It is shallow and suitable as an anchorage for small boats. The northern side of Cameleon Harbour and Thurston Bay are marine park areas. Hemming Bay can be seen beyond, on the opposite shore of Nodales Channel.*

## Thurston Marine Park  charts 3312, 3543, 3539

With lots of time available to linger in this area, a pleasurable stop is at Thurston Marine Park on the west side of Sonora Island, on the southeast shores of Nodales Channel. In the park's anchorage a favourite spot to drop the hook is in Cameleon Harbour. This consists of two bays, Piddell Bay and **Handfield Bay**. We like to anchor in Handfield Bay behind Tully Island in about four metres of water. A reef on the west side of the bay dries at low tide exposing a rock that lies north of the island into the anchorage. Take care when setting the anchor to ensure you won't swing over the rock. There is enough room in the bay away from the rock for a dozen boats to lie at anchor, preferably stern tied to shore or the islets in the east side of the bay.

Alternative anchorage, albeit temporary, can be found in **Thurston Bay** where you can drop the hook at the edge of a steep shelf west of the islets at the estuary of the stream that runs into the bay from Florence Lake. The holding ground of the two above anchorages is a mix of mud, shale and stone.

The lagoon at the south side of Thurston Bay is suitable only for small boats that can anchor in the shallow water. The entrance is very shallow at low tide, dropping to less than one metre. An alternative anchorage is in Hemming Bay on the west side of Nodales Channel (see page 32).

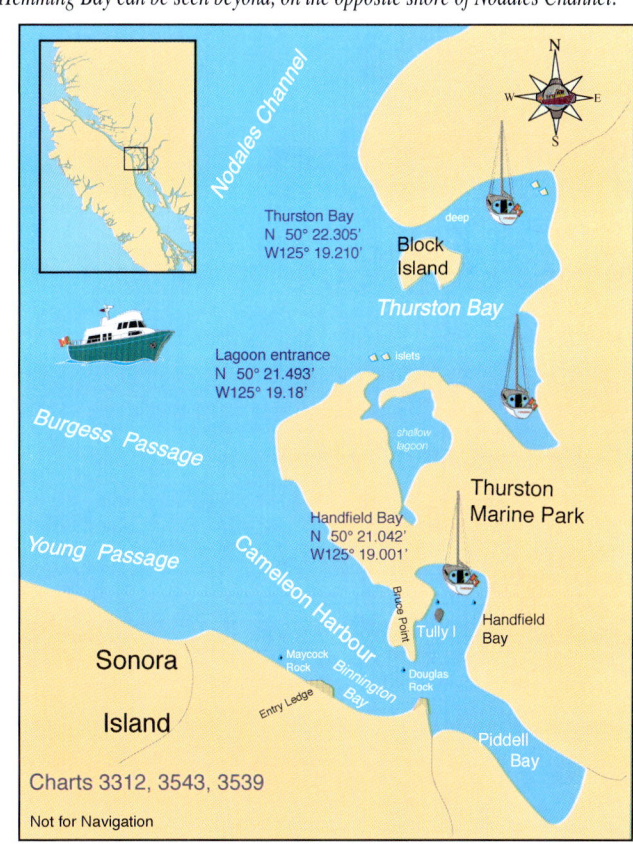

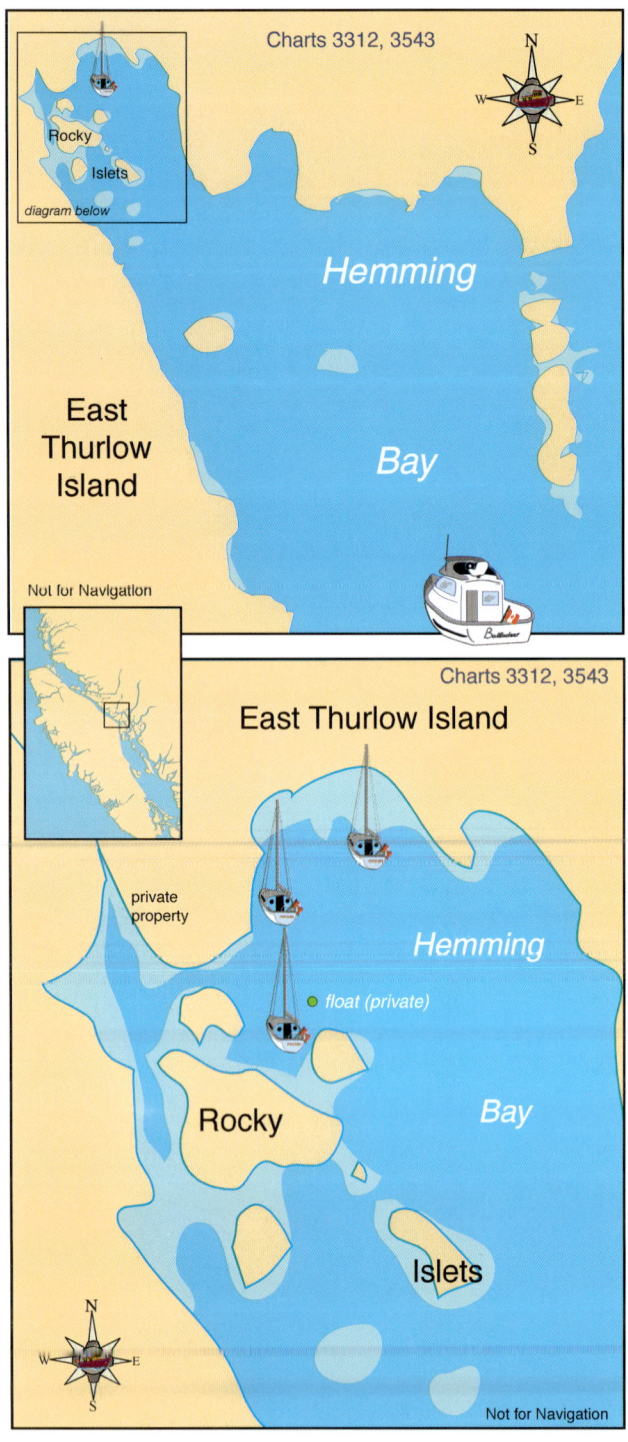

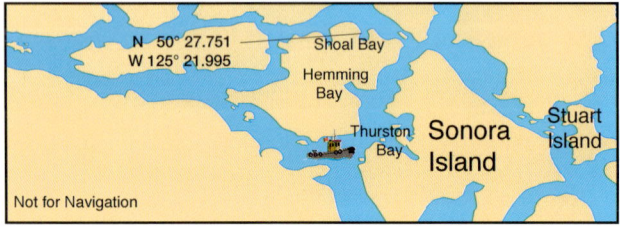

### Fast Planes

On one trip we were enjoying a fast run through these waters and had just passed two large, planing cruising boats at the top of Nodales Channel when we were shocked out of our reverie by the thunderous sound of what at first, and for a fraction of a second, sounded like the engines at the stern of our boat exploding. We had the top of the boat open and I looked up as I turned around and was impacted by the roar of a jet fighter plane as it swooshed overhead. The shock had not passed when it happened a second time. Two fighter planes were barely more than 30 metres above us. I was shaken, but Carla and I love planes and would have liked them to repeat the exercise, only this time with us watching their approach and enjoying the flypast.

### Fast Boats

In order to assess the water conditions, and observe the rips and whirlpools, we have run through the rapids when the current was running strongly between tide turns. While fast boats can handle the swirling currents serious danger exists in the event of a breakdown or striking a floating object. It is safest to avoid transit through the rapids other than slack tide or near slack for all manner of water craft.

## Hemming Bay  charts 3312, 3543, 3539

If Thurston Marine Park is too busy for you, try the Hemming Bay anchorage on the west side of Nodales Channel. Entrance to the bay is to the north of Rocky Islets and the private buoy in the fairway. The anchorage lies just west of and to the northeast of the shallows at the head of the bay where a small, private float serves the local community. The adjacent land is private property and mariners stopping nearby should resist the temptation to go wandering ashore.

Some boaters choose the cozy nook in the northern corner of the larger of the Rocky Islets to drop anchor. Stern tying to the smaller islet is essential because of the limited area to swing.

If you are continuing along Cordero Channel the next good place to stop is at Shoal Bay on East Thurlow Island.

*Anchorage in Hemming Bay is indicated by the sailboat icons in the accompanying diagrams (left).*
*Opposite top: Looking north up Nodales Channel, Howe Island is to the right (diagram page 30), abutting Sonora Island with the opening to Thurston Bay just beyond. The entrance to Hemming Bay can be seen on the opposite side of the channel. A tug is passing the south entrance to Nodales Channel, heading for Chatham Point on calm waters in Johnstone Strait.*
*Opposite bottom: There's tranquility lying at anchor in Thurston Bay.*

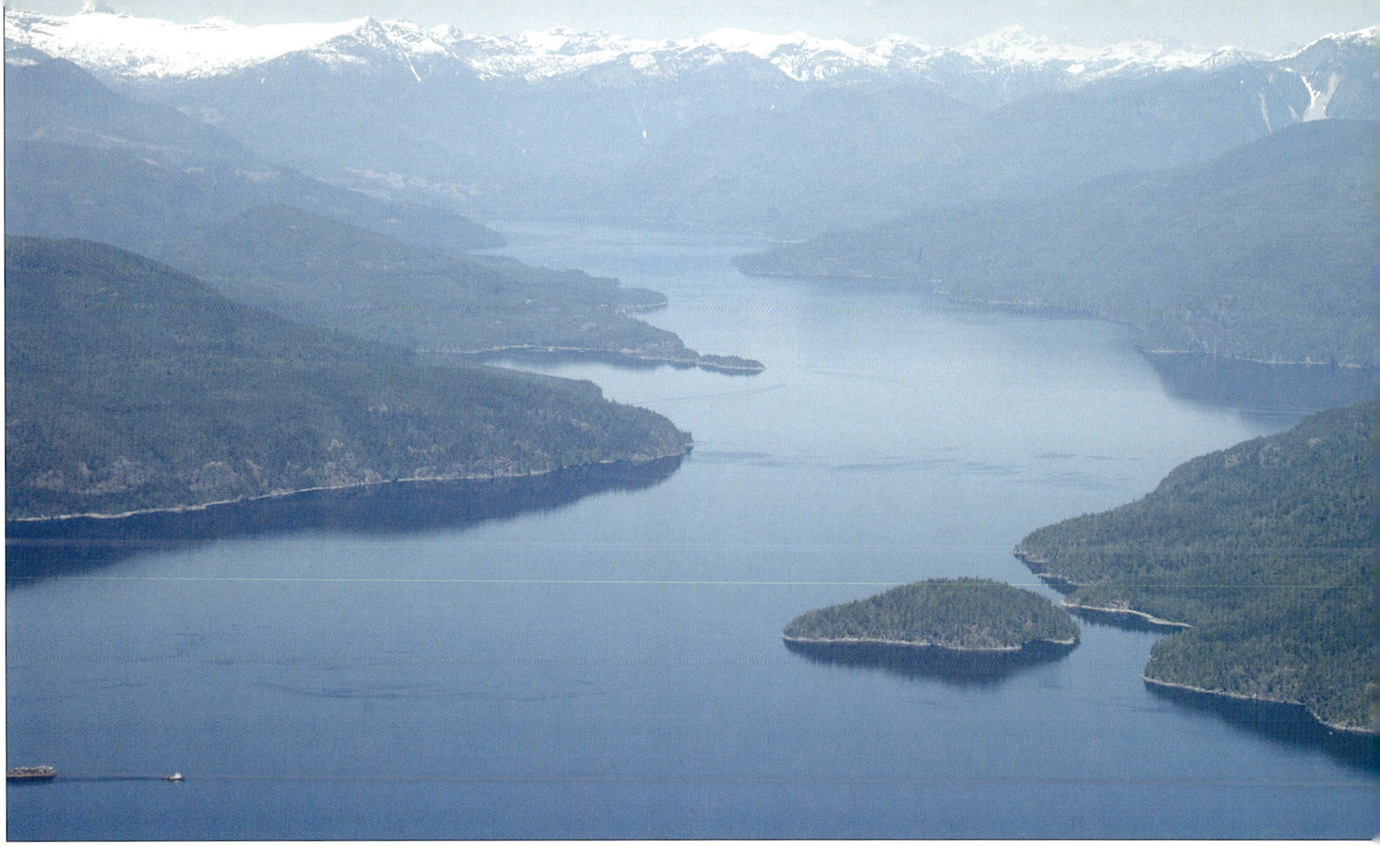

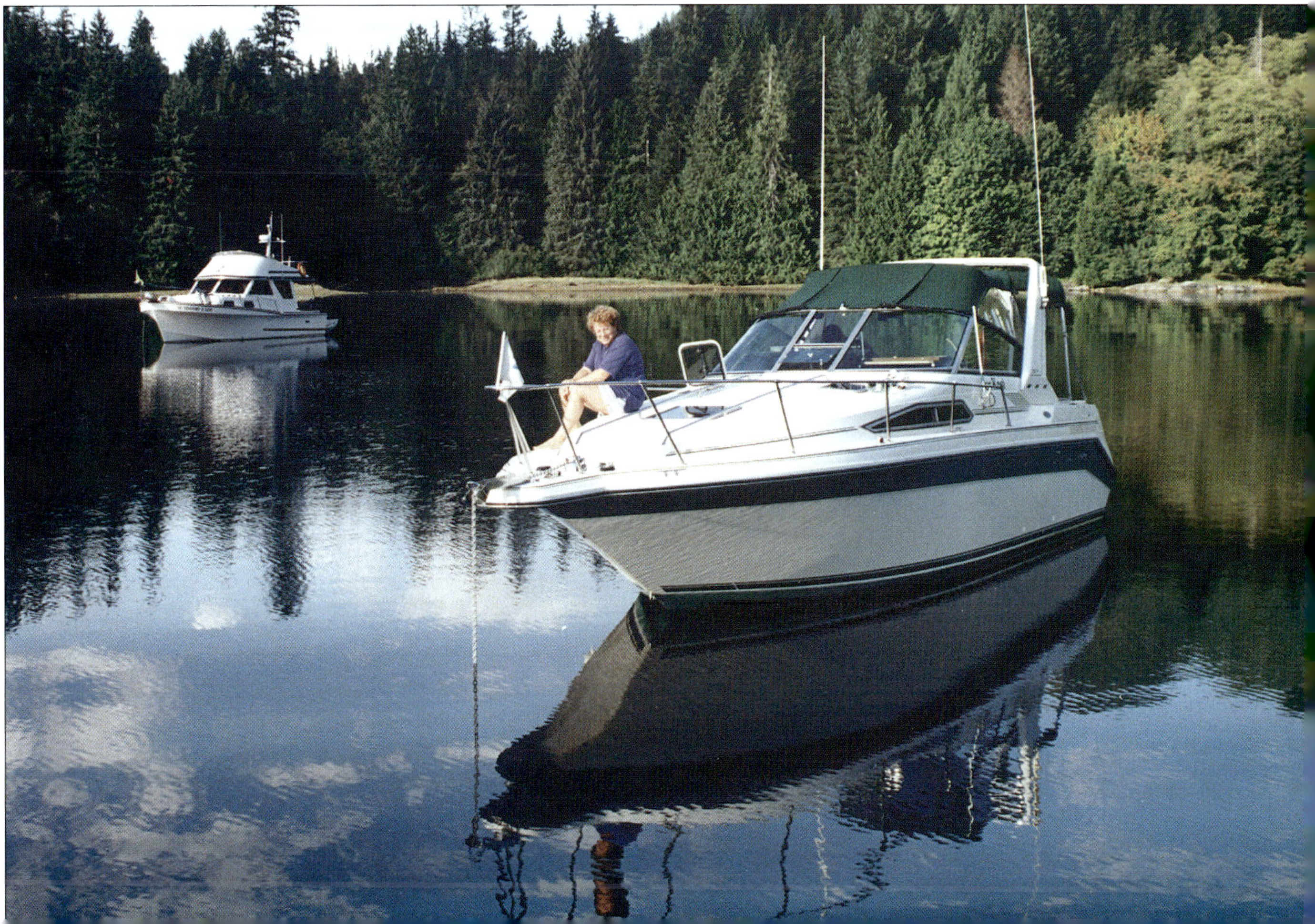

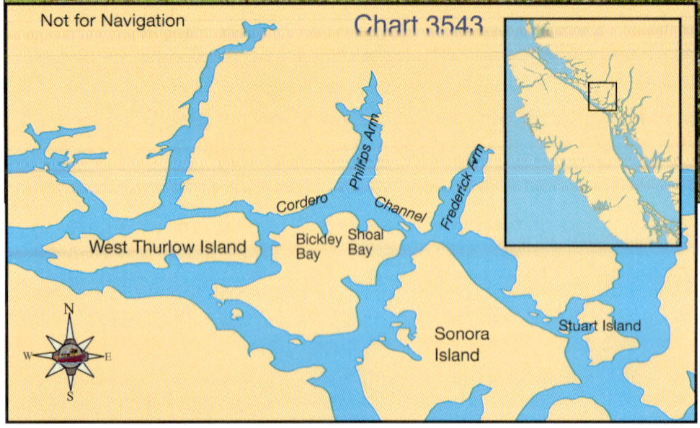

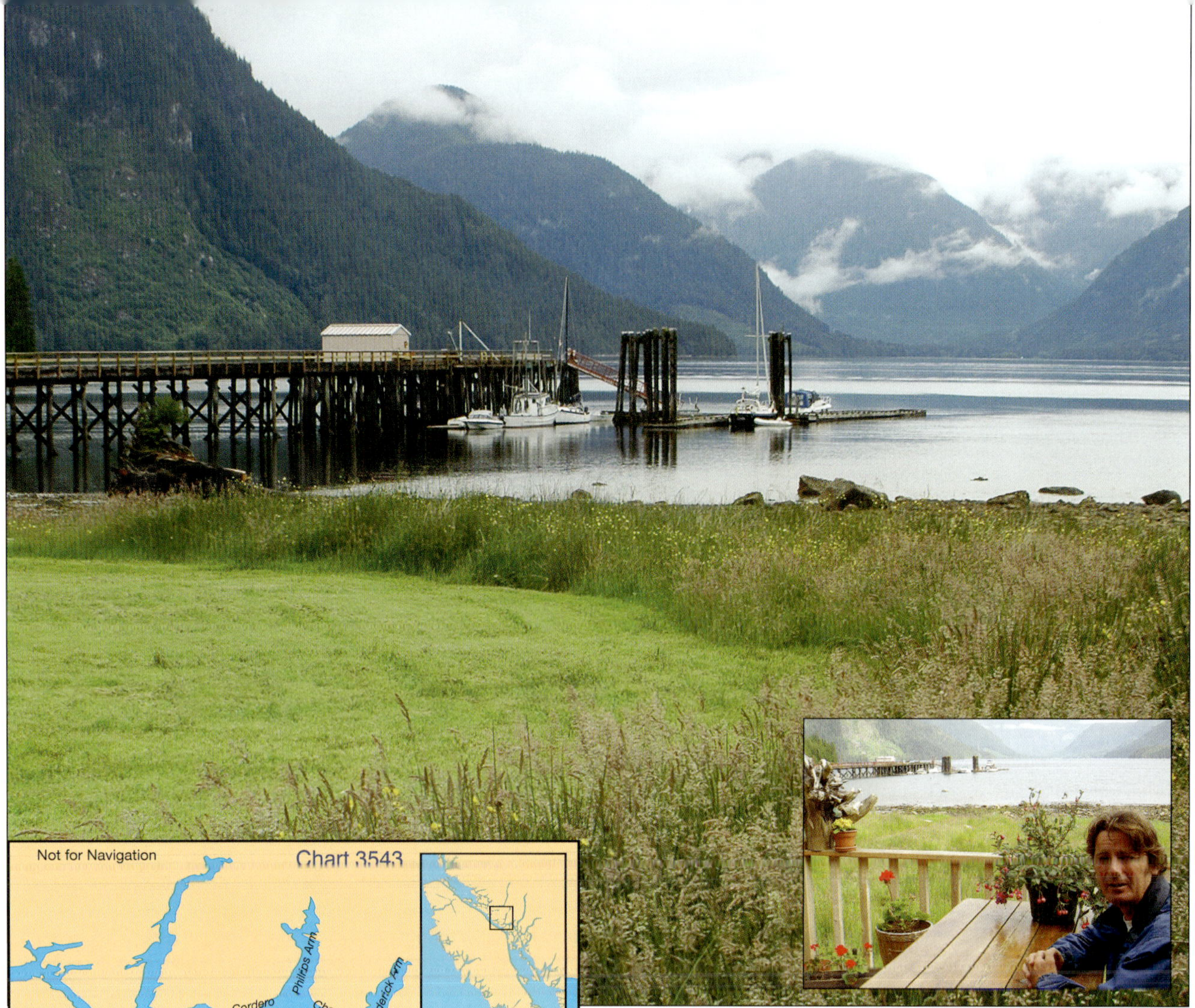

*Shoal Bay was one of the biggest mining towns north of San Francisco at one time, when gold was being extracted from three mines in and near the bay. One site was on the slopes of the mountain at the entrance to Phillips Arm, seen to the left in the photograph. Inset: The owner of Shoal Bay, Mark MacDonald, has been redeveloping the land.*

### Shoal Bay Lodge
Phone 250-287-6818

*shoalbay@mac.com  web.mac.com/shoalbay*

Shoal Bay has moorage at the docks, managed by adjacent property owner Mark MacDonald. Cottages are available for fly-in and other overnight guests. There is free wireless internet access but no power at the dock.

Water is available but there are no other boat services. Pub, coffee bar, laundry, shower and toilets are available at the lodge. Pig roasts, pizza nights, music festivals and other events are offered in summer.

The property boasts a comfortable cabin and patio for group gatherings, and a u-pick vegetable garden. There is an expansive beach and hiking trails with view points

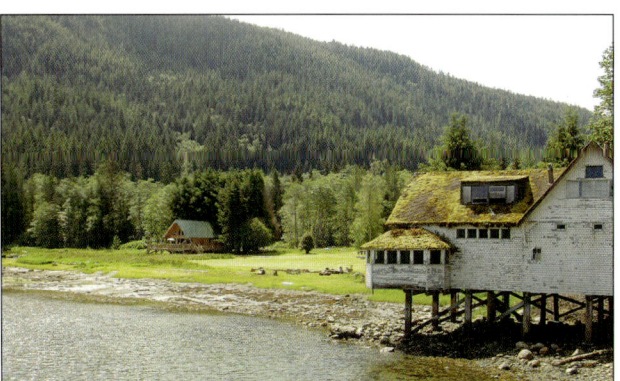

*The familiar old warehouse at Shoal Bay, now demolished, with new structures seen in the background*

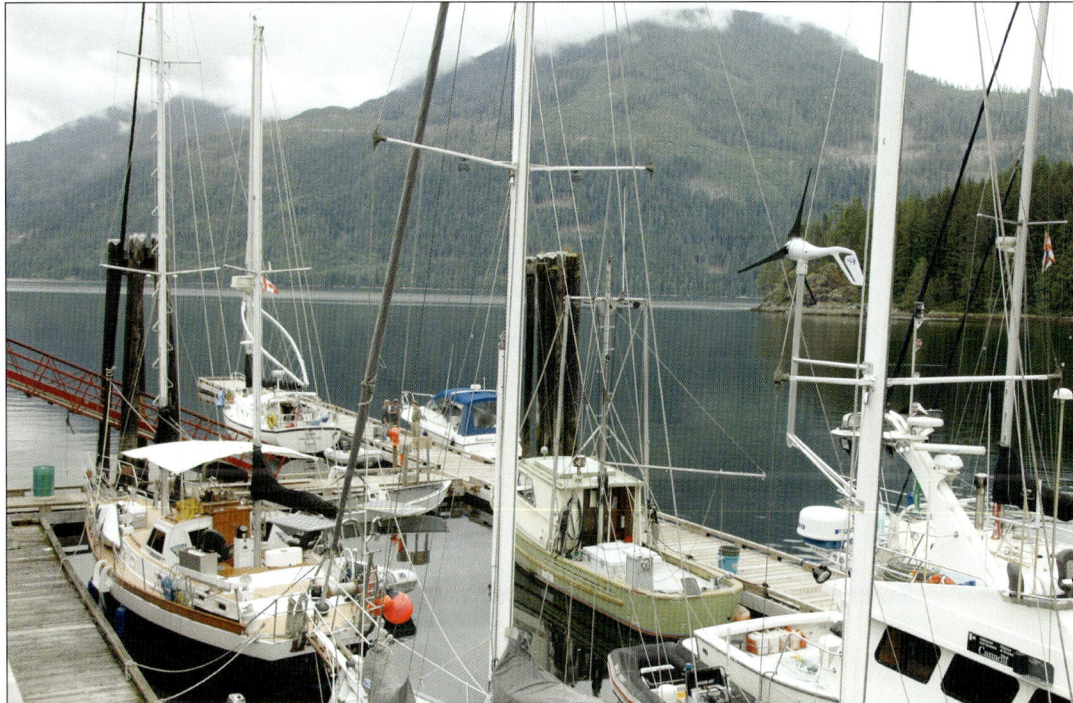

*Opposite and right: Mariners awaiting the tidal changes tie up for the night at the public dock at Shoal Bay. The dock has limited space. It is peaceful in the bay most times in summer and possible to anchor nearby during calm conditions.*

## Shoal Bay  charts 3543, 3312

Cruising up Cordero Channel a fairly straight course leads from Nodales Channel and its intersection with Frederick Arm. Pass on either side of Channe Island (Note: This is the correct name and spelling–Channe). The first shelter to stop at, Shoal Bay, with its large expanse of grassy meadow and shallow shoreline, lies seven miles west of Dent Rapids. This open bay faces north, looking directly up Phillips Arm. The lodge is a family run business welcoming guests to a small pub/cafe and serving as a stop *en route* for whale and bear watching groups out of Campbell River.

Shoal Bay has seen changes over the past quarter century that took it from a lodge and fishing centre to a makeshift inn for transient boaters, and later to an outdoor adventure retreat. Gold mining was prominent in the area in the early years and at one time a large encampment of Chinese workers was established on the property. There were three gold mines in operation, one at the bay and two in Phillips Arm. The largest was the Douglas Pine Mine. The mines brought a lot of attention to the area turning the settlement into one of the biggest mining towns north of San Francisco. It's hard to believe that this quiet bay with its sparse settlement was once a busy town with many floating structures as well as buildings on shore.

Moorage for transient yachtsmen has been available by way of a public dock run by property owner Mark MacDonald. The lodge and property were owned for a while up until about 2001 by Blair and Kevan McLean in Campbell River with resident managers at the site. All of this tenure came to a crashing halt when in 2000 the lodge burned to the ground and the McLeans put it on the market. The property was then acquired by Mark MacDonald, a long time resident of Delta, BC. In recent years the facility has been providing pub fare and light meals to wilderness adventure parties and transient boaters. Anchorage in the bay, to the west of the public dock is subject to possible rolling as boats pass by in Cordero Channel. Wind is not usually a major factor in summer, but monitor the forecast because anything blowing down Phillips Arm could be uncomfortable.

In Frederick Arm, the small floating restaurant, Oleo's, offers space for several boats while dining. Contact the owners at 250-203-6670 or on VHF 66A.

## Bickley Bay  charts 3543, 3312

Continuing along Cordero Channel beyond Shoal Bay the next shelter, at Bickley Bay. There is no public dock in Bickley Bay. Many mariners stop there overnight, although the anchorage is generally regarded only as temporary. Be mindful of Peel Rocks at its western entrance. Passage may be made either side of these rocks if you carefully identify their location. Drop anchor at its head in about 6 metres. The bay is open and without any formal settlement. Fishing boats and tugs sometimes use it as a stop between the rapids when timing necessitates doing so. In Cordero Channel the currents reach about three knots outside Bickley Bay. Don't let this fool you. At Dent Island they are running at up to 11 knots and a turbulent 5 knots at Greene Point, to the west. (Diagram page 37.) A fish farm was present on its NE side in 2011.

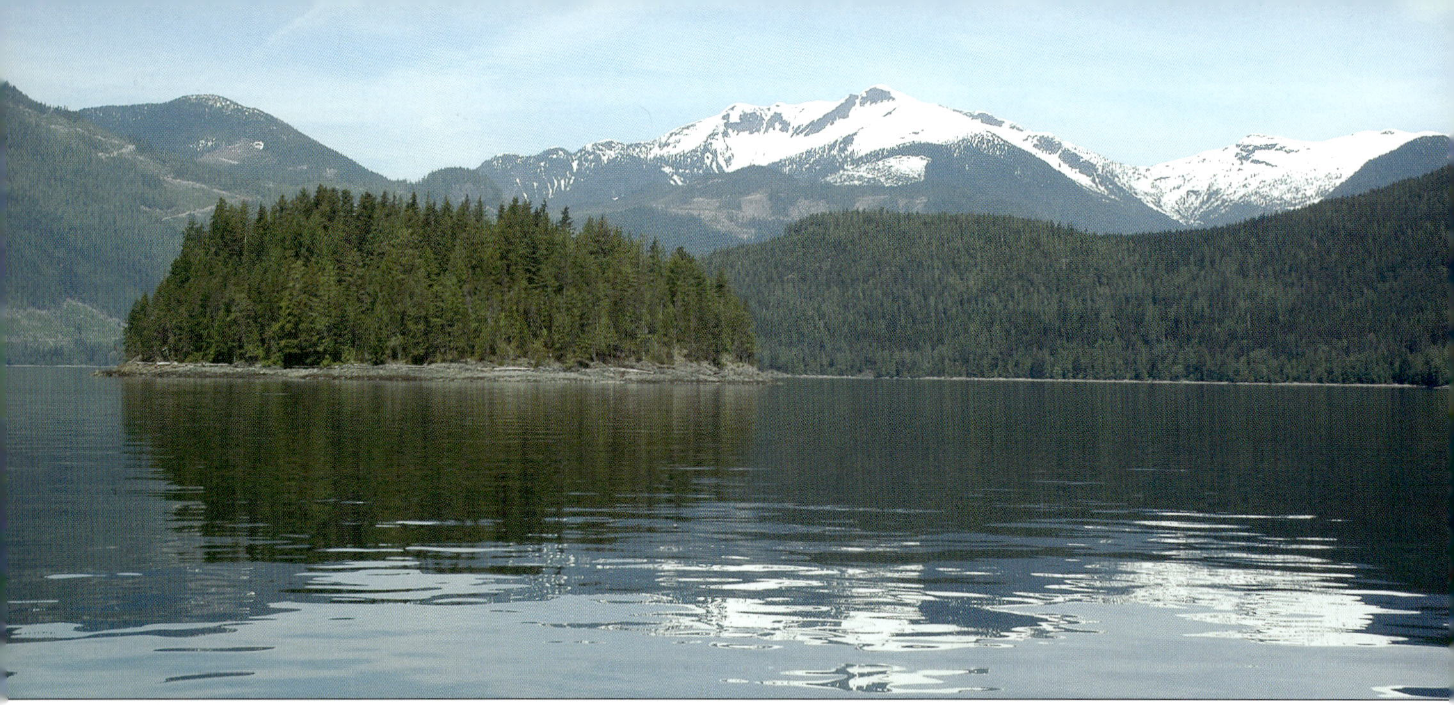

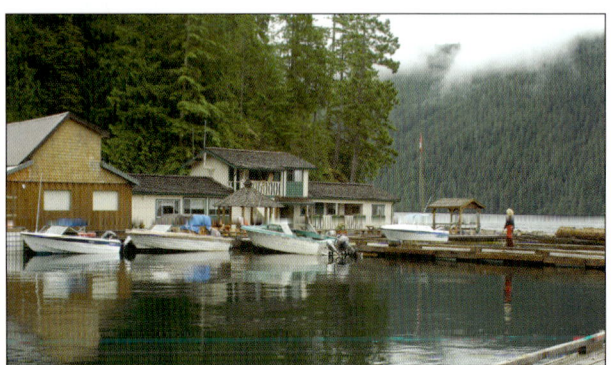
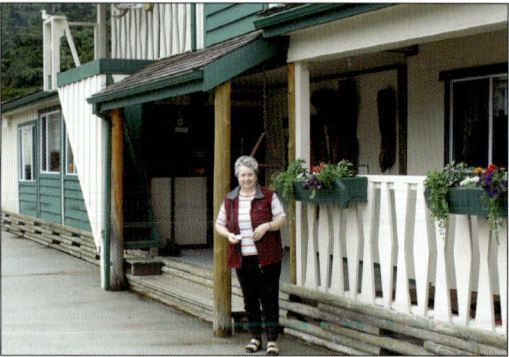

*Left: Cordero Lodge docks and cabins and lodge owner Doris Küppers at Cordero Channel.*

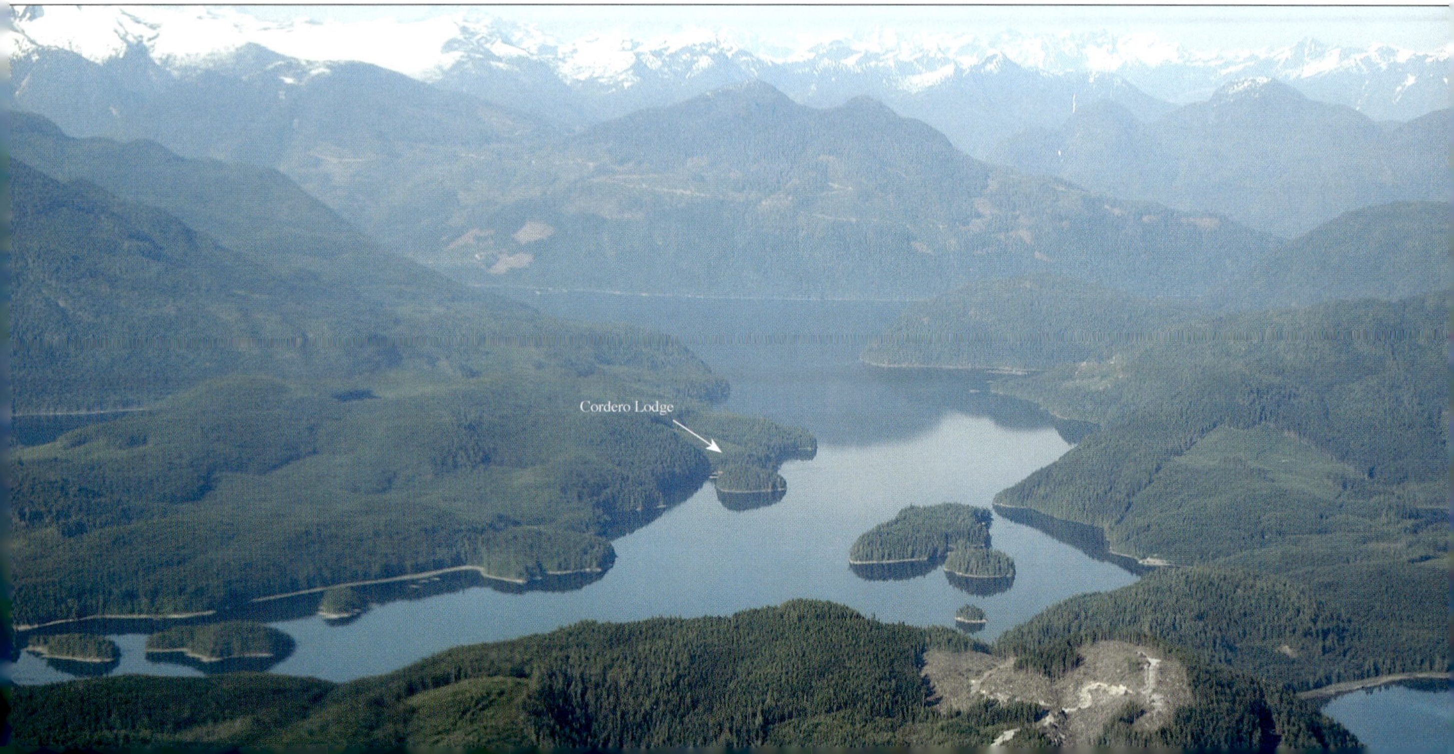

Cordero Lodge

# Cordero Channel  charts 3543, 3312

There is an anchorage tucked in behind the **Cordero Islands**. The flood tide does not affect the anchorage until it is half way through its cycle. Then it can be felt throughout the sheltered nook. It is affected by most wind conditions and therefore should be used only as a temporary stop. Enter between the eastern island of the group and the two on the west. Be mindful of the reef to starboard as you enter. Drop the hook well over in the western end in about 20 metres. The mud and sand bottom provides quite good holding.

You may consider a temporary stop at **Crawford Anchorage** behind Erasmus and Mink Islands, but this anchorage has turbulence and a strong flood current running through it, funneled by the narrow opening at the east end of Erasmus Island. If you are pushing on through the Greene Point Rapids you should be cognisant of the turbulence potential on the east side of Griffiths Islet during a flood and the west side during the ebb. Other anchoring options include **Tallac Bay**, a small cove opposite Erasmus Island that is guarded by a reef protruding southeast into Cordero Channel. Keep clear of this reef because its pinnacles are less than 2 metres at low tide. Inside the bay drop anchor in about 8 metres off the west shore. The bay dries to the northeast but the entrance and the bay are out of the swift current in the channel.

If you want to stop in the most protected overnight place in the area continue down Mayne Passage to Blind Channel where a safe moorage can be found at the **Blind Channel Resort** marina. If you are intent on anchoring you could use the relatively sheltered spot opposite Blind Channel Resort in **Charles Bay** (diagram page 39). It is a shallow bay with Eclipse Islet, surrounded by boulders, in the centre, and is suitable for smaller vessels only. Entrance is to the south of Shell Point. Another possible anchorage is in about 4 metres at low tide in the south portion of the bay, but the bottom is muddy with eel grass and not the best of holding grounds.

Passage through the Greene Point Rapids is subject to a 7 knot current. Overfalls, whirlpools and eddies accompany the stream and it is best to avoid the area until slack tide or near slack. Use Tide Tables Volume 6 for Greene Point Rapids' secondary station referenced on Seymour Narrows.

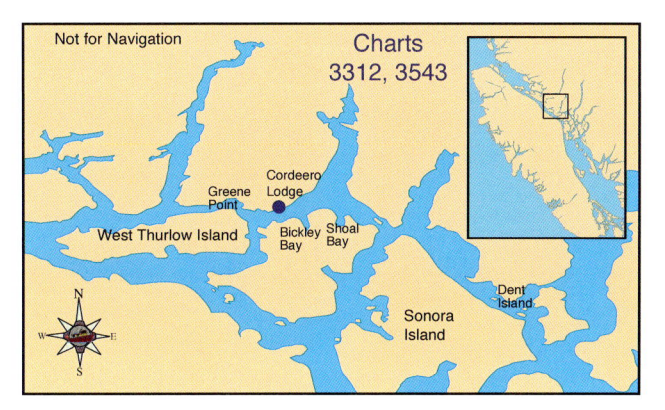

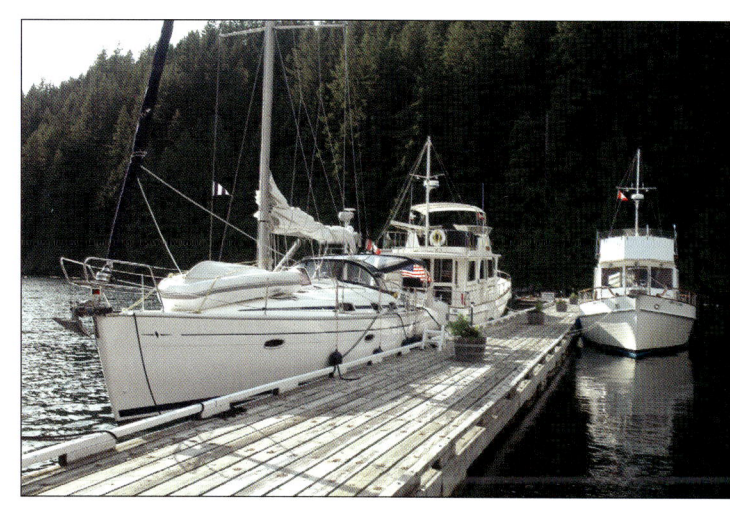

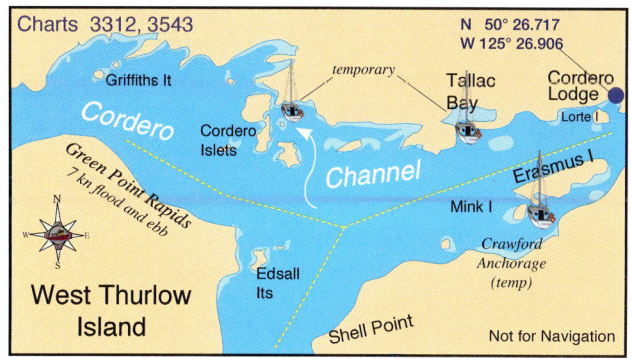

## Cordero Lodge

Cordero Channel. Phone 250-287-0917
info@corderolodge.com  www.corderolodge.com

For several decades a popular stop for many travellers has been at Cordero Lodge east of Lorte Island. Here Reinhart and Doris Küppers and daughter Kellie have been running a restaurant and lodge, catering to an international mix of regular and new customers. For the boating crowd, there is usually limited overnight mooring space for those dining at the restaurant. VHF is not monitored.

Just beyond this floating lodge is the anchorage behind the Cordero Islets or in Tallac Bay in which yachtsmen may find refuge during the tidal change when the Greene Point Rapids are flowing too fast for comfort. There they await the next approaching slack to continue through Wellbore Channel and Whirlpool Rapids. Or they go to Blind Channel.

*Top: Visiting boats at Cordero Lodge docks. Opposite top: Beautiful ocean and mountain vistas greet the mariner in Cordero Channel. Bottom: Looking east along Cordero Channel from West Thurlow Island. Erasmus Island is in the centre. Bickley Bay lies off Cordero Channel on the right.*

*Cordero Lodge is located in the lee of the island abutting the shore to left of Erasmus Island.* **As you approach Cordero Lodge slow down to create no wash. Even passing by a distance off, the channel is narrow enough for a large wash to cause damage to the docks and buildings.**

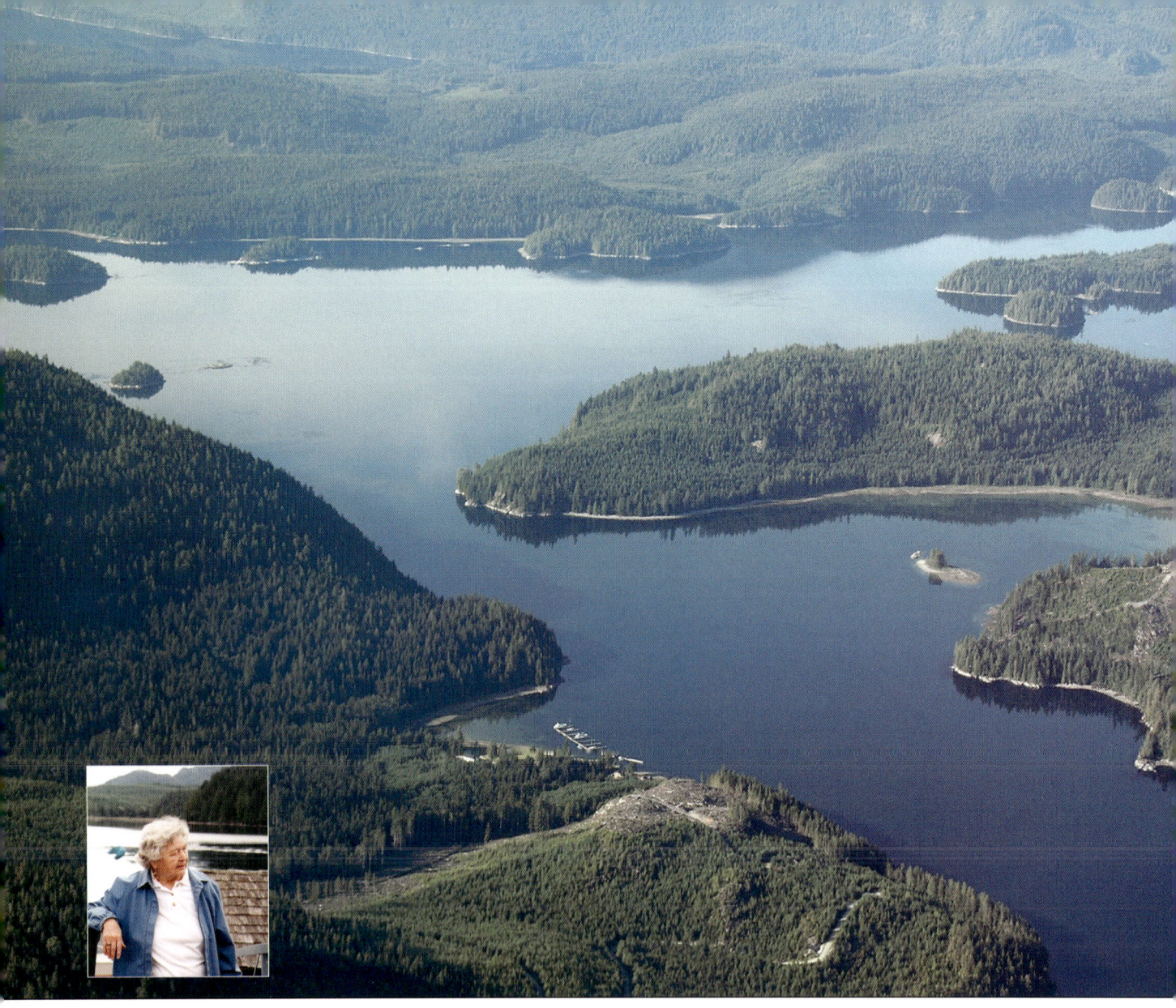

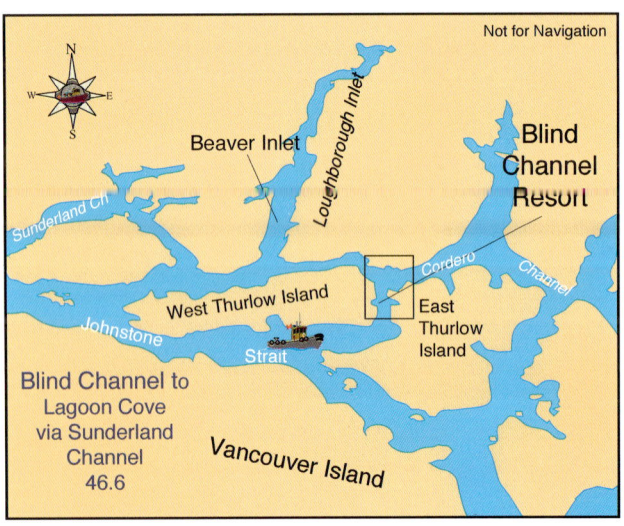

## Blind Channel Resort

Blind Channel BC V0P 1B0
Phone 250-949-1420
toll-free 1-888-329-0475
email: info@blindchannel.com
www.blindchannel.com

This is a well-founded marine facility. It offers transient moorage, showers, laundry and washrooms. It offers fuel–gas, diesel and kerosene. Water and power–15, 20 and 50 amps, are available at the dock. There is a large sunny patio overlooking the marina, with restaurant for fine dining, a hamburger stand, gazebo featuring movie nights on Tuesdays, a store, post office and rental cottage.

Blind Channel Resort is a good place also to replenish ice and propane and pick up charts, books, tackle, bait, groceries, fresh baked goods, frozen foods and other supplies.

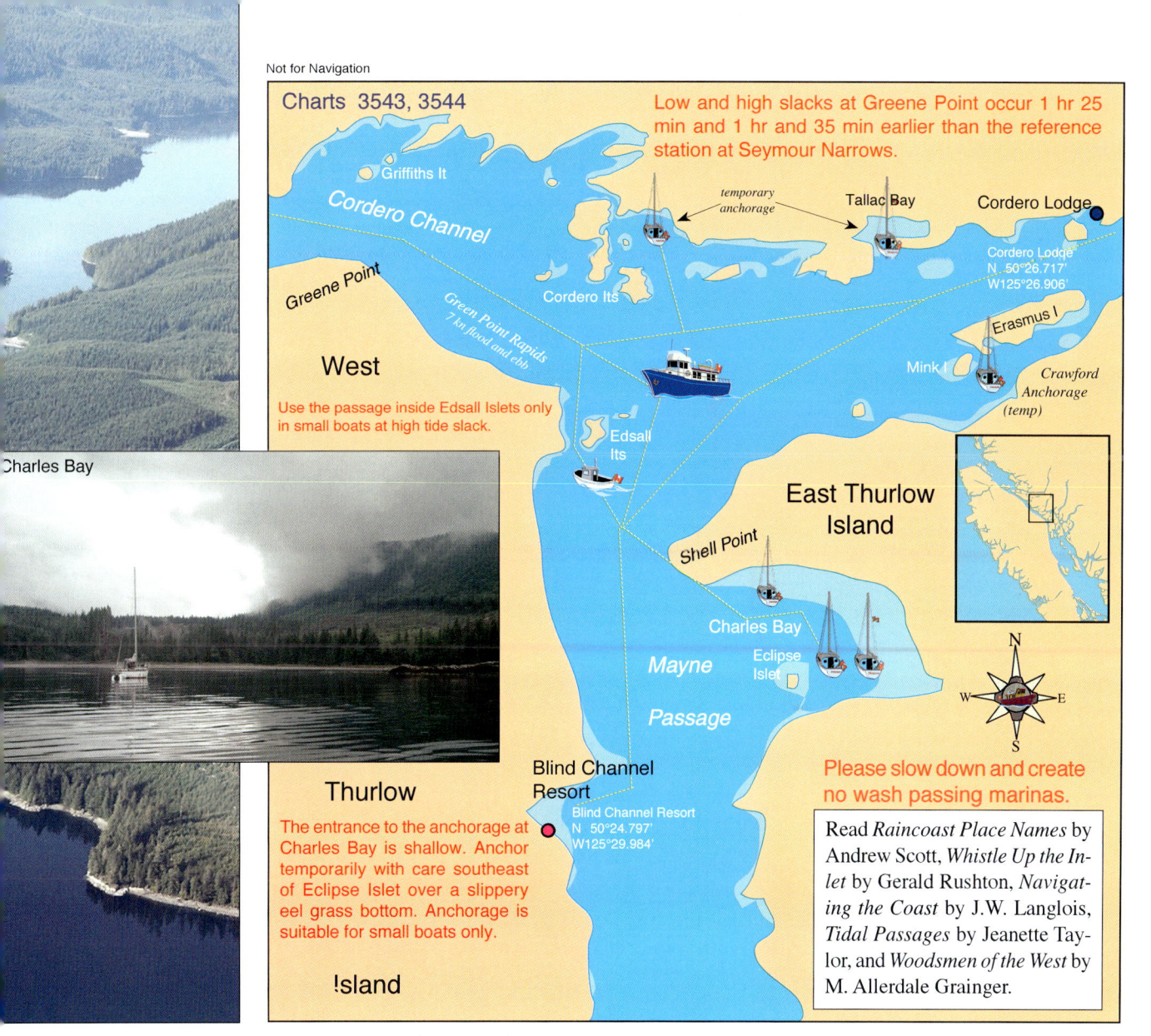

Not for Navigation

**Charts 3543, 3544**

Low and high slacks at Greene Point occur 1 hr 25 min and 1 hr and 35 min earlier than the reference station at Seymour Narrows.

Griffiths It
Cordero Channel
temporary anchorage
Tallac Bay
Cordero Lodge
Cordero Lodge N. 50°26.717' W125°26.906'
Greene Point
Cordero Its
Green Point Rapids 7 kn flood and ebb
Erasmus I
Mink I
Crawford Anchorage (temp)

**West**

Use the passage inside Edsall Islets only in small boats at high tide slack.

Edsall Its

**East Thurlow Island**

Shell Point

Charles Bay
Eclipse Islet

*Mayne Passage*

Blind Channel Resort
Blind Channel Resort N 50°24.797' W125°29.984'

**Thurlow**

The entrance to the anchorage at Charles Bay is shallow. Anchor temporarily with care southeast of Eclipse Islet over a slippery eel grass bottom. Anchorage is suitable for small boats only.

**Island**

Please slow down and create no wash passing marinas.

Read *Raincoast Place Names* by Andrew Scott, *Whistle Up the Inlet* by Gerald Rushton, *Navigating the Coast* by J.W. Langlois, *Tidal Passages* by Jeanette Taylor, and *Woodsmen of the West* by M. Allerdale Grainger.

Charles Bay

Anchorages in the vicinity of Blind Channel should be considered temporary, such as the one at Charles Bay on the opposite side of the channel from the resort (inset photograph, above). The marina offers fuel and protected moorage with facilities that include a fine restaurant and a well-stocked store, including a selection of gifts and souvenirs. Below: Members of the Richter family at Blind Channel Resort. Inset the late Annemarie Richter.

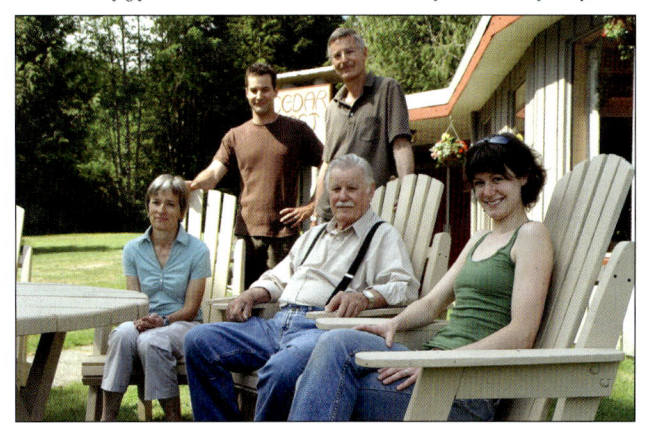

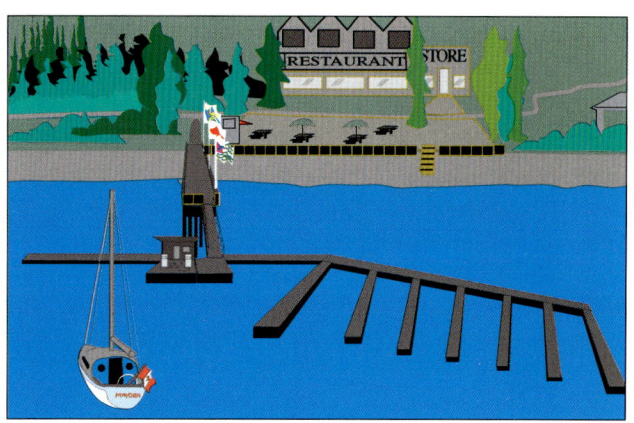

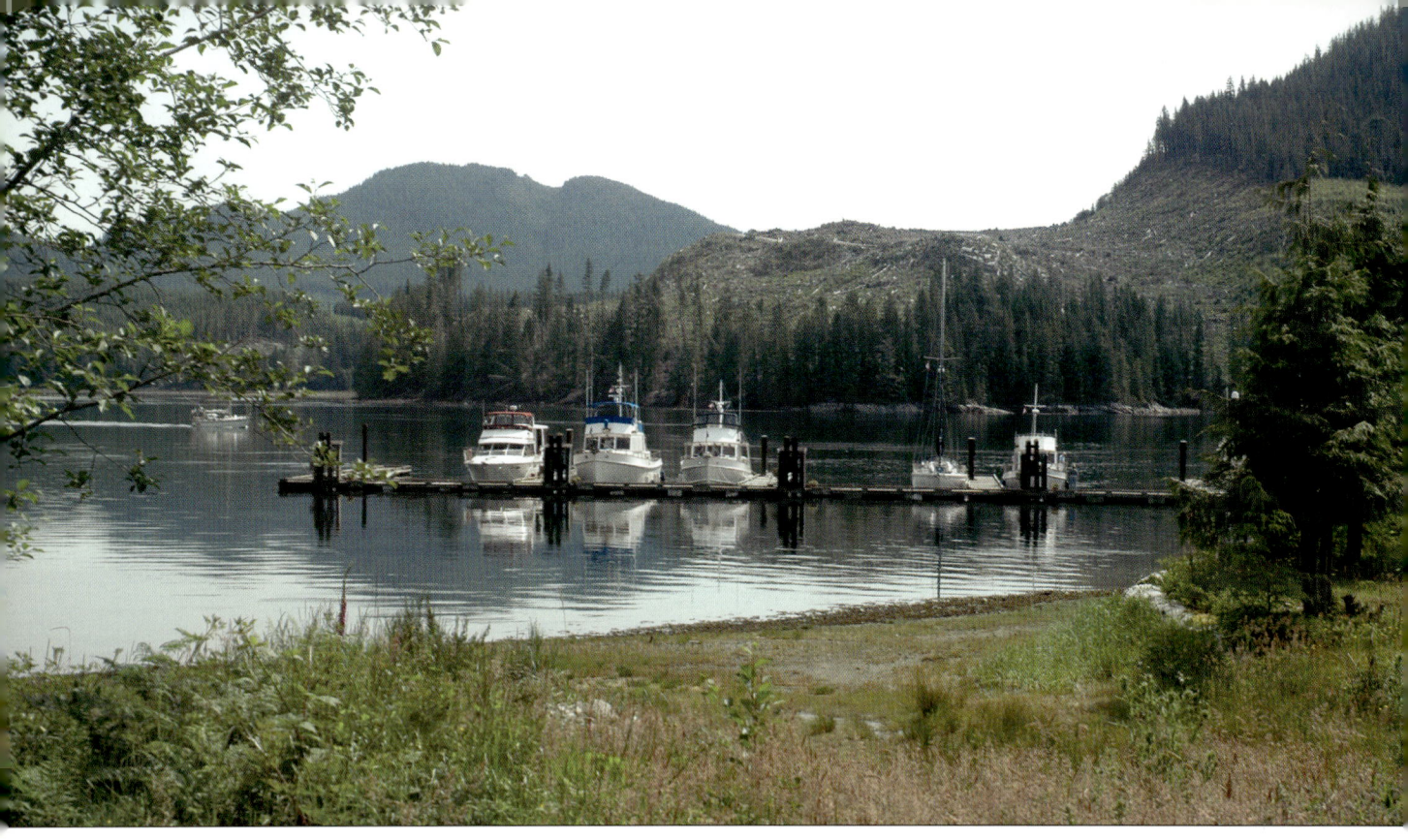

## Blind Channel  chart 3543

Blind Channel Resort is a home away from home to many mariners familiar with these waters north of Desolation Sound. The dock at the resort accommodates small to large yachts and provides amenities ashore which include post office, store and restaurant. The marina offers moorage, fuel, water, propane and shore power service. Other services include showers, laundry, ice and liquor agency.

For many years, decades in fact, the Richter family at Blind Channel has been welcoming visiting mariners at their docks. On our first visit to this tranquil spot on the coast we found a warm welcome and a place to stay rather than a desire to keep going.

There was fresh garden grown produce in the refrigerator in the family home and fresh bread at times. That was the only family building on the property for a while until in later years a store and restaurant building were added.

Today you will find a large sunny patio and a gazebo overlooking the marina. The restaurant provides a fine dining experience to please a variety of tastes. Four generations of the Richter family can be found busy and active around the property when guests are moored at the marina. The welcome is just as warm as ever it has been.

Philip Richter manages the business that his parents established. His father Edgar, continues to be involved with planning and preparing further additions to the property. With the assistance of son Eliot and daughter-in-law Laura, Philip manages the store while his wife, Jennifer, can be found preparing fresh bread and other delectables for the store and restaurant. They also attend a productive vegetable garden and maintain landscaping on the property.

Step off your boat and socialize with other guests moored at the marina. We always stroll along the dock to admire the handywork with the use of pottery and glass shards. The dock pilings supporting the main float are decorated with window boxes with these works.

One of the best known and loved hiking trails on the coast exists behind Blind Channel Resort. Nature lovers and hikers will enjoy these hiking and forest trails that were established by a large logging and sawmill company on West Thurlow Island. The trails, which begin about 300 metres from the Resort, are designed to show the features of a second growth forest. Be prepared for a refreshing walk on the trail into the adjacent woods.

There are three different trails, one to a spectacular viewpoint overlooking Mayne Passage and East Thurlow Island, a second to the Big Cedar, an 800 year old tree with a diameter of over 5 metres, via a forest of 80 year old second growth, and the third through a thinned western hemlock stand that was established in 1964. Years ago the Richters lobbied to have the first growth Thurlow cedar preserved when the logging company intended to log the hillside. The family persuaded them it would be more advantageous to establish interpretive trails. The final segment of the second trail descends through 100 years of old second growth.

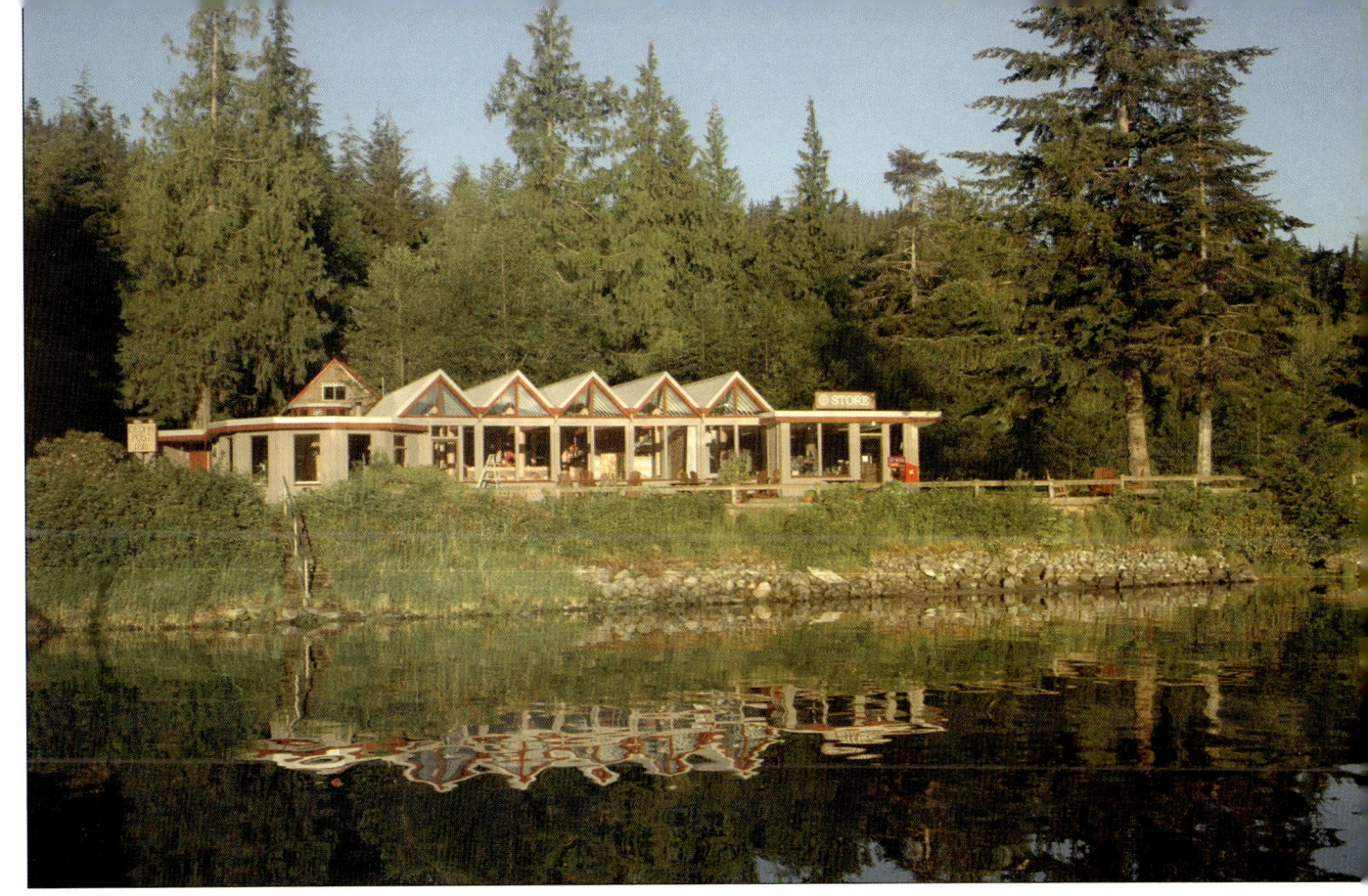

*Above: Early morning sun on the restaurant and store at Blind Channel. Right: In addition to the marina's fine restaurant, the patio (far right) has a burger stand for light lunches. Opposite: The marina at Blind Channel Resort from the patio in front of the store. These photos show a relatively quiet day early in the season.*

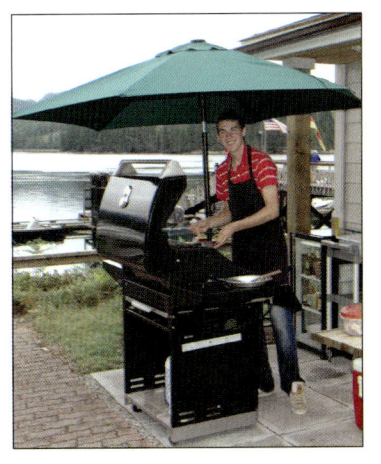

Blind Channel Resort is located in Mayne Passage. In fact, mariners often refer to Mayne Passage as Blind Channel, something that has always been somewhat of a puzzle to me. We refer to the passage as Blind Channel, although when we do we are usually talking about the resort and marina that bears the name. The passage connects Johnstone Strait with Cordero Channel and can be used as an optional route when travelling either direction.

If you continue along Cordero Channel northbound you have another chance at linking up with Johnstone Strait instead of turning up Wellbore Channel. The advantage of not turning into Johnstone Strait at either of these junctures is to avoid possible rough conditions off Kelsey Bay, where wind and wave often combine to create a nasty chop.

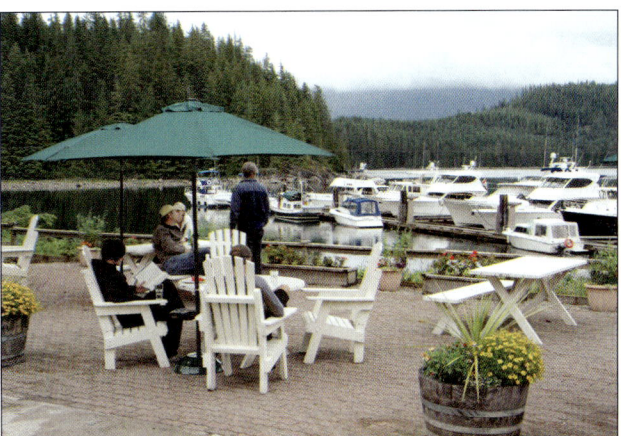

We use these alternatives sometimes if the wind is dead calm and it is slack at Kelsey Bay. However, the speed of your boat may be the deciding factor. The Wellbore Channel route offers an anchorage option in Forward Harbour which you may prefer over Kelsey Bay or nearby anchorages in Johnstone Strait.

At the south end of Mayne Passage you may notice an anchorage indicated on your chart. This was meant for large vessels. There is no suitable anchorage in this area for small craft other than those described earlier.

The route from Blind Channel to Forward Harbour requires passage through the Greene Point Rapids as well as Whirlpool Rapids. By leaving Blind Channel Resort approaching high slack, a slow boat should make it through Greene Point Rapids as well as Whirlpool Rapids without great difficulty before the currents in Wellbore Channel reach uncomfortable speeds.

**Note: There is a reef off Cosby Point that should be given a wide berth.**

Blind Channel to Forward Harbour 14.9

Charts 3543, 3544, 3555
Not for Navigation

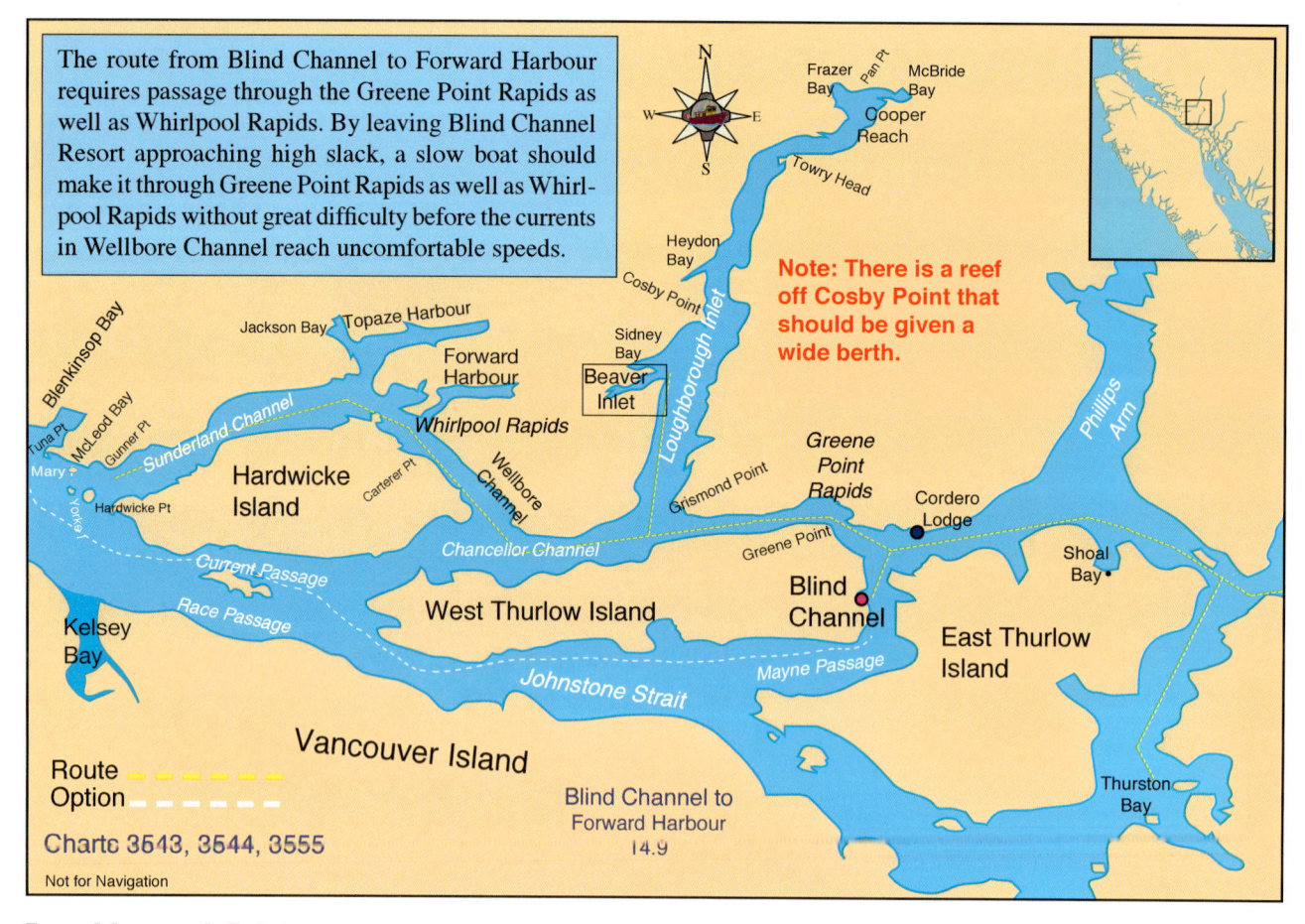

## Loughborough Inlet  charts 3543, 3555

When you depart Blind Channel for the continued trip west and north it is possible for a small boat to cut through the narrow, shallow passage inside of Edsall Islets. Use caution and don't do it unless the currents are slack.

You will soon find yourself at the junction of Cordero Channel and Loughborough Inlet. We normally bypass this deep, nearly 30 kilometer-long fjord in favour of a continuation to our final destination. We usually feel it can wait until the return trip, when, if we have the time, we will explore it and other waterways and inlets more leisurely.

If you do travel up Loughborough Inlet you will find several places to drop anchor, mostly temporarily. The most favourable is in **Beaver Inlet** (see diagram opposite), regarded as well protected against most conditions unless it is blowing hard from the west. Another quite acceptable day anchorage is located in the tiny **Edith Cove** tucked behind Hales Point, a bight on the south shore. Here you may find a temporary anchorage against easterlies near the floats of a long-time resident of the Loughborough area, who has taken up a permanent form of occupation of the cove. There are two other anchorages in the inlet, one in a shallow bay on the opposite shore just west of Dickson Point and the other down in the head of Beaver Inlet.

Small craft usually have it quite easy cruising in Loughborough Inlet in summer due to its relative shelter from most winds. By the time the seasonal westerlies or southeasterlies reach into the inlet, they are usually weakened to a point of comfort and diminished almost completely up Cooper Reach beyond Towry Head. Skip Heydon Bay and Sidney Bay if you wish to find shelter in Loughborough Inlet.

Farther up the inlet there is the possibility of temporary or overnight anchorage in good conditions a short distance beyond Towry Head. Do not choose this anchorage in the event of possible strong southeasterlies. Anchor at the head of the inlet in **Frazer Bay**. Points of interest up the inlet include Pan Point and McBride Bay at the end of Cooper Reach.

Poking around the area you will find booms, a former logging camp site and private landings. Fishermen have homesteaded in the area for many years and were known for their hospitality to visiting boats, sometimes even inviting mariners to tie up to their private floats for the night. If you are gunkholing around McBride Bay and Pan Point watch for the rocks, shown on chart 3543, off Cosby Point. I often wonder what it is about deep, one-way, routes like Loughborough Inlet that appeals to mariners. Besides the craggy surrounding mountains, the tranquil ambience of the place

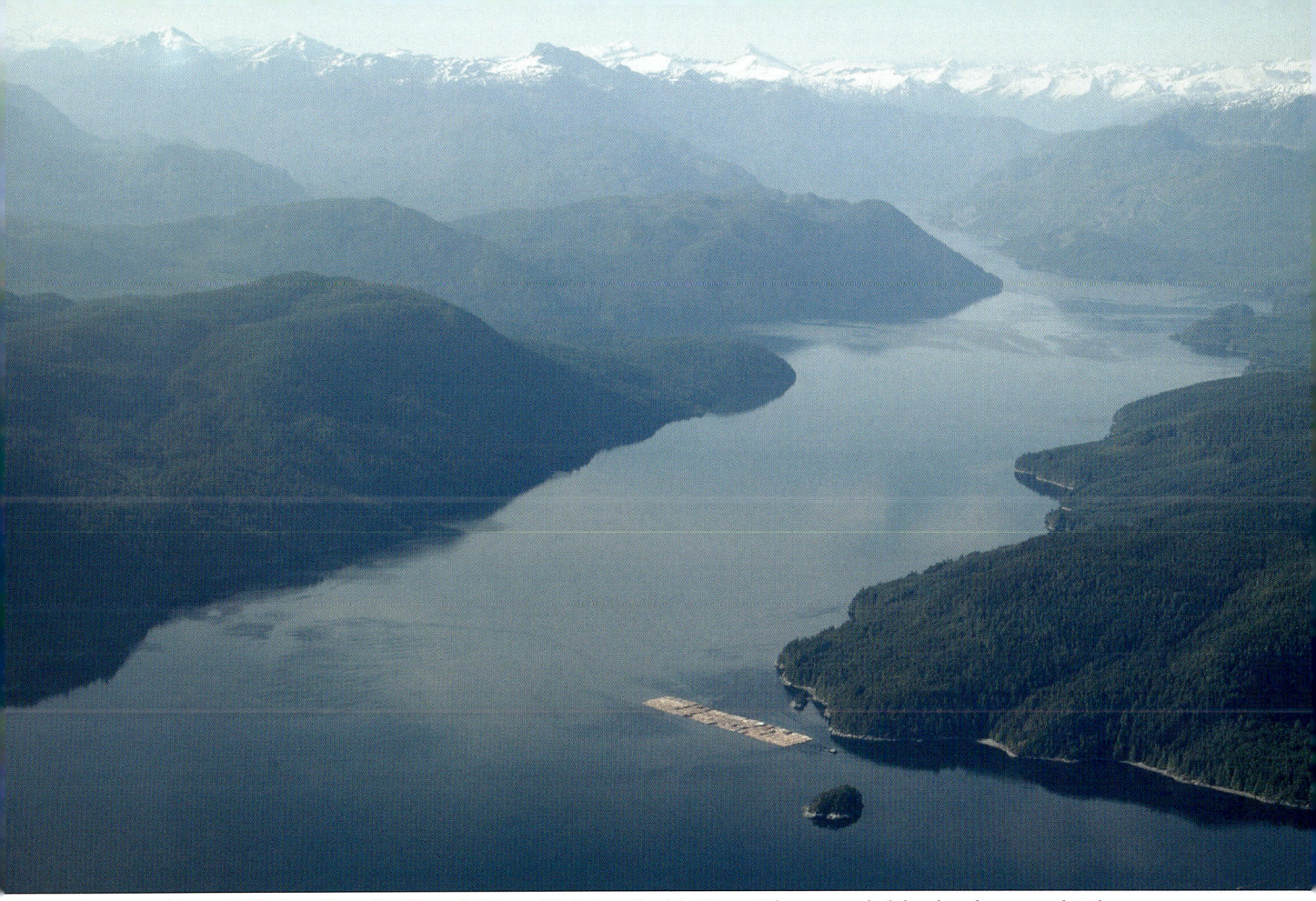

*Above: Loughborough Inlet from Chancellor Channel. Grismond Point is to the right. Beaver Inlet opens to the left a short distance up the inlet.*

and the unbeatable scenery, it must be the incredible prawns caught in its depths.

Boaters who have vast experience on this coast have referred to Loughborough Inlet very fondly. John Chappel was one of these, long-time marine businessman Dennis Binstead of Vancouver, another. Such visitors get caught up in the history of the area, of the whole coast really, and are fascinated by the era of logging camps, homesteaders and visiting ships in recent past years. Dennis Binstead is one of several people who have not only spent many hours boating in the area but also flying in by float plane.

What fascinates those of us who visit the area frequently is the remnants of life and industry that opened up the coast. These isolated communities are exemplified by the likes of a former owner, Pete McDonald, who operated the store and hotel at Shoal Bay; the loggers who rowed small boats through current-swept waters to pick up supplies for their camps from passing coastal freighters; the paddle wheeler *Beaver* that steamed around these inlets in the 1800s; the logging camps and the more recent venturing sailors; and the people of the First Nations who lived off the land and sea.

*Right: Private float home in Edith Cove, Beaver Inlet.*

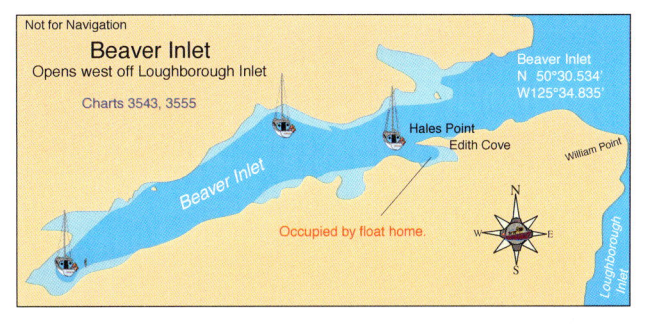

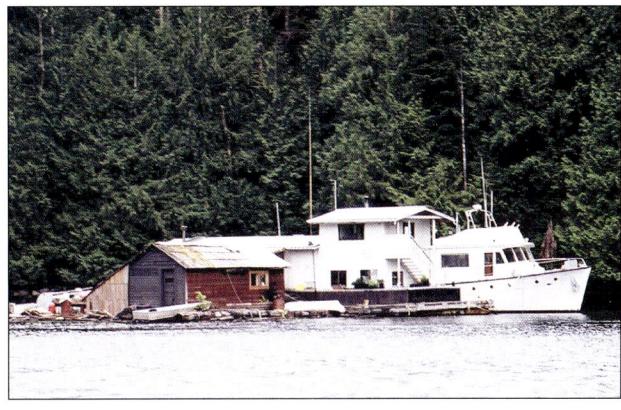

43

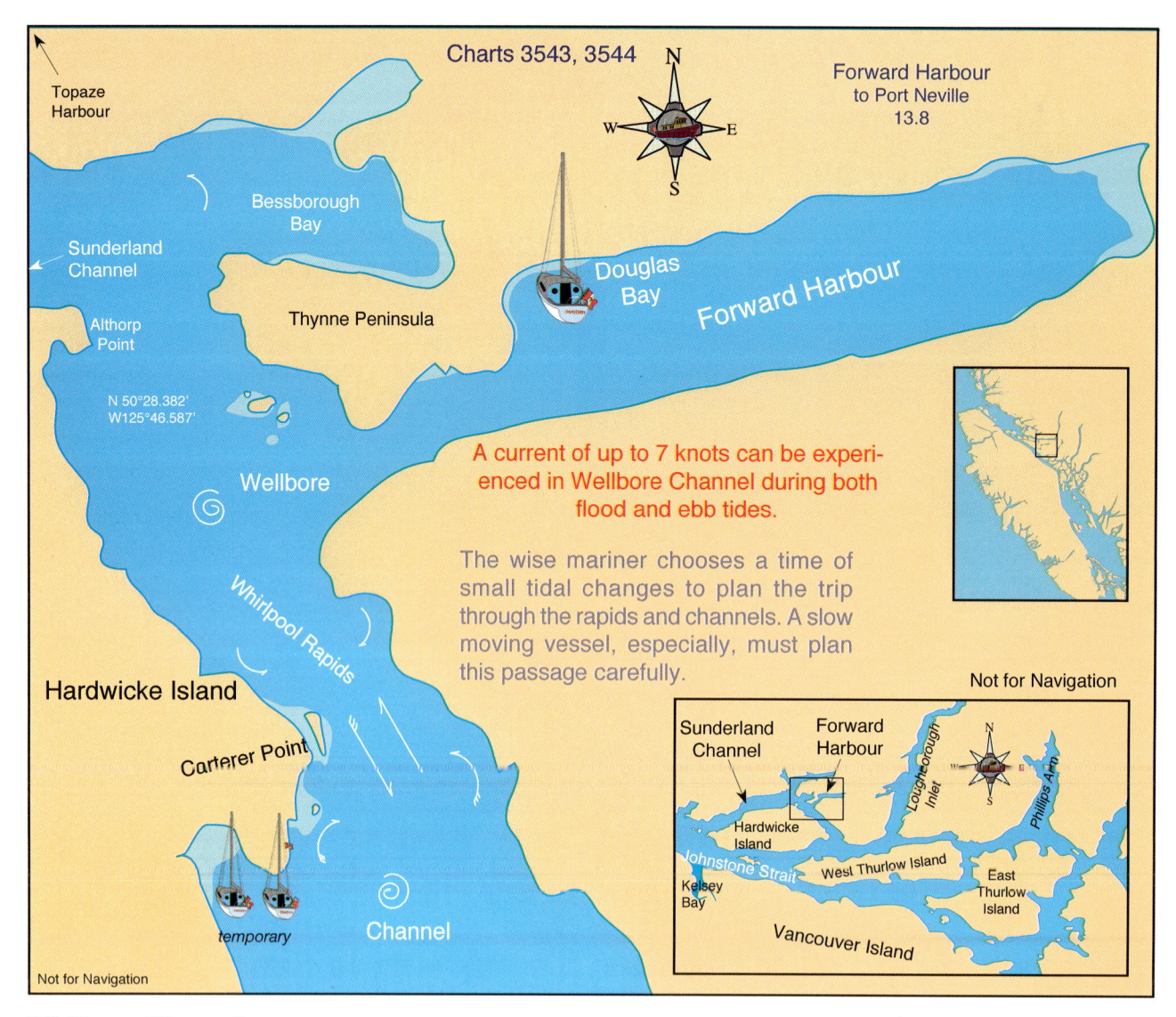

## Wellbore Channel  chart 3544

If you have bypassed Loughborough Inlet or have stopped there awhile and are continuing northbound, you have the choice of cruising along Chancellor Channel, that you entered from Blind Channel (Mayne Passage), or turning up Wellbore Channel. This latter route is the one of choice if you want to avoid Johnstone Strait's Current and Race Passages off Hardwicke Island near Kelsey Bay, which may be why you came the inside route in the first place.

A current of up to 7 knots can be experienced in Wellbore Channel with its respected Whirlpool Rapids, during both flood and ebb tides.

One year I misread the tables and kept motoring north up the channel in calm, flat water. After passing Carterer Point I realised my mistake. The strength of the flow in the ebbing tide increased perceptibly and it was too late to turn back. A huge whirlpool opened in front of us and I altered course rapidly to try to avoid it. The boat rolled heavily into it as I applied full throttle. We dipped our port sheerline into the hole as the boat groaned against the swirling, swift current, righted itself and came over the edge of the pool. To avoid more of the boiling, swift water we turned into Forward Harbour to await the real slack before continuing our trip into Sunderland Channel and then Johnstone Strait.

## Forward Harbour  charts 3543, 3544

Immediately east of Whirlpool Rapids, Forward Harbour can be entered through its narrow passage at any time. Anchorage is taken near a lovely sandy beach in **Douglas Bay** just to the north of the entrance. Winds are mostly westerly in summer and generally allow safe overnight stops but occasionally a watch has to be maintained if easterly winds pick up.

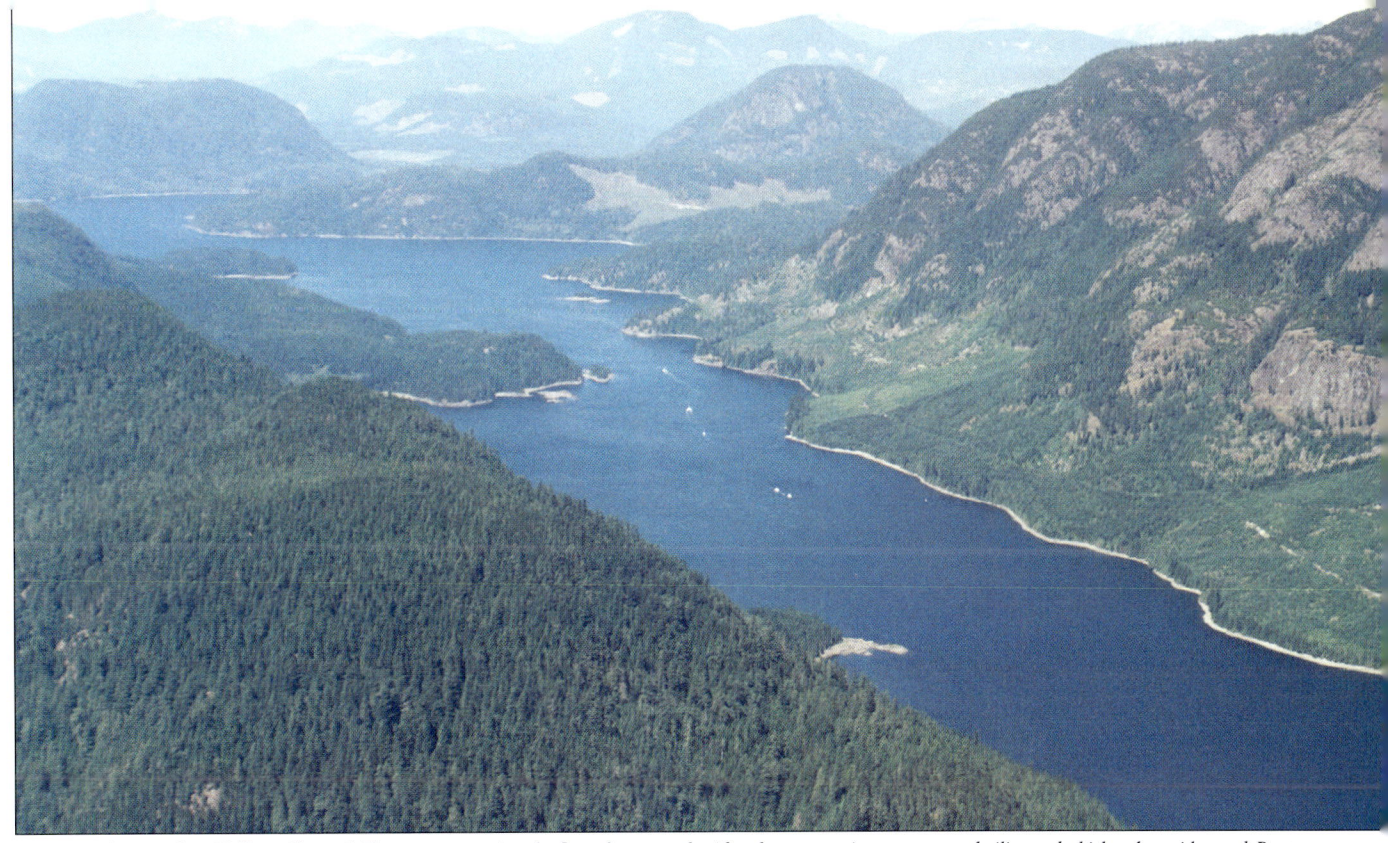

*Above: Looking north up Wellbore Channel. The narrows restricts the flow of water as the tides change, causing some severe boiling and whirlpools at either end. Boats can wait temporarily at anchor in the lee of the point. Below: Forward Harbour. Best anchorage is in Douglas Bay, the nook to the left just inside the basin.*

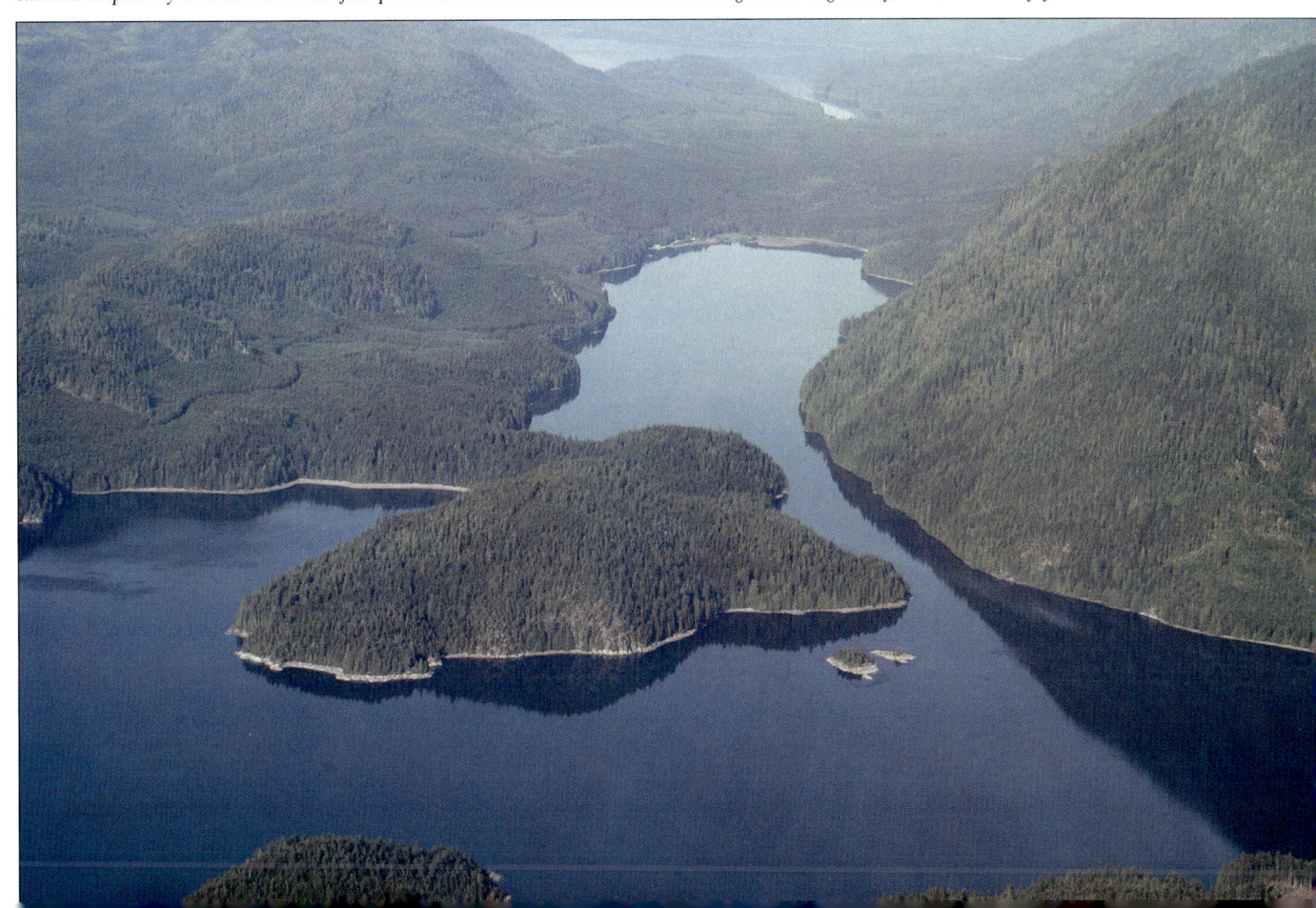

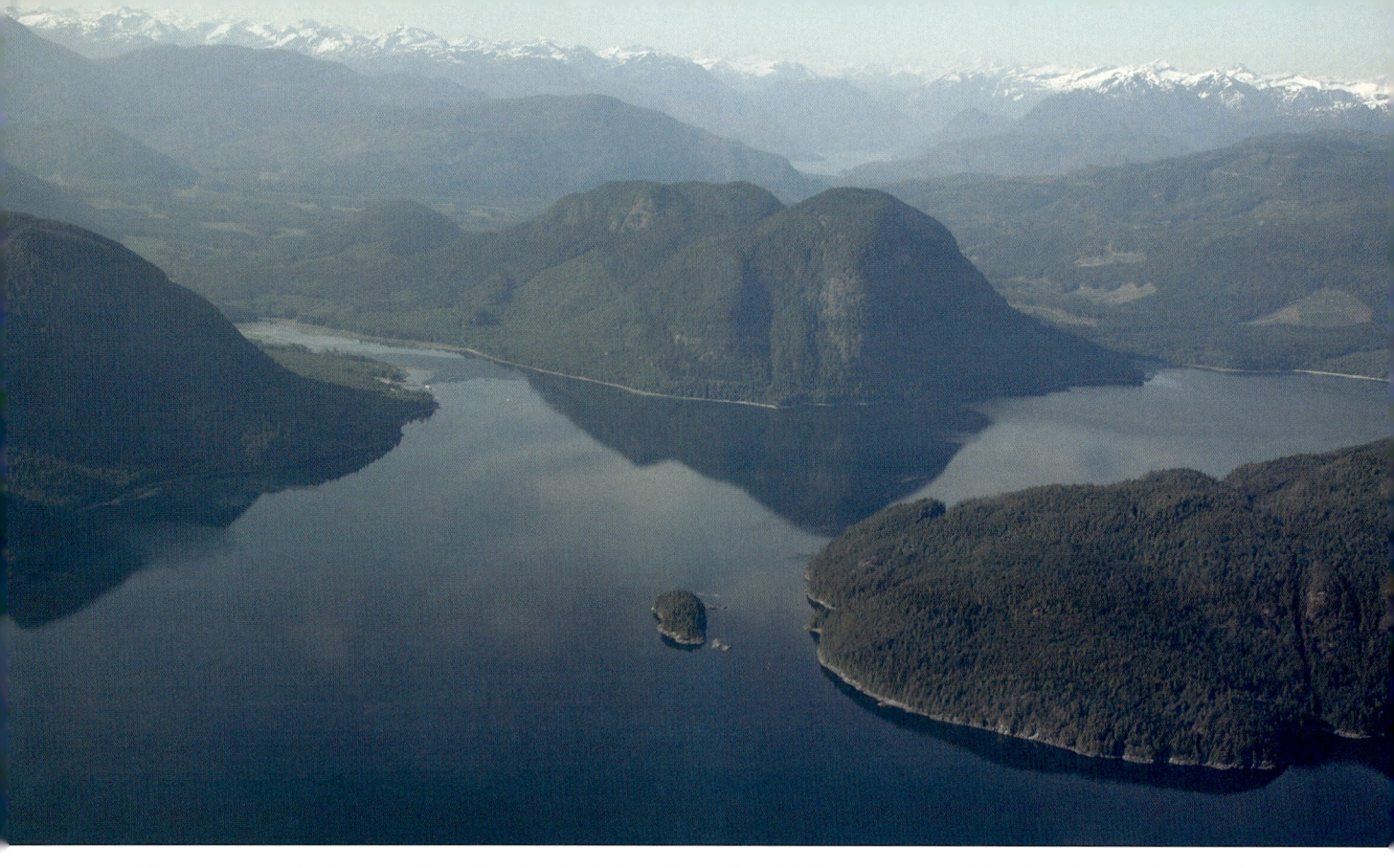

On our return trip that year I again misjudged the tide. Carla was keen to wait, but I insisted that I had read the tables correctly. Furthermore, looking at the water ahead I had never seen it so calm. It was calm all right, until we were in the middle of the narrows at Carterer Point. But by then the water was streaming down into the lower part of Wellbore Channel, and we were fully committed. The water boiled and tumbled, swirled around and threw the boat from side to side. It was not dangerous, just hard work, spinning the wheel one way then the other to counter the rolling of the boat. It took only a few minutes, which seemed a lot longer, then we were through into the calmer waters at the confluence of Wellbore and Chancellor Channels. Several boats were anchored at the temporary stop south of Carterer Point where they had been waiting for the tide to let them through Whirlpool Rapids.

As we were entering the lower reaches at the south end of Wellbore Channel, we slowed down to watch an eagle swooping towards the surface. It plunged its talons into the water and then tried to fly away. But something it had taken hold of was preventing it from getting clear of the water again. The big bird settled on the surface and then with a flapping of wings began to paddle its way towards the shore. We watched it struggle with the large salmon it had caught as it made its slow, laborious way across Wellbore Channel. Eventually it reached the beach and landed its catch. The tide was in our favour so we did not stay to watch the eagle enjoy its hard-won prize. Eagle talons cannot release until they have fully closed. Many are drowned by choosing too large a salmon or cod and being unable to let go when the big fish sounds.

One year we set the anchor in **Douglas Bay** in Forward Harbour, amidst several other anchored vessels. It was early in the day and we were planning to continue later when the tides changed and the current abated. An easterly wind was freshening but we felt confident of our security. Carla and I slipped off to explore the shoreline in our inflatable while my daughter Lianne remained aboard, reading. When we returned about an hour later, the wind, which had been increasing in strength, was catching the boats in Douglas Bay. Our boat had dragged anchor and was moving dangerously close to shore.

We reached the boat quickly, boarded her and immediately started the engine. The depth sounder showed us to have dragged from about 10 metres into two. We checked that it was approaching slack in Whirlpool Rapids, raised anchor and continued our journey. We had considered alternative anchorages in the area for an overnight stay, but after the dragging experience in Douglas Bay decided not to stay there, nor at nearby Bessborough Bay which, as an anchorage, is exposed and only temporary although it is protected somewhat from the currents in Wellbore Channel.

At one time there was a dock along the north shore near the east end of Forward Harbour where mariners could stay overnight when they dined at an adjacent lodge. It was called Forward Harbour Lodge and while the building is still there it

46

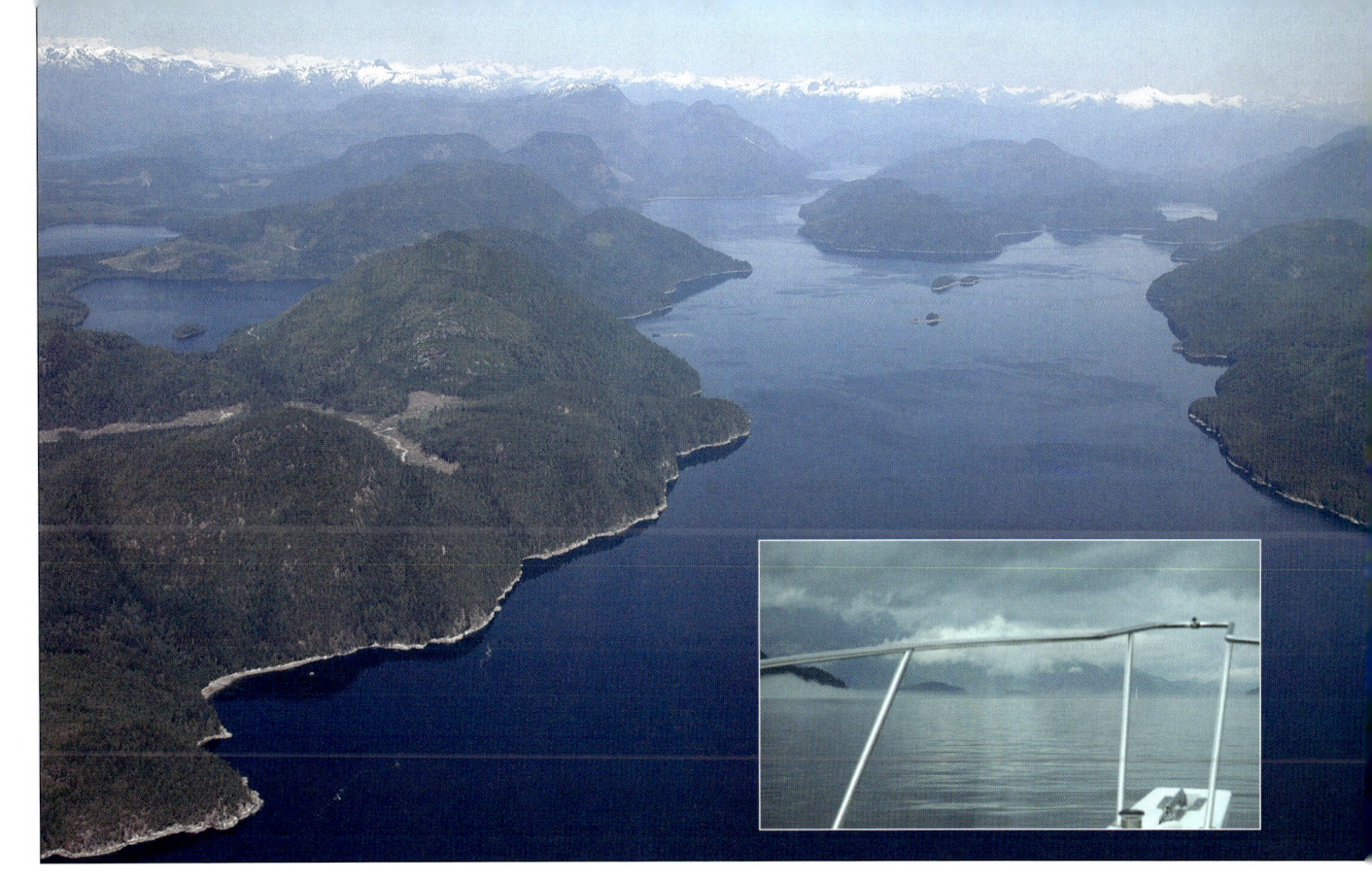

is not advertising any services. The dock was quite solid and the lodge was in operation in the mid 1990s. The kitchen was run by a chef who had worked at some of the finest restaurants in Vancouver. He left to open Oleo's floating restaurant located in Frederick Arm.

## Sunderland Channel chart 3544

The only possibility of anchoring or finding good shelter that ever interested me in Sunderland Channel is in **McLeod Bay**, a small cove between Gunner Point and Blenkinsop Bay. Jackson Bay off Topaz Harbour where Sunderland and Wellbore Channels meet, is of little interest from an anchorage standpoint.

Without a logboom present McLeod Bay would be inadequate to anchor in, unless just one boat did so in calm conditions. When it is calm enough go for Port Neville or beyond while you can.

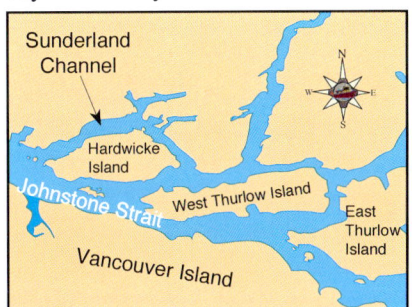

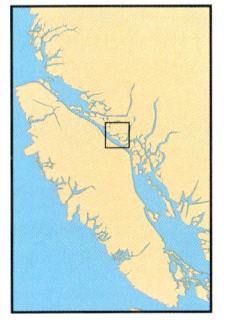

The bay beyond McLeod Bay has no name but anchorage can be found in the western portion sheltered by Tuna Point from westerly winds and sometimes southeasterlies too. Pass Mary Island and head for the inside of Tuna Point to avoid the rocks around the centre of the bay. Our earliest trips past Tuna Point revealed the remnants of a house inside the bay. As for Blenkinsop Bay, it is just too exposed as an anchorage for small boats.

We usually prefer to continue into Johnstone Strait and make for Port Neville or beyond if the Strait is calm. In more recent years we always stopped at Port Neville to visit the Hansen family who ran the post office.

Travelling down Sunderland Channel late one afternoon, we were headed for an overnight stop in either Port Neville or the Minstrel Island area. However, after a bumpy run down Sunderland Channel we wound up spending an interesting night at McLeod Bay rather than continuing to Port Neville. The wind had come up stronger than expected in Johnstone Strait. It was rough as we approached Gunner Point, to the extent that we wanted to find shelter and not round the point into the strait. As it was, the seas we were in were already pretty rough. We later discovered, rounding that point in

*Opposite: Just beyond Whirlpool Rapids is Bessborough Bay and the east end of Sunderland Channel–the route to Johnstone Strait. Above: Sunderland Channel from above Johnstone Strait. Inset: Calm seas in Sunderland Channel usually indicates a calm Johnstone Strait.*

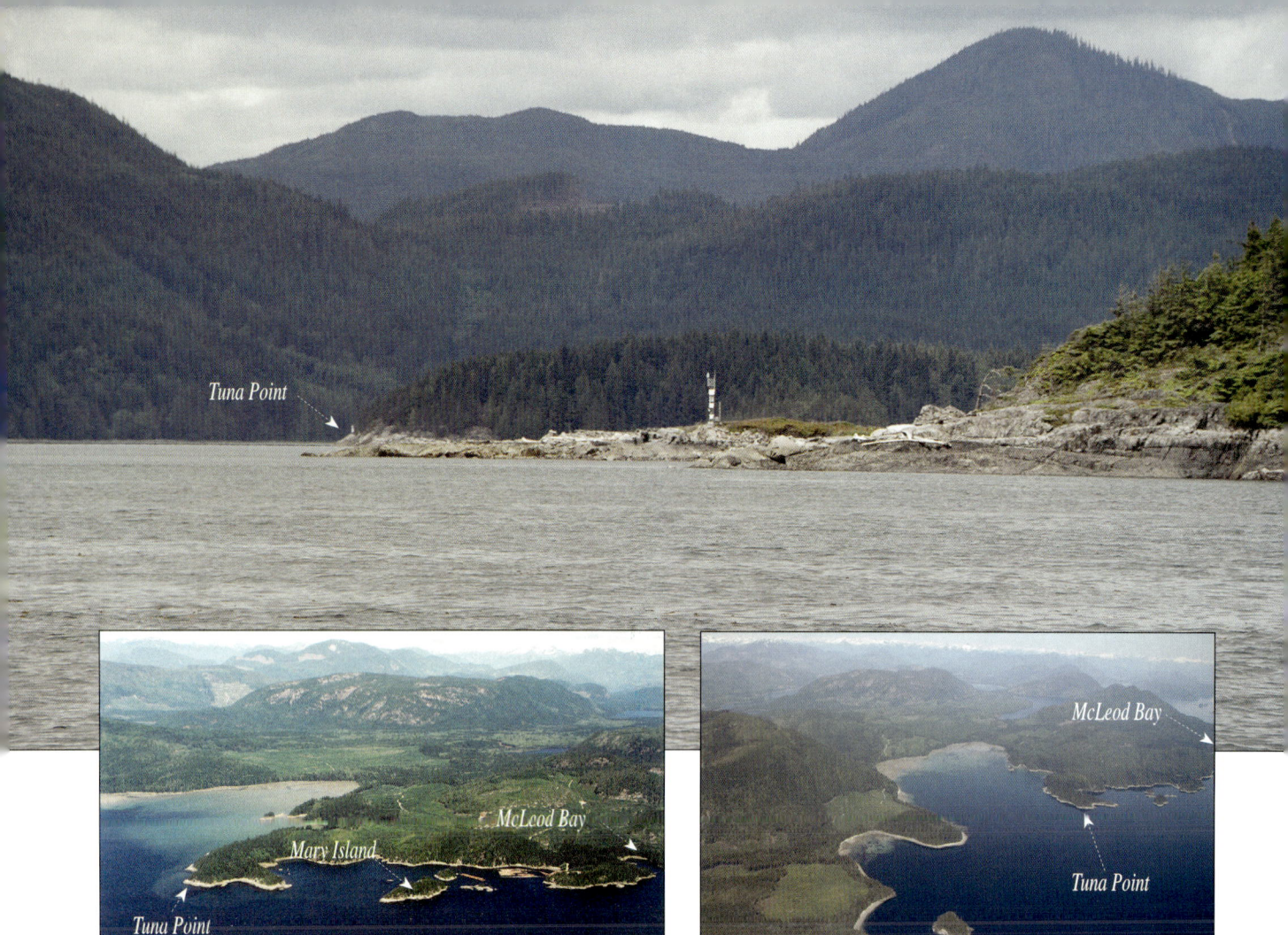

subsequent years, Gunner Point can become snarly when the tides are contrary and the wind is up.

We noticed a log boom just inside **McLeod Bay** and decided to put in there. It was sheltered enough inside the bay and so we tied up to the logs, with some cruising friends in two other boats rafted alongside us.

The three vessels, ranging in size from 11 to 13 metres, rode peacefully alongside the logboom. We watched the waves sweeping by outside and were satisfied that we had made the right decision not to continue that day. Our boat was closest to the logboom. That night we were awakened by the sound of something bumping against the bottom of the boat. I lay awake listening for the sound. There it was again. It was more than a sound–it was the boat riding up and down and occasionally bumping heavily onto something solid. With flashlight in hand I climbed onto the logs. On inspection I saw that one of the logs had slid out of the boom and was angled slightly downwards beneath the hull of our boat. We were coming down on it with a fairly solid thump as the slight rise and fall of some of the waves rippled into the cove.

I decided to try to move without having to disturb the crew in the other boats. It was necessary to slide the boats farther back on the logboom. I untied the lines thinking I could just walk them backwards and re-tie them.

It did not work. There was enough breeze coming into the cove that the bows began to swing out making it impossible for me to hold them and soon they would be beam on to the incoming wind, adrift in the cove and headed for the beach.

I yelled for the others to wake up, received a sleepy response from a head poking out of a window and then, with alarm, a scrambling to start the engines to power assist me with the move.

*Top: The light on Fanny Island to the west of Kelsey Bay. There are gun emplacements on adjacent Yorke island. Names of points and islets, such as Artillery Islets, reflect the one-time use of the islands as a strategic joint Canadian and US military point. When travelling via Kelsey Bay, cross the southern end of Sunderland Channel and continue along Johnstone Strait for Port Neville.*
*Above left and right: Blenkinsop Bay (McLeod Bay –not seen– is beyond to the far right). Tuna Point is seen just to the right of Blenkinsop Bay, with Mary Island at centre in the photograph to the left.*

# Discovery Passage to Knight Inlet

## via Kelsey Bay and Johnstone Strait

Charts 3539, 3312, 3543, 3544, 3545, 3564

Travelling up Johnstone Strait, mariners compete with commercial traffic and with cruise ships in the summer months. Whale watching operators are busy carrying passengers back and forth and in all probability pleasure craft in transit up the Strait will slow down or stop as a pod of killer whales is sighted in the area. These beautiful creatures move up and down the Strait and branch off at several passages, especially near the north end in their daily hunt for food. Where they travel to, coincidentally, are places mariners love to explore in the close proximity of Johnstone Strait. Bear watching trips too have become an important facet of tourism in the region and black bears and grizzlies can be seen on the beaches of nearby mainland fjords.

Cruising by private yacht from Campbell River, a major hub for marine activity, follow Discovery Passage as it wends its way northwards to link up with the eastern extremity of Johnstone Strait at Chatham Point.

The voyage begins with a passage through Seymour Narrows just north of Campbell River. This passage was notorious for its extremely dangerous Ripple Rock that lay just beneath the surface with water swirling and boiling during the tidal changes. It gained fame when in 1958 engineers tunneled beneath the passage and up into the twin peaks of Ripple Rock to blast it out of the water. It was the biggest nonnuclear explosion recorded to date at the time and left the passage a much safer place to navigate.

> Our second route north is via Seymour Narrows. This route bypasses Desolation Sound altogether. However, the close proximity of Campbell River to the Sound is convenient for an easy side trip into the western edges of Desolation Sound, where numerous anchorages and several marinas provide shelter and pleasurable destinations. It is also where interesting and beautiful passages lead through a maze of islands back to the other routes.
>
> Leaving Campbell River northbound it is wise to make sure the currents in Seymour Narrows are mild. They can reach 16 knots on the flood tide and 14 knots on the ebb, so please consult the tide tables.

Large cruise ships, local tugs and barges and other commercial traffic use this waterway as the main route north and south of Campbell River. But they are warily mindful of the tides at Seymour Narrows even with the removal of Ripple Rock.

### Brown's Bay chart 3539

Some mariners may stop just north of Seymour Narrows at Brown's Bay, for fuel and overnight accommodation. The marina has mostly permanent mooring customers, but has some room for transient guests. A restaurant on the docks provides a pleasant ambience afloat with a view of the passing traffic in Discovery Passage. Call Brown's Bay Marina at (250) 286-3135. Fax 286-0951.

### Kanish Bay chart 3539

Continuing north along Discovery Passage, a fine temporary anchorage can be found in Kanish Bay on Quadra Island, just behind the Chained Islands or better yet tucked in near Bodega Point. There is a small island off Bodega Point with a low lying isthmus connecting it to Quadra Island and an exposed rock to the east of the island forming an additional breakwater. Another rock lies to the south of the first rock, forming the entrance to a horseshoe-shaped cove. A log float has created a lagoon just beyond the anchorage. Some backeddies make their way into this anchorage from Discovery Passage, but it is usually safe enough for a single vessel to remain there overnight.

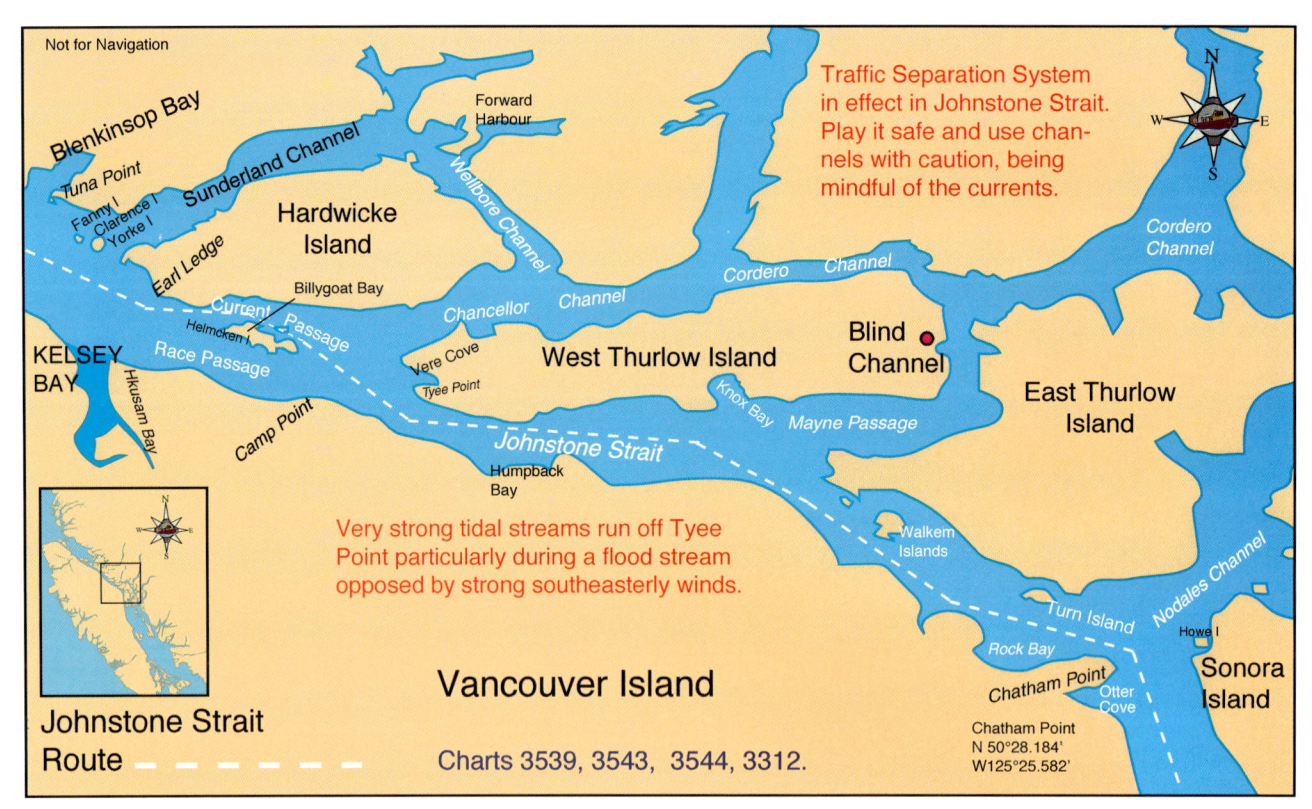

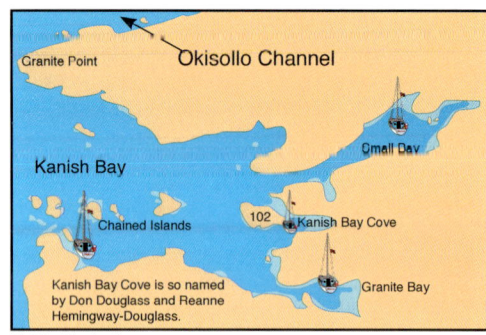

## Johnstone Strait Route

Charts 3539, 3543, 3544, 3312.

**Traffic Separation System in effect in Johnstone Strait. Play it safe and use channels with caution, being mindful of the currents.**

**Very strong tidal streams run off Tyee Point particularly during a flood stream opposed by strong southeasterly winds.**

Chatham Point
N 50°28.184'
W125°25.582'

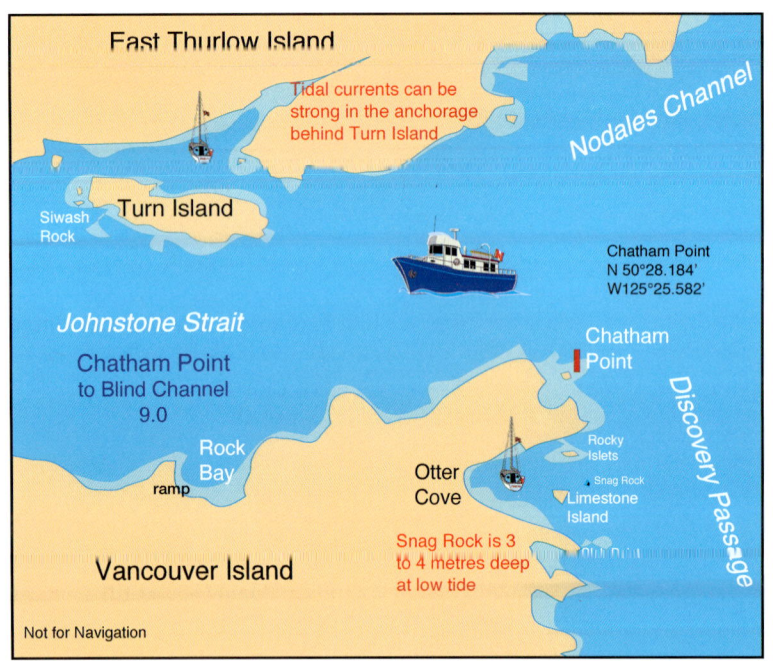

### Chatham Point to Blind Channel 9.0

Tidal currents can be strong in the anchorage behind Turn Island.

Snag Rock is 3 to 4 metres deep at low tide.

Kanish Bay Cove is so named by Don Douglass and Reanne Hemingway-Douglass.

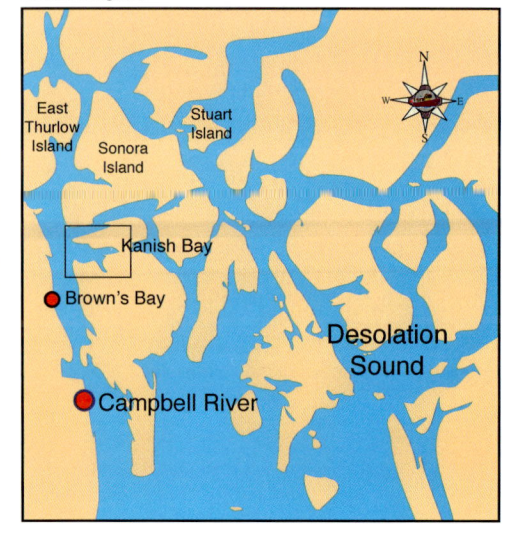

*Kanish Bay on Quadra Island, above right, is indicated in the diagrams to the right. It is located just before entering the waterways of the area in the diagram at top of page. Above, right: Diagram shows Otter Cove and Rock Bay either side of Chatham Point and the confluence of Nodales Channel and Discovery Passage at the entrance to Johnstone Strait.*

**Emergencies: Call Comox on channels 6, 78 and 16 on VHF**

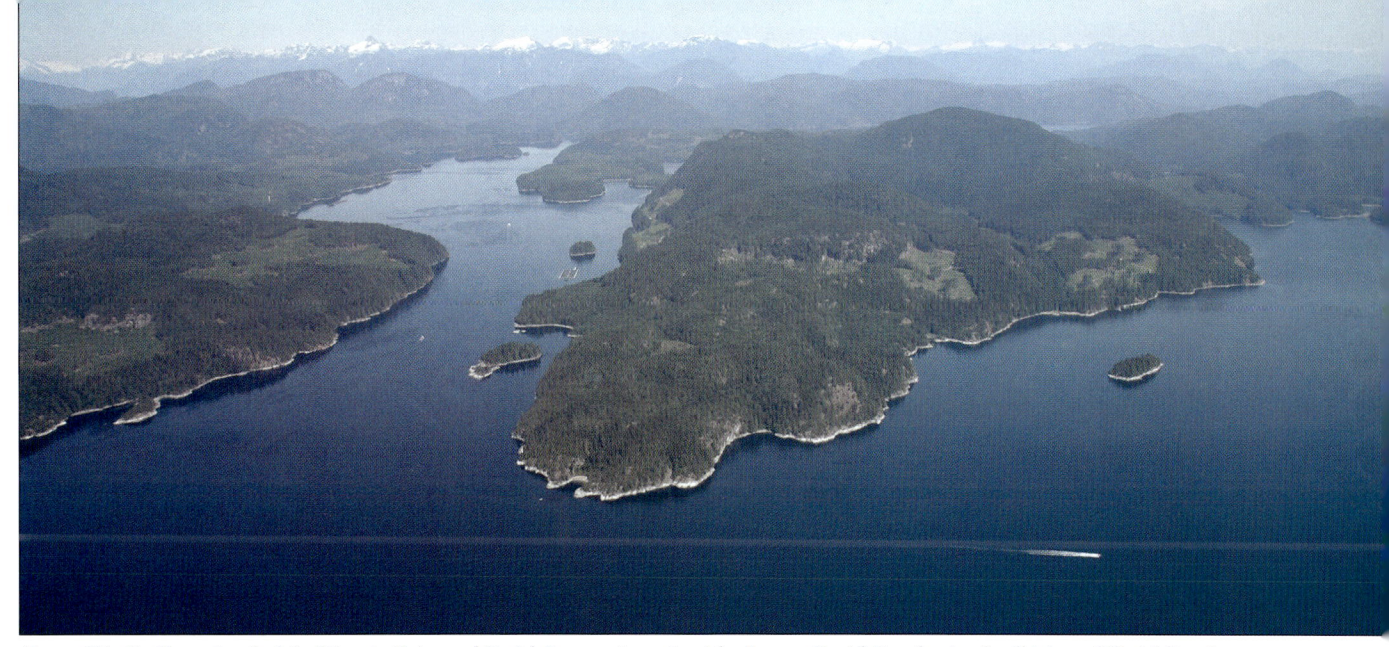

*Above: Okisollo Channel to the left of Granite Point, and Kanish Bay opening to its right. Bottom: Kanish Bay showing Small Inlet and Kanish Bay Cove.*

Deeper inside Kanish Bay, Granite Bay provides protective shelter while another, in a small cove behind the island to the north of Granite Bay recommended by Bill Wolferstan (*Desolation Sound and the Discovery Islands–Cruising Guide to British Columbia volume II*), has since been occupied by a fish farm pen. There is a fish farm also in the lee of the easternmost of the Chained Islands.

**Granite Bay** is a sometimes windy anchorage with a muddy bottom. A community float serves the small-boat owners of homes along the shore and nearby on Quadra Island. A sandy launch ramp runs into the bay at its southwest corner. There is a dilapidated float at the low water edge of a drying mud flat that once served as a government dock. Last time we looked we determined that one small boat may still tie up at the remnants of the dock.

**Small Inlet** lies adjacent to a Provincial Park's protected area inside Kanish Bay. The narrow entrance to this inlet reaches a depth of less than 3 metres at low tide so should be avoided by larger craft. Take it in the centre and expect to brush against the kelp lining the passage. Inside there is questionable anchorage for several craft, with winds known to blow through at times. Best shelter is against the north shore. The inlet comprises a larger outer basin and a small inner basin. The latter basin is good for one boat to swing comfortably on a short anchor rode in just over 2 metres at low tide–perfect for our shallow draft Monaro 27. Entrance to this inner anchorage requires careful navigation between the small islands and the rocks dividing the two basins. This is easiest at low tide when the rocks are exposed,

There were numerous First Nations villages located in Kanish Bay on Quadra Island at one time. Raids by rival bands from the north eventually drove the resident band out of them. Whites arrived later and tried to establish themselves in the area but today there are merely remnants of logging settlements and some archaeological evidence of former attempts to settle. A portage trail from Granite Bay, once used by aboriginals, leads to **Waiatt Bay** on the east side of the narrow neck dividing the northern and southern parts of Quadra Island. Newton Lake, ideal for warm bathing lies south of Small Inlet and a path to it branches off the Waiatt Bay trail. Mind Nixon Rock south of Nixon Island as you leave Kanish Bay.

Proceeding towards Kelsey Bay and beyond, cross Discovery Passage to the western shore and follow a course towards Chatham Point where it meets Johnstone Strait and Nodales Channel. Tidal currents up to 6 knots occur in Johnstone Strait.

If the currents are strong around Chatham Point you might want to wait awhile in **Otter Cove** on the Vancouver Island side of Discovery Passage, where the water remains quite calm despite the fast currents off Chatham Point. Read more about Brown's Bay, Otter Cove and Kanish Bay in the author's ***Cruising to Desolation Sound***.

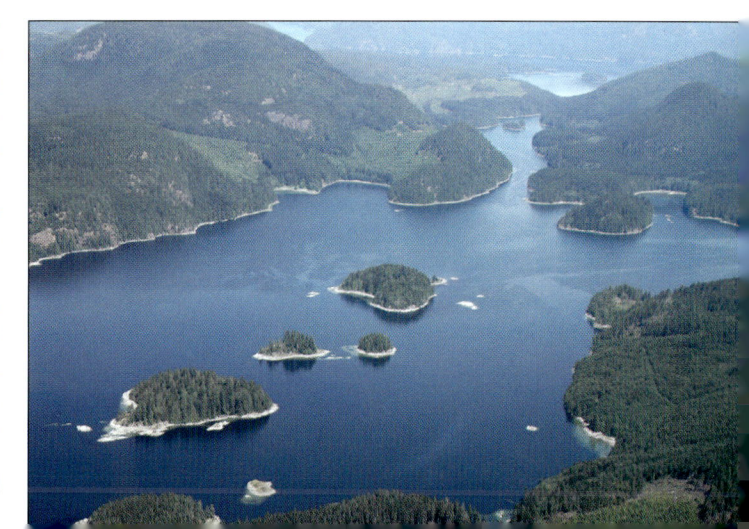

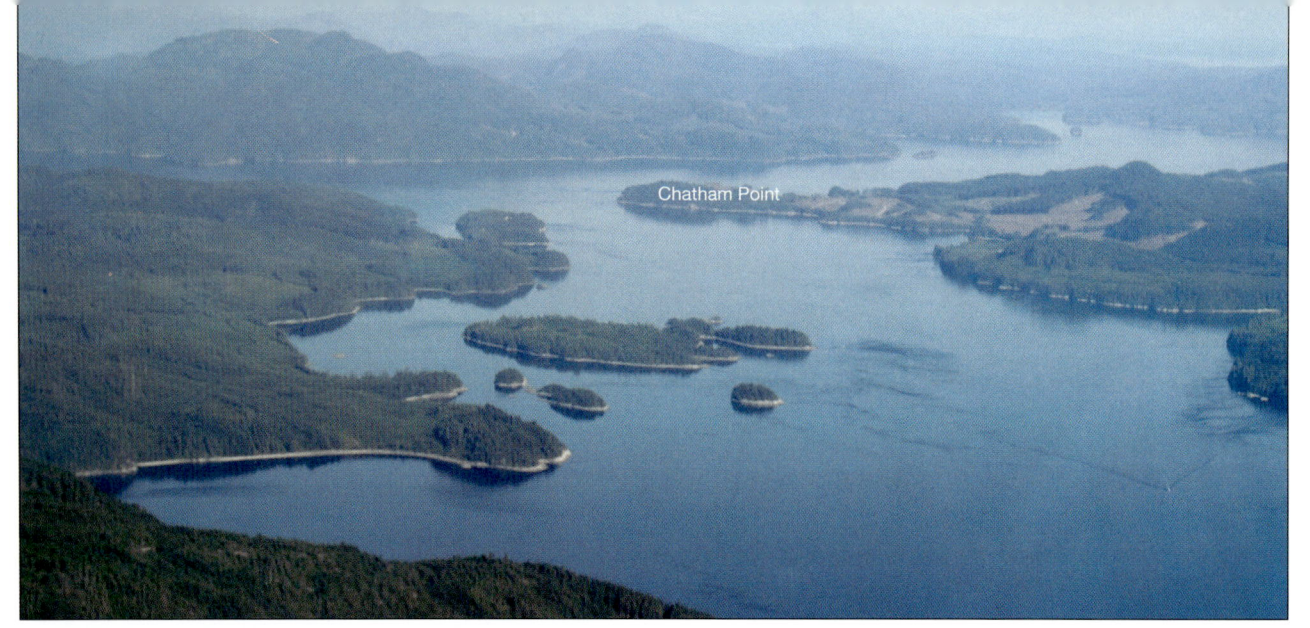

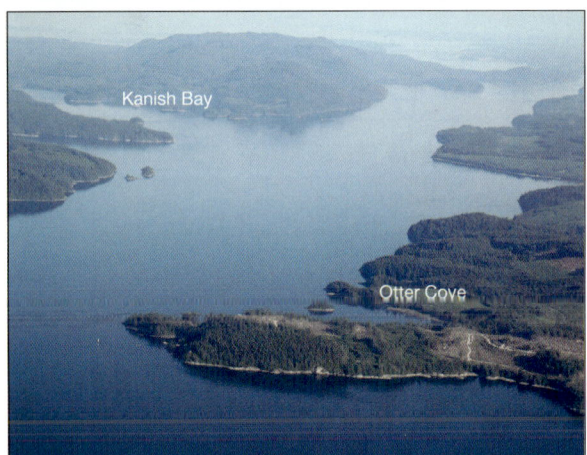

*Above: Looking east along Johnstone Strait with the Walkem Islands in the foreground. The only anchorage is on the east side of the two larger islands. Chatham Point and Discovery Passage lie beyond. Photograph taken from above the entrance to Mayne Passage.*

*Left: Discovery Passage south from Chatham Point to Seymour Narrows in the distance. Otter Cove is in the lee of Chatham Point. Kanish Bay opens off to the east side of the passage in the upper left of the photograph.*

*Below: Rock Bay faces onto Johnstone Strait directly opposite Turn Island. Beyond Turn Island to the right Nodales Channel leads to Hemming Bay and Thurston Bay marine park. There is possible anchorage behind Turn Island. This was the site of a busy logging camp, and submerged equipment remnants have been known to snag anchors. Rock Bay affords some temporary shelter, but if you are looking for a reliable anchorage in the vicinity of Chatham Point, the best bet nearby is Kanish Bay.*

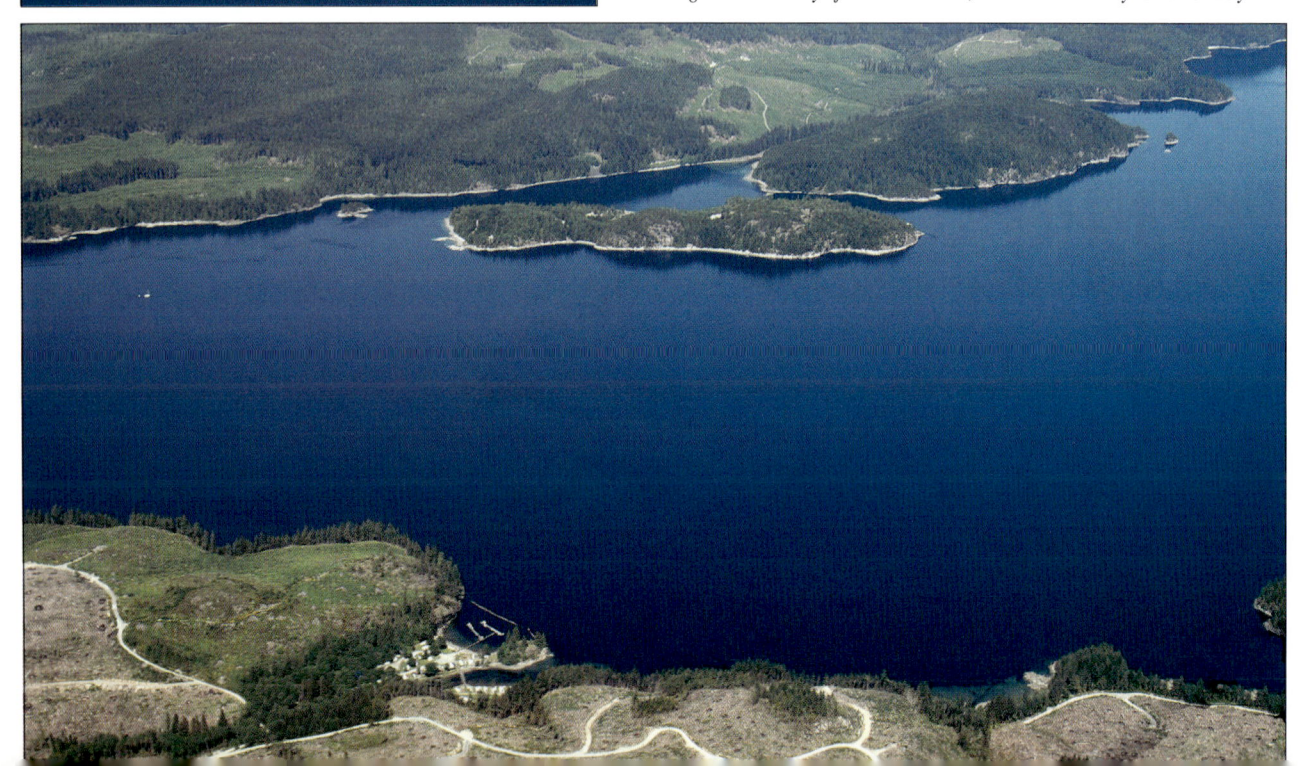

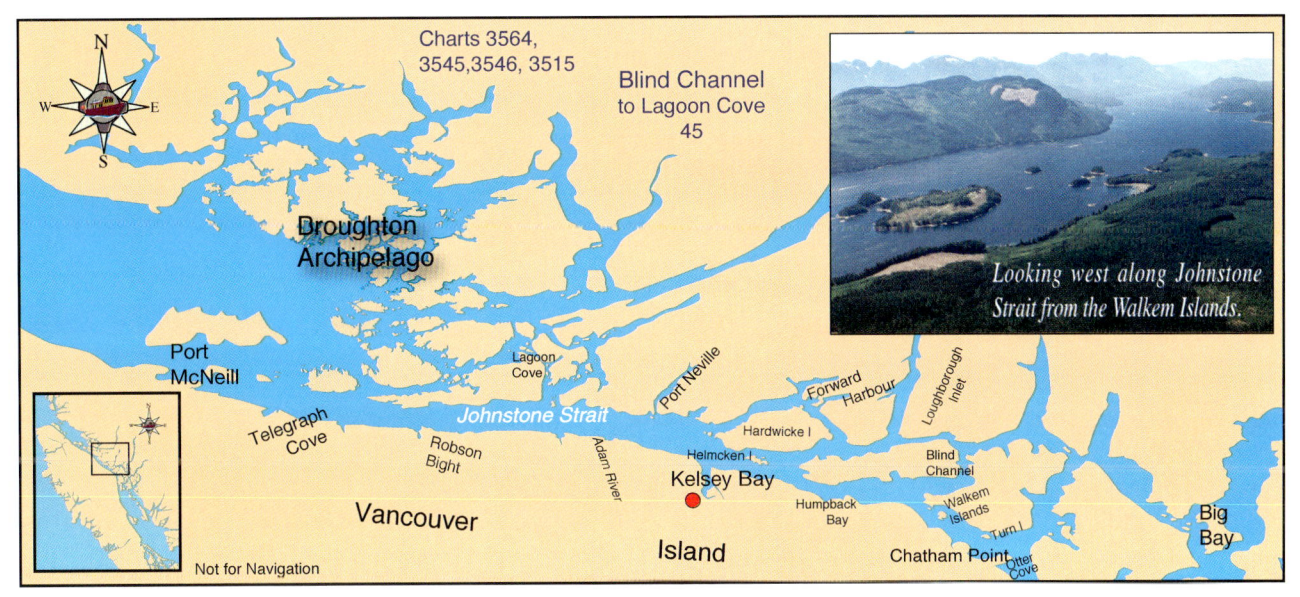

*Looking west along Johnstone Strait from the Walkem Islands.*

## Otter Cove  charts 3539, 3543

Enter between Rocky Islets and Limestone Island and anchor off the beach at the head of the cove. It has a muddy bottom and you can anchor in about 12 to 14 metres. If it's blowing from the east it's best to keep going, or wait in Kanish Bay.

North of Otter Cove there may be some protection from the wind in **Rock Bay**. Pass Chatham Point and Beaver Rock and enter Johnstone Strait.

You may find fog in Johnstone Strait and adjacent channels in summer months due to the cold sea surface temperatures. It is 10° colder in the Strait than in Desolation Sound and 3° colder than at the north end in Queen Charlotte Strait.

Rock Bay Marine Park (est 1996) includes Otter Cove and Rock Bay. See diagram page 50.

> Johnstone Strait is the direct route of large passenger liners. It is also the preferred route of commercial boats and other vessels that cannot negotiate the curves and narrows of some of the inside channels, or that do not have the time to do so.
>
> Slow moving craft using the main Johnstone Strait route, time their passage through the Seymour Narrows and Kelsey Bay area with great care.

reasonable anchorage is behind an exposed rock on the east side of the two larger islands in about 7 to 8 metres.

The *Sailing Directions* advises mariners "to keep 0.2 of a mile distant" from the Walkem Islands because of the tidal streams. Nearby **Knox Bay** is good for a brief stop to escape westerly winds. It is no great distance, once past Chatham Point, to run into Mayne Passage and pull into the marina at Blind Channel. This leads you to the alternative passage between Stuart Island and Port Neville, which you could choose to join at this juncture rather than the shorter but more challenging Kelsey Bay alternative.

## Turn Island  charts 3539, 3543

There are some possible temporary anchorages in the eastern portion of Johnstone Strait that we normally run past without a second thought. The shelter behind Turn Island looks inviting on the chart and could provide temporary anchorage away from the current. It has a narrow entrance with a rock guarding the eastern side and anchorage is possible in about 6 metres. Stopping there is not recommended, because of remnants from a logging camp strewn on the bottom.

## Walkem Islands  chart 3543

Farther along the Strait, it may be tempting to look for anchorage in the shelter of the Walkem Islands, but do so with caution because they are subject to strong currents. The only

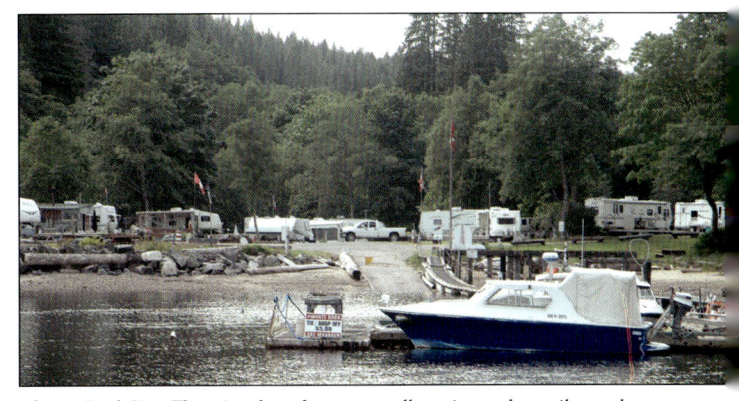

*Above: Rock Bay. There is a launch ramp, small marina and a trailer park. This is where many residents of nearby islands launch small boats or access Campbell River for supplies.*

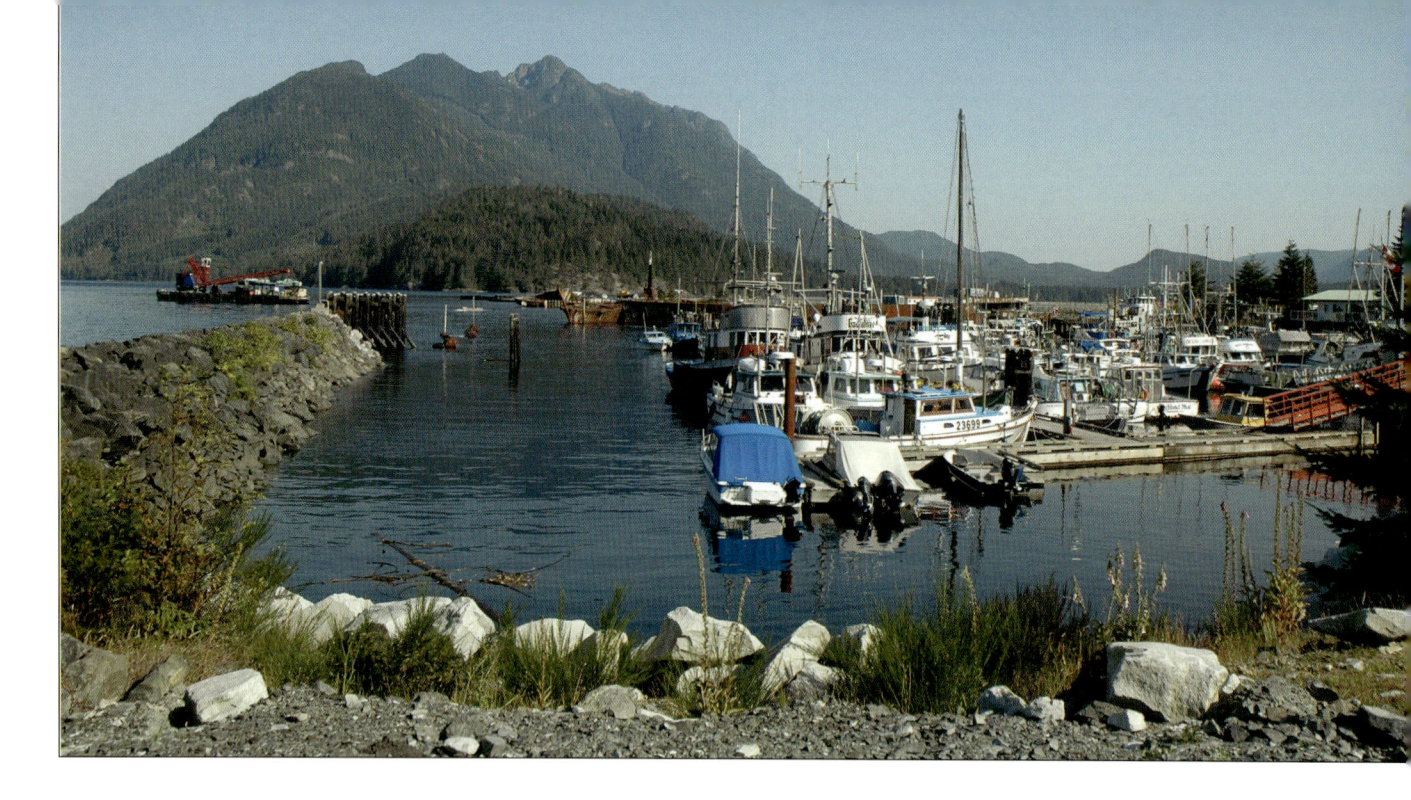

## Kelsey Bay  chart 3544

Kelsey Bay lies on Vancouver Island at the west end of Salmon Bay at the mouth of the Salmon River. It is wise to travel through this area early in the day when winds are calm, and then during slack tides. People who keep their small boats at Kelsey Bay have agreed with my expressed concerns about boating into the area. They do insist, however, that if you read the current and tide tables and monitor the weather you will be comfortable enough boating in and out of the bay. They launch their trailerable boats at a ramp at Kelsey Bay but during summer you will find some tied up at the small craft docks behind the rock breakwater just south of the former fuel dock and its breakwater. There were once large fuel storage tanks on the shore behind the old fuel dock but these have since been removed.

Just to the east of the entrance to the small craft harbour is a breakwater of several ship hulks serving the adjacent log booming ground. A floating breakwater has been installed and the docks in the main basin were extended. Some summers on shore there is a small cafe. Also available in summer are toilets and showers.

The loading area has an electric winch for handling heavy equipment. The main wharf has a gift shop with a variety of art and crafts and adjacent to it is a small-craft landing, tucked away between it and the shore. Beyond these basins is the old ferry dock inside of which is a private dock for a whale watching outfit. The RCMP patrol vessel ties up at Kelsey Bay when it is working in the area and occupies one of the slips in the basin. The onetime government dock and marina is now run by the local community.

If you have to go into Kelsey Bay do so cautiously and be mindful of the currents. If not, keep going while favourable conditions permit you to do so.

## Approaching Kelsey Bay

Continuing northwest along Johnstone Strait to Kelsey Bay follow the south shore of West Thurlow Island or cross over to Bear Point if you want to anchor temporarily in **Humpback Bay** or the small cove just beyond it. Either of these anchorages has a depth of about 6 metres. In Humpback Bay approach the house on shore between the gravel bar and the islet to the west of it and drop anchor near the beach. The unnamed cove just to the east offers sheltered anchorage away from the tidal stream.

Beyond Camp Point on Vancouver Island, the next leg between Current Passage and Race Passage can be taken on either side of **Helmcken Island**. The currents in these two passages reach 6 knots, and the standing waves that occur can be significant.

Your choice of which passage to take is restricted by the traffic separation scheme that extends from about Vansittart Point to the west end of Hardwicke Island. Although small craft usually enjoy a self-appointed exemption from traffic separation, here in particular it should be observed, especially when there are large vessels and commercial traffic moving through the area. In a small, fast boat, in calm conditions, we normally choose our passage subject to what traffic is moving through the area. Be mindful of large vessels. If you have come this far and need to stop to wait for tide changes you could pull into **Vere Cove** just beyond Tyee Point, West Thurlow Island. This will shelter you from the tidal currents although very strong tidal streams run off Tyee Point, particularly during a flood stream opposed by strong southeasterly winds. There is a drying rock on the south side of the cove and anchorage is best in the centre in about 15 metres. It is exposed and subject to westerly winds but will provide temporary shelter from easterlies.

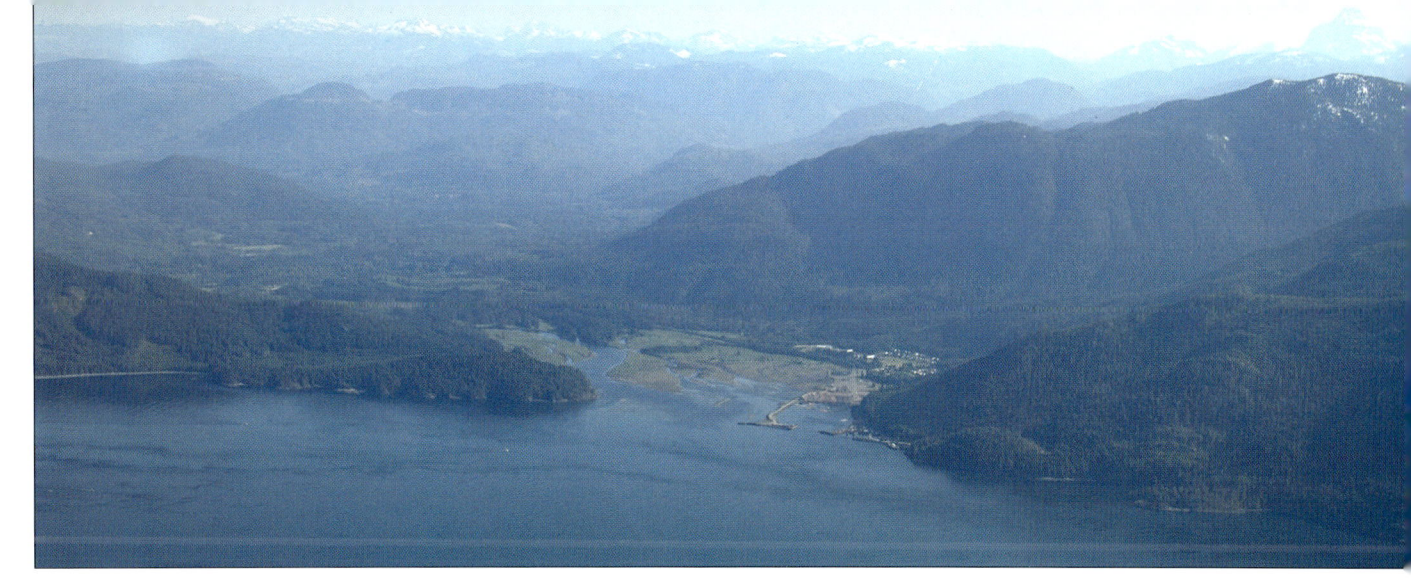

You will generally find some uncomfortable eddies off Earl Ledge. Hardwicke Point and Fanny, Clarence and Yorke Islands can also present rough water. But when it is calm and the tide is slack this is a beautiful passage northbound into Johnstone Strait.

If you use this route do so at absolute slack. We have used both of these passages and have found mostly that Current Passage has been kinder to us. Follow the western curve of the end of West Thurlow Island past Tyee Point keeping well away from Ripple Shoal then proceed along the south shore of Hardwicke Island swinging out into the mid channel off Earl Ledge. Keep at least half a mile away from the east side of Earl Ledge. Rip tides occur directly adjacent to the ledge

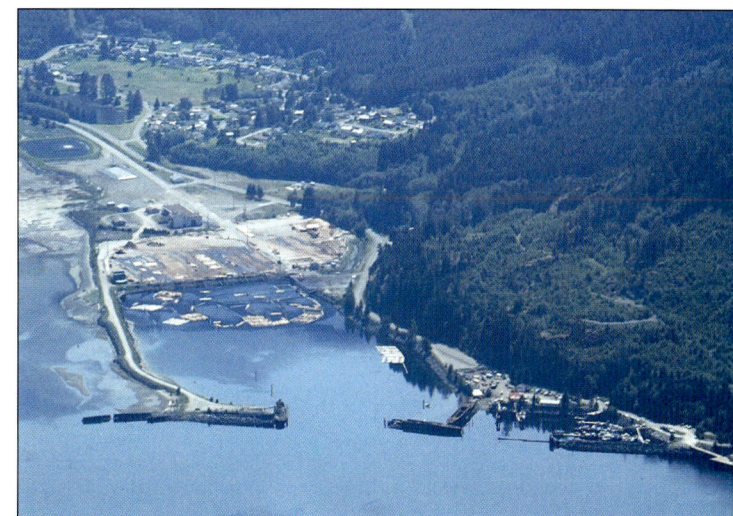

*Top: Salmon Bay at the mouth of the Salmon River, with Kelsey Bay harbour to the right. Above: The entrance to the harbour is to the west of the large, open bay. Below: A tug with its charge heads in the direction of Discovery Passage and Campbell River. Opposite: Kelsey Bay small craft harbour.*

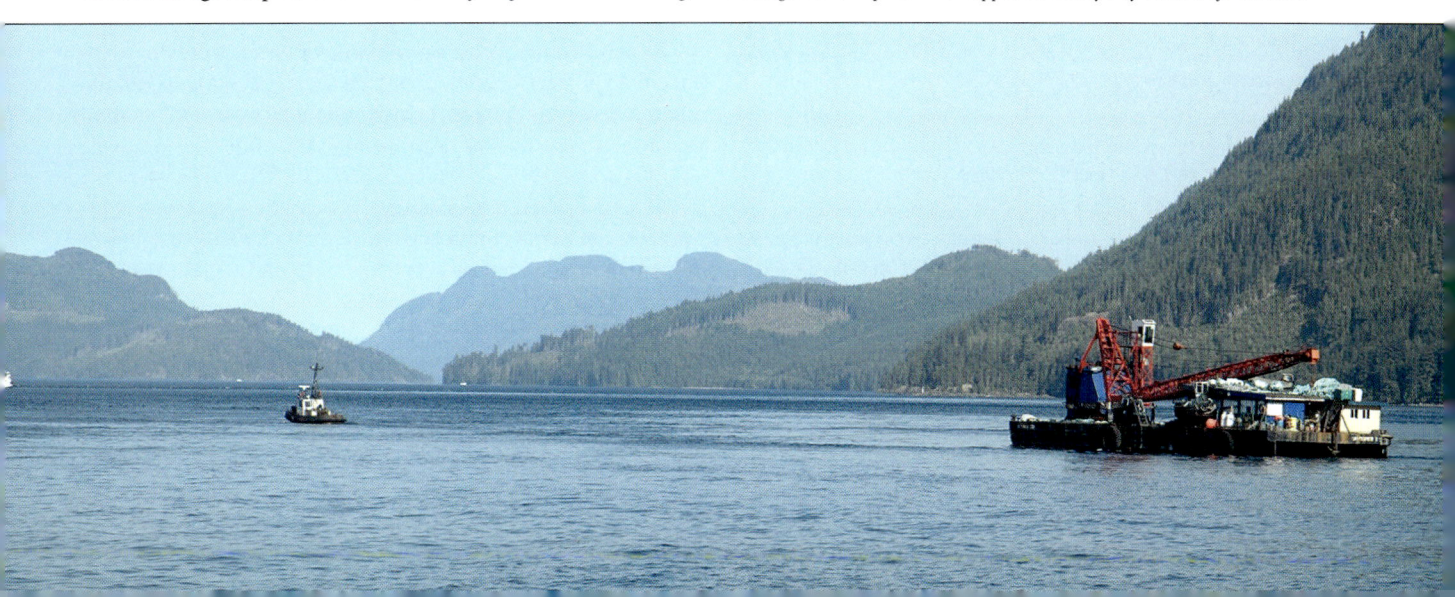

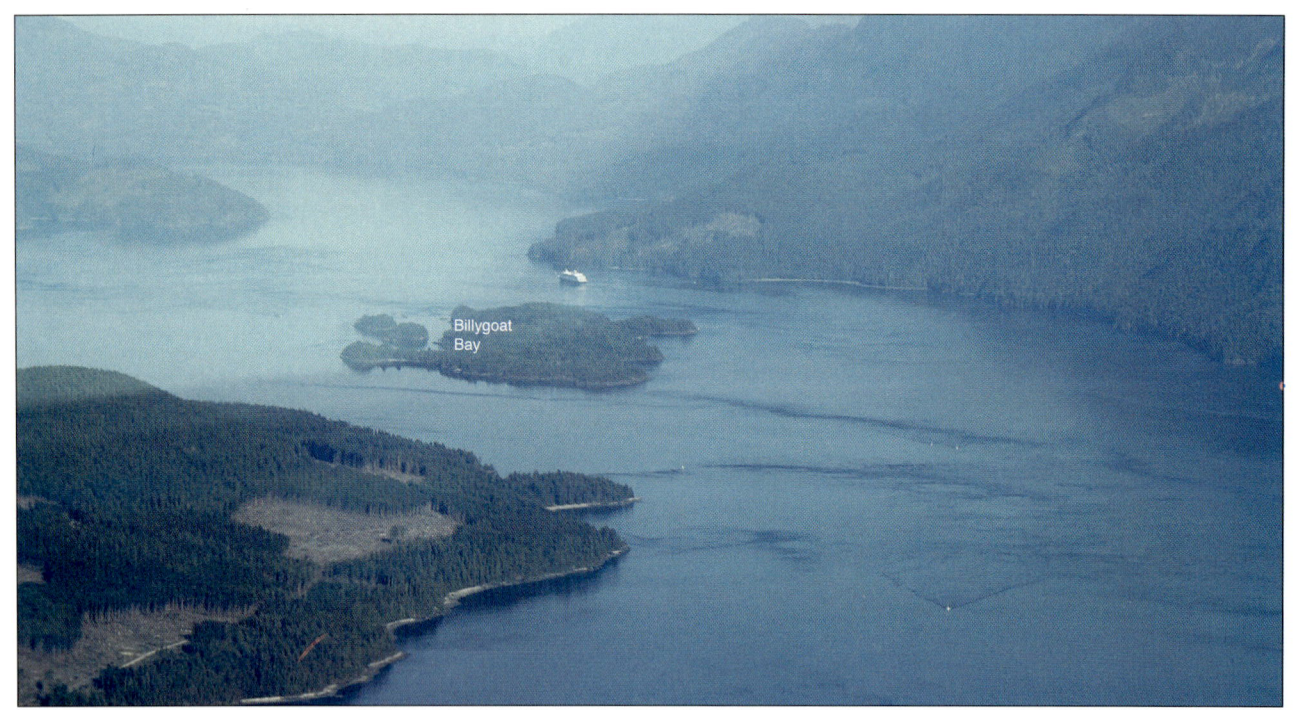

as well as midway between it and the Vancouver Island shore. Refer to the BC Coast *Sailing Directions* for concise information about sea conditions in this area.

Stay north of the centre of Johnstone Strait to avoid possible short steep waves that can occur even at slack tide. The tides ebb and flood in confusion throughout this area and studying the charts will provide some information on where the currents are. The flood currents run just off the south end of Earl Ledge and ebb just west of it. It is important to consult your tide tables for passage through this waterway, but do not be intimidated by it. It is an ideal exercise in seamanship.

At one time there was a logging settlement at **Earl Ledge**, which was also the site of the Hardwicke Island Post Office. The settlement is now privately owned and the float is not available for public use. Why anyone ever thought to establish a landfall here, with the swirling currents sweeping the shore, is a mystery to me.

## Billygoat Bay   chart 3544

Billygoat Bay is a deep indentation in the northeast side of Helmcken Island. It has been recommended by some and considered uncertain by others. The bay is protected by two islets off the entrance and a drying rock in the centre. To avoid this rock the best access to the anchorage is between the two islets. Anchor in about 12 metres. Several boating friends and I choose to keep travelling while the going is good, rather than stop in this cove only to find the currents have become stronger later, when trying to press on.

After the stretch from Chatham Point and Discovery Passage to Kelsey Bay, Johnstone Strait links up with Sunderland

*Johnstone Strait, looking southeast over Earl Ledge and Helmcken Island with a cruise ship off Camp Point.*

Channel. Continuing on to Port Neville takes you past Yorke Island, Clarence Island and Fanny Island. Tide rips can be steep mid channel between Fanny Island and the wide mouth of Blenkinsop Bay so keep going in a straight line for Port Neville. If the currents are not strong but the wind is coming up you may cross Johnstone Strait to the anchorage tucked in behind **Tuna Point**. This is a very small anchorage in that you will have to compete for space with kelp and sunken logging debris. But it will shelter you from some wind. Once you have passed Fanny Island however, you are probably best off running for Port Neville, or beyond.

Whichever direction you have travelled to the junction of Johnstone Strait and Sunderland Channel, you will soon arrive at the entrance to Port Neville. You have navigated the currents and challenges of the tidal streams and entered a realm of boating that takes you back in time.

Ahead lies scenic Johnstone Strait and the adjacent waterways to the Broughton Islands. Beyond lies Alert Bay, Port McNeill and Port Hardy. The nearly 50 nautical miles from Chatham Point in the east, to its western end at the Blinkhorn Peninsula, provide the shortest route between Campbell River and the Broughton Islands.

Despite the majestic, snow-capped mountain peaks on Vancouver Island and the beautiful valleys and streams abutting the shores, the channels described previously, with all of the rapids to be negotiated, are still the routes of choice for owners of small recreational boats.

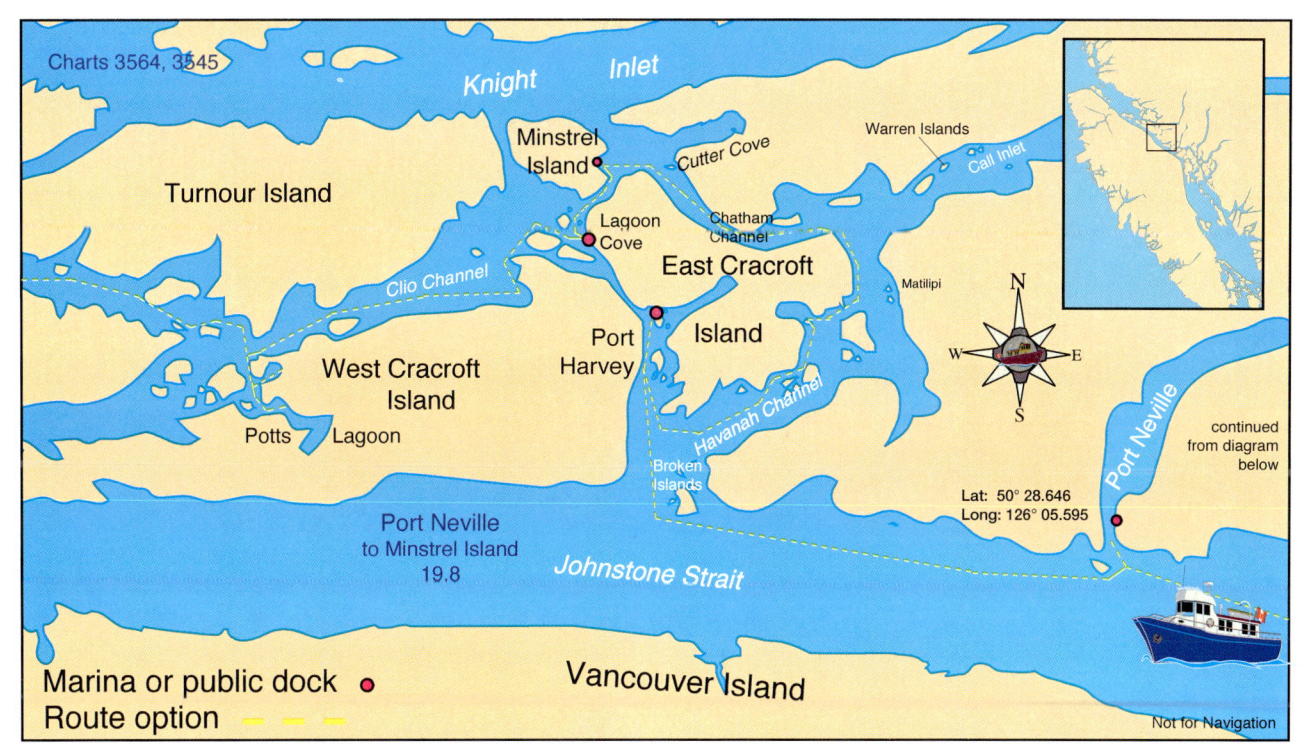

Before reaching Kelsey Bay you will pass Hkusam Bay, another spot where the location of the former landing defies logic. It is a shallow bay with a rocky approach and best left to port as you cruise on by. If you are interested in local history and want to understand the past existence of places like Hkusam you will find interesting reading in a number of reference books at the BC Provincial Museum in Victoria, UBC and local libraries. The village was occupied until 1914. It had a store, post office and hotel built in the 1890s by a white settler named Theodore Peterson. After the village was abandoned the buildings decayed and before long there was nothing left.

*The Sayward-Kelsey Bay Saga*, a book by Frances Duncan details life and settlement at Sayward and in the nearby Kelsey Bay area. It discusses early families of the area and their relationship with the First Nations people and of the coming and going of traders and coastal steamers.

A government dock was built at Kelsey Bay in the early 1900s and a float was added in 1905 by the Hastings Logging Company for the convenience of the Union Steamship Company. Steamships stopped calling at Kelsey Bay in the 1970s and since then the facilities have dwindled until today there is not much left to stop for. Kelsey Bay was named after a handlogger, William Kelsey, formerly of Topaze Harbour at the top end of Sunderland Channel. Other settlers in the Salmon River area farmed cattle and logged timber.

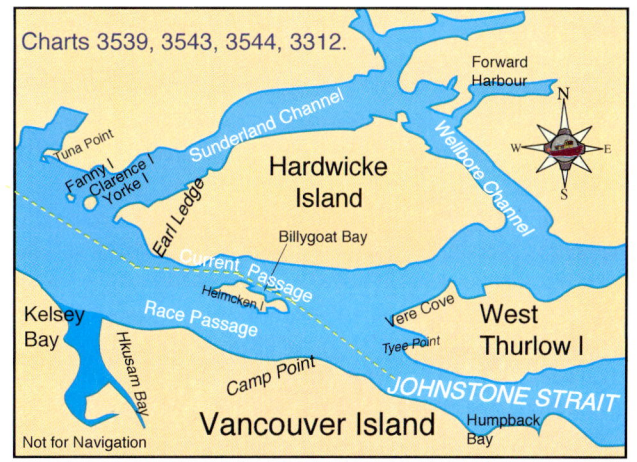

## To Port Neville  charts 3545, 3564
Link up with the Big Bay route. Continues from page 48.

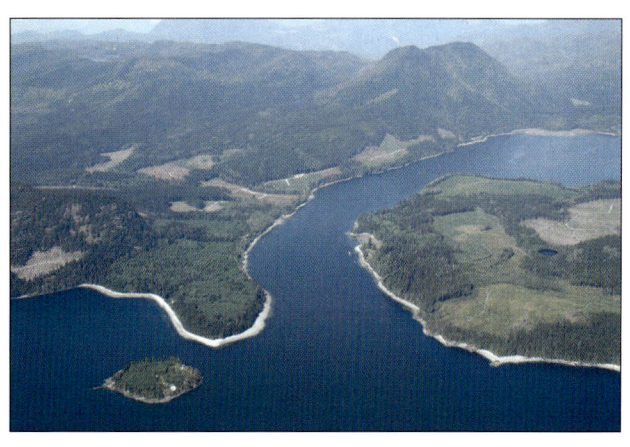

**Map annotations:**

Not for Navigation

Charts 3564, 3545

The entire port is subject to wind. Most boats anchor over a mud bottom in the shallows opposite the Port Neville landing for protection from westerly winds.

Mind the drying area immediately adjacent west and east of Robbers Nob.

Baresides Bay

Robbers Nob

logging camp

Petroglyphs behind the high tide mark on Robbers Nob

Port Neville

Baresides Bay is also called Rock Bay by some local residents. Beware of westerlies and of rocks in the shallows.

Port Neville to Minstrel Island 19.8 to Echo Bay 29.3

Note: the mileages given are always from the first named place.

Channel Rock

Port Neville

ruins

Don't anchor in the centre of a port, channel or bay where there is possible tug traffic. In Port Neville anchor clear of tugs towing log booms.

Port Neville Historic store and landing

A current of up to three knots runs past the dock at the Port Neville landing. Take care when docking. Tie up securely.

Point Neville

Ransom Point

Port Neville N 50°28.646' W126°05.595'

Point George

Blenkinsop Bay

Tuna Point

Johnstone

Milly Island

Strait

Jesse Island

---

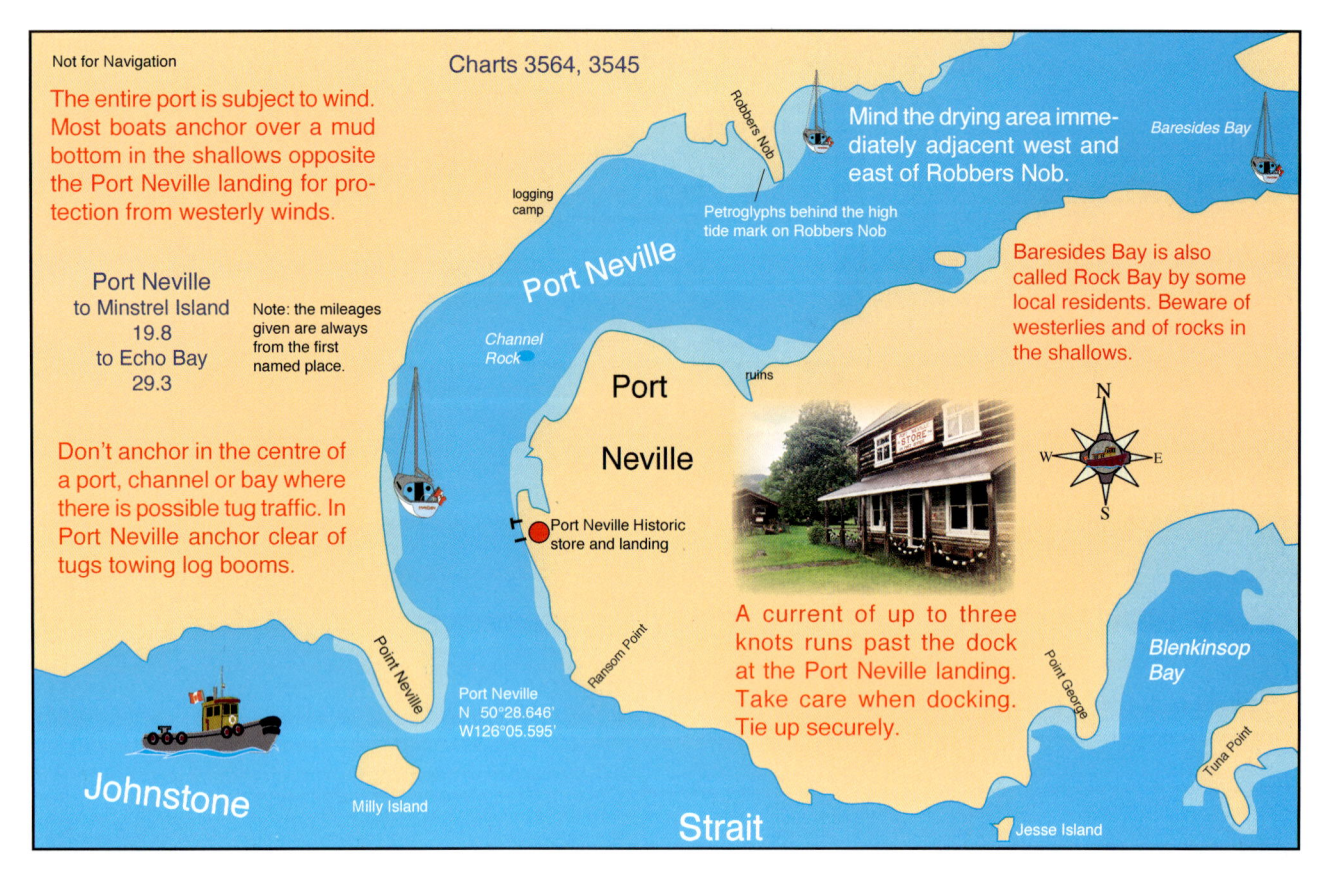

## Port Neville  charts 3564, 3545

Port Neville has a small dock with no facilities. It has 34 metres of docking space (rafting permitted), and provides access to historic Port Neville. The Hansen family were pioneering settlers here. Today Lorna Hulm (Chesluk-Hansen) or a caretaker opens the small store located in the historic old family building when they are present on the property. The building houses a gift shop with local art and a book and magazine exchange. Like other visiting mariners, we enjoyed the warm hospitality of Lorna and her daughter Erica for many years. They would not only welcome guests warmly but also put on a nice spread of homebaked treats, or invite guests to join in on a potluck dinner. This latter practice can be found at many of the marinas as you wander through the islands beyond Port Neville.

The post office, which served the local community as well as passing mariners, is now closed. While at Port Neville there are things to do other than to view the historic store building. It is probable that you will encounter wildlife in the vicinity of the homestead. Most visitors have seen deer, which have become quite tame and spend time in the garden. Cougars and bears are a factor and incidents of them foraging in the garden and adjacent meadows have been recorded. Spend some time exploring the port and look for the petroglyphs at Robbers Nob.

The only reason to skip Port Neville en route northwards, is if the forecast calls for an impending change, and if the current sea conditions in Johnstone Strait are favourable for a continued passage to Havannah Channel and the protection of the inside channels and islands.

Of course, if conditions are to remain good, then stop in at Port Neville for a while. On the return voyage a stop in Port Neville is also likely because it is closer to the end of the trip down Johnstone Strait. And if conditions are getting rough and your timing for the tides at Gunner Point is not good, then a wait at Port Neville makes sense. Moreover you can view windy conditions in the Strait from the vantage point of the dock, the homestead or an anchorage in the port. The government dock can hold several small to medium sized boats comfortably, or more when rafted up. Expect that as a possibility. There is deep water even at low tide on the inside of the dock, where boats have been known to raft three deep.

During westerlies the dock and adjacent shoreline can be uncomfortable and it is best to anchor on the west shore in the shallows opposite the landing. Some larger yachts drop the hook temporarily farther up the port in the questionable protection of **Robbers Nob**. Mind the drying area immediately adjacent west and east of this point. Unsettled weather can reduce the reliability of the anchorage, making it wise to plan for a stay in a sheltered place other than Port Neville. In the port, **Baresides Bay** is probably the most sheltered anchorage.

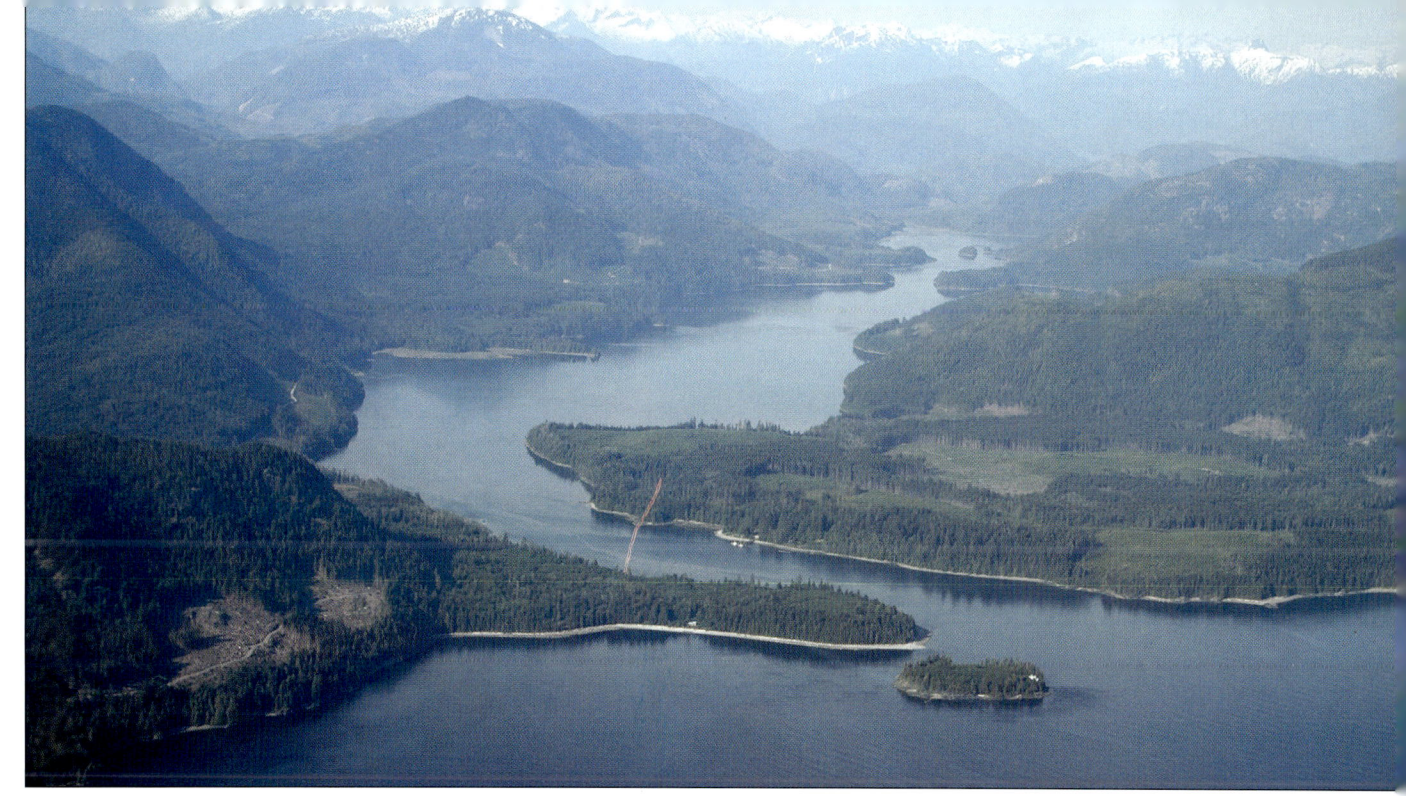

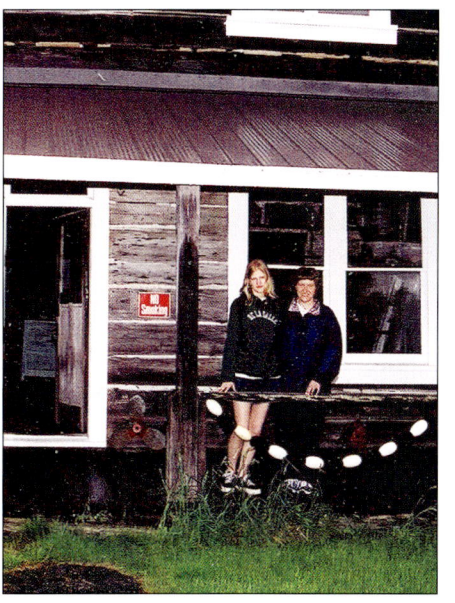

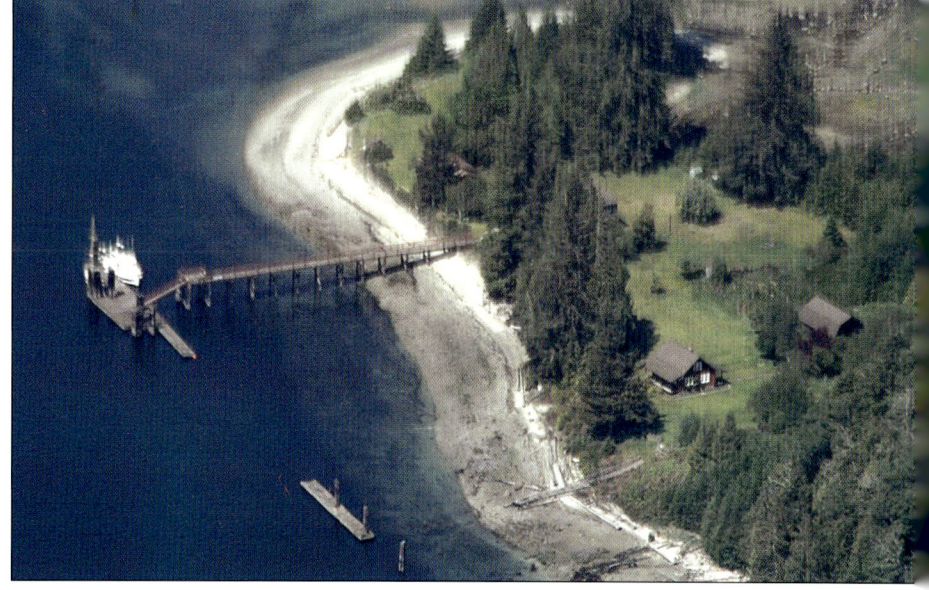

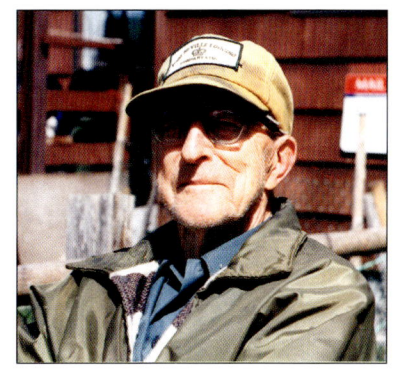

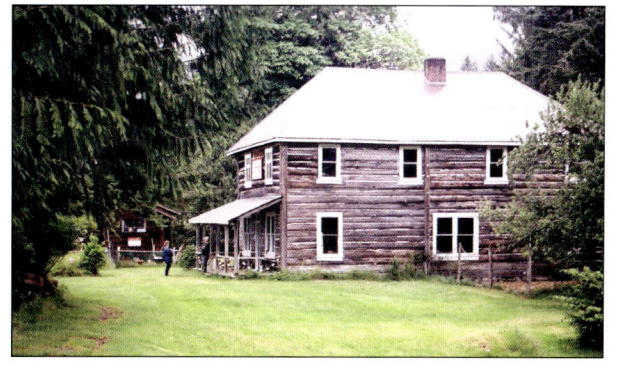

*Top and above: Port Neville. Left: The old general store and residence of the Hansen family. Lorna and Erica, circa 2002. The late Olaf Hansen, photographed in 1995. There is a museum inside the old building that is open when someone from the family is visiting the property.*

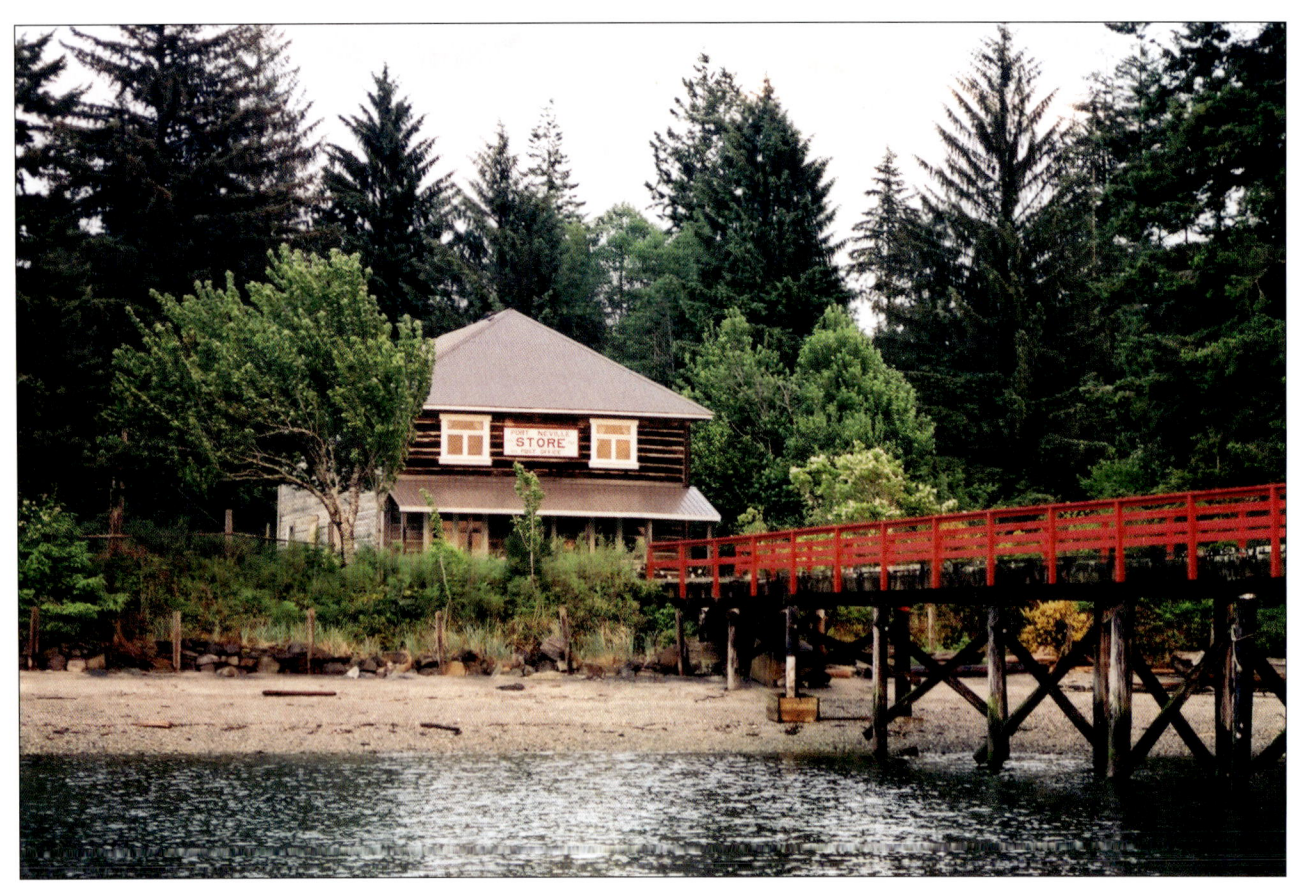

*The historic general store at Port Neville. The dock serving this landing is not officially managed. Land with care, noting the tidal current at the dock.*

From Port Neville to Port Harvey boats may encounter a build up of seas and wind coming down Johnstone Strait, from the west. This build up continues all the way to Yorke Island and beyond in certain tidal and wind states. It is wisest to find shelter either side of this area if the forecast is not favourable. If you are continuing along Johnstone Strait you may find temporary shelter from westerly winds in **Forward Bay,** or in **Boat Bay** with a little more difficulty due to a rock at the entrance. Boat Bay lies opposite Robson Bight, favourite rubbing grounds of orcas (killer whales), and about six miles to the west of Forward Bay.

The preferred route into the cruising waterways of Broughton Archipelago is via Havannah Channel. This popular route out of Johnstone Strait to Knight Inlet is wide and usually calm. When entering the channel some boats use a passage behind the largest of the Broken Islands. Careful navigation is required for this. Use the large scale chart 3564.

> Watch for red tide warnings and be wary of eating shellfish. Not all red tides (algae blooms) are toxic. Many are, and clams, mussels and oysters can retain the poisons, with sometimes fatal results for those who have eaten them. One should always check with Fisheries and Oceans before harvesting any shellfish seafood in local ocean waters.

Most mariners choose to cruise around these islands entering Havannah Channel well clear of them, which means remaining in Johnstone Strait a little longer before turning into sheltered waters.

## Havannah Channel  charts 3564, 3545

Some mariners may opt to use Port Harvey as an overnight destination after the long trek down Sunderland Channel and the first portion of Johnstone Strait. Then, instead of continuing along Johnstone Strait westwards, take the inside route via Havannah Channel.

Port Harvey is tranquil and the anchorage inviting enough to stay a while as a destination in its own right. The recently established Port Harvey Marine Resort offers overnight moorage. George and Gail Cambridge have been building a facility to accommodate mariners overnight, at the dock or in cabins. The owners can be found at the resort year round and their marina has services for transient visitors.

There are also several options for anchoring (diagram page 62). **Open Cove** at the entrance, between Harvey Point and Transit Point provides anchorage in about 10 metres. The favoured anchorage is in the shallows, behind **Range Island**

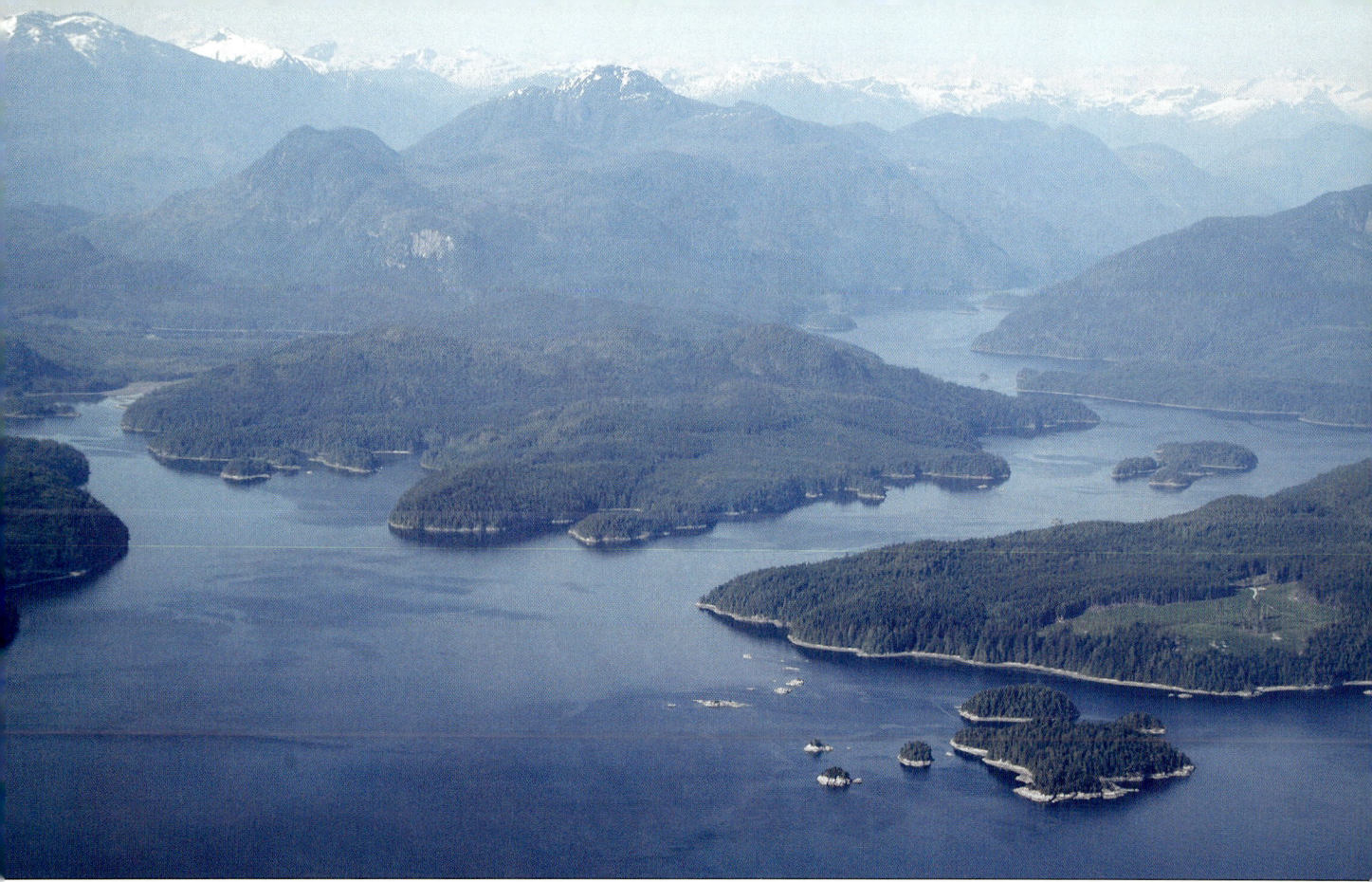

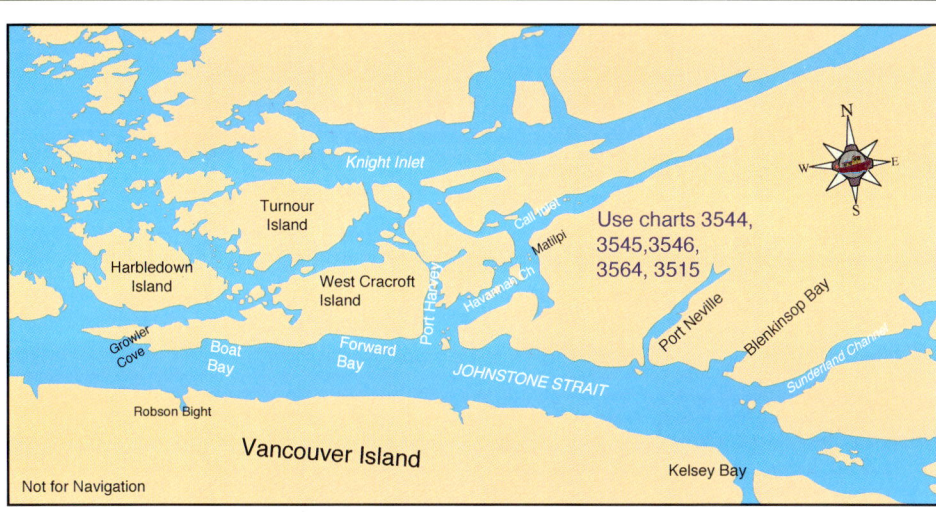

*The passage up Havannah Channel to Chatham Channel is easy after leaving Johnstone Strait. The view is north past the Broken Islands with Port Harvey to the left.*

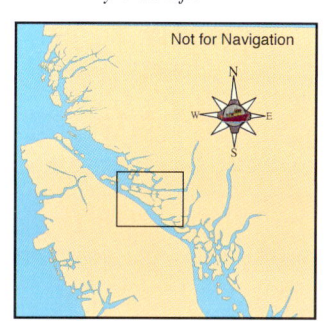

in about 6 metres at low water, but northwesterly winds are known to blow down between the islands and can make this anchorage uncomfortable. Two other anchorages in the port, one behind the outer of the **Mist Islets** and the other tucked in north of them, are considered temporary to excellent depending on wind conditions. A public dock once stood at the end of the bay and provided easy access to shore where an old cedar cabin stood in ruins for many years.

The muddy, marshy canal at the head of Port Harvey between the two Cracroft Islands (East and West) is not a suitable passage for boats, although it was used as a canoe pass by First Nations people at one time.

This area can be pleasant when the mosquitoes are not swarming. Walk the trails or beaches starting with the meadow off the shallows. In the past couple of decades mariners anchored in the port would comb the area for wild fruit and scour the beaches for clams. A long time resident of the area, Doug Gordon, well known in the logging industry, has a house in Port Harvey located near the site of a one-time hotel and public dock. Today the port's main feature is the marina.

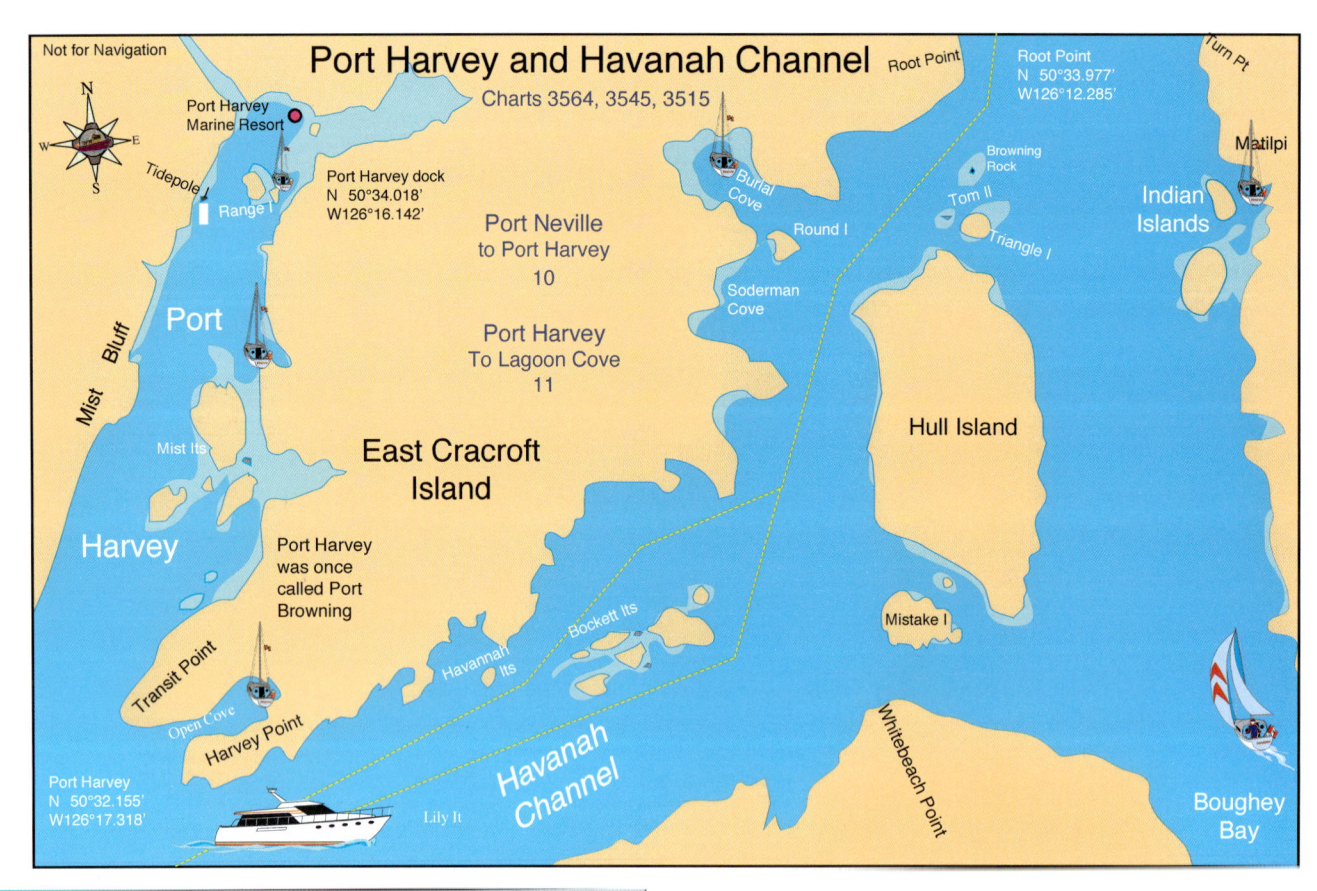

## Port Harvey and Havanah Channel
### Charts 3564, 3545, 3515

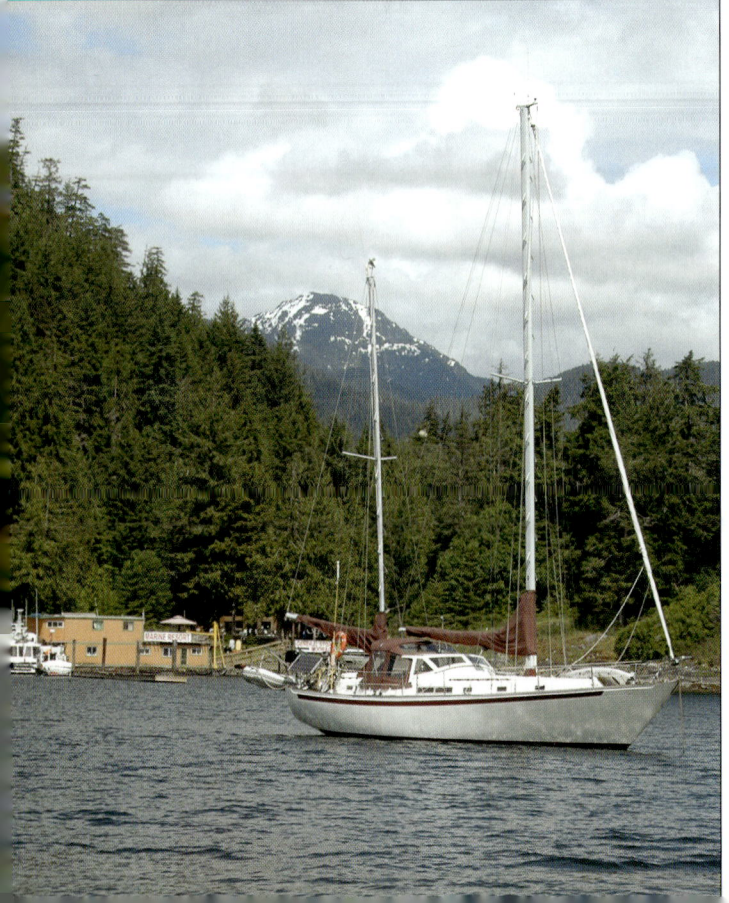

## Port Harvey Marine Resort
PO Box 40 Minstrel Island BC  V0P 1L0
Ph: 250-902-9003          VHF 66A
email: cambridge@xplornet.com
www.portharvey.blogspot.com

Established 2009. The facilities, in the lee of Range Island, at Port Harvey include docks for transient visitors that will accommodate large boats.

Power and water are available at the dock.

Facilities include washrooms, laundry and showers. There is the *Red Shoe Pub and Restaurant* and a store that supplies groceries, baked goods and hardware. Look for the fresh cinnamon buns, ice cream and coffee. There is no fuel, with the nearest being available at Lagoon Cove. There is wifi and good cellular phone reception at the resort.

There is a fire pit and an outdoor games area, as well as nearby hiking trails.

Owners George and Gail Cambridge are the hosts and are at the resort year round. Check with them about available cabins and camping sites.

A post office is located in Chatham Channel near Minstrel Island.

*Left: Anchored at Port Harvey. Part of the marine resort can be seen in the background beyond the anchored boat.*

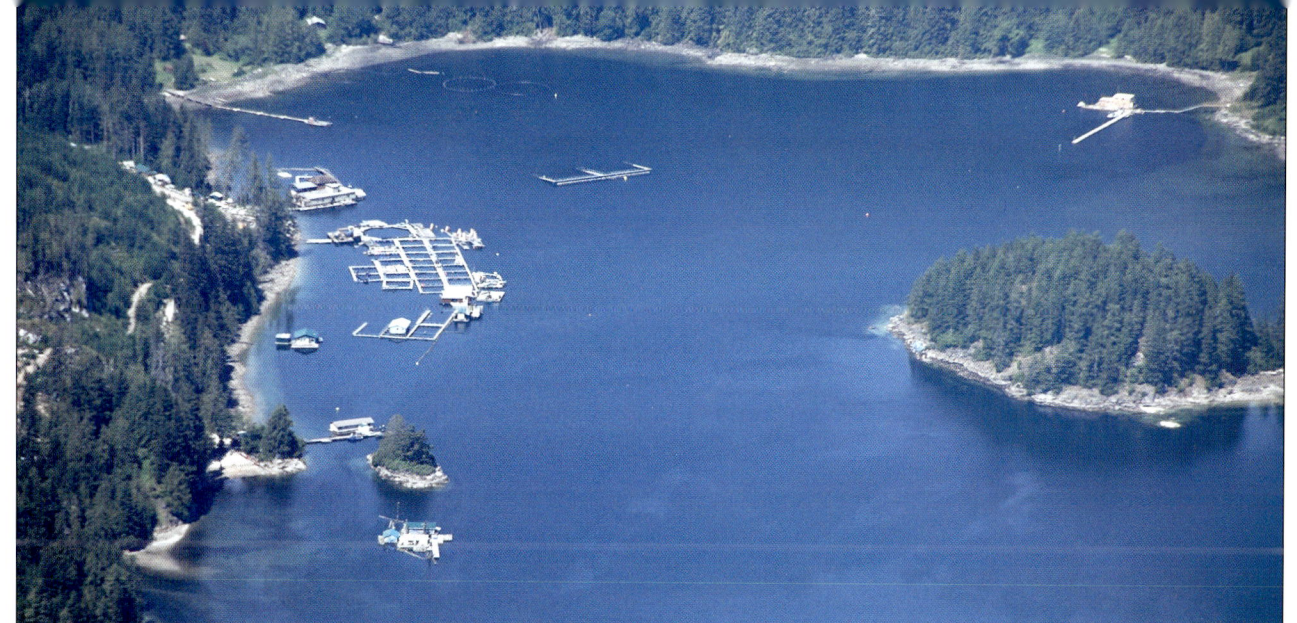

Port Harvey, above, is a wide harbour but with reasonable protection behind the islets and at its head.
Right: The Port Harvey Marine Resort docks have been expanding and the facility includes accommodations and pub/restaurant. It can be seen in an early stage of construction at the upper right in the photograph above. Look for petroglyphs on the edge of the Mist Islets.
Below: A view of Port Harvey including Mist Islets in the foreground and the marina beyond Range Island at the head of the port.

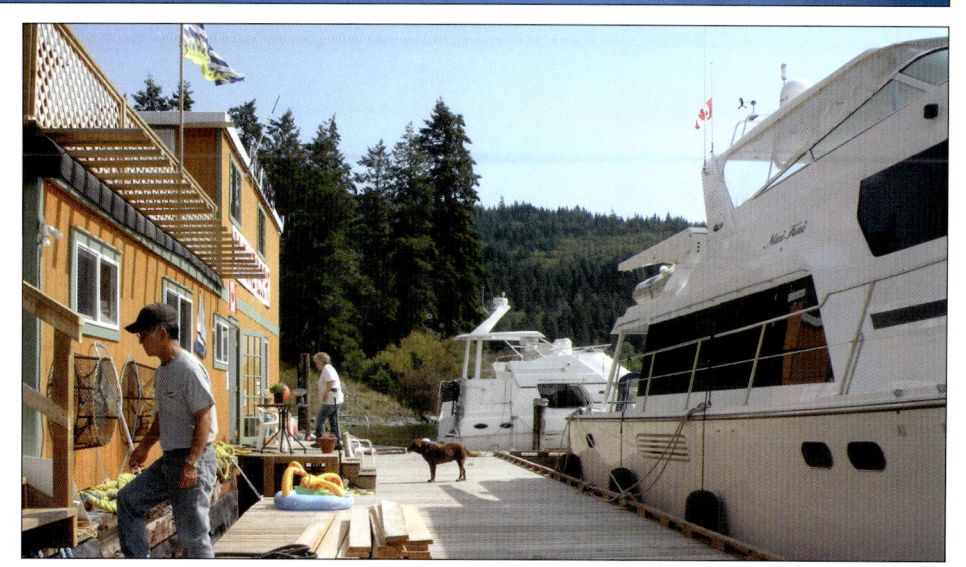

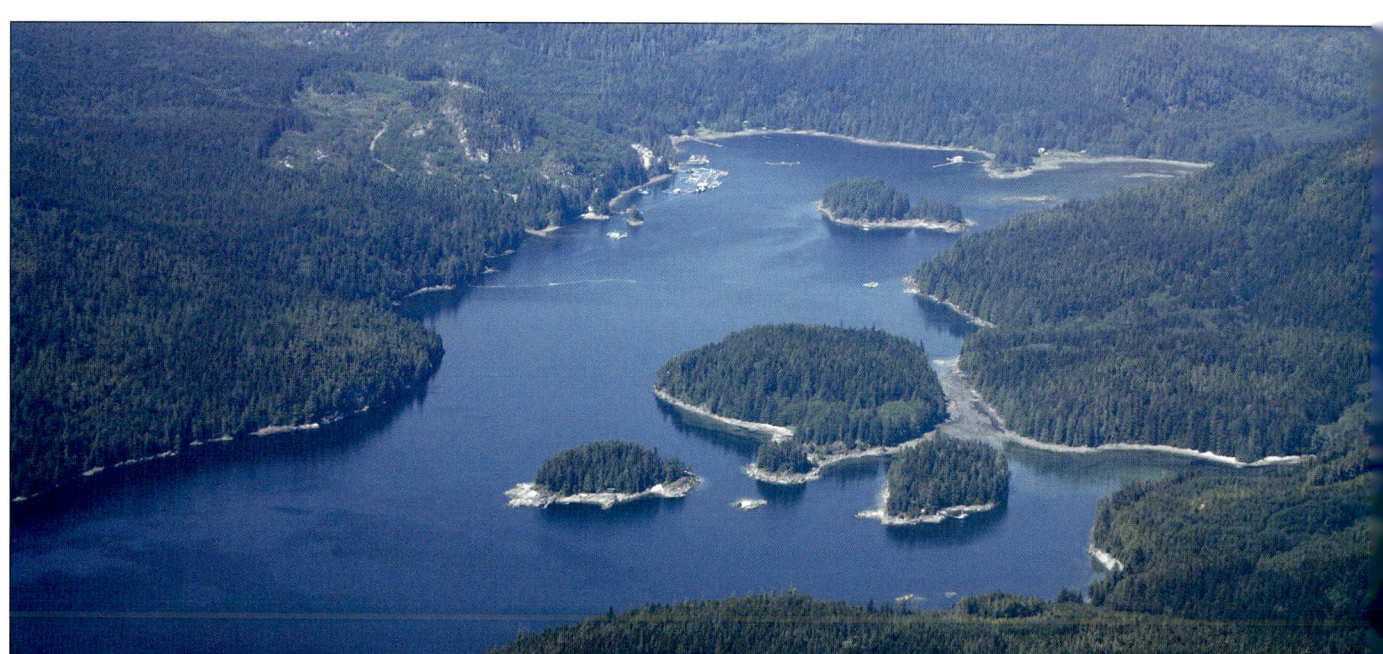

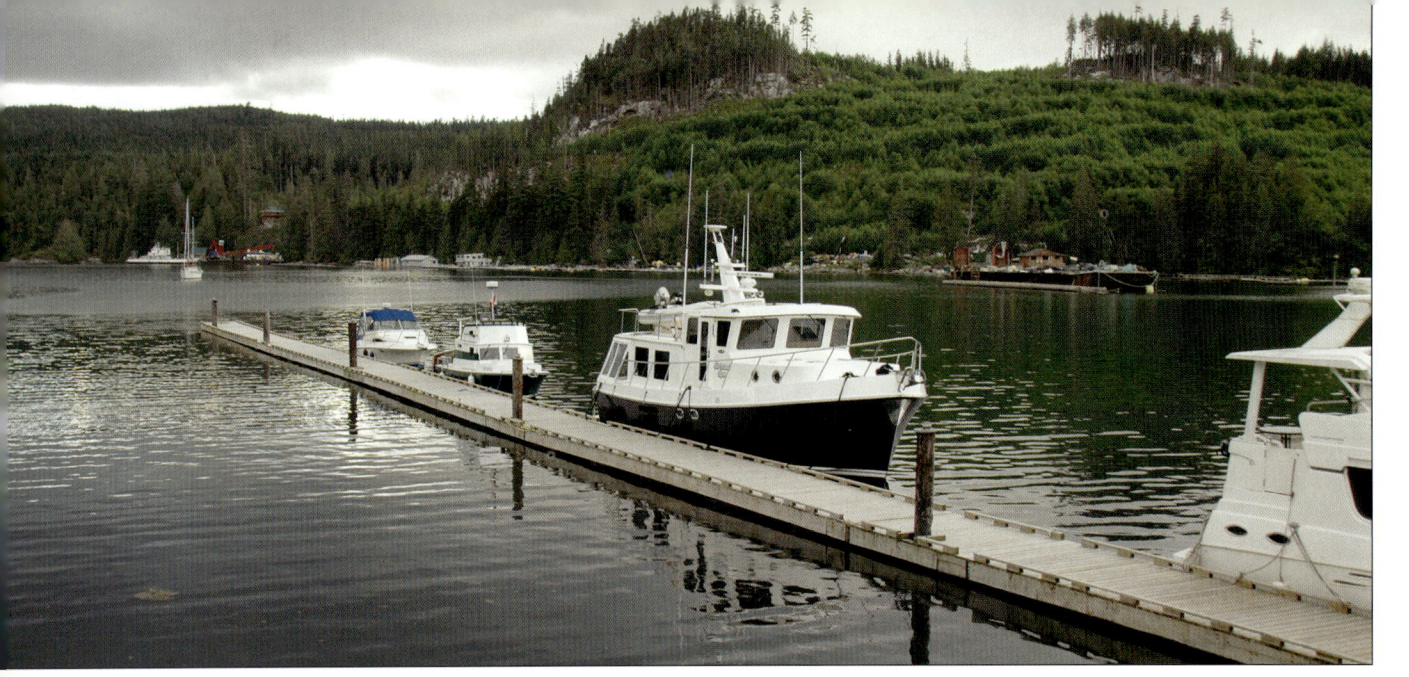

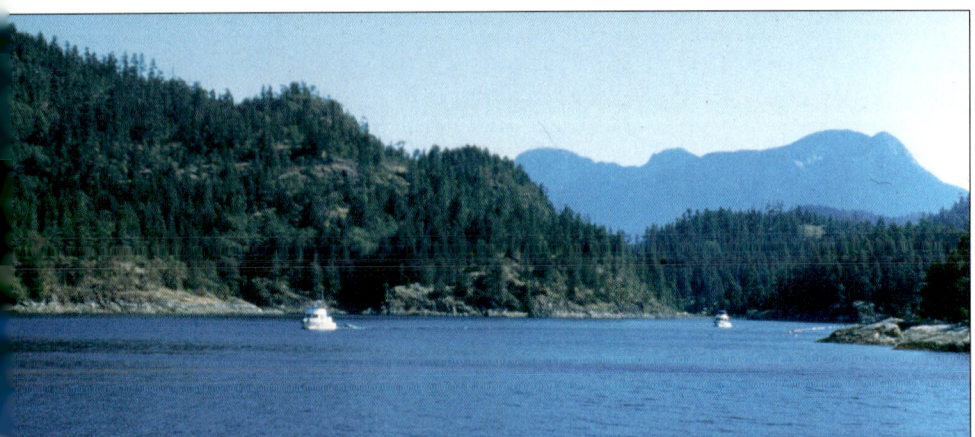

*Above: Tied up to the dock at Port Harvey Marine Resort. Left: Cruising up Havannah Channel near Minstrel Island. Below: Anchored at Matilpi in the lee of the Indian Islands. They lie to the east of Hull Island at the north end of Havannah Channel. Another anchorage can be found in the Warren Islands at the entrance to Call Inlet. Both are temporary anchorages best in calm conditions. Call Inlet is known to be windy. Opposite: Boughey Bay off Havannah Channel is open and unprotected.*

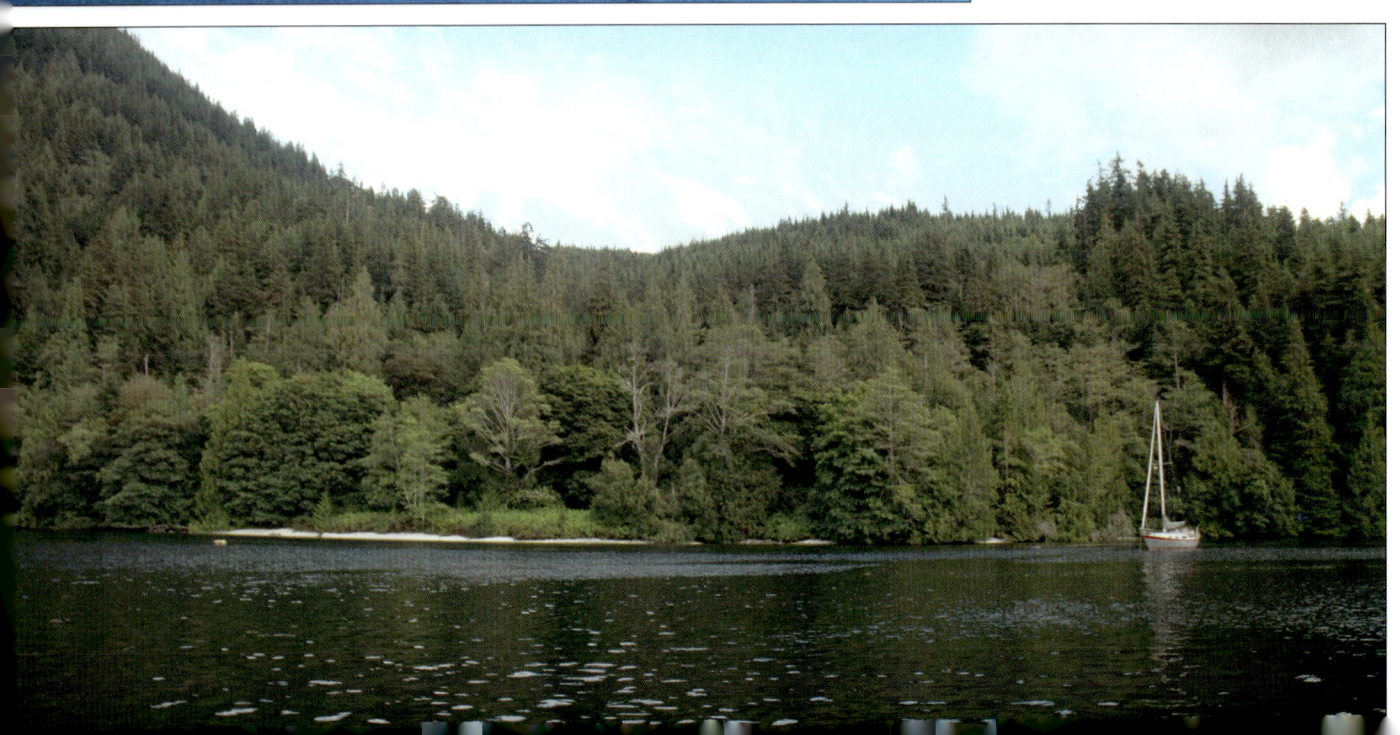

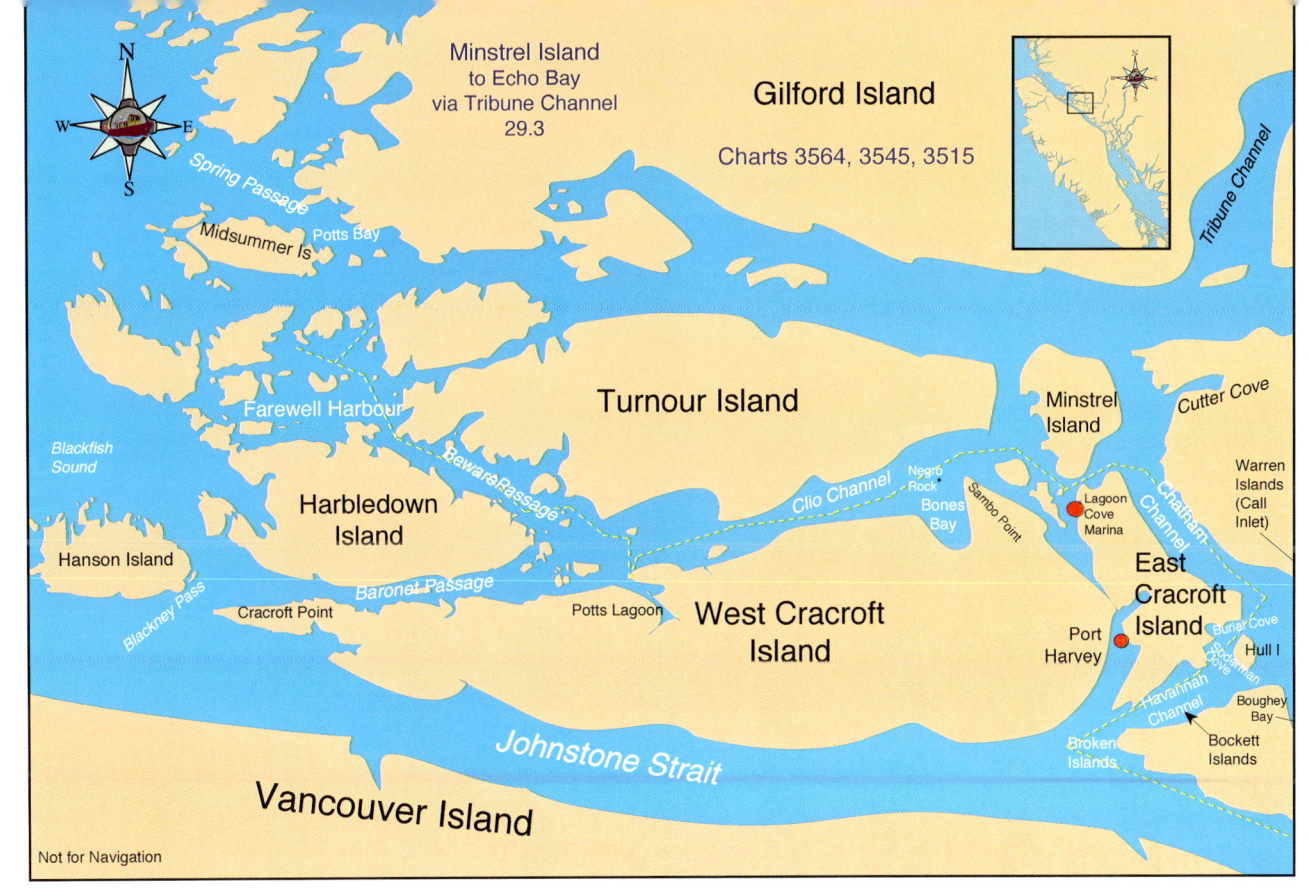

## Chatham Channel–Port Harvey to Knight Inlet via Minstrel Island
**Charts 3564, 3545, 3515**

Passing Port Harvey to your port continue northwards past the Bockett Islets and Hull Island. Soderman Cove and Burial Cove open off the west side of the channel but do not offer particularly good anchoring. **Burial Cove** is the the better protected of the two. Private residences have been appearing in and near Burial Cove.

Following the chart through these waterways one could study the inlets and speculate on alternative routes. If you have time, poke around and see what they have to offer.

The cove behind **Indian Islands** east of the northern tip of Hull Island offers a good day anchorage for one boat. It has been pointed out that this is a good all round anchorage, but some mariners disagree. It is about 18 metres deep over a mud bottom and lies opposite the abandoned village of **Matilpi**. Most mariners continue to Minstrel Island and Lagoon Cove. Bypass the long and potentially windy Call Inlet. The **Warren Islands,** in Call Inlet, look inviting, but here again, stop for a short while, being cautious about anchoring overnight due to the easterlies that blow down the inlet. Northwesterly winds too, often disturb the quiet and solitude of these islands.

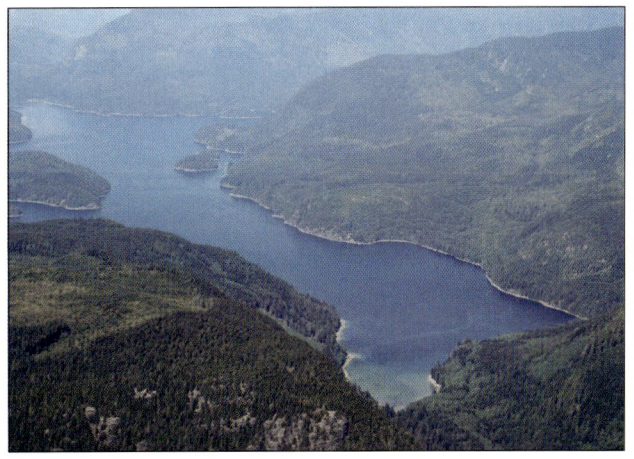

### Chatham Channel  chart 3564

There's a particular joy in navigating a narrow, shallow channel. Chatham Channel is one of those. The channel divides East Cracroft Island from a mainland peninsula that parallels Knight Inlet for a long distance. It has range markers at either end and it is quite simple to follow a straight line between them, at high or low tide. Depending on the tides, some current, about five knots, runs through the channel. The worst time is during spring tides. Kelp marks the extreme shallows in summer. Operators of power boats that leave big wakes should be considerate of smaller craft and the post office dock as they pass by in Chatham Channel.

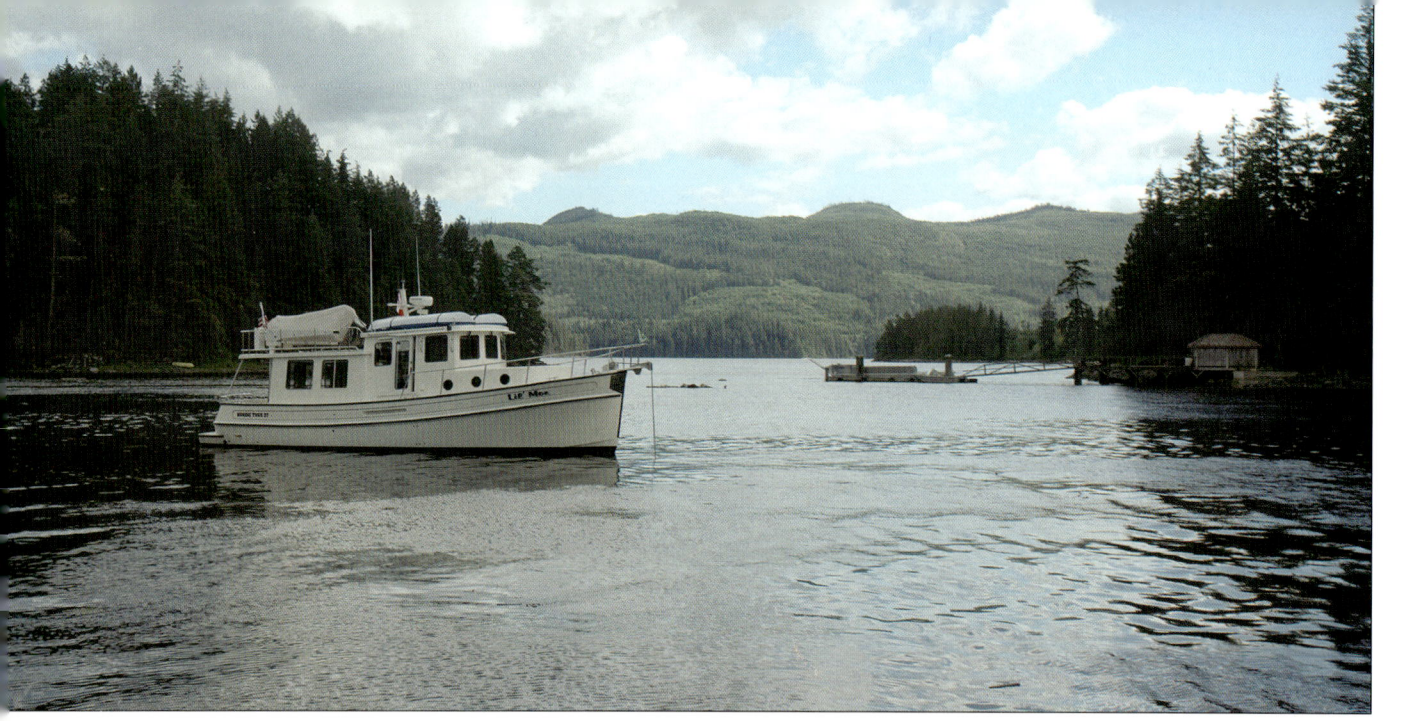

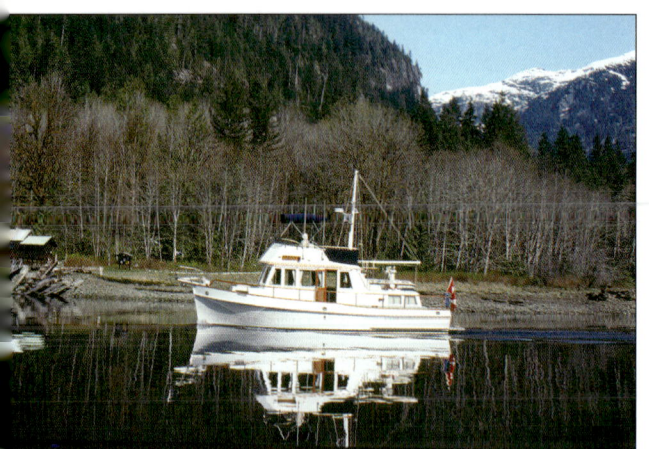

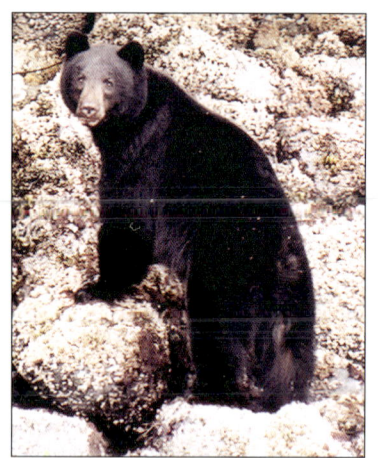

*Above and centre left: Anchored in Burial Cove on a calm day in summer. Left: In previous summers we watched black bears foraging for food along the beach on the Cracroft side of Chatham Channel. Below: Burial Cove off Havannah Channel. Stop in the area at places such as this or Lagoon Cove then continue down Clio Channel to the native villages, or continue your trip northwest to Kwatsi Bay and Echo Bay by following Tribune Channel.*

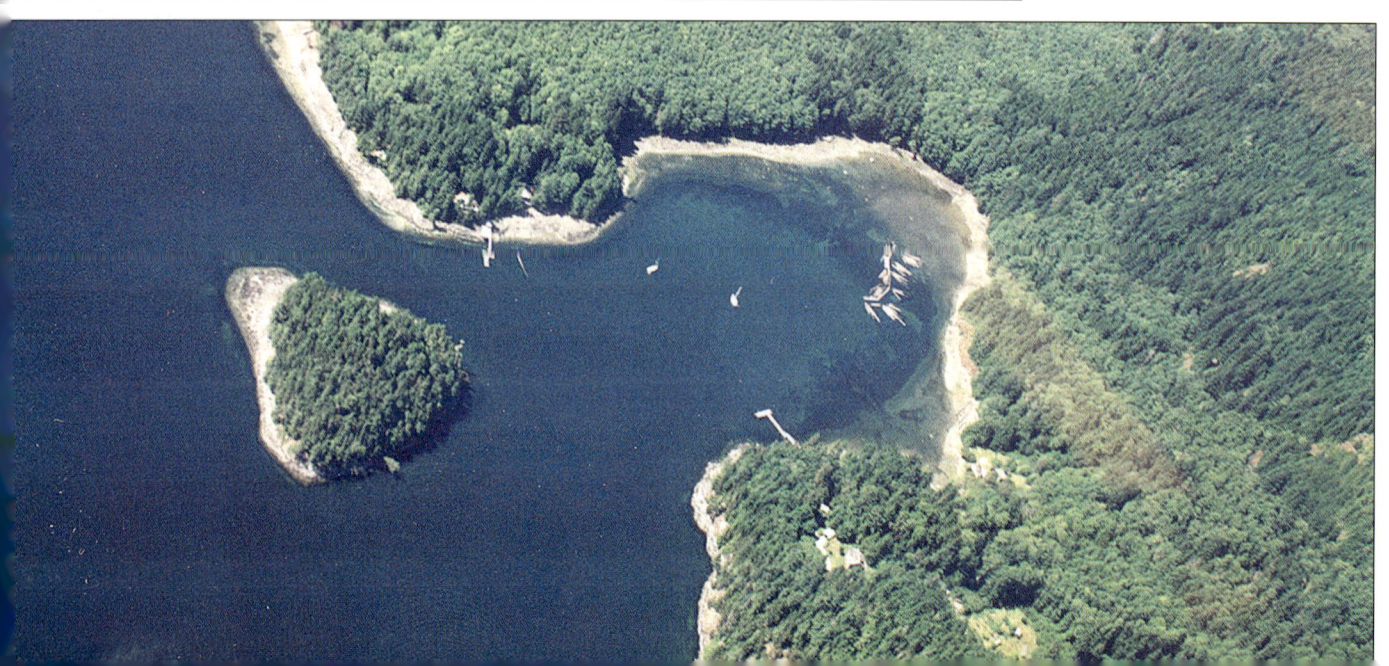

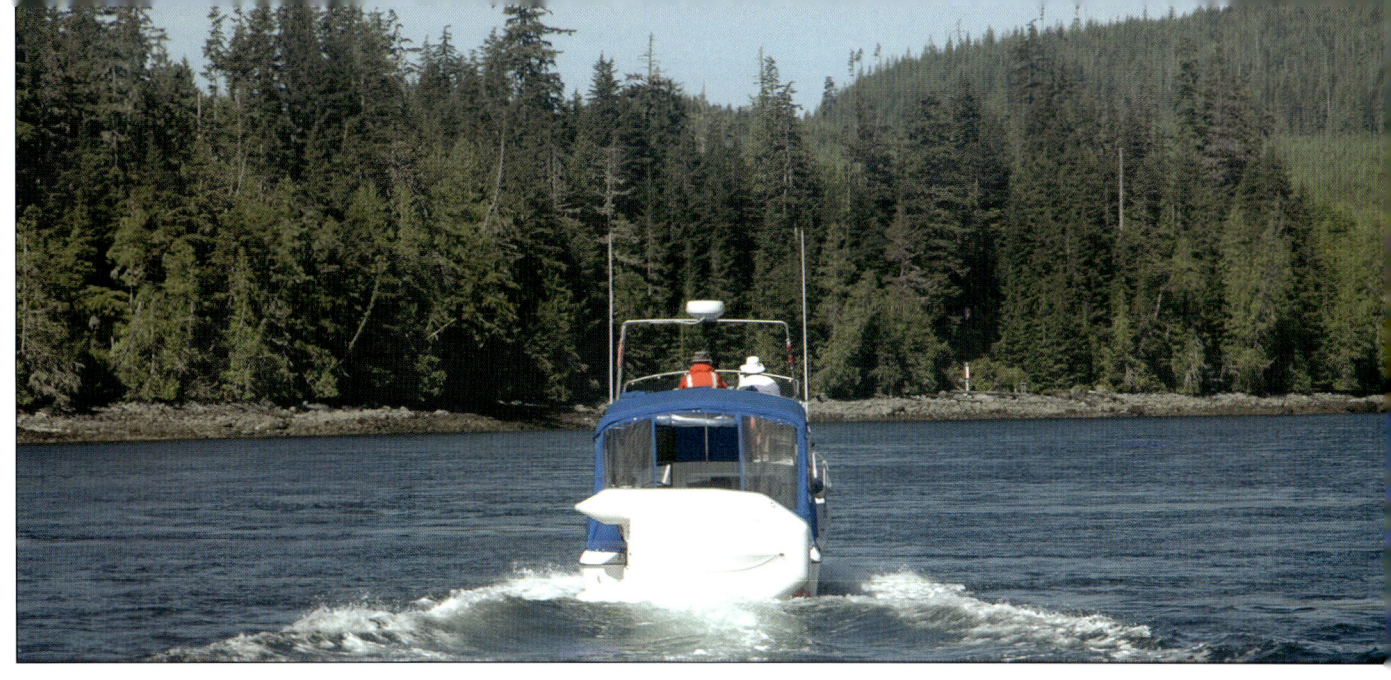

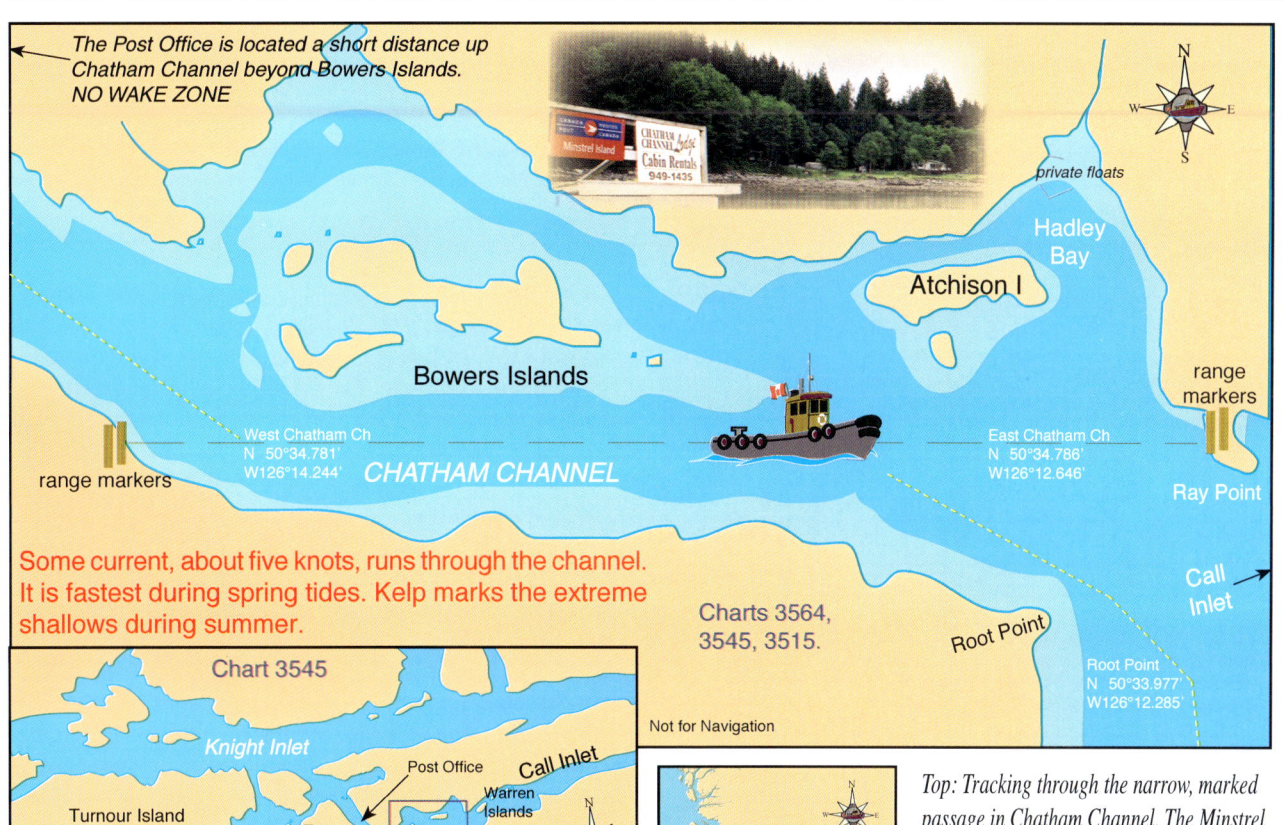

The Post Office is located a short distance up Chatham Channel beyond Bowers Islands. **NO WAKE ZONE**

private floats

Hadley Bay

Atchison I

Bowers Islands

range markers

West Chatham Ch
N 50°34.781'
W126°14.244'

East Chatham Ch
N 50°34.786'
W126°12.646'

range markers

CHATHAM CHANNEL

Ray Point

Some current, about five knots, runs through the channel. It is fastest during spring tides. Kelp marks the extreme shallows during summer.

Charts 3564, 3545, 3515.

Root Point

Call Inlet

Root Point
N 50°33.977'
W126°12.285'

Not for Navigation

Chart 3545

Knight Inlet

Turnour Island

Post Office

Call Inlet

Warren Islands

East Cracroft Island

Chatham Channel

West Cracroft Island

Port Harvey

Johnstone Strait

*Top: Tracking through the narrow, marked passage in Chatham Channel. The Minstrel Island post office is located in the upper reaches of Chatham Channel, beyond the shallows shown in the diagram. Manager Jenny Rücker runs a bakery, gift store and rental cabins on the site. The small dock was due for upgrading on the author's most recent visit.*

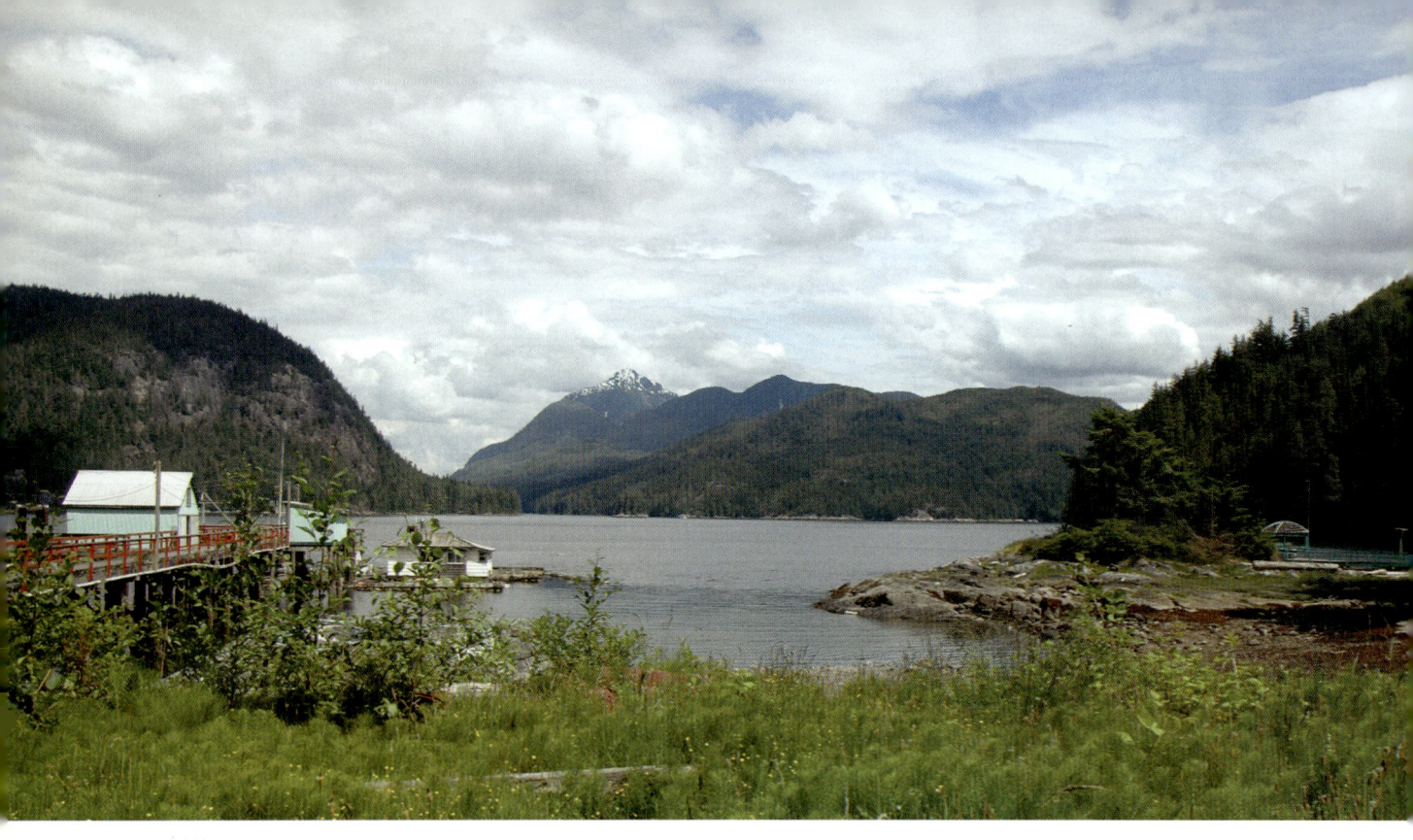

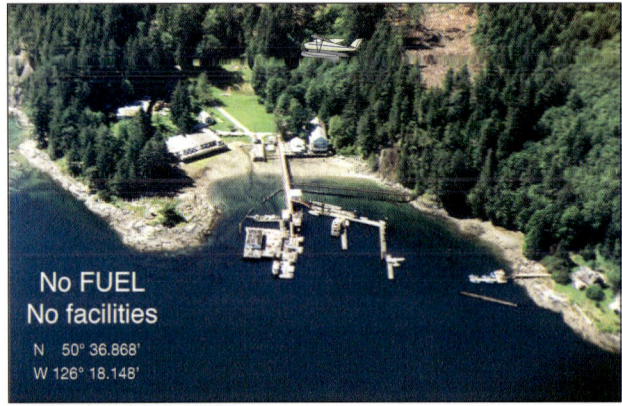

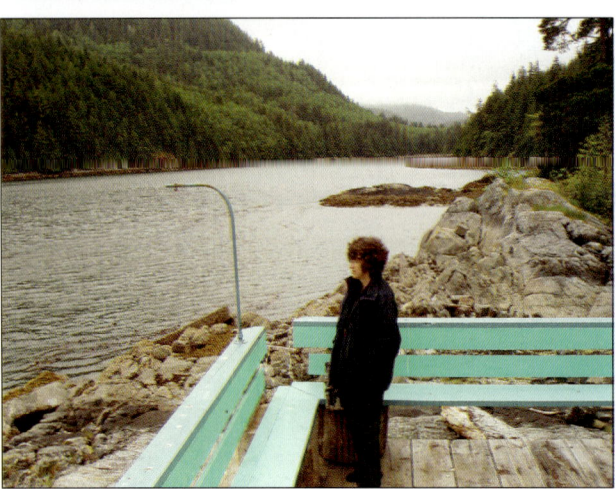

## Minstrel Island  charts 3564, 3545, 3515

Minstrel Island has been the centre of these cruising waters for decades. This is where logger Oscar Soderman became one of the first people at the settlement when he built himself a home just after the turn of the 20th century. It was a humble home, a shack. Nearby was the hotel and general store run by another logger, Tom Bennet, and a partner by the name of Armstrong. Bennet also owned a store that once stood in Port Harvey.

Minstrel Island is well named for its association with a minstrel ship from the USA that stopped in at the island, prompting a survey crew to call the island by that name. Other places nearby bear names reflecting the association with minstrels: Sambo Point, Negro Rock and Bones Bay in Clio Channel. Minstrels were brought in to perform at a once bustling dance hall at Minstrel Island settlement. It's a great pity that the hall no longer stands, as it would produce enough interest among visiting mariners to make it a focal point.

We entered the old hall in the 1970s, on that first trip with Chappel's book in hand, and were in awe of the aura of what had been a popular old west styled entertainment centre. We could almost hear the sound of an old honky tonk piano and laughter as the minstrels performed on the stage, now (on that first visit) a dusty, weather-worn platform with its steps leading up from the audience. It's a memory we were pleased to be able to carry away with us considering it was no longer there on our following visit. Nor was Ed and Margit Carder's

68

### Cutter Cove

This seemingly sheltered bay is deceptive. Often touted as an alternative anchorage in the Minstrel Island area, it has been the scene of late night disturbances for weary mariners, being that it is exposed to prevailing winds. Unless you have carefully monitored the wind forecast and are convinced that it will be accurate, look for overnight moorage elsewhere. Wind from the east dictates that you take shelter on the south side of the cove. Winds from the west require taking shelter on the north side. While this guide prefers to overlook coves and bays that afford little or no overnight protection from wind, this cove can be used as an option provided mariners check forecasts and use it wisely.

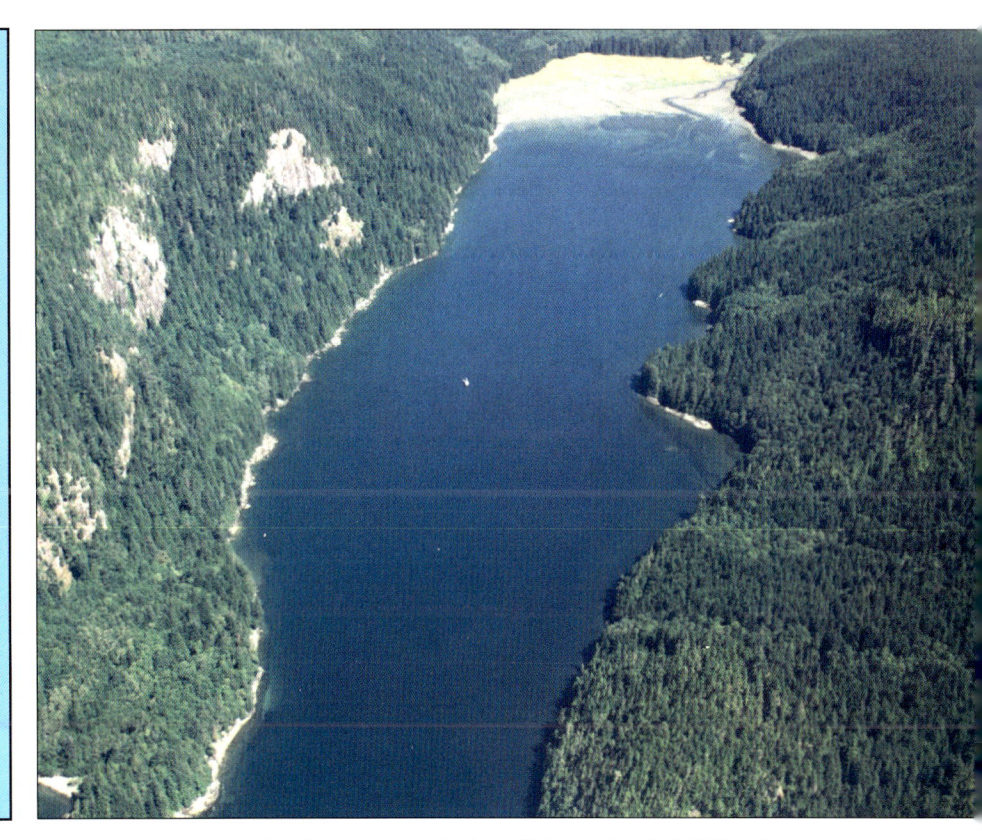

old general store that once stood on pilings alongside the wharf. It had burned down in a fire leaving the area without the convenience of a source of groceries and supplies in a onetime crucial location. On later visits the store was gone, then a small convenience store was established in the old hotel building. It has since been abandoned as a store with the change of property ownership.

One former owner was Jean Sherdahl, who with her husband Perley owned and operated the hotel, until Ed and Margit Carder purchased part of the property. It is believed that Perley bought Minstrel Island after an incident in the bar in which he was declared *persona non grata*. Perley Island in Lagoon Cove must have been named for Perley Sherdahl.

One of the more recent owners, Ed Carder, a pilot, left Minstrel Island one day and never returned, and although he is believed to have crashed in Knight Inlet, rumours have it that he never crashed at all but rather left BC and took up a new life somewhere in the south.

In more recent years Sylvia Douglas and her husband Grant ran a resort at Minstrel Island. At one time it was the hub of the area with large American boats crowding the busy docks, fishing and canning their catch, flying in guests and enjoying the island's facilities. Minstrel Island was also a major stop for float planes. Fuel and supplies were available to mariners as well as pilots and it was a very busy station renowned for its aviation and maritime role in the community.

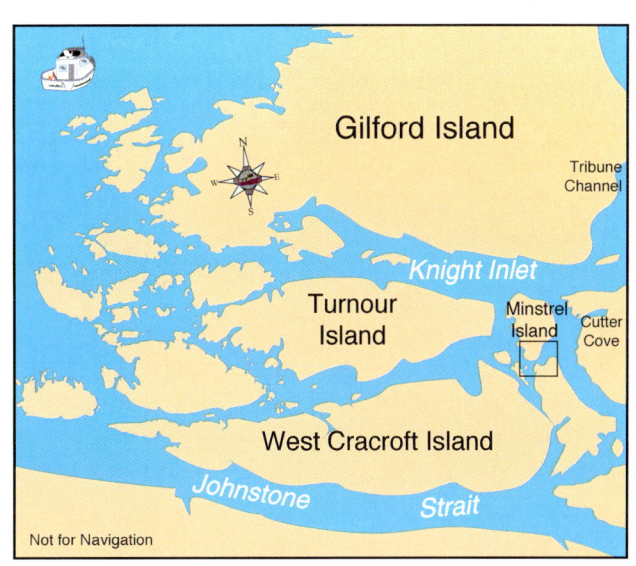

*Above: Cutter Cove, an anchorage that can be windy at times. Previous page, top: The view from Minstrel Island towards Cutter Cove. Centre: The docks from the air. Once a busy marine destination, it is now privately owned. Changes have taken place since the photograph but the dock layout remains much the same. Bottom: View from the Minstrel Island lookout at the entrance to The Blowhole.*

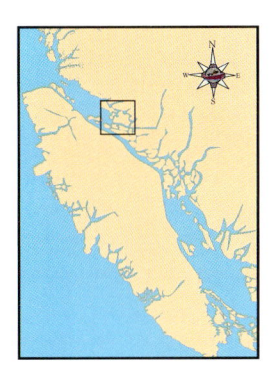

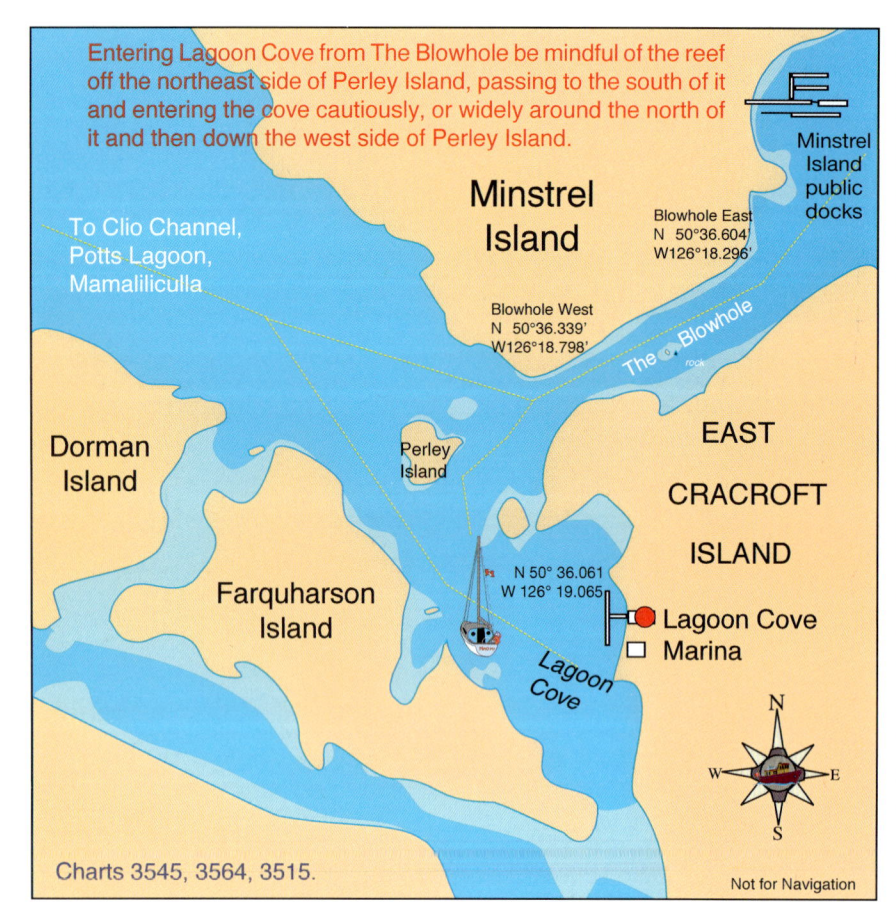

Entering Lagoon Cove from The Blowhole be mindful of the reef off the northeast side of Perley Island, passing to the south of it and entering the cove cautiously, or widely around the north of it and then down the west side of Perley Island.

Minstrel Island public docks

Minstrel Island

To Clio Channel, Potts Lagoon, Mamalilicula

Blowhole East
N 50°36.604'
W126°18.296'

Blowhole West
N 50°36.339'
W126°18.798'

The Blowhole

Dorman Island

Perley Island

EAST CRACROFT ISLAND

Farquharson Island

N 50° 36.061
W 126° 19.065

Lagoon Cove Marina

Lagoon Cove

Charts 3545, 3564, 3515.

Not for Navigation

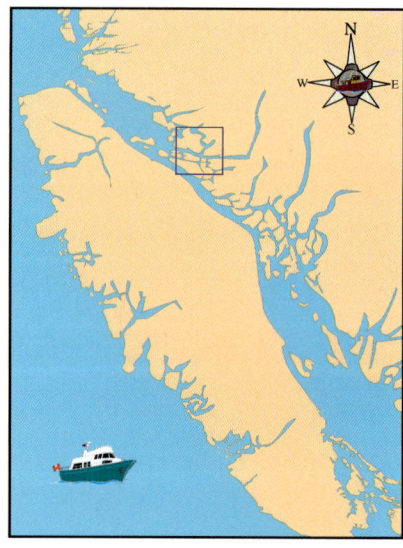

*Left, below: Bill Barber sorting through his catch for the regular afternoon prawn feast at Happy Hour.*

*Opposite: Lagoon Cove and The Blowhole waterway from Chatham Channel near Knight Inlet via Minstrel Island.*

*Opposite bottom: The Happy Hour is a popular, regular event at Lagoon Cove Marina.*

## Lagoon Cove  charts 3564, 3545

This semi protected anchorage with its popular marina is sandwiched between East and West Cracroft Islands. Sharing this wedge of water are three islands, two large and one small. They are Farquharson and Dorman Islands, the larger, and Perley Island, the smaller. Entering the cove from The Blowhole be mindful of the reef off the northeast side of Perley Island, passing to the south of it and entering the cove cautiously, or widely around the north side and then down to the west of Perley Island.

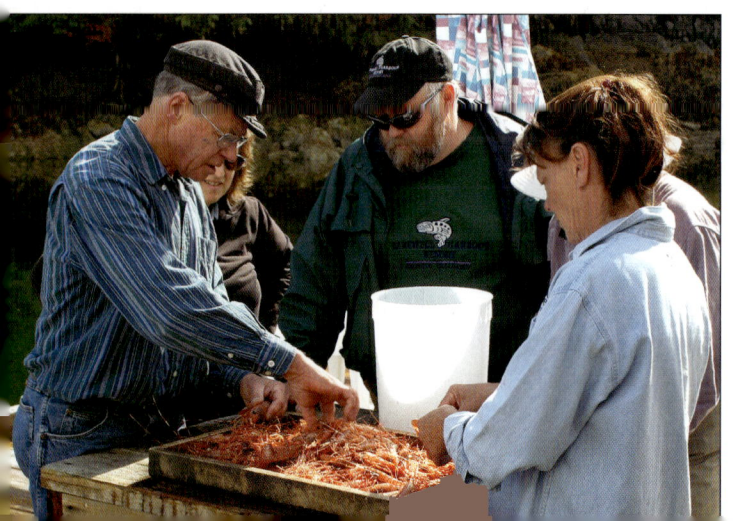

The wind can blow uncomfortably in the Lagoon Cove anchorage, funneling down The Blowhole from the east. Winds from the southwest are not known to be a problem, however. So take anchorage in the cove with a keen eye on approaching wind conditions. Or check into the marina for a secure overnight stay and the possibility of some good socializing with fellow mariners.

Bill and Jean Barber run the popular facility at Lagoon Cove. They took over a marina that was beginning to deteriorate rapidly after a former owner, David Sedgley, passed away and another owner, Jan Laan, decided to move along after only a short duration, selling the property to the Barbers. The Barbers set about restoring the buildings and grounds and turning it into an attractive destination for mariners on cruising vacations. Soon it became a focal destination in the area with regular visitors appearing every summer, joining the Barbers in social evenings around the barbecue and at the old shed on the wharf for happy hour. Overnight guests meet for a potluck social hour on summer evenings. When the weather is favourable visitors gather after happy hour at the barbecue pit where marshmallow roasts are a favourite event, with occasional sing-alongs to the accompaniment of Lagoon Cove resident, Ron Dillon, on the guitar.

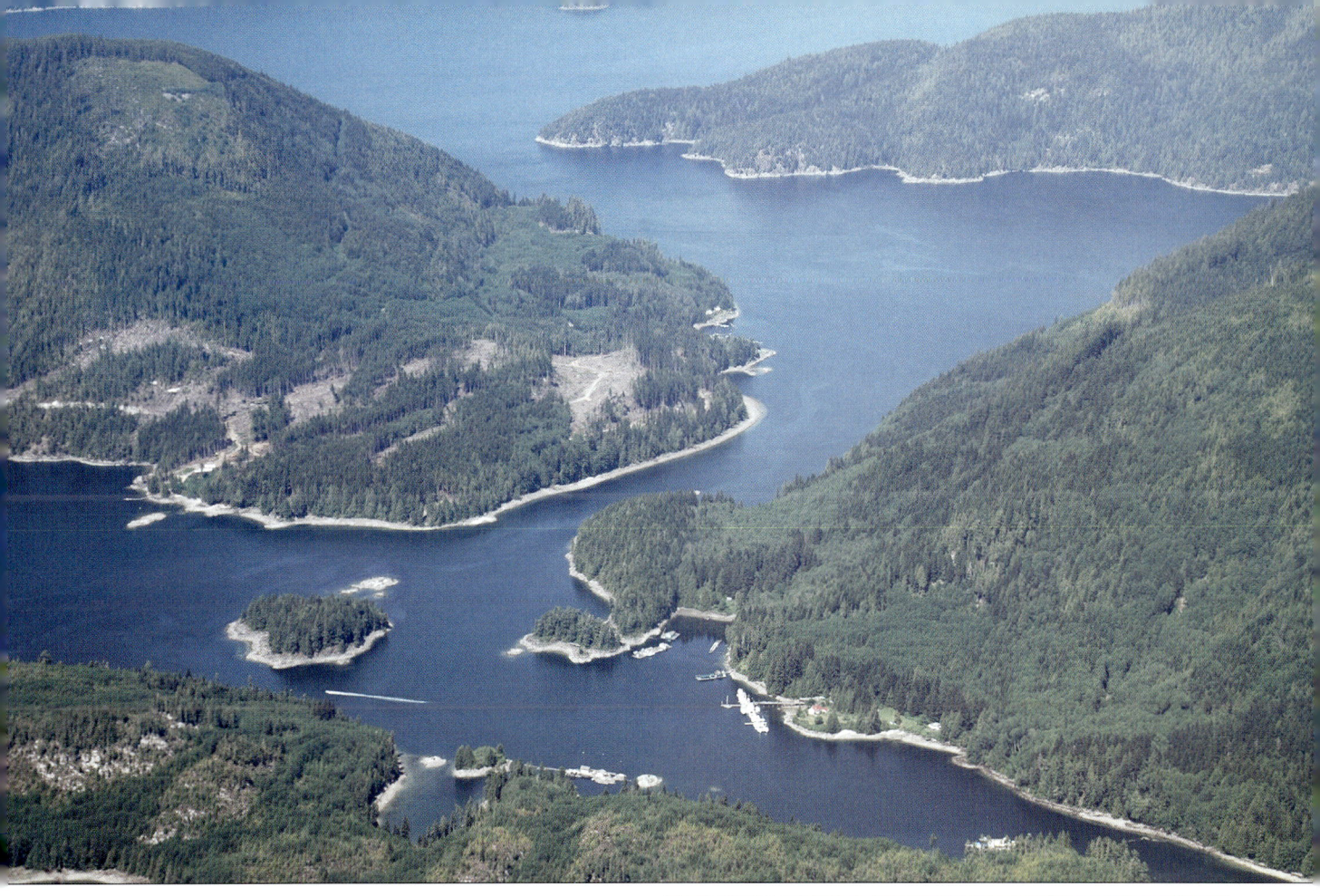

## Lagoon Cove Marina

General Delivery, Minstrel Island BC V0P 1L0
VHF 66A

Enter Lagoon Cove cautiously through the Blowhole between Minstrel Island and East Cracroft Island. It is quite an easy passage but use chart 3564 to negotiate it safely. The owners, Bill and Jean Barber, have established a routine that visitors enjoy. Happy hour every evening on the patio, at the old shed on the wharf, is followed some evenings with a group barbecue and potluck appetizers at the Crab Cooker Cabana.

The marina caters to many regular visitors and welcomes newcomers. Services include DSL internet, potable water, power at the dock, diesel, gasoline and propane. Some oils are available as well as charts, books, fishing tackle, licences, ice, some supplies and snacks.

Facilities include showers and washrooms.

Invariably Jean Barber has a selection of gifts and clothing in the *Edgewater Emporium* gift shop on the dock.

There is a fish cleaning station and a pet path. Enjoy hiking local trails and viewing wildlife.

There are magnificent sunsets and views to be seen from the marina docks and adjacent property or from atop the hillside above the resort.

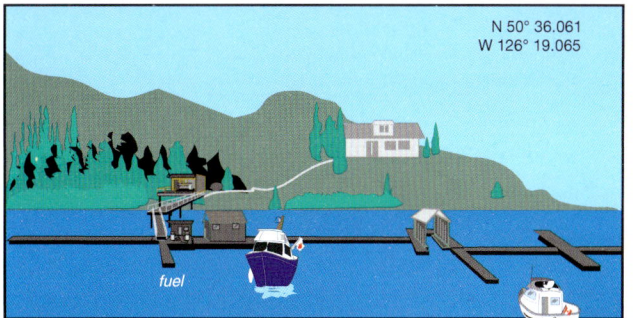

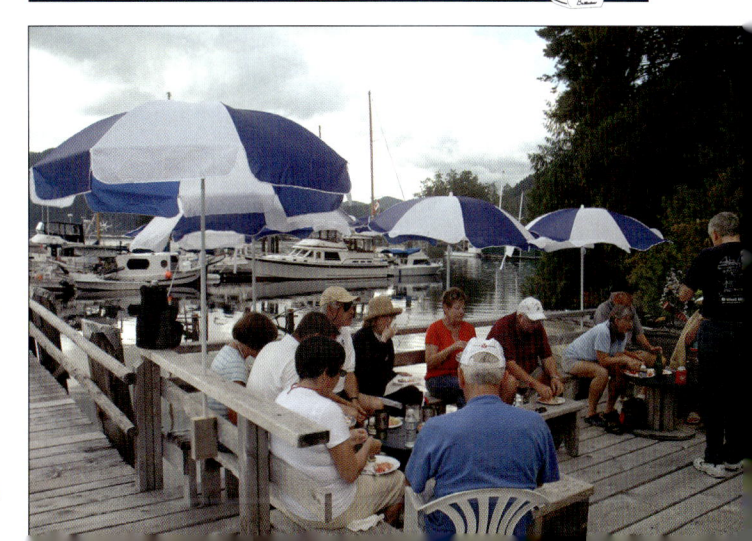

N 50° 36.061
W 126° 19.065

71

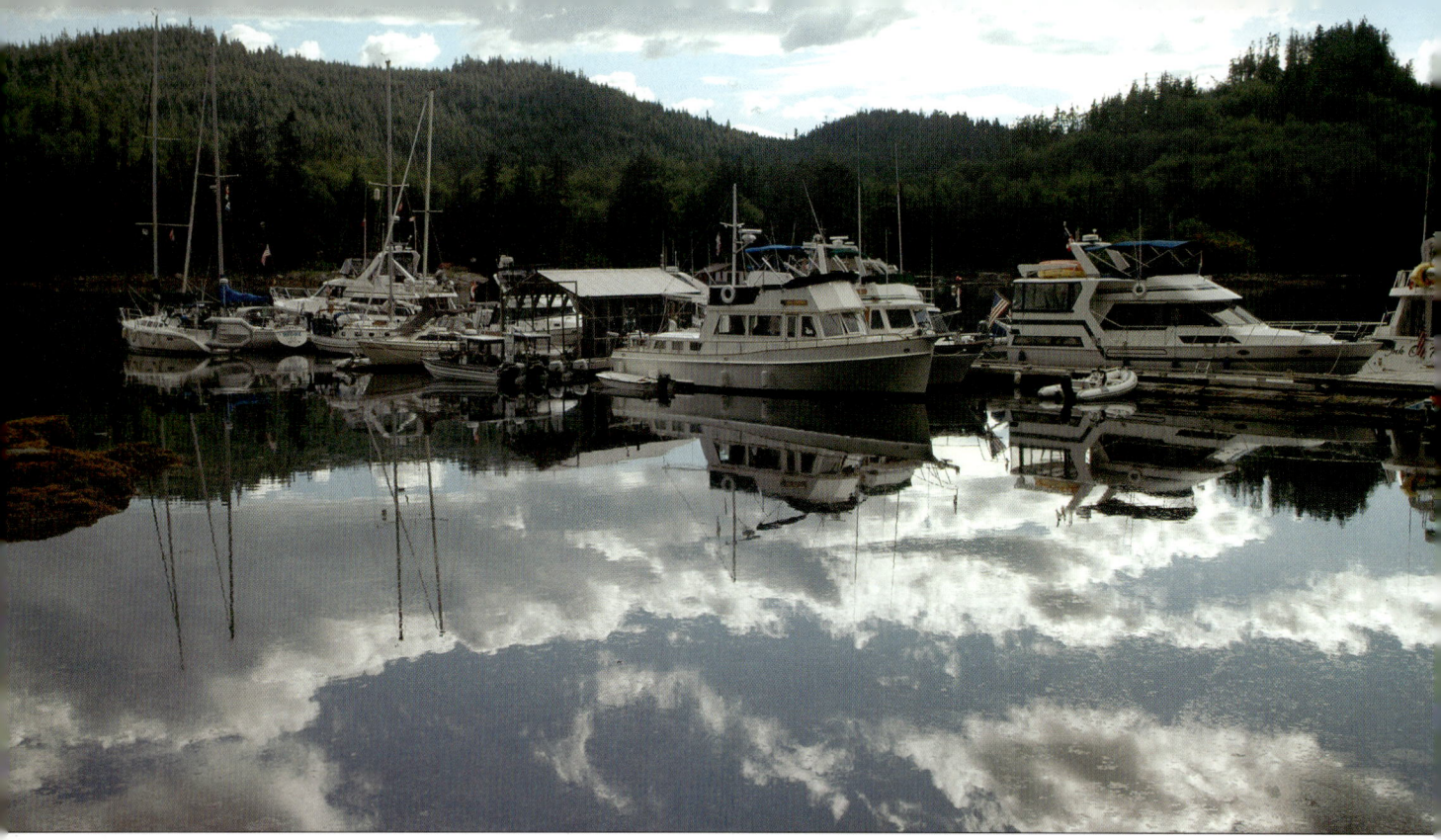

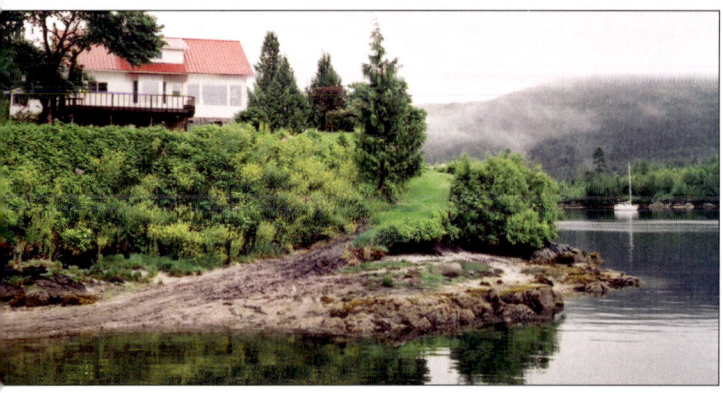

Don't worry about the lyrics. They are all in a sizeable songbook which you'll find being thrust into your hands.

When David Sedgeley and his wife Laurel owned Lagoon Cove Marina it went by the name of Cracroft Marine Service. Here the Sedgeleys offered a marine ways that could haul 15 tons, a workshop and service–particularly to wooden boats. They had a policy in those days of one night free moorage and then the princely sum of 10 cents a foot for any following nights. Guests could tie up and look after themselves with the only marina provisions being water, fuel and some fishing supplies. David showed me his workshed with great pride on more than one occasion. He pointed out some projects he was working on and described how the adjacent ways had been very busy at one time. But in the latter days of his tenure they were called on less frequently and the maintenance cost was on the rise. Some of the buildings fell into disuse just before he died. The old shed was full of rusting equipment and discarded supplies when the Barbers moved in, left there even by the interim owner. Sedgeley also left behind several trunks that had carried his possessions when he migrated to Lagoon Cove from Australia in the 1960s. Some of those belongings are still in the trunks inside the old building.

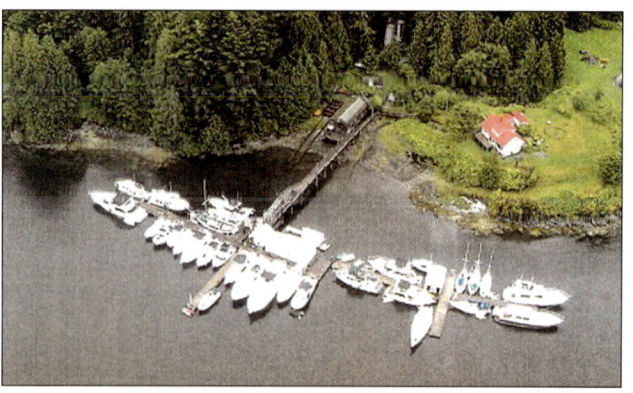

*Top: Boats tied up at Lagoon Cove Marina in early summer.*
*Above left: Owners' residence overlooking the marina and the anchorage in Lagoon Cove. Above right: Aerial photograph shows the layout of the docks, busy with many visiting boats, in the early part of summer. The ways and shed can be seen in the upper centre of the photograph. Its patio is the place where overnight guests gather for happy hour and where Bill Barber joins in to tell his amusing stories of coastal life.*

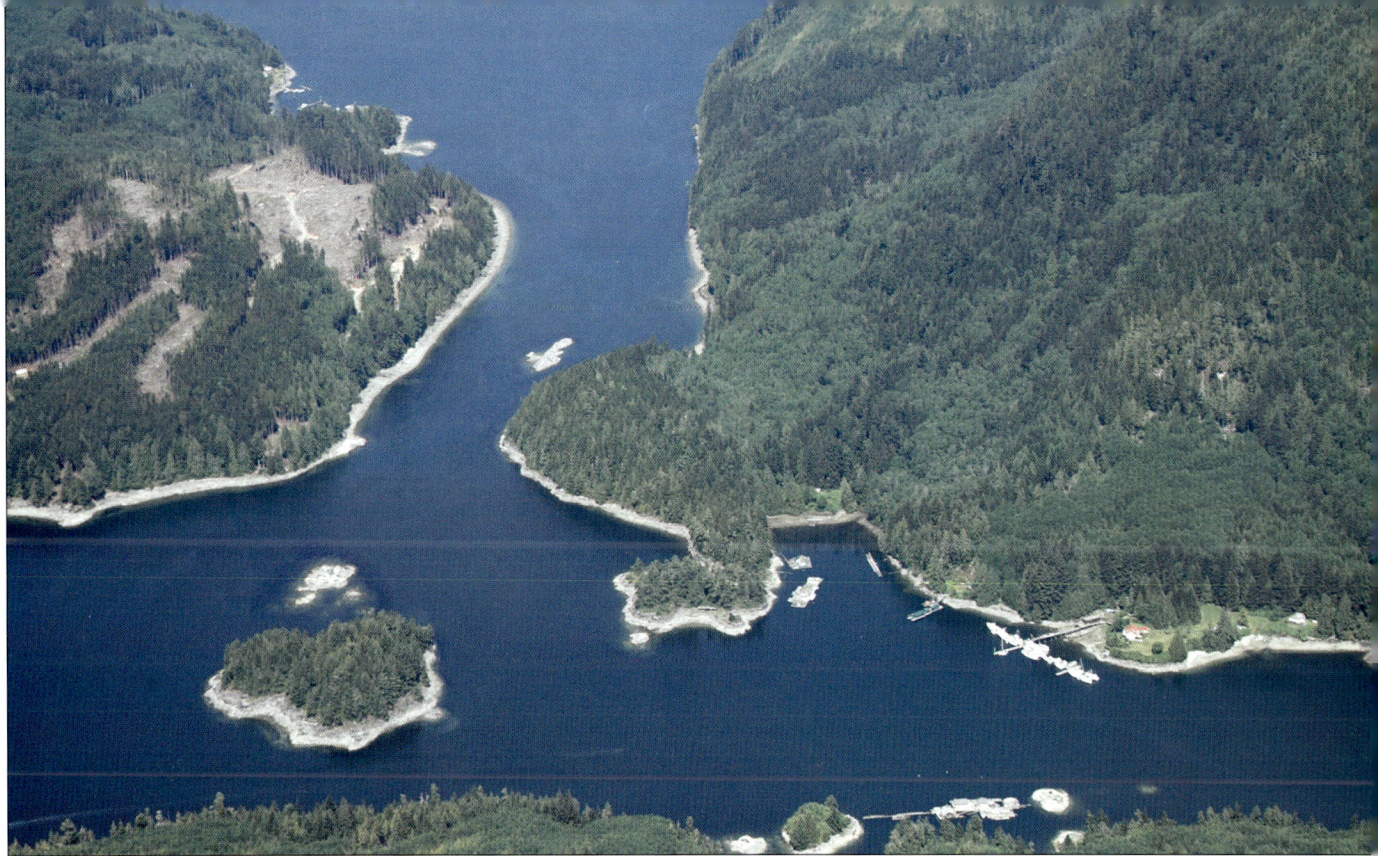

*Above: View of Lagoon Cove entrance from The Blowhole. The marina and the anchorage in calm conditions. Some winds disturb the anchorage and boats anchored out are advised to check in at the marina when adverse weather is forecast. Below: The fuel dock landing at the busy marina. The old marina office at the fuel dock, once a Union Steamships ticket office at Minstrel Island, has since been replaced with a new building.*

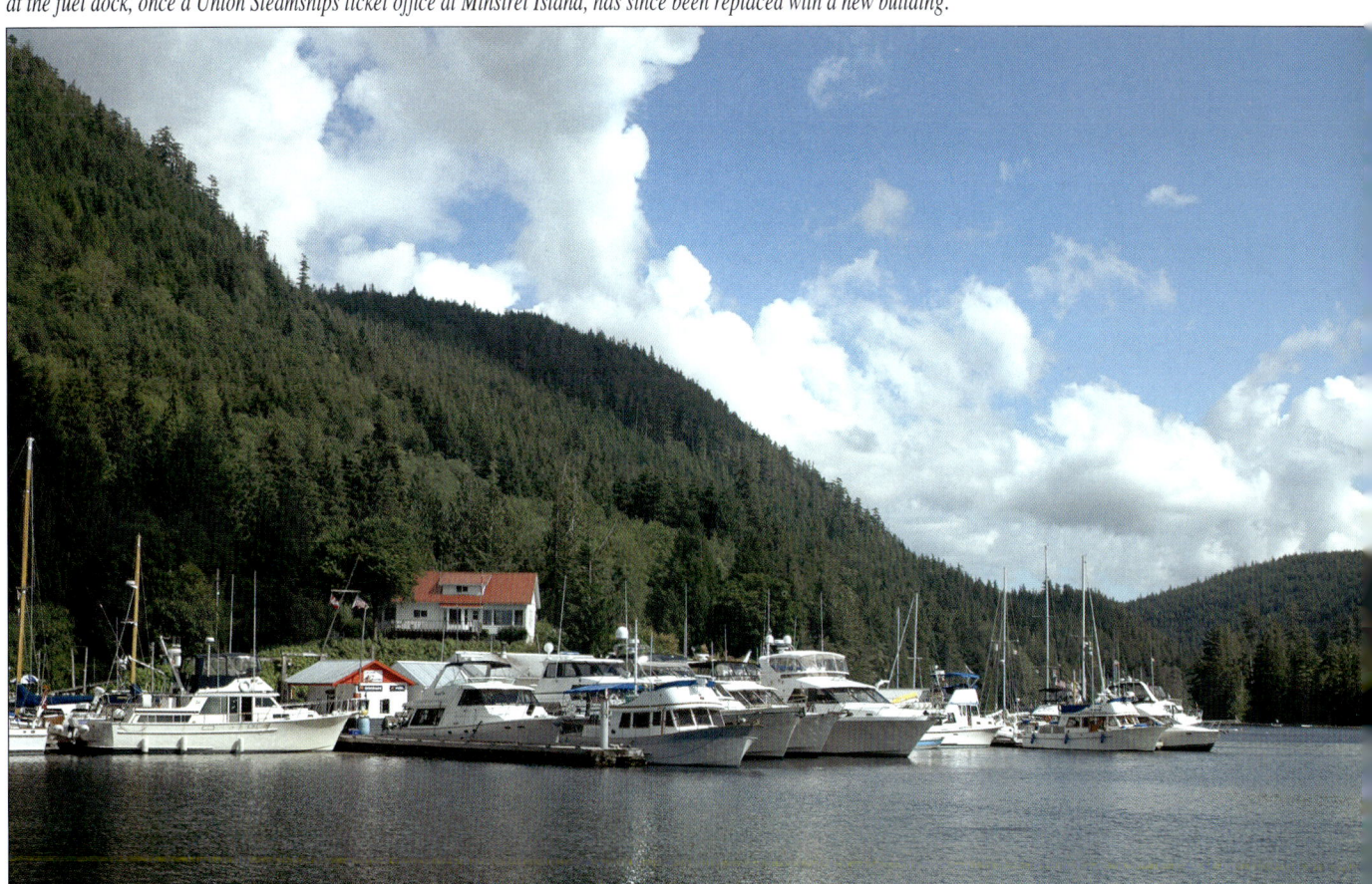

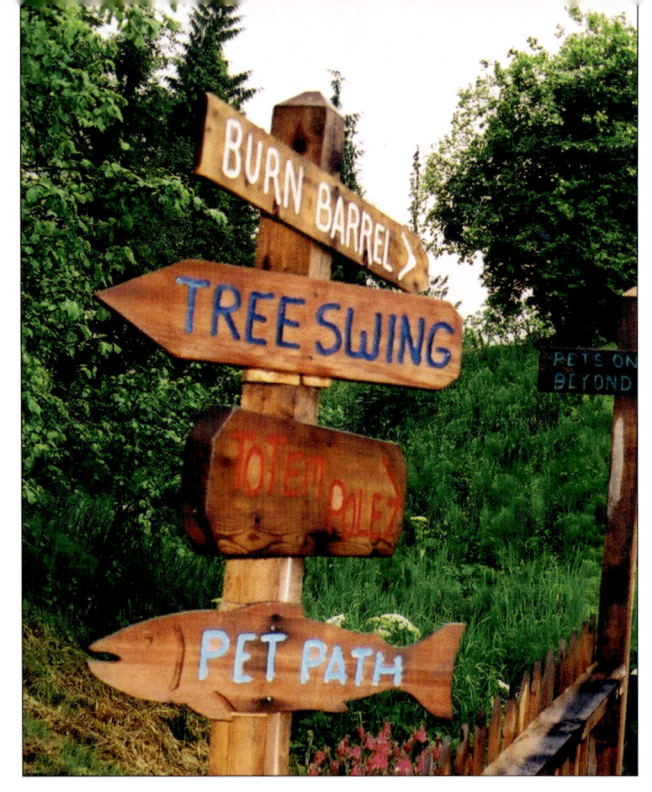

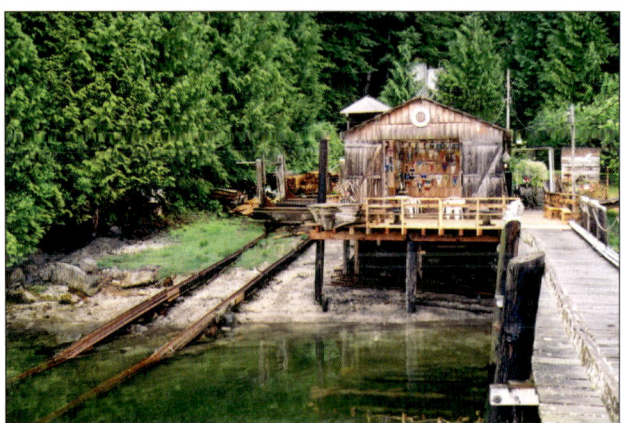

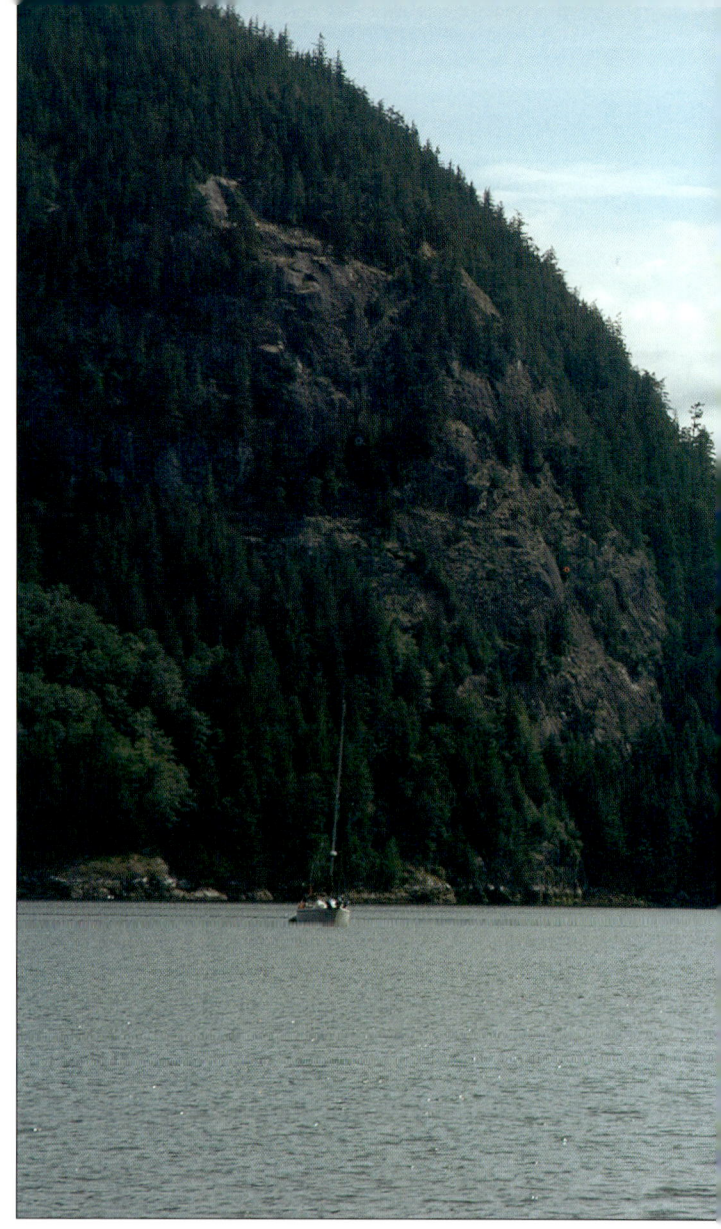

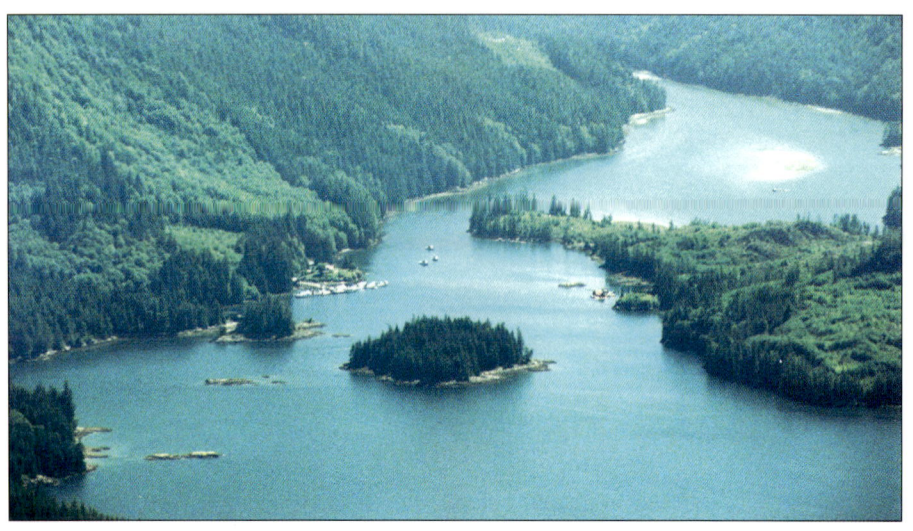

*Above:* A tranquil waterway with a view south down Chatham Channel in the direction of Havannah Channel and Port Harvey.
*Top, left:* Directional sign, just for fun, at Lagoon Cove. *Centre:* The old ways and shed. This is where the evening happy hour takes place and where a collection of artifacts is displayed.
*Left:* Lagoon Cove looking over Perley Island with the marina, the anchorage and the lagoon beyond.

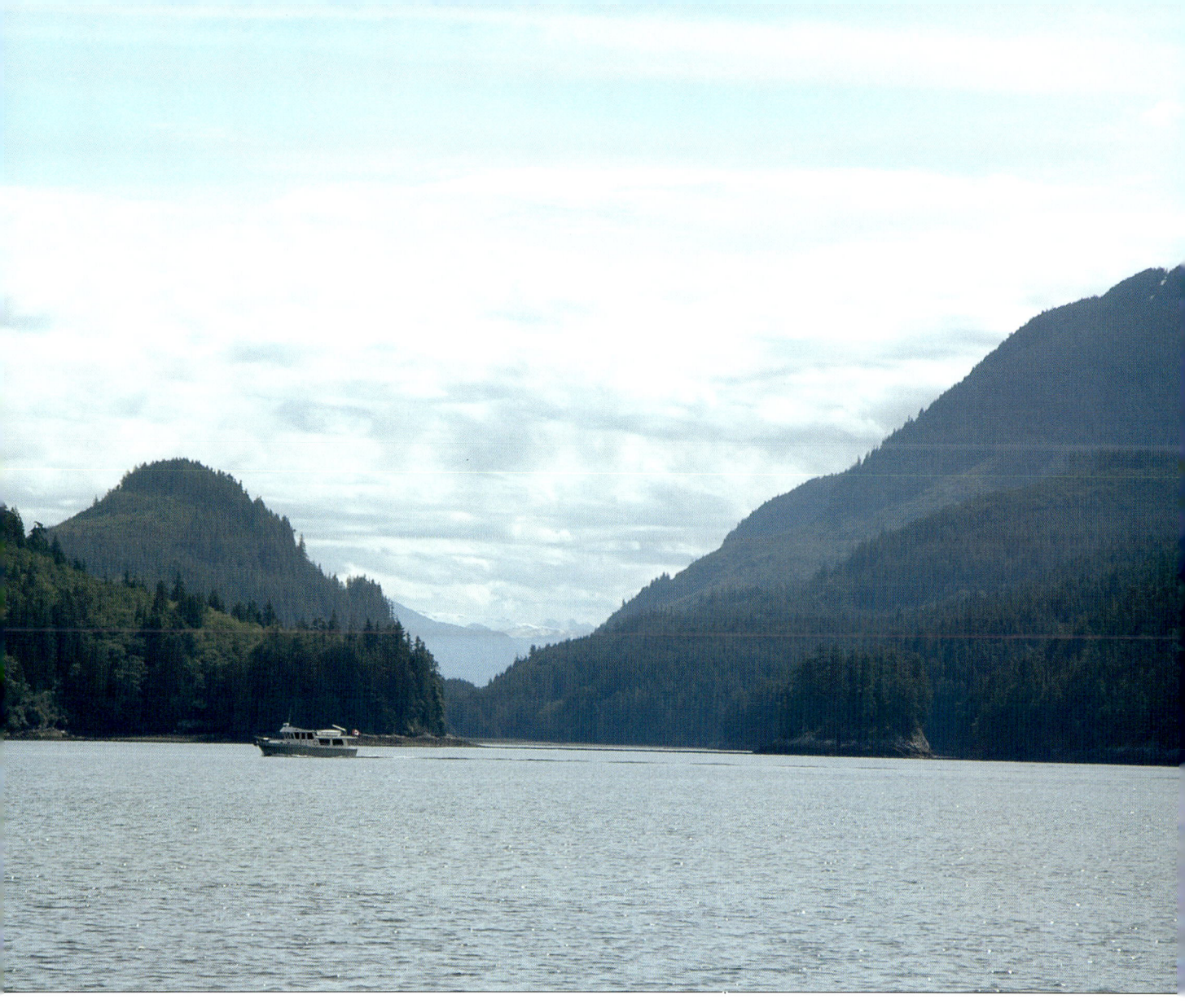

## Lagoon Cove trails

Trails wind up the hillside above the cove on East Cracroft Island. They ascend to a lookout near the summit, one to a view of The Blowhole. The trails are known as *Hillside Loop Trail* and *Deer Trail*. They begin separately at a pet path that leads from behind the marina workshop along the waterfront and link in the forest high behind the marina owners' home.

The trails are easily accessible but all guests are cautioned to beware of black bears. They are known to be in the area and may be using the same trails. While hiking, it is advisable to carry a pop or beer can with a few stones inside or some other noise-making device to alert the bears to your approach. They will usually move away from the noise.

## From Minstrel to Potts Lagoon

After stopping at Minstrel Island and Lagoon Cove the option is to travel to Echo Bay via Tribune Channel, which we do in the following pages. Continuing to Potts Lagoon requires easy navigation down Clio Channel following chart 3545. The passage carries you through Bones Bay past Sambo Point and Negro Rock.

You can put into Bones Bay and view the remains of the old cannery on the east shore. This was a regular steamship stop at one time so imagine how busy the area used to be.

Continue west along Clio Channel to Bend Island for a temporary anchorage or beyond to Potts Lagoon where you will find well protected moorage.

## Beyond Potts

The passage down Clio Channel to Potts Lagoon and Village Island continues on page 87.

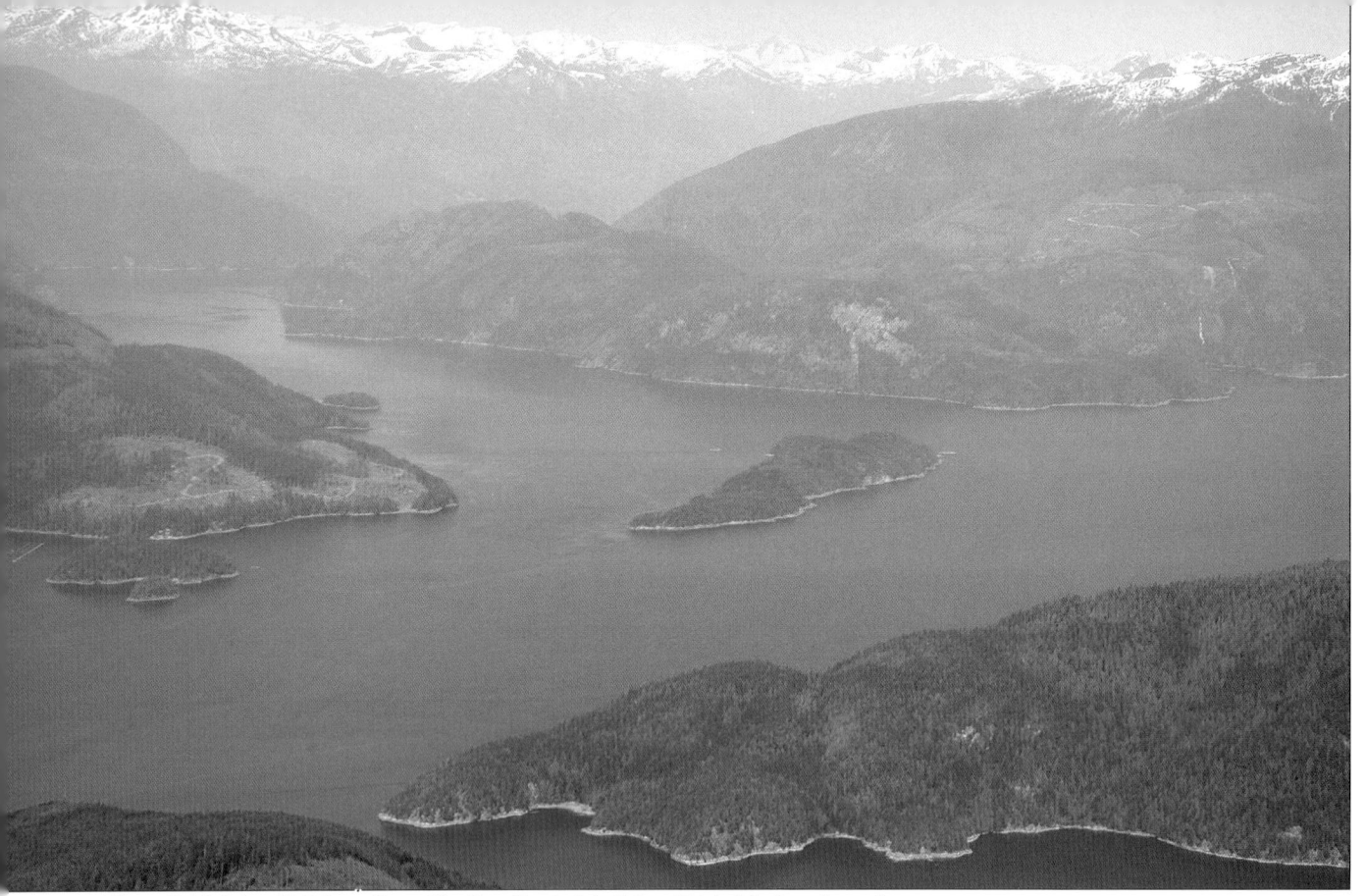

*Above: Knight Inlet with Tribune Channel leading off to the left. Below: Knight Inlet from the northeast.*

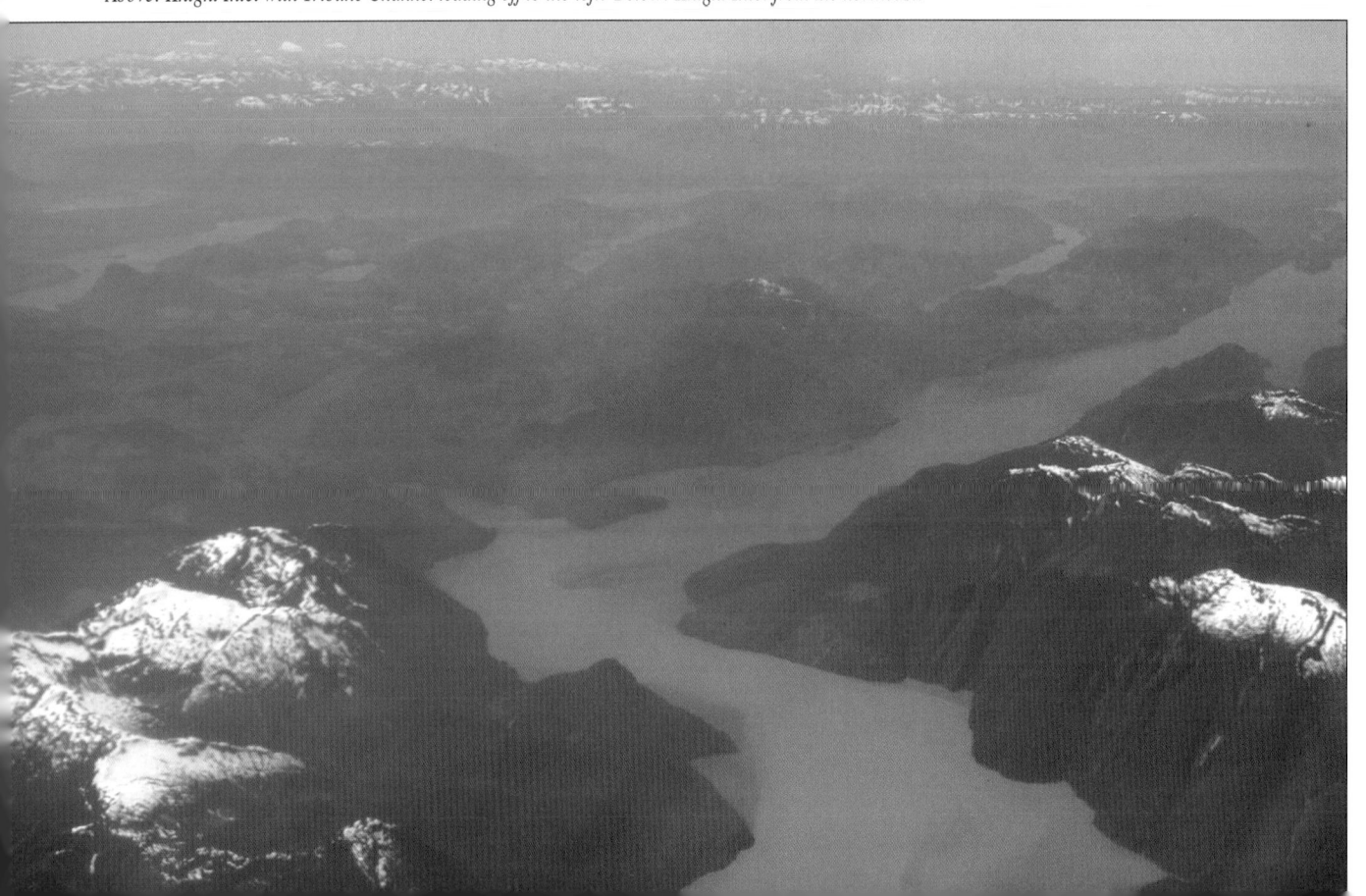

# Tribune Channel

## The alternative, direct route to Echo Bay from Minstrel Island to Broughton Island

Charts 3515, 3545, 3564

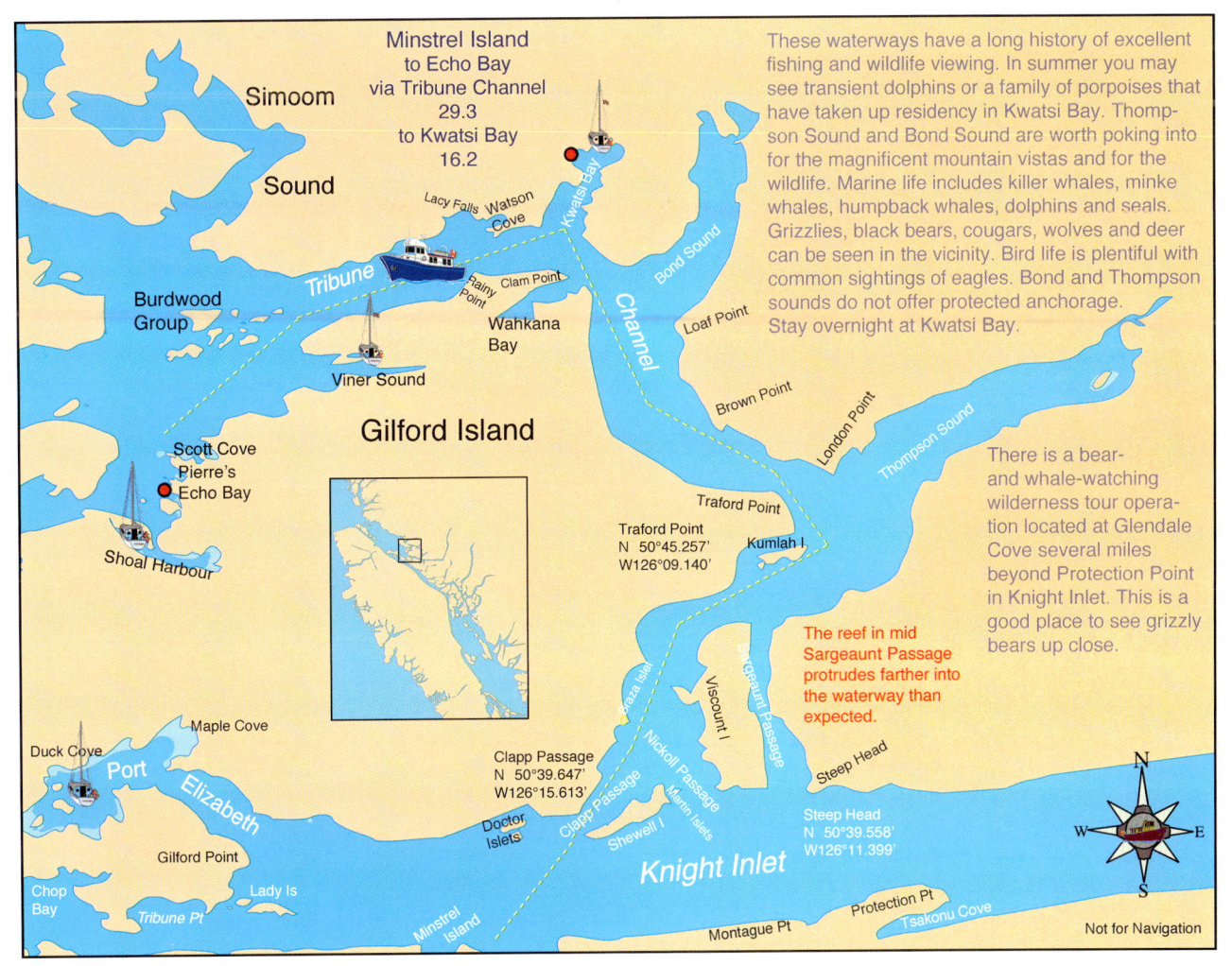

*Minstrel Island to Echo Bay via Tribune Channel 29.3 to Kwatsi Bay 16.2*

These waterways have a long history of excellent fishing and wildlife viewing. In summer you may see transient dolphins or a family of porpoises that have taken up residency in Kwatsi Bay. Thompson Sound and Bond Sound are worth poking into for the magnificent mountain vistas and for the wildlife. Marine life includes killer whales, minke whales, humpback whales, dolphins and seals. Grizzlies, black bears, cougars, wolves and deer can be seen in the vicinity. Bird life is plentiful with common sightings of eagles. Bond and Thompson sounds do not offer protected anchorage. Stay overnight at Kwatsi Bay.

Traford Point N 50°45.257' W126°09.140'

There is a bear- and whale-watching wilderness tour operation located at Glendale Cove several miles beyond Protection Point in Knight Inlet. This is a good place to see grizzly bears up close.

**The reef in mid Sargeaunt Passage protrudes farther into the waterway than expected.**

Clapp Passage N 50°39.647' W126°15.613'

Steep Head N 50°39.558' W126°11.399'

Not for Navigation

## Tribune Channel to Echo Bay  chart 3515

Tribune Channel is the most direct one to Echo Bay from Minstrel Island. This beautiful passage with its magnificent scenery is the gateway to the Broughton Islands from their northeast. Crossing Knight Inlet enter Tribune Channel at Shewell Island using either Clapp Passage or Nickoll Passage and follow it north and west as it curves between towering snow-capped mountains and deep adjoining inlets.

We like to cross Knight Inlet from Chatham Channel and enter Tribune Channel passing northwest of Shewell Island in Clapp Passage, or sometimes on the return voyage we make our way through Nickoll Passage and go south of the island, depending on sea conditions. A small cove between Shewell Island and the Martin Islets provides temporary anchorage. Sometimes we travel by way of Sargeaunt Passage, a delight-

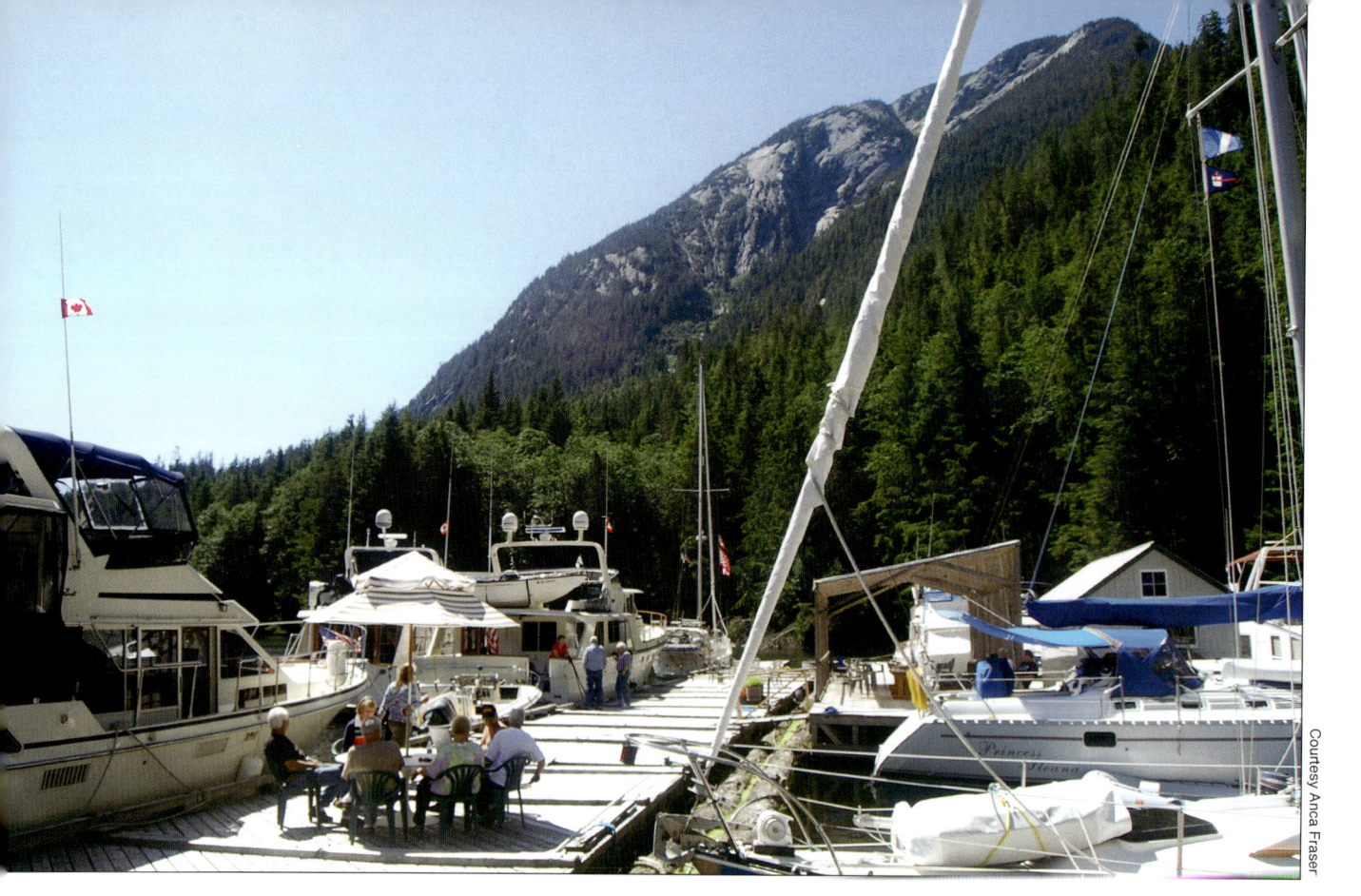

*Above: Gathering for happy hour on the dock at Kwatsi Bay. This 'potluck' event is held at most marinas in the Broughtons every day during summer. On the opposite page, the view from the docks is one of tranquility and remoteness.*

ful, narrow channel with tall, steep sides. Don't be intimidated by its narrow appearance on the chart. Use chart 3515 (1:80,000) and navigate carefully to avoid the shallows that protrude into the channel. Larger craft will fare more easily during higher tides. We find that the reef at the south end of the narrow passage protrudes farther into it than expected, so we swing wide to the east side to avoid it, even though the reef is quite well marked by kelp. Travel close to Bamber Point keeping clear of Humphrey Rock. Round the north end of Viscount Island and proceed up Tribune Channel, passing either side of Kumlah Island off the east tip of Gilford. Continue up the channel, passing the entrances to Thompson Sound and Bond Sound on the starboard side and then turn into **Kwatsi Bay** for a pleasant stay overnight or longer.

## Bond Sound  chart 3515

A wide inlet that ends in a shallow logging ground, this body of water offers no sheltered anchorage. It was the home to loggers through many years of the early days on the coast. Then and now good fishing has been reported in the area. Streams feed a muddy lagoon and there is va tract of First Nations land at the head of the sound.

## Wahkana Bay  chart 3515

Opening off Tribune Channel on the south shore just before Watson Cove on the north side is Wahkana Bay. Anchor near the shore in 15 to 25 meters on the east side of this cove. Otherwise the depth in the inner basin is 35 meters. There is a narrow shelf before the water drops off steeply. The bay is not very far across a valley from Viner Sound and breezy conditions in Viner Sound sometimes funnel westerly winds into Wahkana Bay.

## Kwatsi Bay  chart 3515

This is a tranquil place, in a peaceful setting. Stop at Kwatsi Bay for a spectacular vista of tall mountains, a comfortable anchorage and a pleasant stop at the marina. The friendly welcome will prompt you to stay awhile and visit the marina and then return in future seasons.

The marina owners Max Knierim and Anca Fraser have set up home on land adjacent to the float at the foot of a tall steep mountain with waterfalls and deep gorges in their backyard. While marina amenities are rudimentary, the facility does offer showers. Anca Fraser runs a small store on the floats in which she offers preserves, gifts, books and other items.

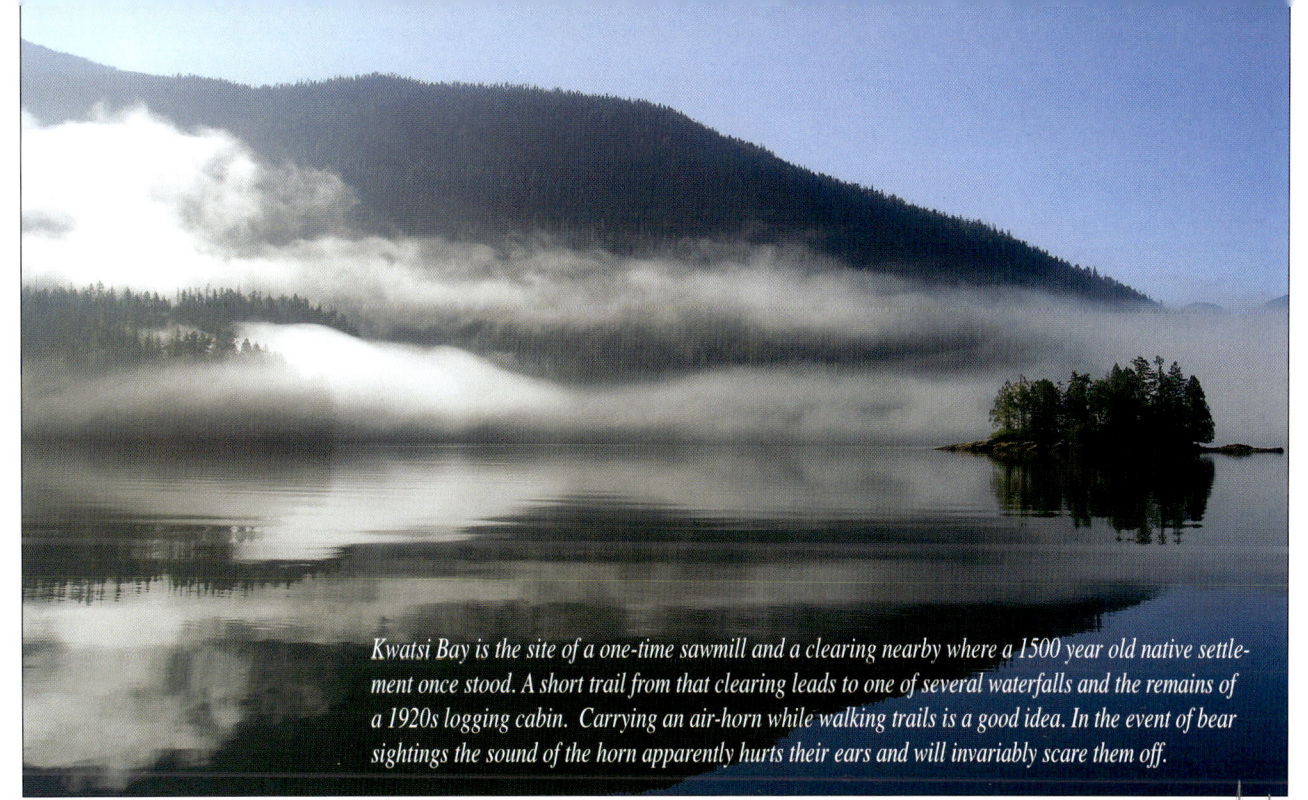

*Kwatsi Bay is the site of a one-time sawmill and a clearing nearby where a 1500 year old native settlement once stood. A short trail from that clearing leads to one of several waterfalls and the remains of a 1920s logging cabin. Carrying an air-horn while walking trails is a good idea. In the event of bear sightings the sound of the horn apparently hurts their ears and will invariably scare them off.*

Courtesy Anca Fraser

Visits by wild animals are frequent, with bears coming out of the woods and the occasional cougar showing up. The family knows how to deal with the situation and there is no need for concern, other than to respect wildlife and stay as far away as possible.

If you choose to anchor in Kwatsi Bay the most popular location is adjacent to the shore opposite the marina, in about 20 metres off the beach near the point. The rest of the bay, although shown as shallow on the chart, is about 27 metres deep except for a ledge close to the beach, and most of that is rocky with poor holding ground in adverse winds. The best anchoring point is just beyond view of the marina.

Kwatsi Bay with its looming, tall mountains is a place to experience the coast at its natural best.

## Kwatsi Bay Marina

General Delivery,
Simoom Sound BC  V0P 1S0
Phone 250-949-1384    VHF 66A
*email: kwatsibay@hughes.net    www.kwatsibay.com*
Parallel tie up at the dock. Water is available in plentiful supply—you can usually fill your water tanks at the dock. Hot showers are available. There are no marine or boat services. Your hosts are Anca Fraser and Max Knierim. Join in a daily happy hour at the gazebo or on the dock when other overnight boats are present. A small store and dock office is located on the floats. Some products are for sale—including local art, preserves, books and gift items.

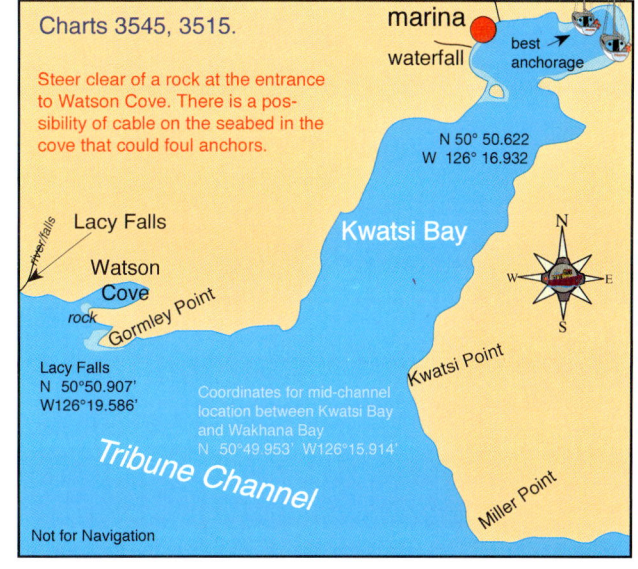

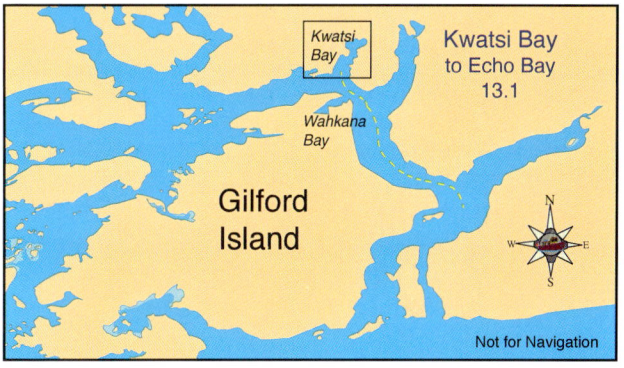

Charts 3545, 3515.

Steer clear of a rock at the entrance to Watson Cove. There is a possibility of cable on the seabed in the cove that could foul anchors.

marina
waterfall
best anchorage

N 50° 50.622'
W 126° 16.932'

Lacy Falls
Watson Cove
rock
Gormley Point
Kwatsi Bay
Kwatsi Point

Lacy Falls
N 50°50.907'
W126°19.586'

Coordinates for mid-channel location between Kwatsi Bay and Wakhana Bay
N 50°49.953'  W126°15.914'

Tribune Channel
Miller Point
Not for Navigation

Kwatsi Bay
Wahkana Bay
Gilford Island
Kwatsi Bay to Echo Bay 13.1
Not for Navigation

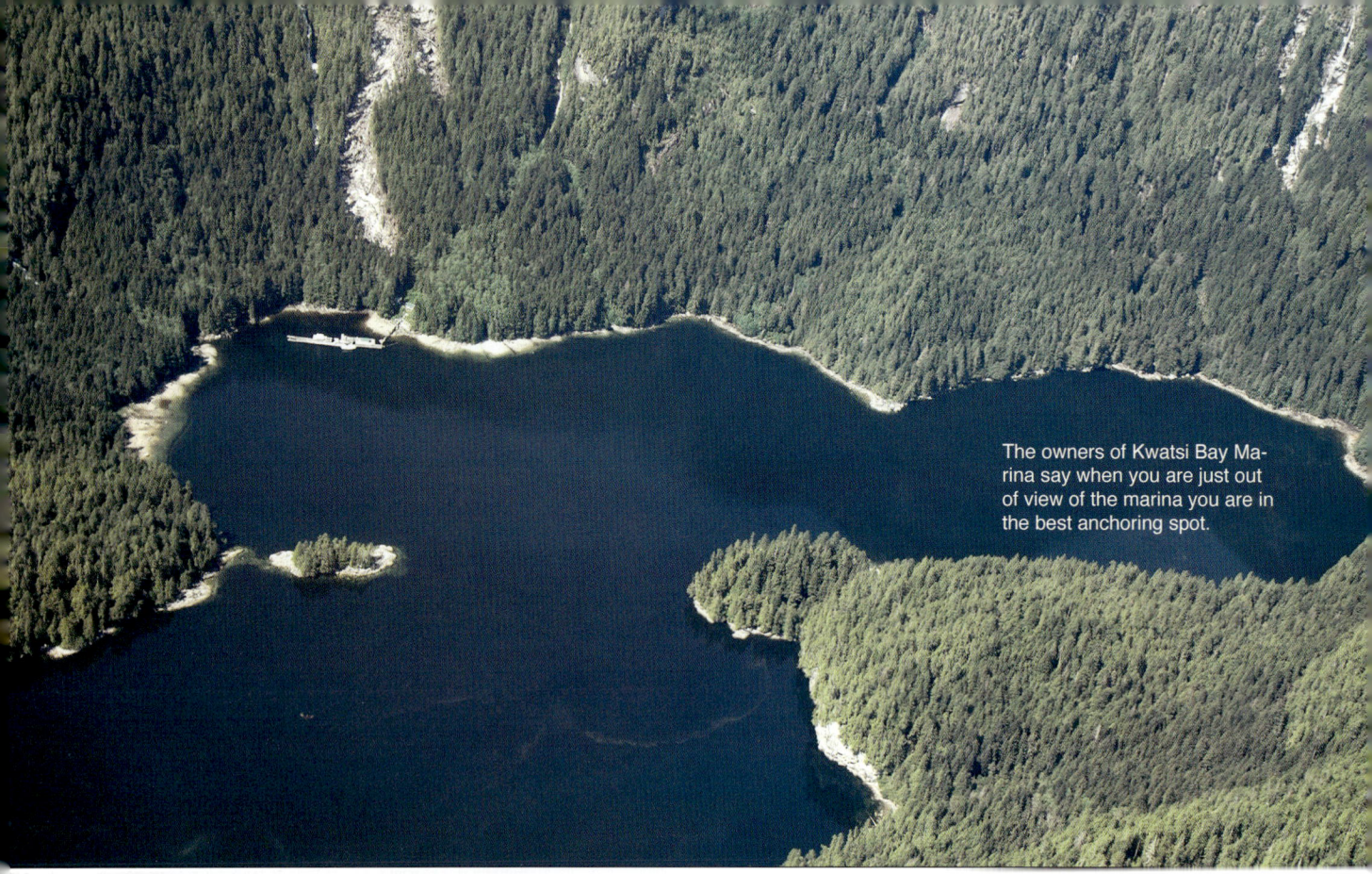

The owners of Kwatsi Bay Marina say when you are just out of view of the marina you are in the best anchoring spot.

Chart 3515 — Not for Navigation

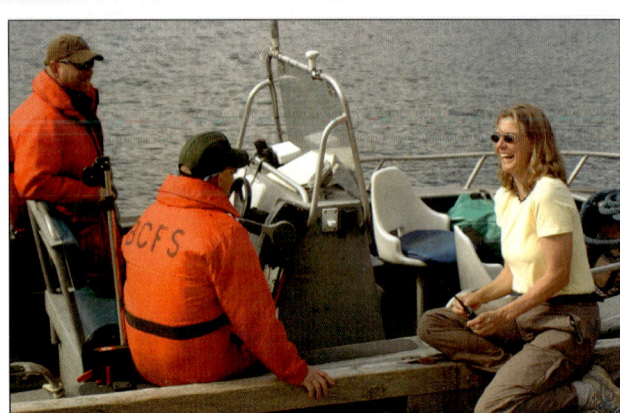

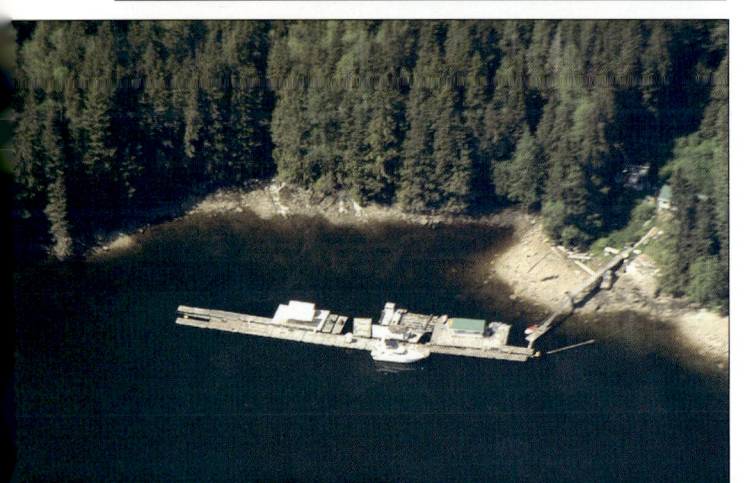

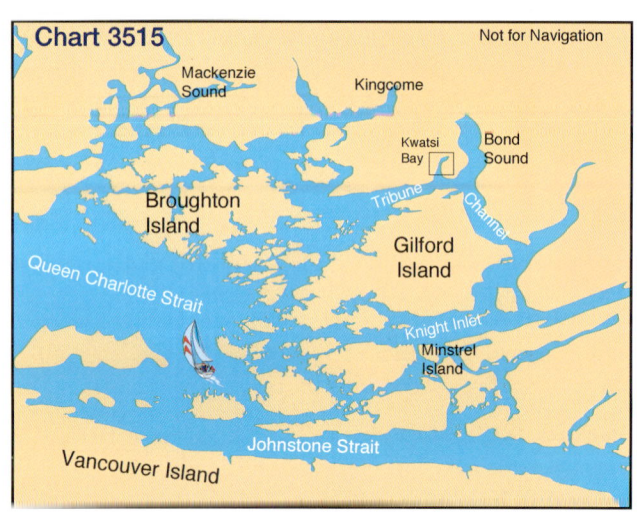

*Top: View from above tall peaks on a tranquil day in Kwatsi Bay.*
*Left: Anca Fraser greets the crew on a BC Forestry Service boat.*
*Left: The docks at Kwatsi Bay on a quiet day in the month of June.*
*Opposite: Kwatsi Bay and the dock at the marina, courtesy Anca Fraser.*
*Overleaf (pages 82-83): Anchoring at the entrance to Kwatsi Bay. A suitable spot in calm weather. Best bet is to check in at the marina or anchor on the opposite side of the bay, just out of view of the floats.*

80

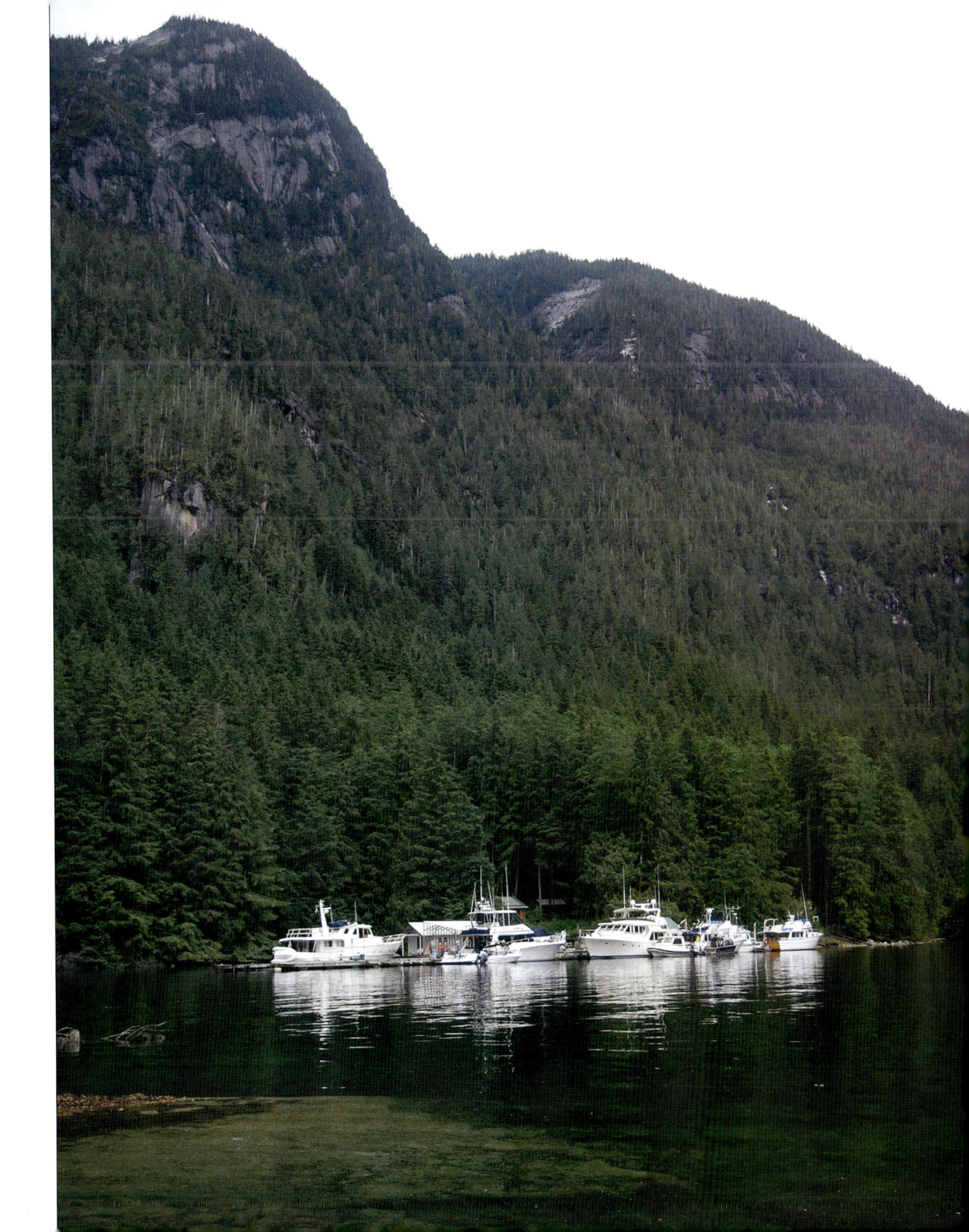

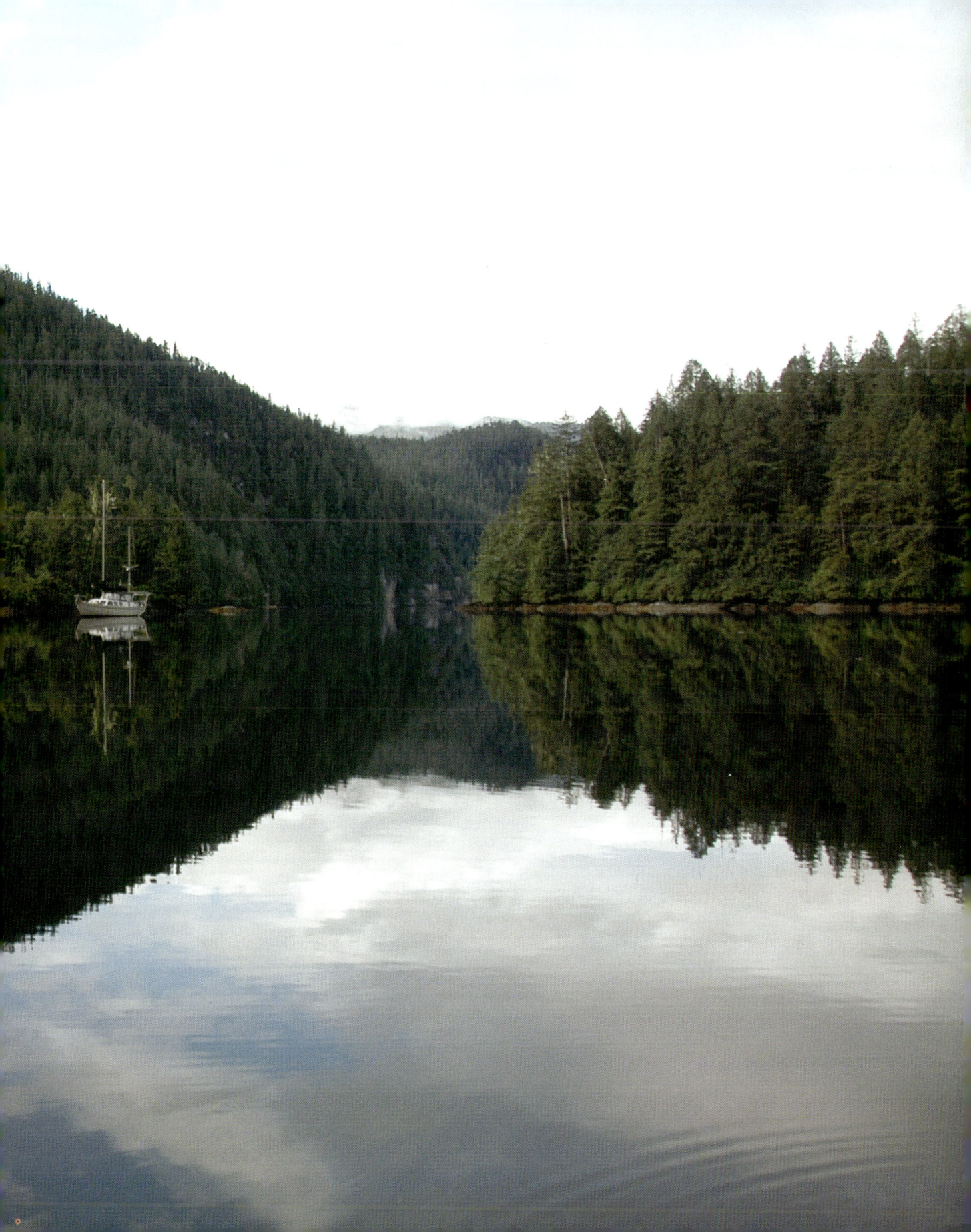

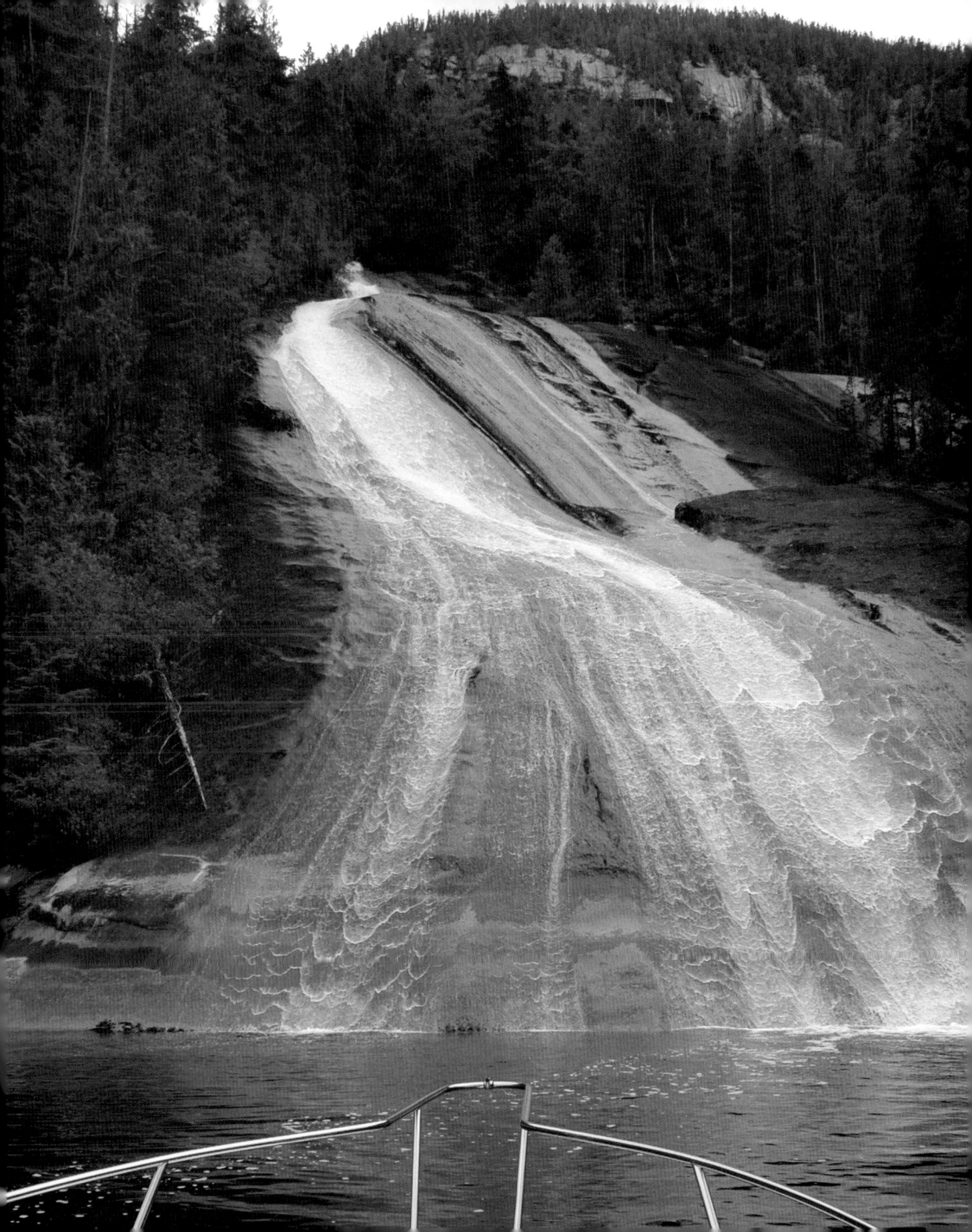

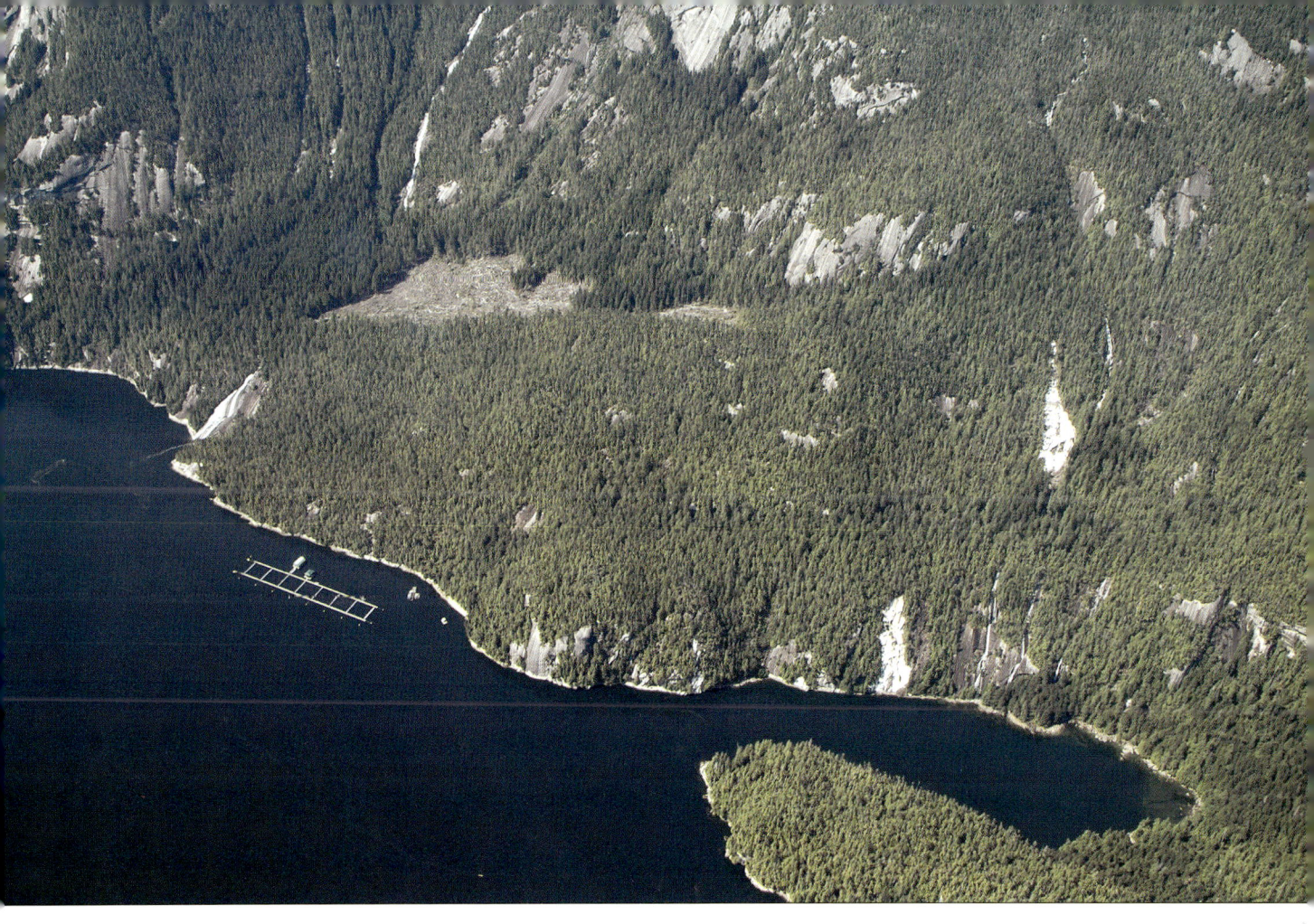

## Watson Cove  Chart 3515

Leaving Kwatsi Bay the cruise along Tribune Channel is one of the finest on the coast, with more tall mountains and spectacular waterfalls. One waterfall in particular puts on a show that will amaze you, in springtime or early summer. That is when Lacy Falls flows at its peak. It is possible to nose right up to within a couple of metres of the tumbling water as it cascades down a steep, mineral-discoloured granite cliff.

The waterfall tumbles steeply to the channel immediately west of Watson Cove. This small bay has been occupied in recent years by fish farming equipment and a floathouse. Fish farm pens have been located in and out of the cove at times. Entrance to Watson Cove is along the north shore staying clear of the rock near the opposite point. Anchoring may be a challenge when you come to lift the anchor because of logging debris on the seabed. But if you do stop in the cove you will be rewarded with beautiful scenery of the surrounding terrain and the magnificent waterfall.

Tribune Channel is the route we prefer when travelling directly from Johnstone Strait to Broughton Island, largely because of Kwatsi Bay and the view of the waterfall. At the west end of the channel lies the Burdwood Group, Simoom Sound and Viner Sound.

*Opposite: The spectacular Lacy Falls in Tribune Channel, unofficially named by Don Douglass and Réanne Hemingway-Douglass.*
*Above: Watson Bay and Lacy Falls showing the sheer rise of the mountains in Tribune Channel. Right: Nosing up close to the falls, the water is deep and the dropoff steep but there is a small ledge at the base of the rocky slope. It is advisable to stay clear of the base by at least a couple of metres.*

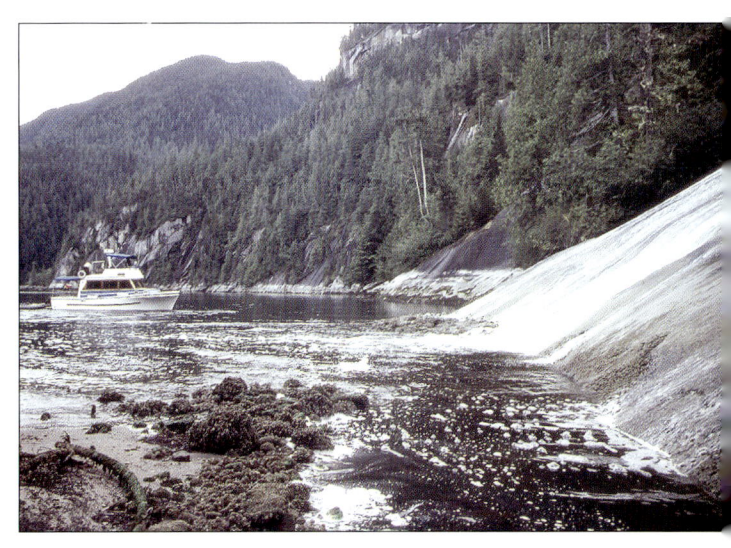

86

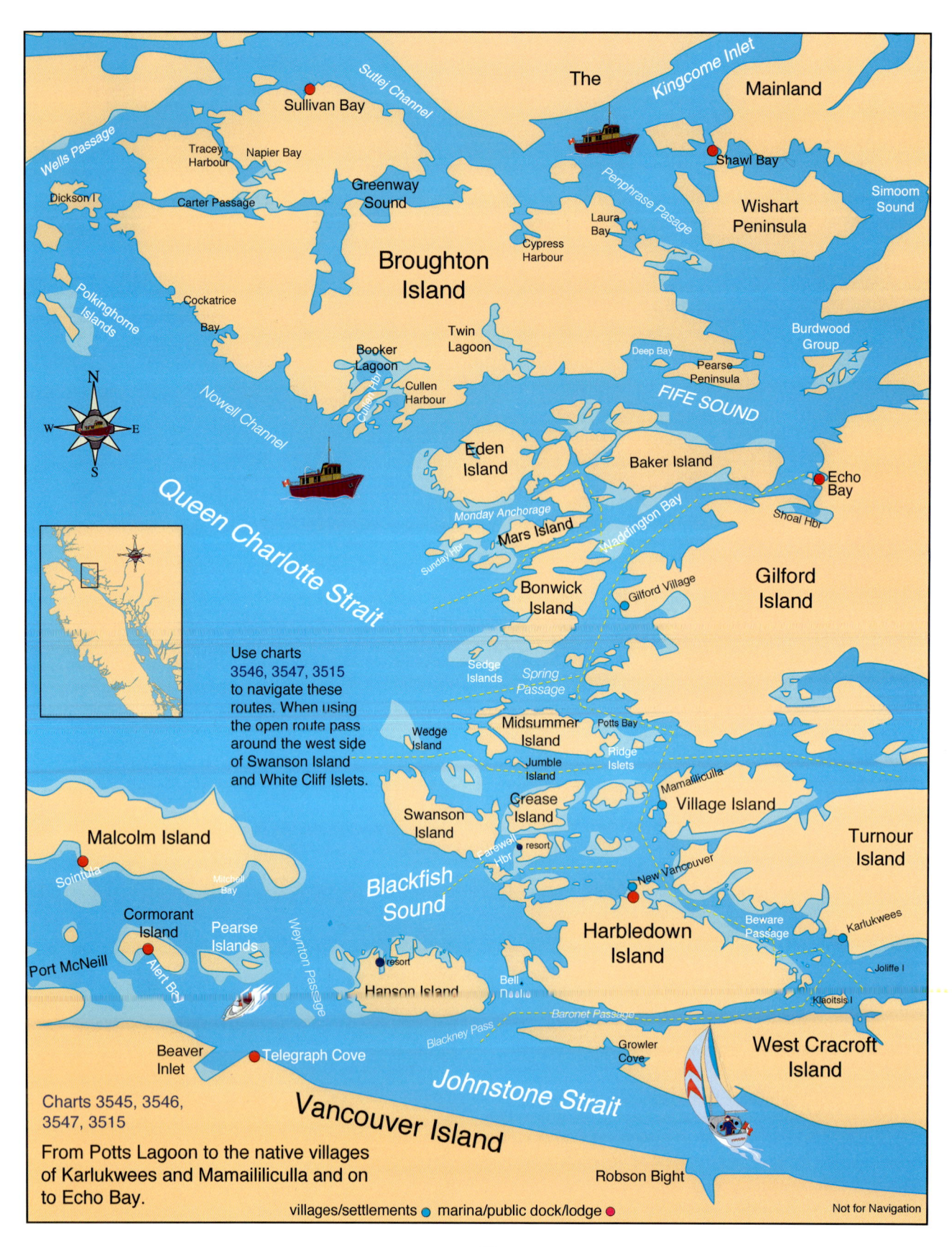

# Havannah Channel to the Broughtons
## First Nations villages and welcoming destinations

You can enter the Broughton Archipelago via Knight Inlet or Blackfish Sound for a scenic voyage to 'The Mainland'

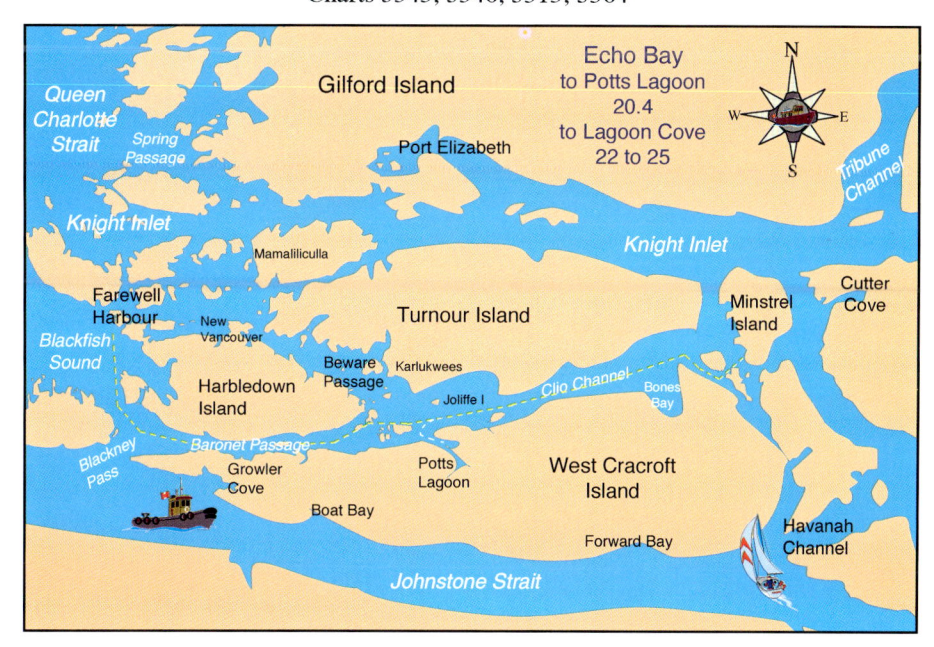

Charts 3545, 3546, 3515, 3564

From Havannah Channel and Minstrel Island you could choose one of several routes to the various ports, islands and settlements of the Broughton Archipelago. The options are to continue along Johnstone Strait, or from Minstrel Island go west down Clio Channel to Potts Lagoon. Then by way of Beware Passage continue to the native villages of New Vancouver, Mamalilaculla and Karlukwees.

From Minstrel Island an optional route to the Broughtons is across Knight Inlet to Tribune Channel and Echo Bay which was discussed in the previous chapter. One may, of course, travel north by one route and return by the other. Now we follow the Johnstone Strait and Potts Lagoon routes.

Had you not turned off Johnstone Strait at the Broken Islands and Havannah Channel to go to Minstrel Island, and instead travelled along the south shore of West Cracroft Island you may use the lower end of Baronet Passage via Blackney Pass to reach Potts Lagoon. Blackney Pass is also the route via Blackfish Sound to Farewell Harbour and the First Nations villages in the south of the Broughton Islands.

From Minstrel Island down Clio Channel to Potts Lagoon is about 8 miles. The Lagoon opens into the north shore of West Cracroft Island about midway between Johnstone Strait and Minstrel Island. Travelling from Minstrel Island approach Klaoitsis Island and turn to port to enter Potts Lagoon opposite Joliffe Island near the east end of Beware Channel. There can be strong currents in this area, so be mindful of the tidal streams. Overfalls occur in the passage adjacent to Klaoitsis Island, with westerly flooding down Baronet Passage. Mind the rocks off Klaoitsis Island.

To reach Blackney Passage, Blackfish Sound and Johnstone Strait from Potts Lagoon continue west along the West Cracroft Island north shore by way of Baronet Passage. To reach Village Island and the First Nations villages enter Beware Passage opposite Potts lagoon and carefully make your way between Harbledown Island and Turnour Island to Indian Channel (see page 94).

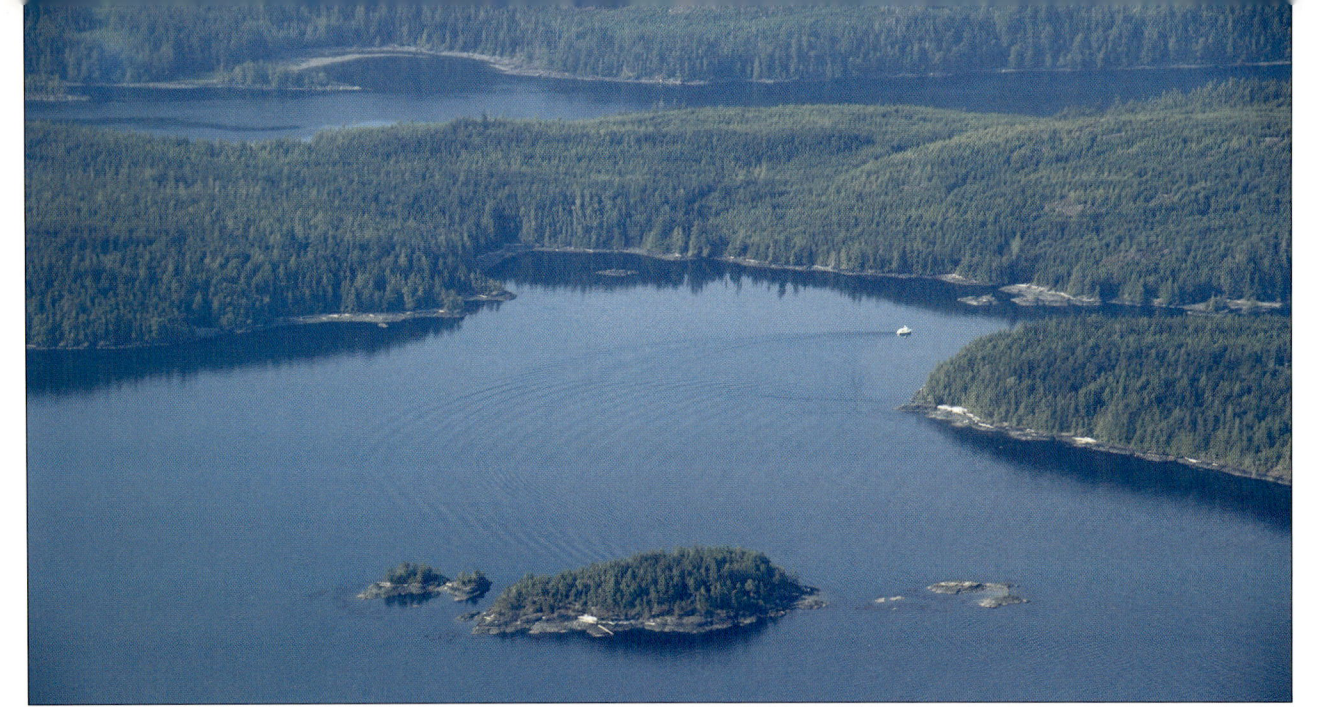

### Johnstone Strait  charts 3545, 3546

Travelling along Johnstone Strait, before reaching Growler Cove and Blackney Pass is **Boat Bay.** It can be entered around the east side of a small island that offers protection from the open waters of Johnstone Strait. Passage may be taken to the west side of the island with caution.

### Growler Cove  charts 3545, 3546

Near Blackney Pass Growler Cove opens into West Cracroft Island in the lee of the Sophia Islands. Mind Baron Reef on the approaches. It is a convenient place to stop and anchor overnight while waiting for suitable conditions in the Strait, or before proceeding up Baronet Passage into the Broughtons. Growler Cove is narrow and dries at its head. It has always been a popular shelter for fishing boats, and small pleasure craft can also find anchorage in 9 to 13 metres. The anchorage shallows out to a sandy beach and is lined on one side by sheer rock cliffs. Stay clear of the rocks close to either shore.

Blackney Pass produces a fair amount of choppy water from the current and wind. The worst tide rips are encountered off Cracroft Point and the opposite islands east of Hanson Island. When travelling through Blackney Pass into Baronet Passage favour the Hanson Island shore to avoid the tide rips, but move away from that side as you approach the two small islands then head for the north side of Cracroft Island keeping well away from Bell Rocks off Harbledown Island.

If you are travelling out of Johnstone Strait heading for Blackfish Sound follow the same procedure discussed above when going through Blackney Pass and head for the south end of Parson Island. Approaching Parson Island turn northwest along the north shore of Hanson Island.

For scuba diving, the water is cold but clear and colourful. Scuba divers have long understood and appreciated the benefits of cold, moving water. The clarity is almost always guaranteed and the colourful, diverse marine life can be seen readily on underwater explorations along current-swept rock walls. The currents in Blackney Passage dictate very careful planning for safe dives around Cracroft Point and divers are advised to visit the area with experienced guides.

### Baronet Passage  charts 3545, 3546

From Minstrel Island, hug the shore of West Cracroft Island and proceed down Clio Channel into Baronet Passage taking into account the tidal current around the islands off Potts Lagoon, of which Klaoitsis is the largest. There is a reef off the eastern corner of Klaoitsis Island so don't venture too far over into the passage. Nearby Jamieson Island and an unnamed island off its southwestern corner are separated from other islands in the group by Wilson Passage. It is best to avoid this area other than at slack or near slack tides because of the narrow waterways with a possible 5 knots of current. This applies equally when navigating into Beware Passage on the way to Karlukwees and beyond to New Vancouver.

Slow boats waiting for reduced currents, sometimes use the two small coves south of Klaoitsis Island as temporary anchorages, particularly when moving towards Potts Lagoon against the flood.

On the east side of Klaoitsis, a white beach area has prompted people from anchored boats in Potts Lagoon to venture ashore for a picnic lunch. Despite the swift waters in the surrounding passages it is fairly calm around the shore of this island. Mind the rocks and reefs as you navigate towards the beach in your small boat.

From Potts Lagoon return to the open waters of Johnstone Strait via Baronet Passage, or use this as an alternative route

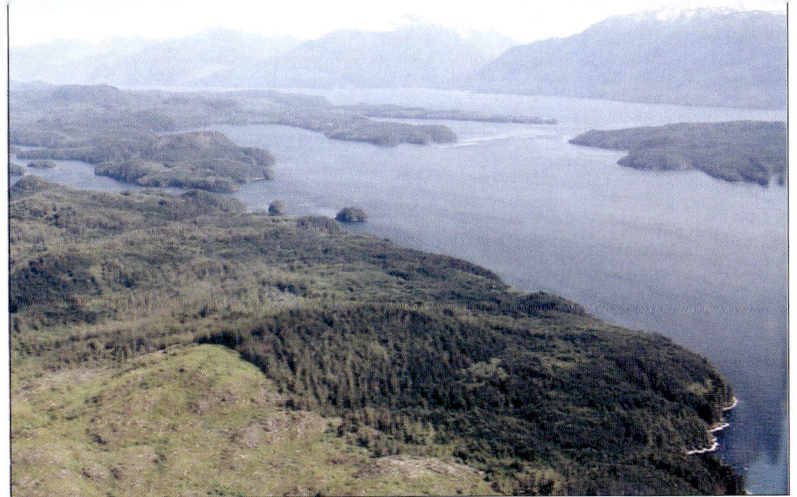

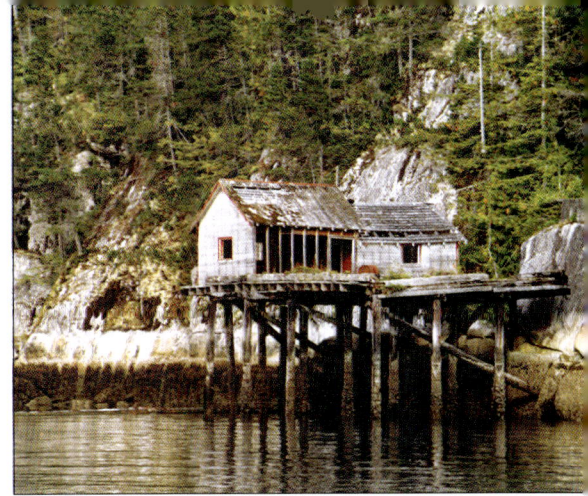

> The current was running quite strongly through Blackney Passage and a small pod of Orcas had just gone through on the way to their favourite rubbing beach in Robson Bight, Johnstone Strait. While we waited for slack water we watched fishermen in their boats catching fish in the lee of the tip of West Cracroft. Three boats were hovering off the shore, and three eagles sat in the branches of nearby trees, lined up with the boats. Each eagle had designated a boat as "theirs" and when a fisherman caught a rockfish and threw it back the respective eagle would swoop down from its perch and grab the fish. The other two eagles remained in their trees moving only when "their" boat had a catch.

to enter the historic lower Broughton group of islands from Johnstone Strait via Blackney Passage.

About half way along Baronet Passage, Walden Island breaks up the relatively good width of the channel, giving mariners a narrow opening off its northern side. A reef and a rock off the east end of Walden require that you approach the island or leave it at that end well clear and favouring the Harbledown Island shore. As you emerge at the west end of the passage you may come across sports fishermen trying for salmon in Blackney Pass.

## Knight Inlet entrance    charts 3545, 3546, 3515

If you have bypassed entrances to the Broughton Islands off Johnstone Strait and decide to stop first at Telegraph Cove and Alert Bay you may choose to cruise into Queen Charlotte Strait en route to Knight Inlet. Here the strait heaves itself against the northwest shores of the islands that form the Broughton Archipelago. If you find yourself looking for anchorage in this exposed region the most recommended places include Farewell Harbour or the closer but smaller **Potts Bay** (not to be confused with Potts Lagoon), tucked into the northeast end of Midsummer Island. This forms part of the entrance to Knight Inlet (see page 113).

*Top left: View southeast to Blackney Pass from above Swanson Island. Above: Growler Cove (also opposite) is in the foreground with Baronet Passage beyond. Top right: Ruins of a former camp in Clio Channel.*

The main entrance to Knight Inlet from Queen Charlotte Strait is through the opening south of Wedge Island. Swing around Wedge Island and curve your way past the south side of Jumble Island, keeping north of the rocks off Twist and Whirl Islands. Alternatively travel north of Jumble Island to ensure a totally clear passage past Clock Rock near the entrance to Eliot Passage and Mamalilaculla. If you are entering Eliot Passage at this stage either steer a course for the northwest shore of Pearl Island and hug it as you enter Eliot Passage, or travel well clear of the east end of Pearl Island at a distance away from Clock Rock and then turn sharply to enter the passage. We usually watch for the large patch of kelp that marks the rock and keep a good distance from it crossing Knight Inlet when travelling between Mamalilaculla and Echo Bay via Spring Passage (diagram page 97).

If you choose to enter the Broughtons by way of Spring Passage and bypass Knight Inlet en route to Echo Bay, be mindful of the reefs and islets off Swanson Island. During high seas this area is swept by fairly large waves.

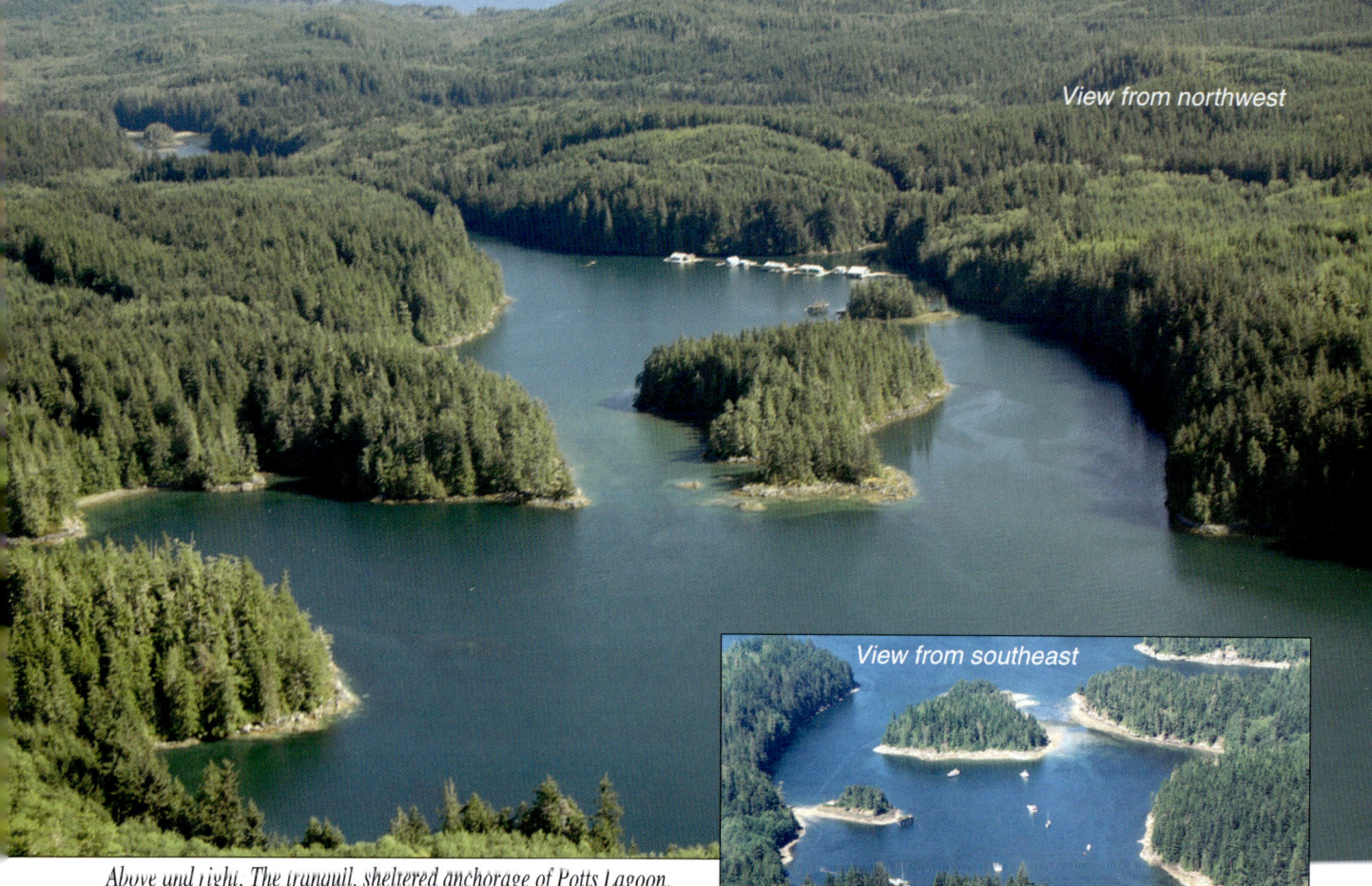

*Above and right. The tranquil, sheltered anchorage of Potts Lagoon.*

View from northwest

View from southeast

## Potts Lagoon  chart 3545

The anchorage in Potts Lagoon became one of our favourites on the coast the moment we first entered it. We choose the south cove in Potts Lagoon over the northern one, the latter of which is the first you would encounter as you enter. Old pilings were all but fallen down inside the lagoon. The preferred anchorage, judging by other boats that were there ahead of us, was beyond these pilings. We dropped anchor in the lee of the 41 metre island that guards the entrance. The northern arm of the lagoon is also suitable and recommended in westerly winds. In easterlies, move to the south side beyond the ruins. Be cautious in the centre of the main cove as there are only one to two metres of depth during very low tides. There is an expansive marshland and meadow beyond the navigable depths of the lagoon, much of which can be explored in a dinghy or kayak.

During high tides and at the tail end of a flood tide careful passage in a dinghy will get you into the upper reaches of the lagoon. Do not linger, because you may find bottom very soon after the tide turns. Also, beware of black bears, which frequent this part of the lagoon in large numbers. As a favourite anchorage it was not surprising to find that Bob Stewart, long time boat builder, for many years occupied a corner of the lagoon with his floating home.

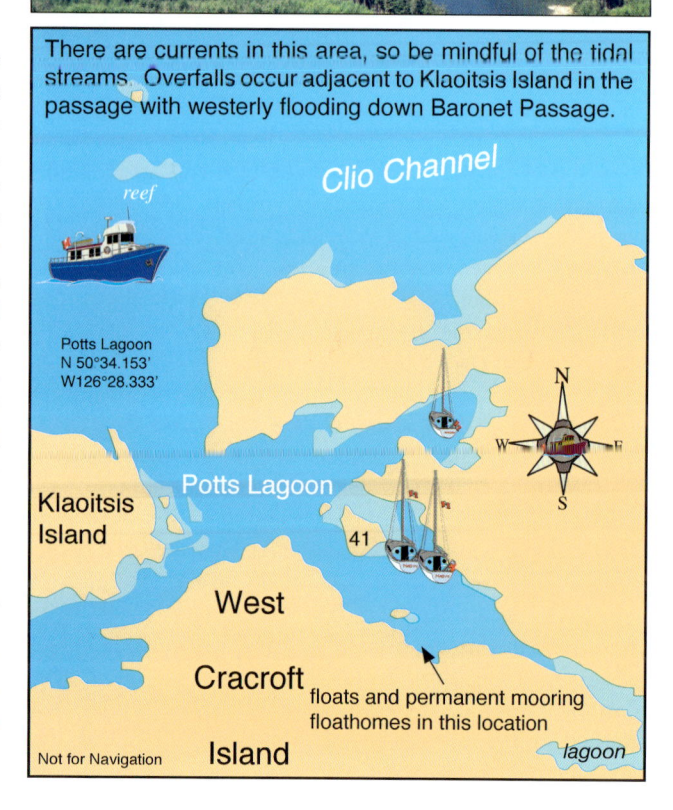

There are currents in this area, so be mindful of the tidal streams. Overfalls occur adjacent to Klaoitsis Island in the passage with westerly flooding down Baronet Passage.

reef

Clio Channel

Potts Lagoon
N 50°34.153'
W 126°28.333'

Klaoitsis Island

Potts Lagoon

41

West Cracroft Island

floats and permanent mooring floathomes in this location

Not for Navigation

lagoon

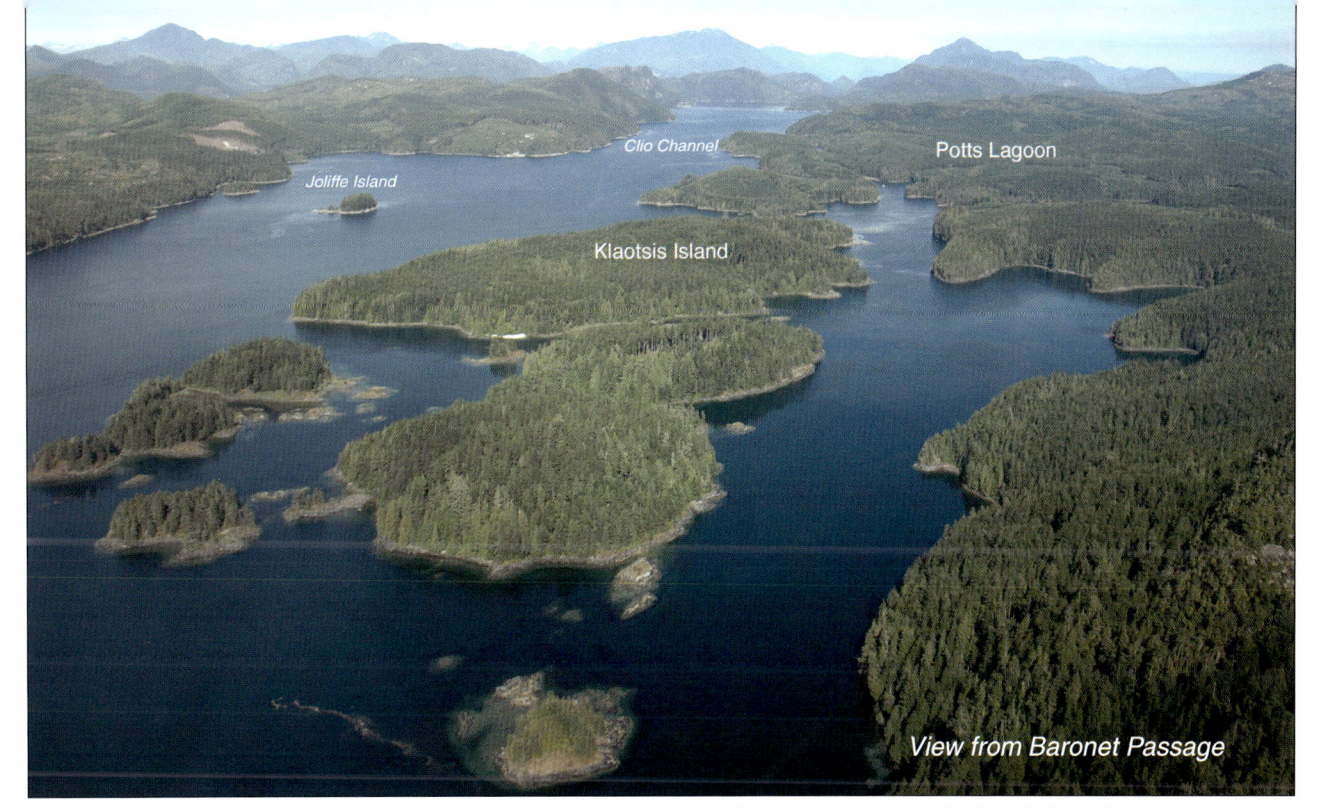

*From Baronet Passage looking over Clio Channel with Klaoitsis Island at top centre and Potts Lagoon opening off to the right, beyond it.*

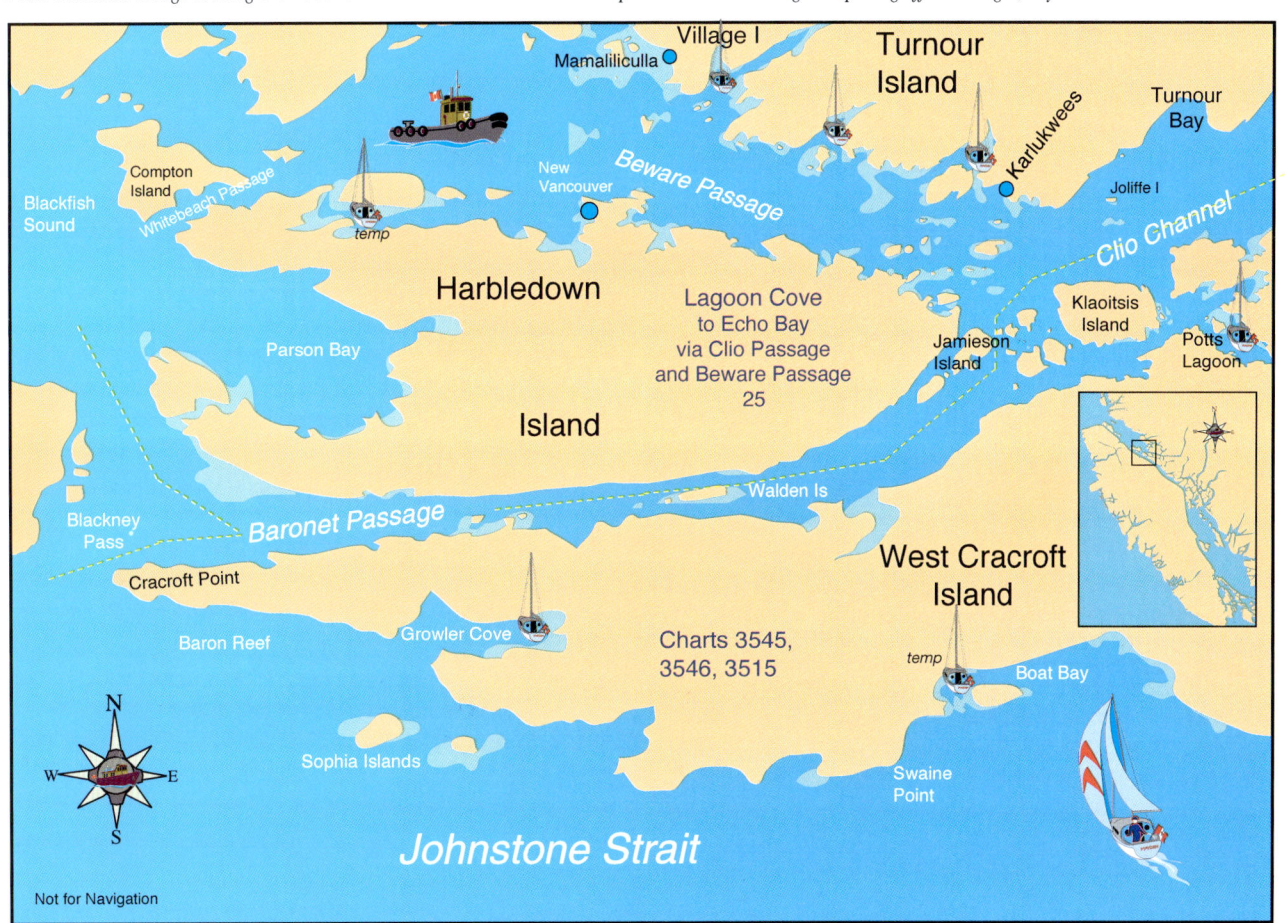

91

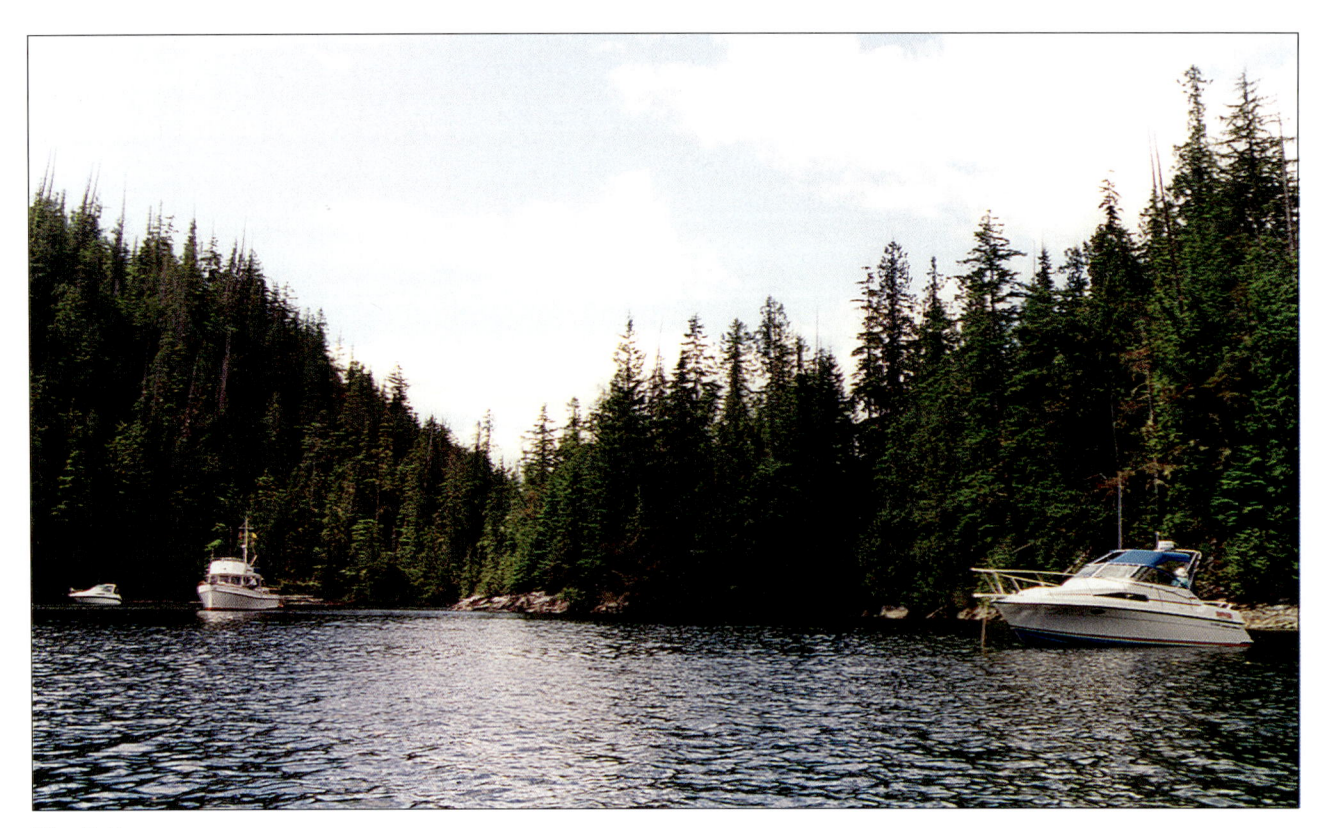

## Karlukwees  chart 3545

In recent years the dock that allowed mariners to stop for short visits and walk ashore crumbled into a dangerous pile of rotting wood, then disappeared. The remnants of the village were boldly standing along the water's edge overgrown by blackberries and thimbleberries. A small house sat on pilings over the white sand and shell beach. And it was possible to venture along the former waterfront access path the length of the village. More recently one had to be satisfied with cruising past slowly taking in the crumbling remains from a short way off shore. Move in towards the dock ruins from Nicholas Point and then turn sharply towards the small island north of Kamano Island passing either side, but being wary of the reef that protrudes east. Use chart 3545.

In the 1970s residents of Karlukwees were planning to return to their village, but as the years wore on it remained abandoned. Through the 1980s the docks became more and more waterlogged and weather worn. In the early 1990s landing became difficult and then impossible. Visitors were not encouraged but many mariners stopped by to walk the beach and among the remains of tumbling down houses along the waterfront trail that was fast becoming overgrown by thick berry bushes. In 2003 it was reported that restoration plans were underway for Karlukwees as well as for New Vancouver, on the north shore of Harbledown Island. New Vancouver has since come a long way but Karlukwees remains an abandoned village site.

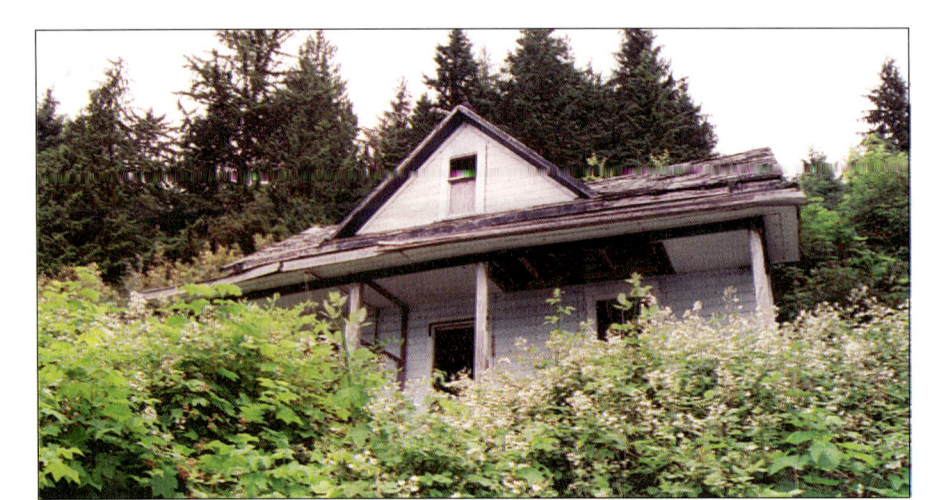

*Top: Anchorage in the outer cove of Potts Lagoon opens into Clio Channel opposite the southeast end of Beware Passage.*

*Left: A house that once stood overlooking the beach at Karlukwees. Photographs left and opposite, top, were taken in the 1980s.*

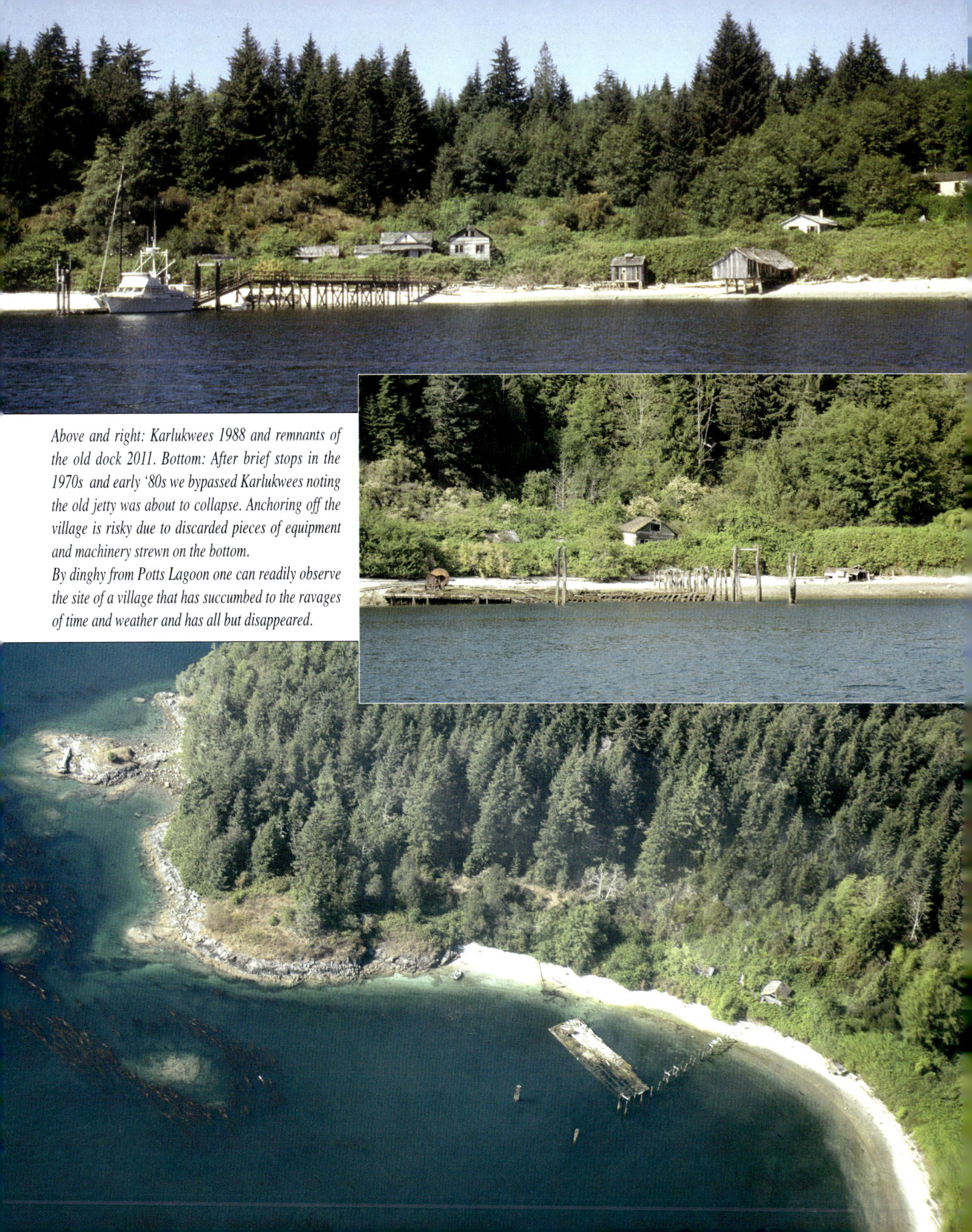

*Above and right: Karlukwees 1988 and remnants of the old dock 2011. Bottom: After brief stops in the 1970s and early '80s we bypassed Karlukwees noting the old jetty was about to collapse. Anchoring off the village is risky due to discarded pieces of equipment and machinery strewn on the bottom.*

*By dinghy from Potts Lagoon one can readily observe the site of a village that has succumbed to the ravages of time and weather and has all but disappeared.*

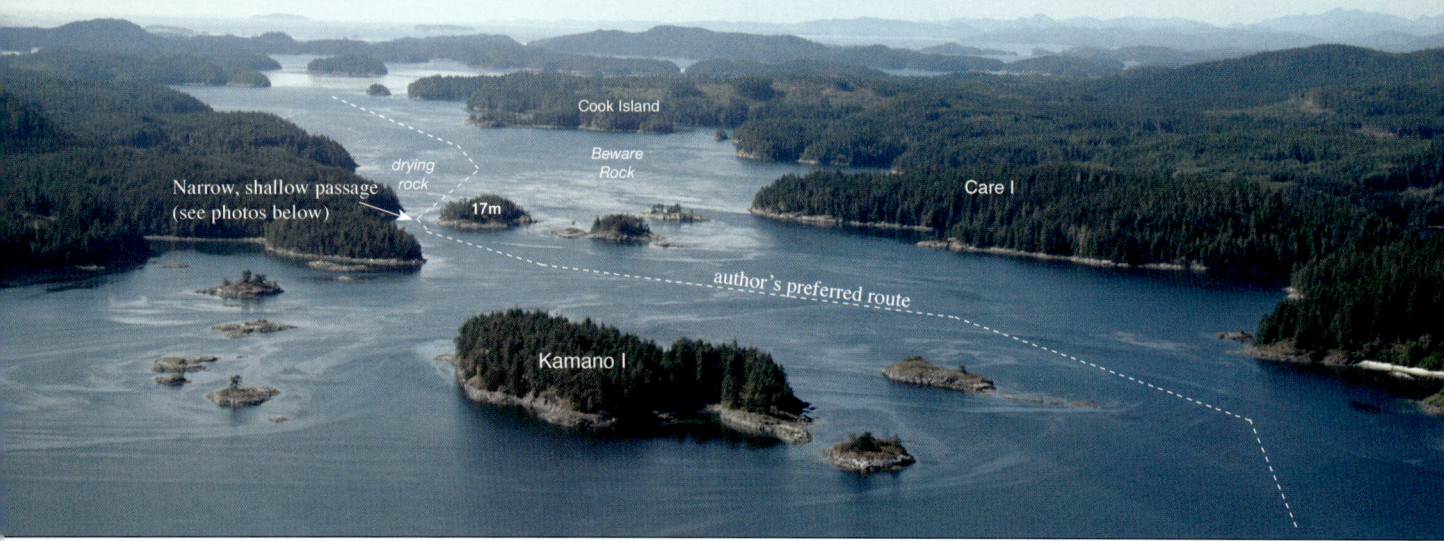

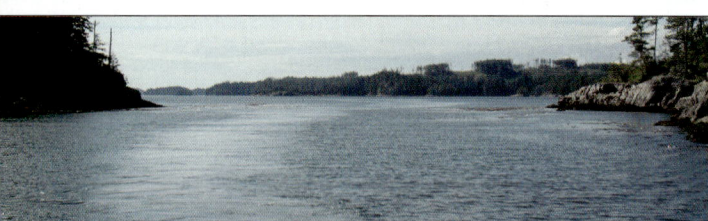

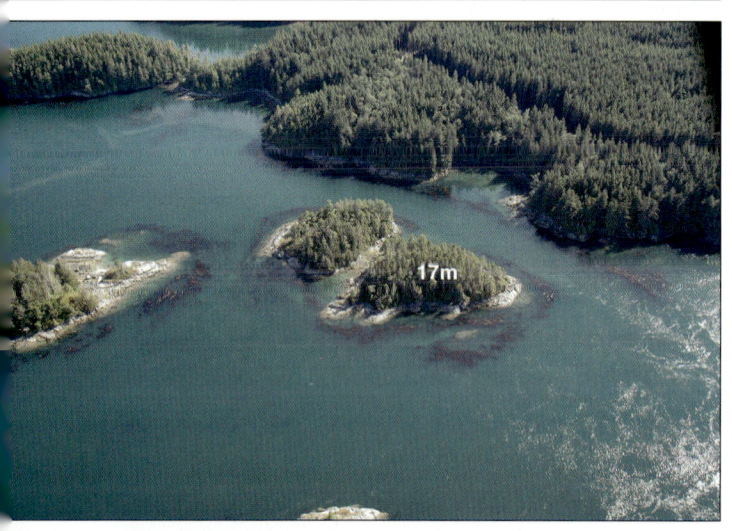

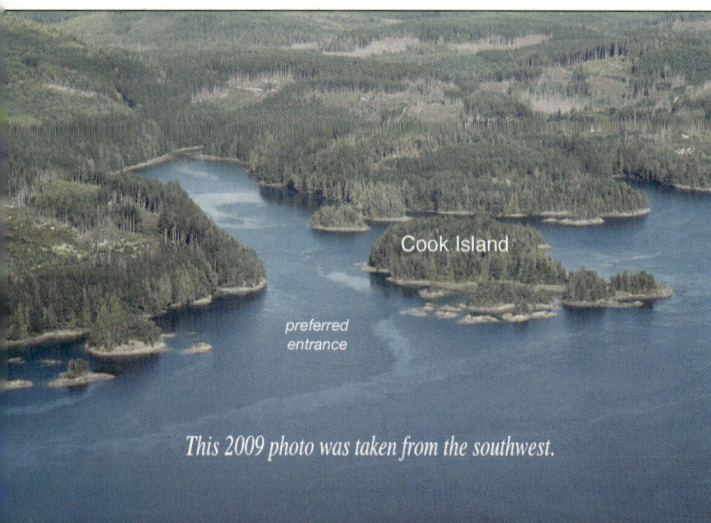

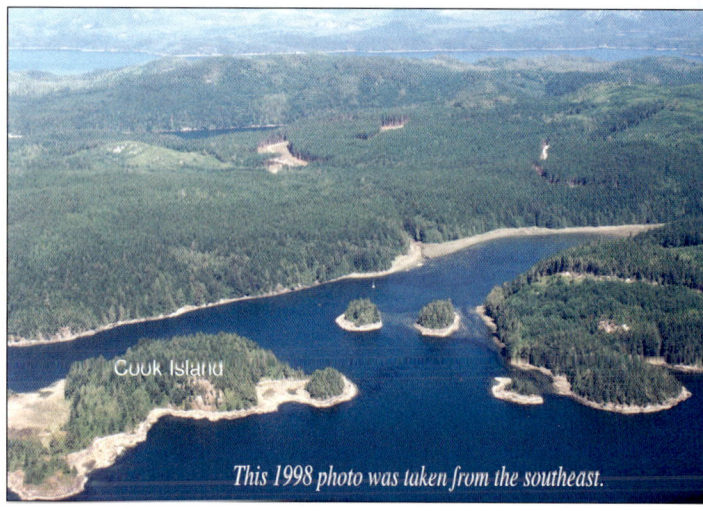

*Image labels (top photo):* Cook Island; Beware Rock; Care I; Narrow, shallow passage (see photos below); drying rock; 17m; Kamano I; author's preferred route

*Image label (middle right photo):* Cook Island — *This 1998 photo was taken from the southeast.*

*Image label (middle left photo):* 17m

*Image label (bottom photo):* Cook Island; preferred entrance — *This 2009 photo was taken from the southwest.*

Top: Beware Passage. At the far end Village Channel runs past the Indian Group and leads into Knight Inlet. Left and above left: A popular route in Beware Passage is lined with kelp but is wider than at first appears. Above right and bottom left: Beware Cove opens off Beware Passage.

## Beware Passage  charts 3545, 3546

From Potts Lagoon, it is a short but interesting run past Karlukwees into Beware Passage. Interesting in that you will need to follow a large scale chart very precisely to navigate through the rock-strewn waterway that begins your cruise into historic native waters. See photos above and on page 97.

Locals use the preferred route, which they have named Towboat Passage, to enter Beware Passage from the east. Pass north of Kamano Island and take a route through the passage between Care Island and the two small islets opposite it, then follow mid channel of Beware Passage keeping clear of the reef that juts into the passage off Turnour Point. Small boats sometimes turn to port and pass the reef off the south side of the 15 metre high island, beyond which lies Care Rock. Then head for the south side of the 17 metre island off Harbledown Island. Take the route that cuts behind the islets off the Harbledown shore. Then head towards Beware Rock bearing north of the drying rock well out into the passage. The passage (photograph opposite) is very narrow but quite navigable in about 6 to 7 metres at low water.

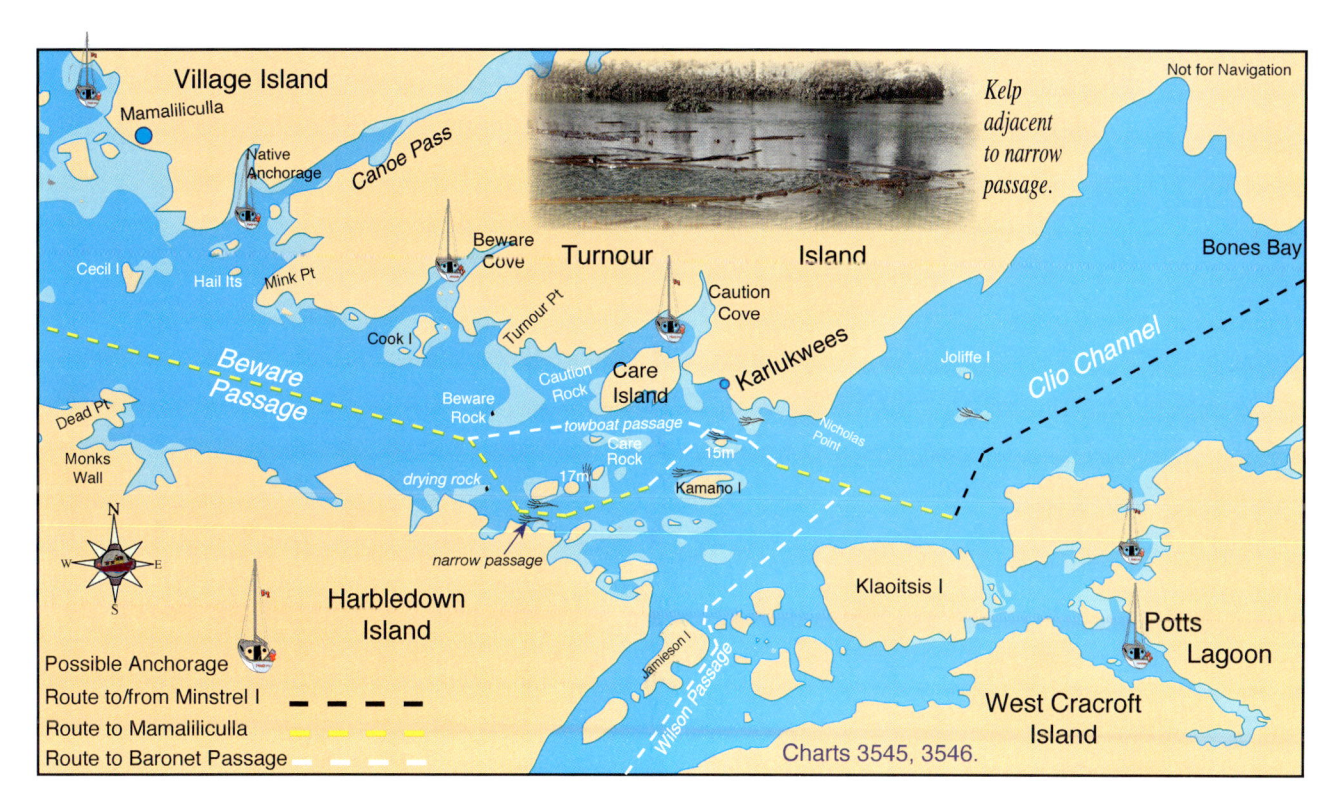

Through this troublesome passage and other waterways I use the presence of kelp as a guide to where the shallow rocks and reefs are located. This is a good method for navigating in shallow, reef-strewn passages, but it is not foolproof, so verify your course by using the largest scale chart available and by keeping a sharp lookout from the bow when necessary. Be aware of the tide and currents through these passages.

## Caution Cove chart 3545

If you like to watch the tidal waters move along Beware Passage, and other boats navigating its precarious route you may want to anchor temporarily in Caution Cove. Be mindful of drying Caution Rock at the entrance and two more inside. Drop the hook temporarily just off Care Island. This was a busy booming area at one time and some remnants of pilings may be seen at the head of the cove.

## Beware Cove chart 3545

As you continue along Beware Passage, similar conditions for temporary anchorage exist in Beware Cove. Mind the rock at the southeast entrance or take the better entrance on the west side of Cook Island. Most of the cove dries.

The best anchorage is just behind the westerly of the two small islets in the cove. On the other side of the passage, just

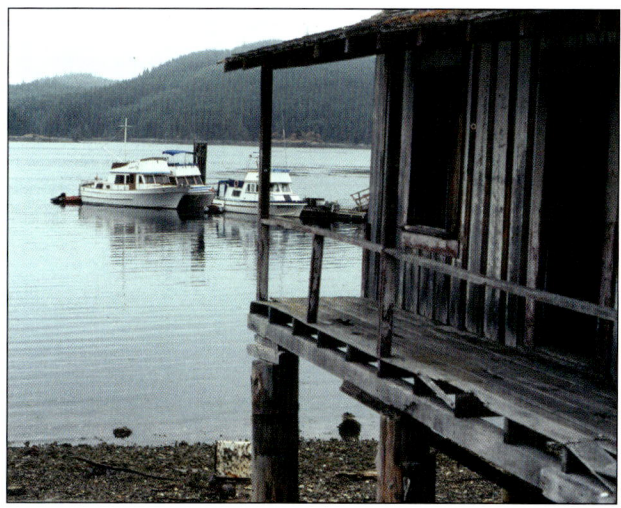

*In the 1980s boats were able to stop at a dilapidated dock at Karlukwees at the entrance to Beware Passage. These docks and structures are now rubble.*

The nearest fuel is at Lagoon Cove, or Telegraph Cove on Vancouver Island (where you will find gasoline but no diesel). If you are looking for diesel in this area plan your stops at Lagoon Cove or Port McNeil.

before reaching Dead Point, there is a cove with a large curve of drying mud flats. Adjacent to this beach, hidden in the thick brush is a wall known as Monk's Wall. This is the remains of a homestead and trading post from the 1800s.

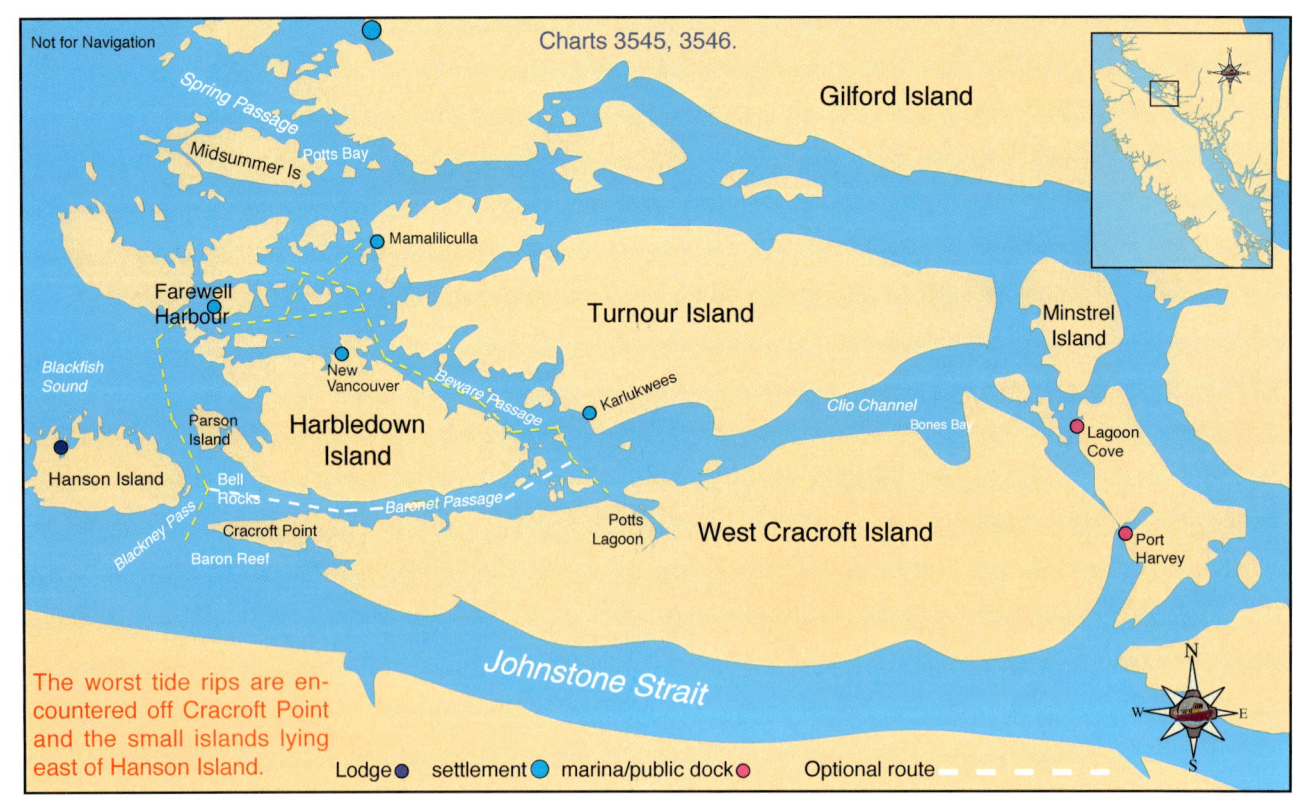

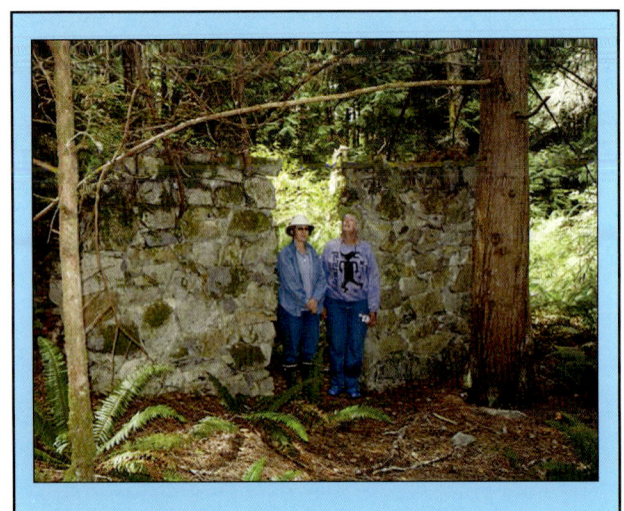

## Monk's Wall

Just before reaching Dead Point there is a cove with a large curve of drying mud flats. Adjacent to this beach is a wall hidden in the thick brush. This wall, known as Monk's Wall was not built by Chinese monks as thought, but by island resident Bill Galley and his wife Mary Anne. They had settled on the island in the late 1800s and established a farm and trading post. The wall was part of their homestead. —*Billy Proctor*

*Into the Broughtons optional routes are through the native village islands via Potts Lagoon or from Johnstone Strait. Left: Monk's Wall. Photograph courtesy of Sharon Allman and Iz Goto. Below: Some islands within the dotted lines are designated marine park areas. See the author's **Anchorages and Marine Parks**.*

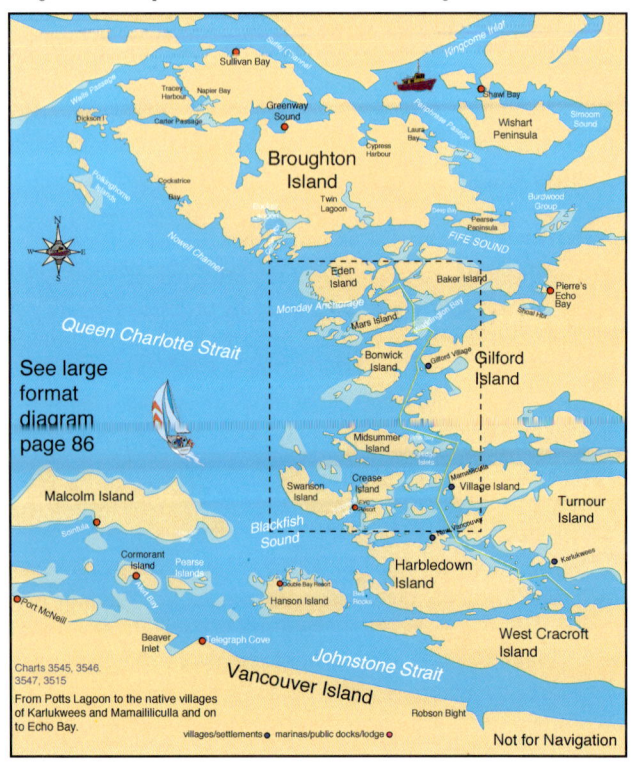

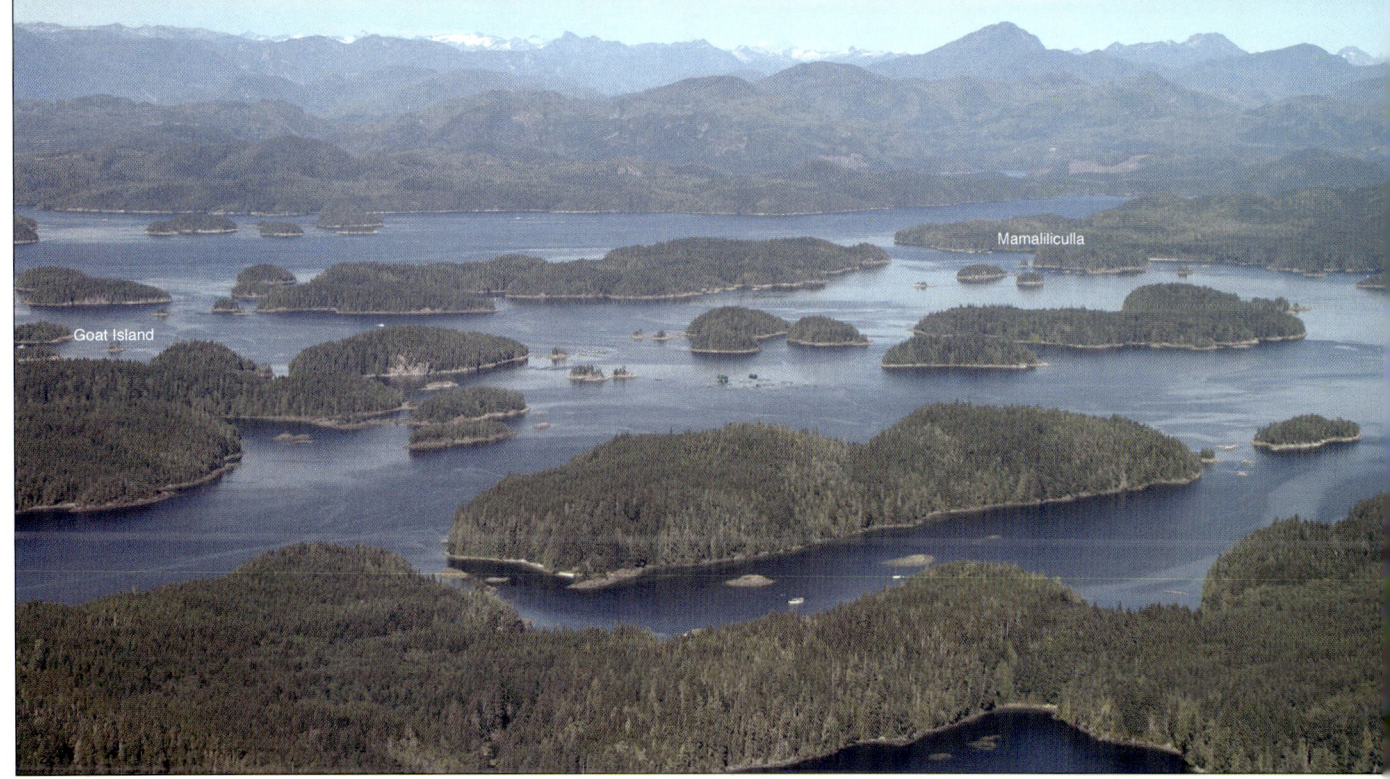

*Above: Looking across Indian Channel towards the Indian Group with Mound Island in the foreground. Goat Island anchorage is to the left, Mamalilliculla to the right. The author refers to the islands and waterways seen here as "The Village Group".*

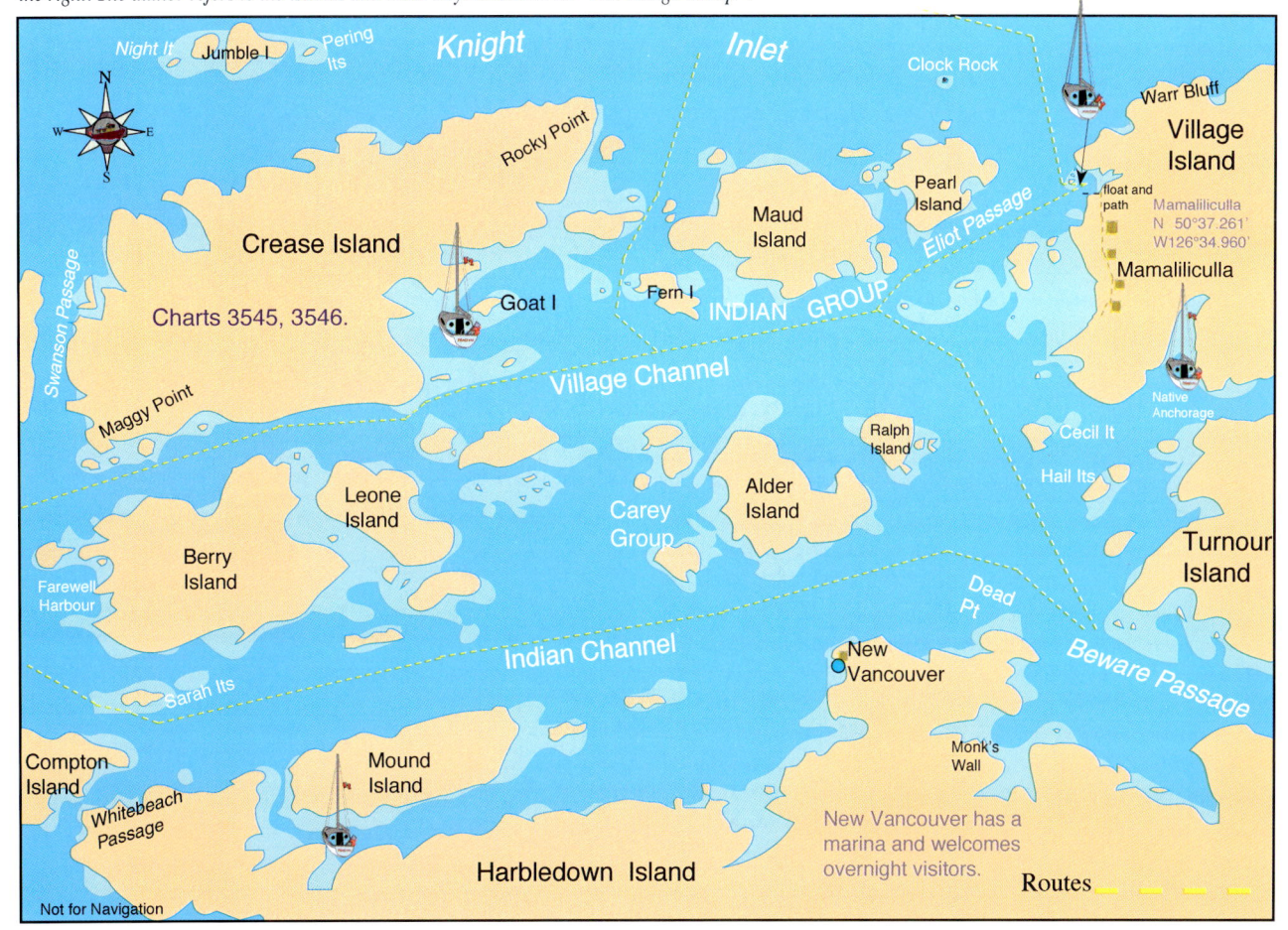

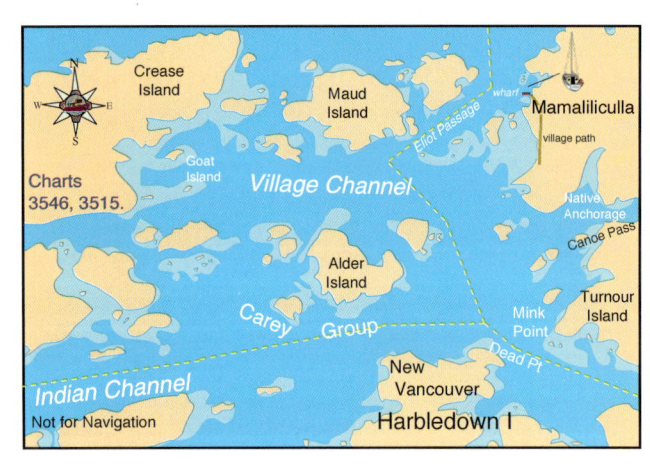

## Mamaliliculla   charts 3545, 3546, 3515

Enter Native Anchorage off Village Channel after passing between Dead Point and Mink Point on Harbledown and Turnour Islands respectively. The shallows off the beach at Mamaliliculla are such that approaching by water is fraught with danger of colliding with the bottom or hitting one of the many craggy rocks and reefs. You can anchor in Native Anchorage if it is not windy–a strong easterly blow comes through Canoe Passage–and go by dinghy to the village of Mamalilaculla. The real name of the village is 'Mi'mkwamlis' while Mamalilaculla was the name given to the people of the village. (Note the various spellings–see page 18.) We prefer to anchor in the small cove adjacent to the old wharf off Eliot Passage on the west side of Village Island. There were two mooring buoys at one time. Like other anchorages in the area, this spot can be uncomfortable in a blow.

Mamaliliculla was a thriving village not very long ago. In her book *The Curve of Time* Muriel Wylie Blanchet records meetings with the villagers and the prediction that the village would be abandoned before long. It was, although in recent years descendants of the original residents hosted tourists some summers, teaching about the history of the village and its people, and telling of the planned restoration of the village, which has not taken place to date (2011).

The first time we visited Mamalilaculla was in the late 1970s. We were able to tie up to a dock off Eliot Passage and walk the path through the brush into an unkempt soccer field surrounded by decaying houses and an old school building. This building was once run as a hospital. We had walked along a path from the anchorage to the edge of the village after clambering over the remaining planks of a crumbling wharf. We wandered among the houses, and examined the remnants of a longhouse along with at least one easily identifiable totem. There were still other significant structures in place, left standing for the ravages of time and nature to take their toll. The pathway is now an awkward stroll beneath overhanging branches of cedar and alder and through an invasion of thimbleberry covering the adjacent ground and throttling the trees in the encroaching forest. We emerged into an open meadow surrounded by cut-back thickets and looming tall evergreens. Several houses still dotted the waterfront and the big structure of the old school building lay immediately ahead. It was falling into decay but still stood firm as though confidently challenging the elements. More houses or their remnants were dotted about what used to be the village site. Poles and fallen house logs and posts were on the ground in some disarray. Today the wharf is only a skeleton.

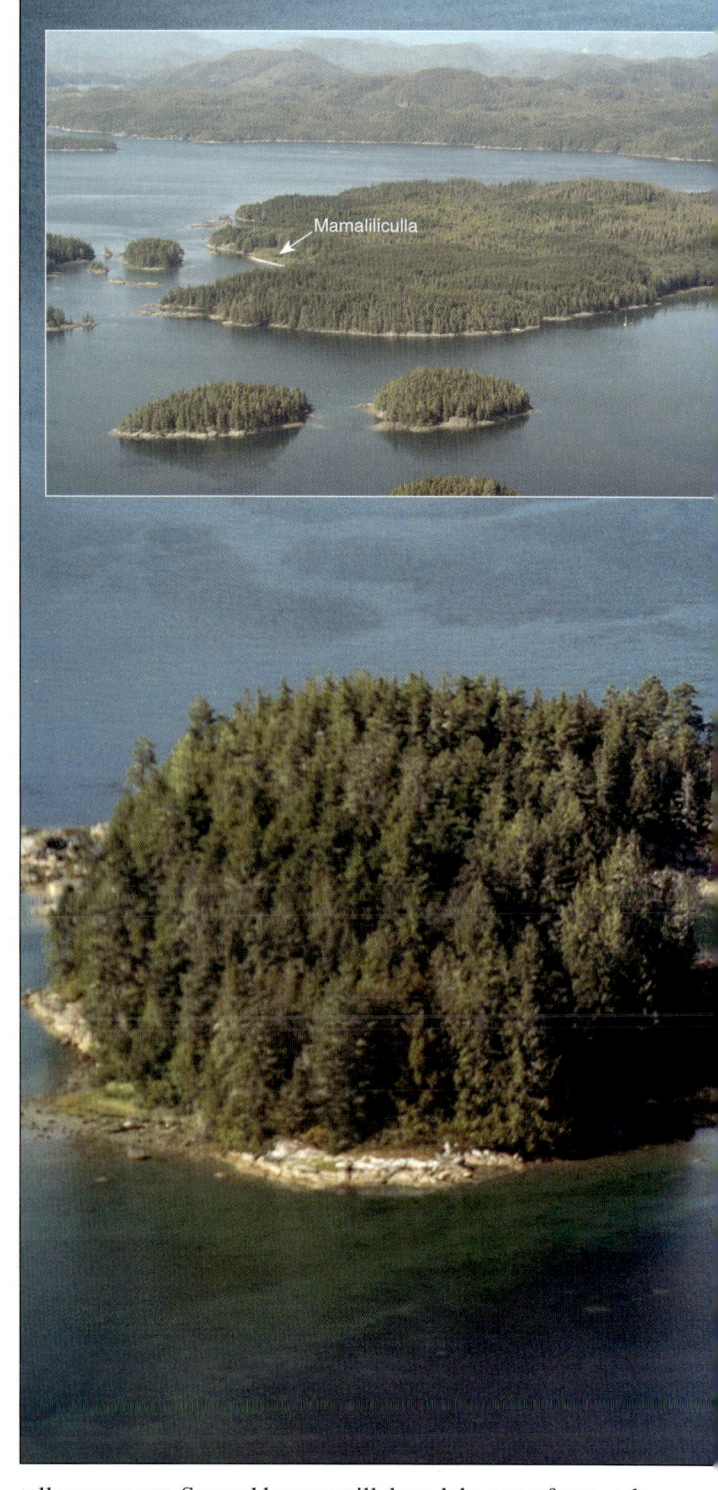

We walked along the beach of white sand and crushed

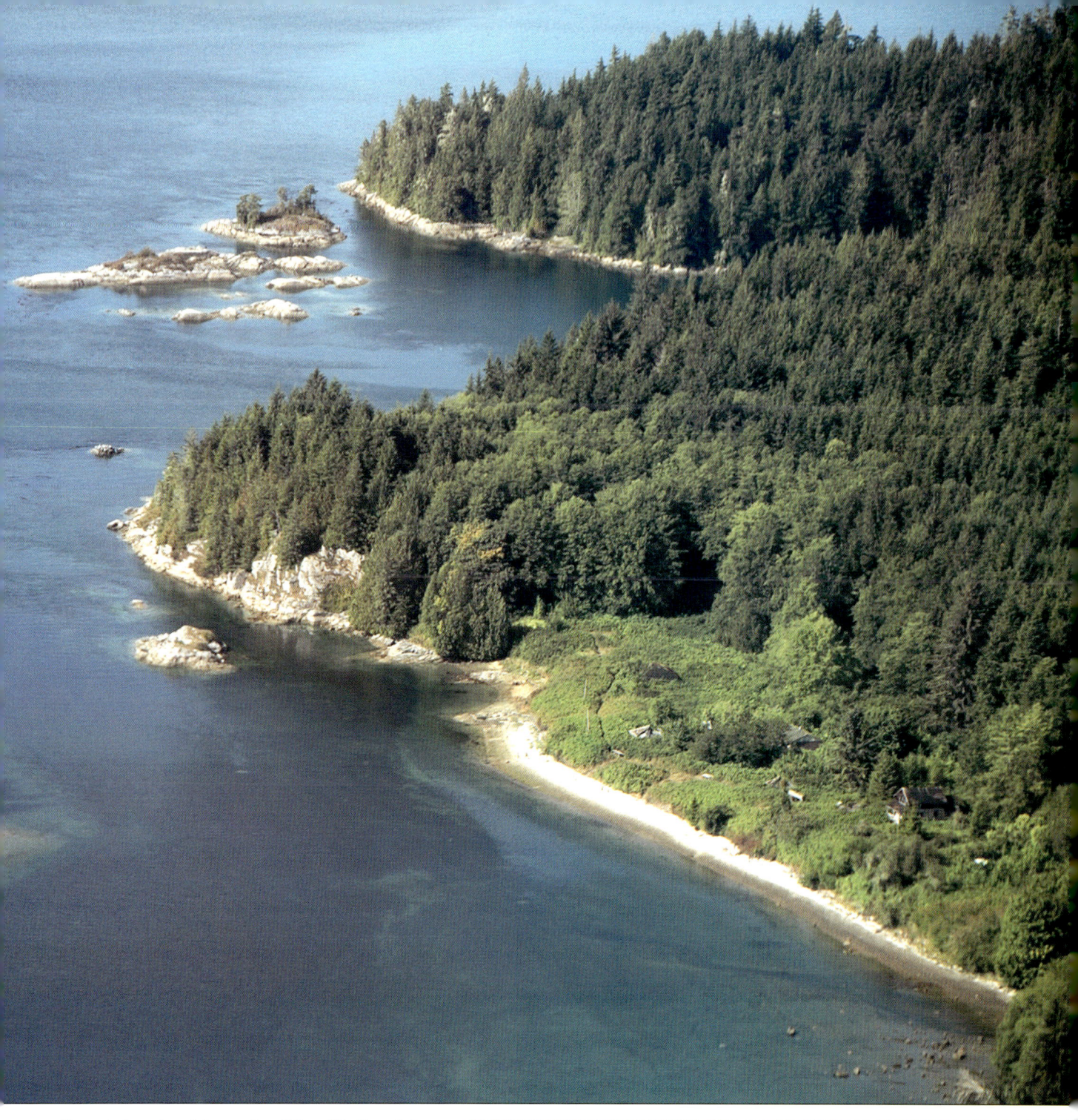

*Above: A close view of the remains of Mamaliliculla and the conditional anchorage beyond. The water off the beach in front of the historic village is shallow and strewn with rocks and debris. Inset: This view shows a boat in Native Anchorage and Mamaliliculla to Knight Inlet with the Hall Islets in the foreground. Right: The photograph of this fallen figure was taken in 1993. It was all but gone ten years later and more recently could scarcely be found.*

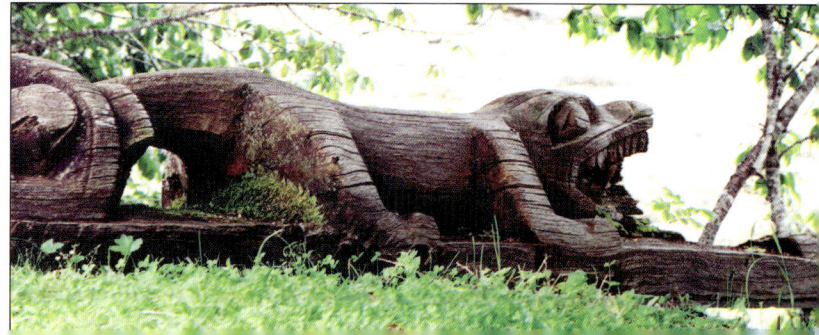

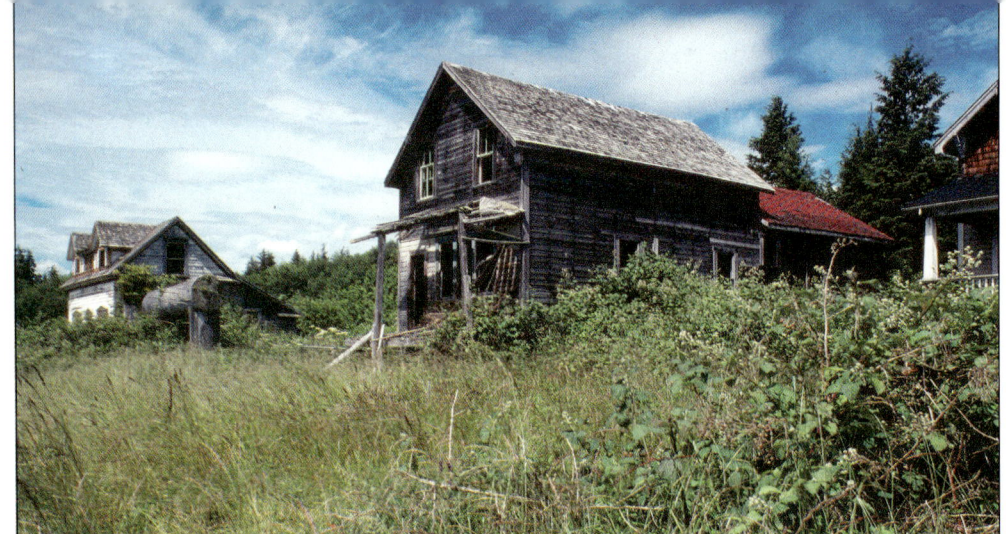

*Left: Buildings at the village of Mamaliliculla in 1979. Photographs this page and opposite, show the village structures in various states of disrepair.*

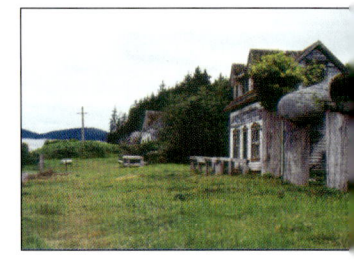

*In 1979 the village of Mamaliliculla was in a state of neglect. But in 1993 it was well on its way to being restructured by tribal descendants.*

*A member of the Village Island band welcomed tourists on and off over several years. The remains of some of the buildings had fallen down by 2003 and more by 2011, and overgrowth had again reclaimed much of the open fields and paths.*

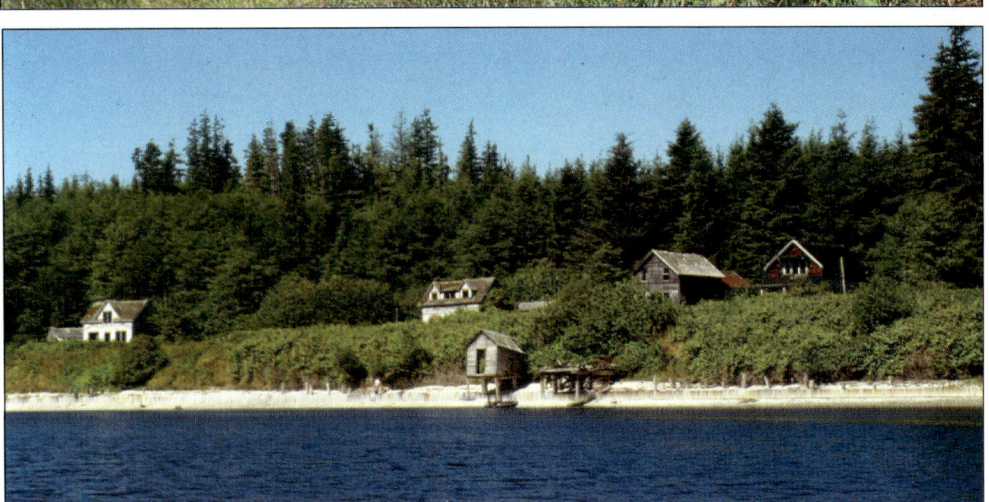

shells, amidst debris of old, abandoned and broken equipment, wondering when someone would show up to reclaim their homes and property. We went into some of the houses and found they had been seriously vandalized. We poked into one of them, still standing intact except for broken windows, doors and ceiling panels. Strewn around were bits and pieces of old equipment ranging from machine parts to domestic furnishings and utensils. Remnants of curtains hung loosely in one window. Some old magazines and newspapers littered the floor.

By 1990 access to the village had become more difficult, necessitating a walk around the beach and over craggy rocks to regain access to the remnants of the buildings. No longer could we walk through the archway of overhanging trees along the path from the old wharf. No longer was it possible to walk across the open field.

Then the First Nations people began cleaning up Mamaliliculla and temporarily returning it to a presentable condition for visitors. A book appeared on the market–*Totem Poles and Tea* by Hughina Harold (Heritage House) that is a fine account of the author's days at Mamaliliculla as a school teacher in the 1930s. It brought back to life the way things

### Village Group

There appears to be no overall name for the groups of small islands and islets north of Harbledown Island that include the Indian Group and the Carey Group and lie between Crease Island and Village Island. I tend to refer to all of them, including these two groups, as the *Village Group*. In his introduction (page 18), Dr Phil Nuytten refers to The Indian Group, the northerly of the two groups of islands. The Indian Group consists primarily of Maud and Pearl Island with the smaller Fern Island and a few others charted without names.

The main features of the area are the two major passages that run through The Village Group east to west. These are Village Channel and Indian Channel, passages that can be taken quickly to move through the islands en route to Farewell Harbour or slowly to enjoy the scenic vistas as you pass by. Either way, use as large a scale chart as possible (chart 3546) and navigate with care.

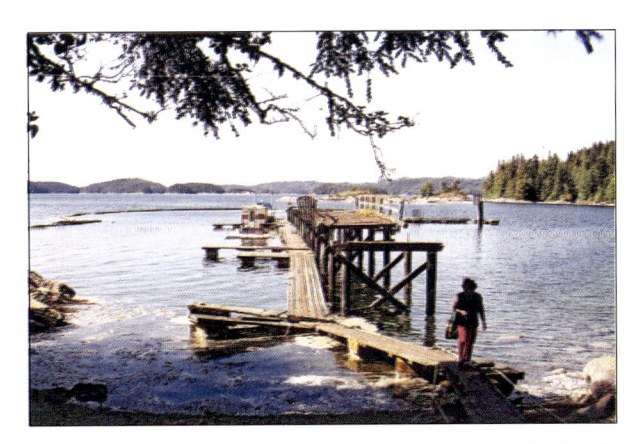

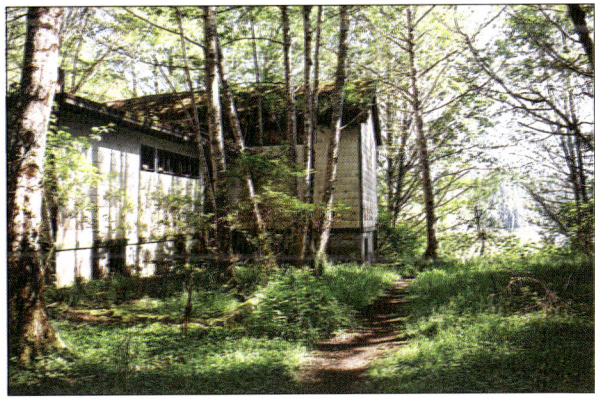

*Right: In 1993–Dsu-no-kwa lurks in the woods at Mamaliliculla–singing with..."red mouth to lure children to be eaten," the legend says. This pole has long since succumbed to nature and has become very difficult to locate in the grassy area beneath the trees.*
*Top: Remains of the dock, and the anchorage at Mamaliliculla in 2003.*
*Above: The old school building at the head of the path to the village from the wharf. Below: A house at Mamaliliculla and houseposts seen in the 1970s, 80s and 90s. In recent years, along with other structures and fallen poles, they have all but disappeared. The posts are remnants of Harry Mountain's Big House at Mem-kumlees (Mamaliliculla).*

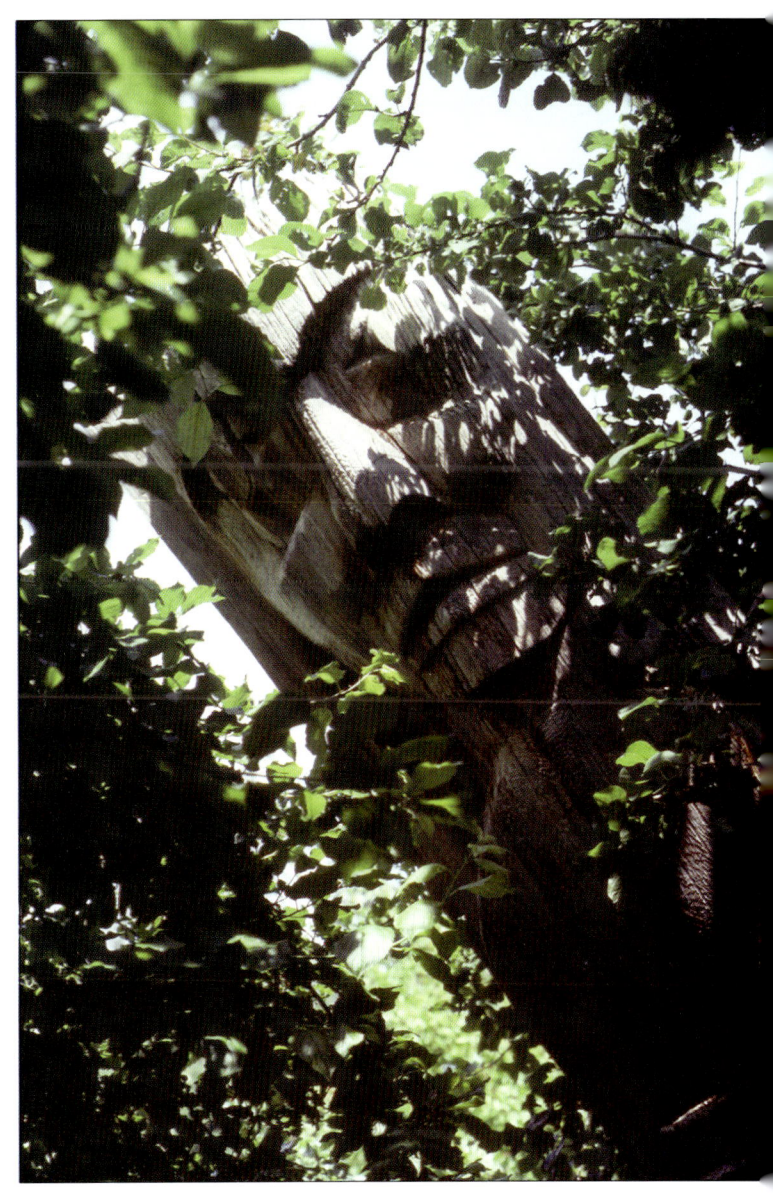

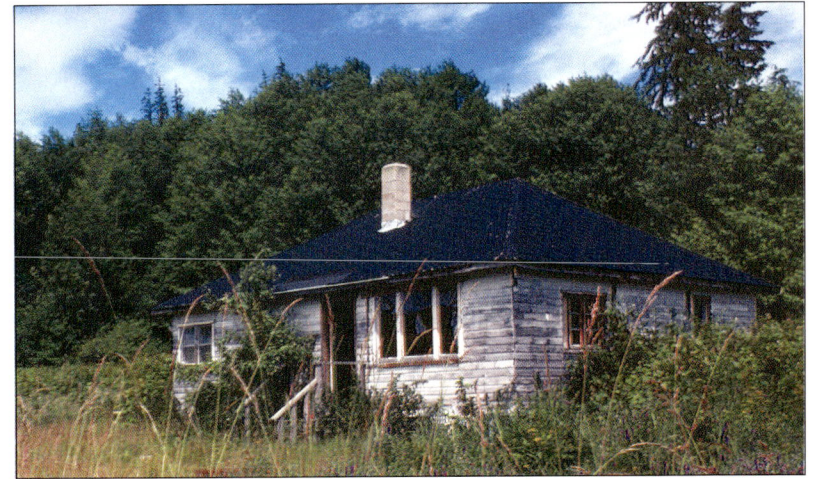

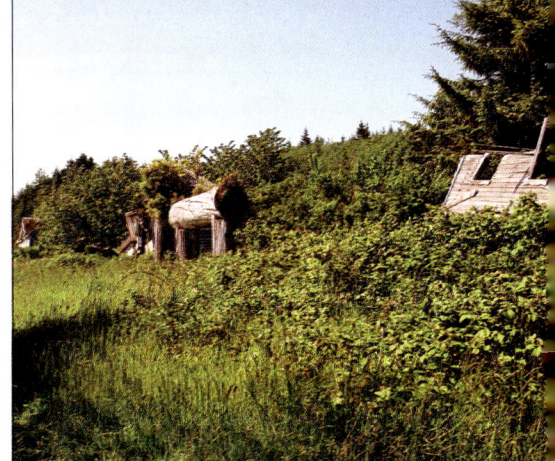

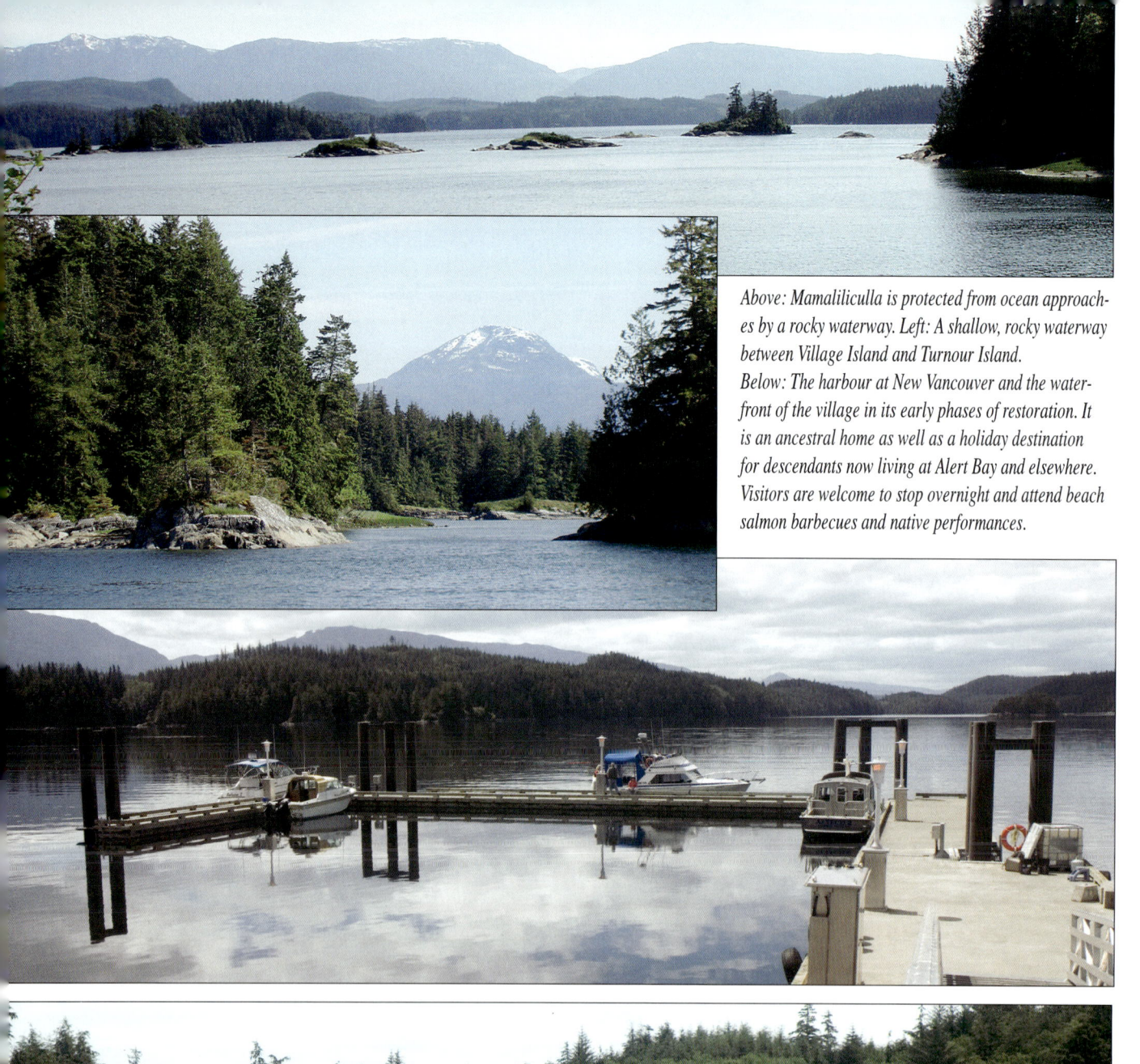

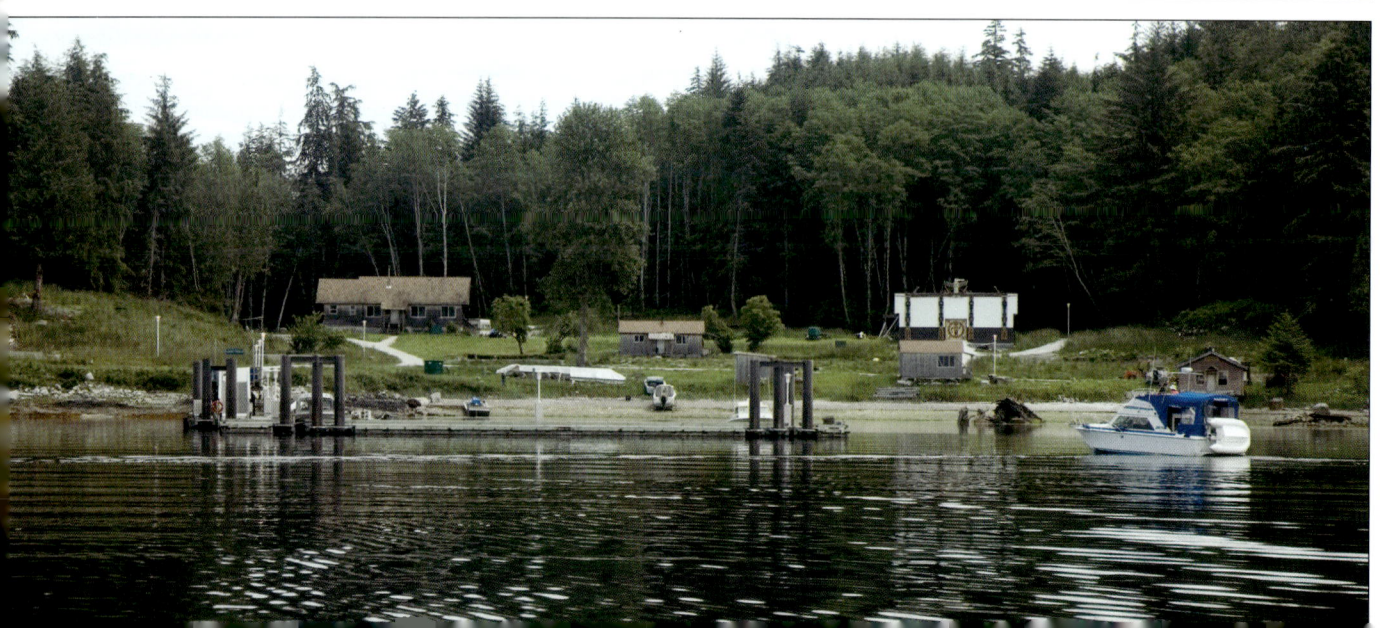

*Above: Mamalilicualla is protected from ocean approaches by a rocky waterway. Left: A shallow, rocky waterway between Village Island and Turnour Island.
Below: The harbour at New Vancouver and the waterfront of the village in its early phases of restoration. It is an ancestral home as well as a holiday destination for descendants now living at Alert Bay and elsewhere. Visitors are welcome to stop overnight and attend beach salmon barbecues and native performances.*

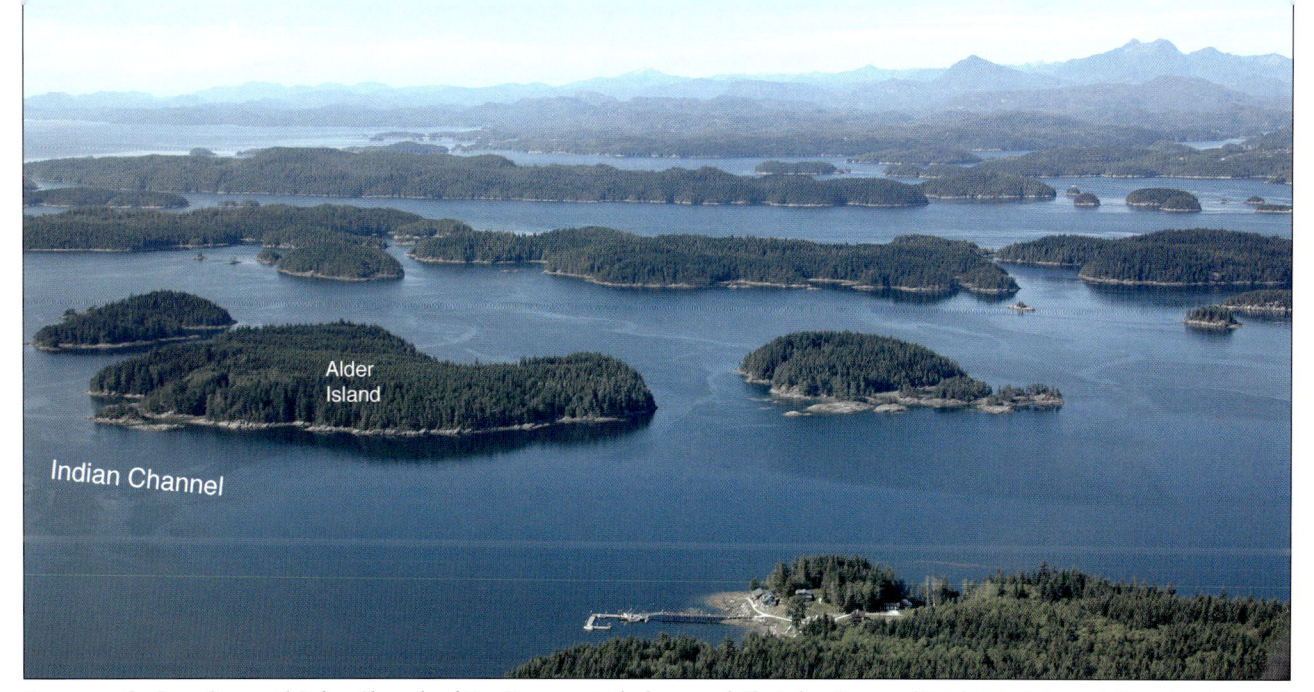

*View across the Carey Group with Indian Channel and New Vancouver in the foreground. The Indian Group and Knight Inlet lie beyond. Since this photograph was taken, in 2009, a floating breakwater has been added off the dock at New Vancouver.*

were in the village in the early 20th century and provided a vicarious experience of being subject to the whims of nature in allowing residents to move about on the waters between the islands and the nearby centre of Alert Bay.

One can stand at the shoreline and look out at the nearby islands and picture the coming and going of visiting natives in their canoes, of passing vessels from the various Missions, of the regular callers bringing mail and supplies and of the emergency evacuation of patients suddenly taken ill. This sometimes involved taking a patient to hospital in a small boat, poorly equipped for the open water conditions between the islands and Alert Bay, and often in stormy conditions, carrying more passengers than safety should have dictated.

One day in the early 1990s we encountered a young band member, back home in his forefathers' village, working at restoring Mamalilicula to a reasonable state for visitors. Once again the field was being cleared and the condition of some of the buildings was being improved. The old, fallen poles were exposed for viewing. During subsequent summers visitors were welcomed and offered tours of the village. Refreshments were available at a seasonal store.

In early 2003 the village houses had all but fallen to the ground and the path was very overgrown again with thimbleberry. A rough dock placed at the anchorage was still there. Conflicting reports on the plans for the village suggested uncertainty as to its future.

In his book *Beyond Desolation Sound*, cruising guide author the late John Chappel referred to 'the totem of Dsoniqua (sic) lurking in the woods nearby,' quoting a legend that says she is 'singing with round red mouth to lure children to be eaten.'

On one trip in more recent years we discovered Dsu-no-kwa (or Dzunuḵ'wa) and took a photograph that appeared on the back cover of *Totems Poles and Tea*. She is featured again in this book (page 101).

Leaving the anchorage at Eliot Passage follow your chart with much care and move down to Farewell Harbour, passing **New Vancouver** on Harbledown Island. You may have noticed the village as you came through the west end of Beware Passage, just beyond Dead Point. Some mariners love to find anchorages in nooks and out of the way places most boaters would overlook. There is limited protection in the lee of Dead Point. But it is sound advice to bypass this spot if the southwest wind is up and settled in for a while. There are many such tiny anchorages dotted around the Village Channel area. Remember that variable tidal currents, and wind that sometimes comes over the low lying islands with considerable force, make these anchorages temporary and ideal for daytime use only, when weather permits. New Vancouver offers suitable shelter in windy weather.

### New Vancouver  charts 3545, 3546, 3515

The village of New Vancouver has been undergoing restoration in recent years. It is inhabited primarily by residents of Alert Bay and serves as a summer getaway for many of them. The village has a Big House and during summer native performances and beach salmon barbecues are offered to visitors. Book in advance. The marina at New Vancouver is well constructed and can accommodate a number of overnight guests. Water and 20 amp power are available at the dock. Contact the office at 250-974-2179 (Bruce Glendale at time of writing–cell: 250-974-8422).

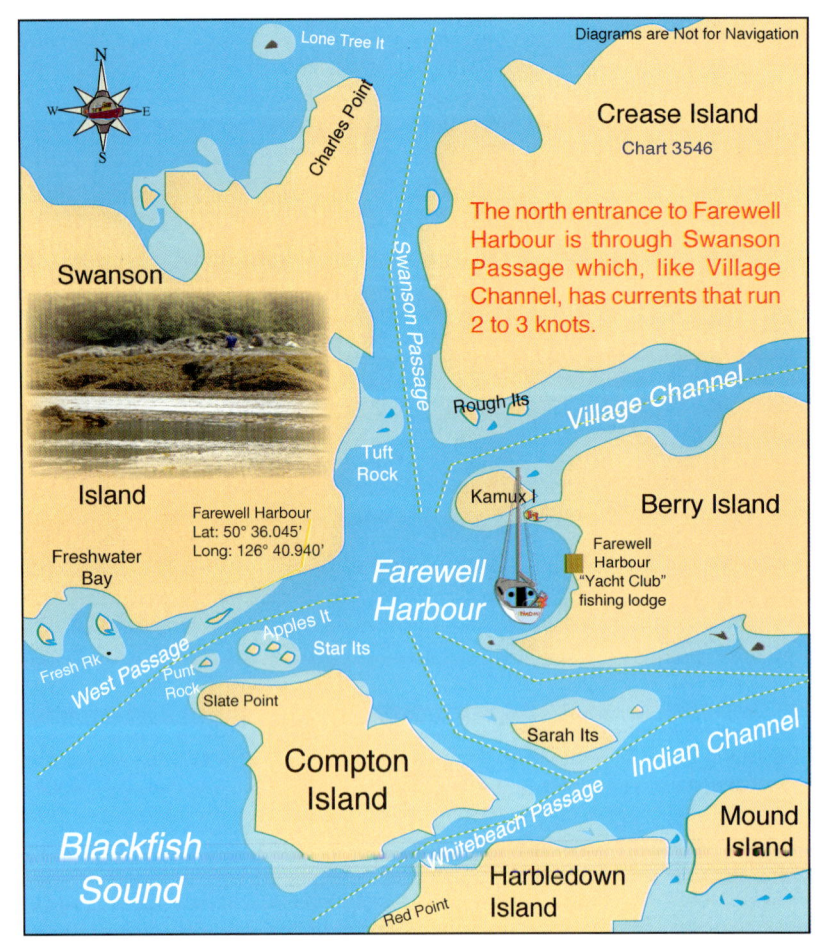

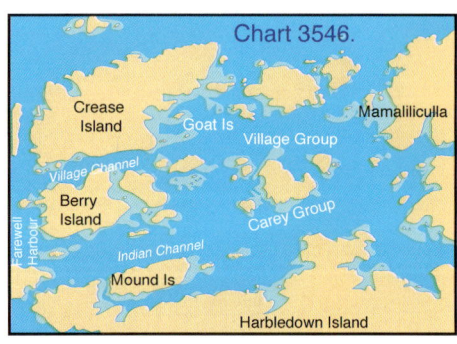

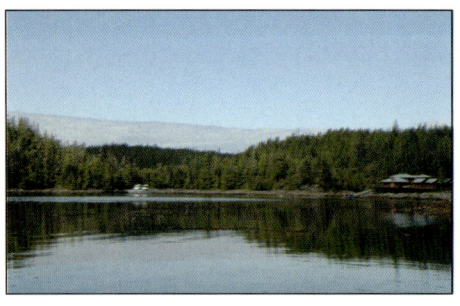

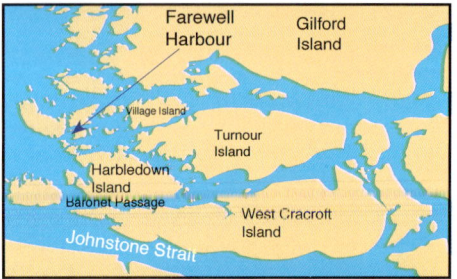

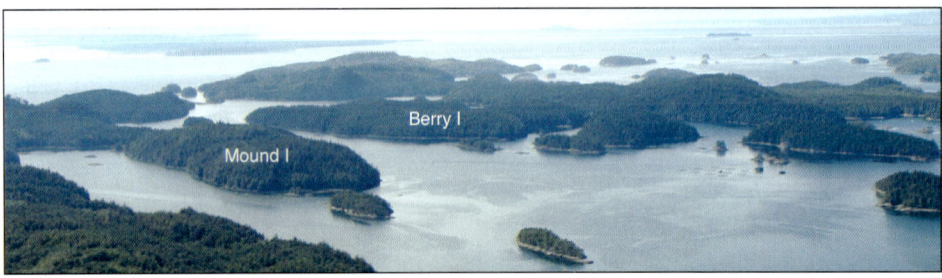

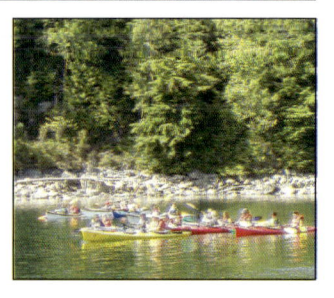

We leave the ghosts and residents of the First Nations villages to their increasing number of tourists and move to other places where we can stop or lie at anchor overnight. Such a place is Farewell Harbour, which is reached by way of either Village or Indian Channel. These channels skirt north and south respectively of the Carey Group of islands and give easy access to Farewell Harbour. The southern one, Indian Channel is obstructed south of Berry Island by the Sarah Islets. However, these do not block the passage to a great extent and pleasure boats are able to pass around them easily.

## Goat Island  charts 3546, 3515

On the way to Farewell Harbour there are alternative nooks at which to stop for further exploration of the area in a small runabout. There is a shallow cove where knowledgeable yachtsmen will readily drop the hook, for example, on the east side of Crease Island (see diagram top right, photo above and opposite) at the edge of Village Channel. This anchorage at Goat Island has a mud and sand bottom and is considered a good spot to spend some time. It can be accessed by taking a centre channel course after passing north of Goat Island.

Using the large scale chart, entrance to the cove can also be made south of Goat Island. Some mariners have said that this cove is a temporary anchorage, but in all excepting strong westerly winds it should be reasonably sheltered. A number of yachtsmen I have spoken to have used it as an overnight anchorage. It was occupied by two mid-sized boats when we stopped by on our previous trip to the Broughtons.

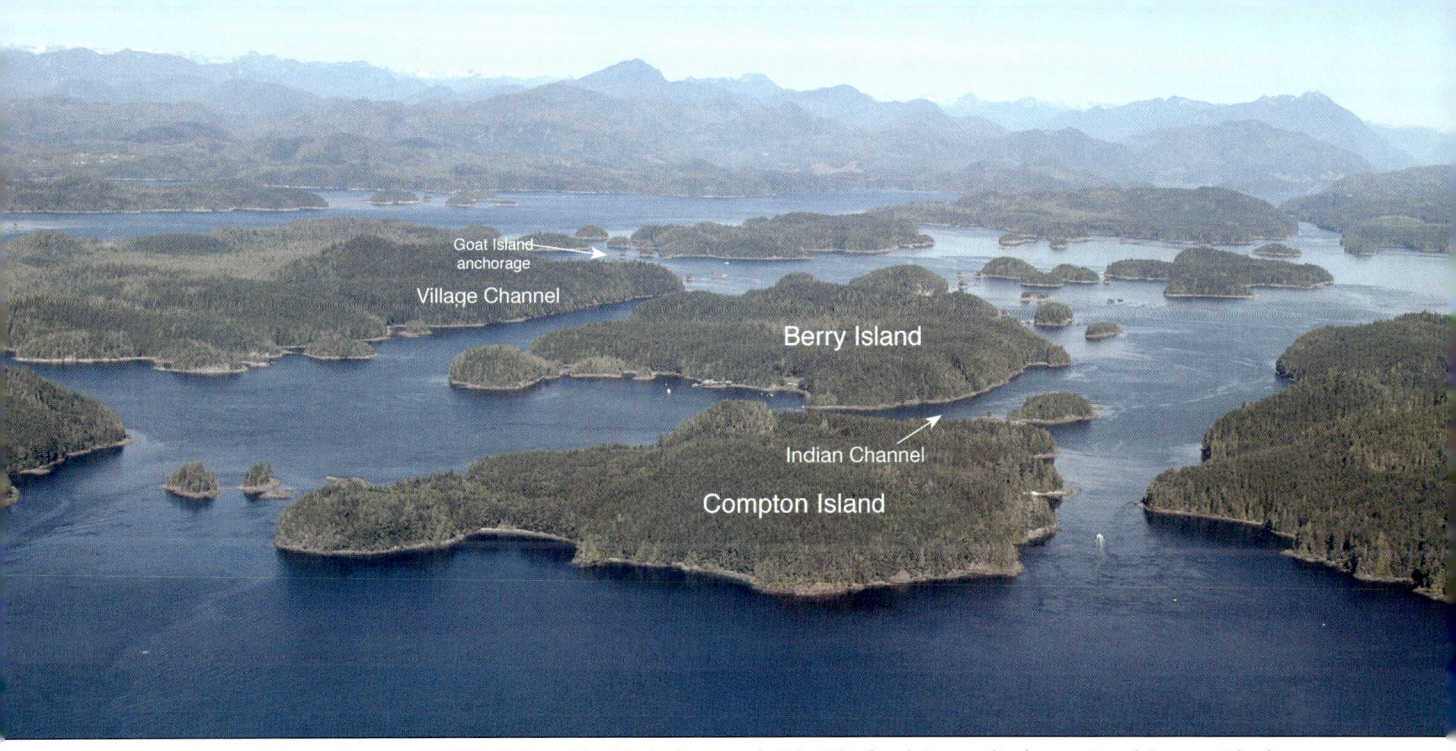

*Farewell Harbour, with the northwestern tip of Harbledown Island in the foreground, right. Whitebeach Passage lies between it and Compton Island, centre. There is a small white beach in the passage. Currents up to three knots run in Village Channel north of Berry Island. Below: The lodge and its small dock can be seen off to the right in Farewell Harbour. A small boat is leaving through West Passage. Opposite page: Anchorage and the fishing lodge building in Farewell Harbour, with a view of Mound Island, Indian Channel and the east side of Berry Island. A popular place for kayking is around Farewell Harbour.*

## Farewell Harbour  charts 3546, 3515

Entering this deceivingly calm enclosure, surrounded by islands, one has the instant gratification of having arrived in nirvana. Particularly if you were flushed through the entrances by the currents and arrived during particularly windy weather. In winter this anchorage could be uncomfortable in strong westerlies. In summer be mindful of all forecast winds. Take shelter against the shore of Compton Island to escape the flood out of the harbour. Waves from Blackfish Sound sweep through West Passage into Farewell during a strong westerly blow. The flood also comes through this passage, which is pretty foul with rocks. In calm conditions the route closest to Swanson Island is straight forward with kelp revealing the location of the rocks. Outside in Blackfish Sound the flood sweeps northwards along the Compton Island and Swanson Island shores and swirls around southwards in the centre of the Sound to pass through Blackney Passage into Johnstone Strait.

Nearby, around the entrance to Baronet Passage, flood currents do a counter-clockwise sweep to clash with water flowing the opposite way down the passage in the vicinity of Bell Rocks.

The buildings of Farewell Harbour Yacht Club, not a club facility at all, but rather a fishing lodge, are located on the east side of the anchorage on the west shore of Berry Island. The lodge has changed ownership from time to time and has been open or closed during our various visits to Farewell.

Rick Bradley of the 32 metre Vancouver motor yacht *Black Tie* says he has no difficulty entering Farewell Harbour in his beamy vessel. On one of our visits a large tug carrying a sailboat on its upper deck had easily entered through one of the passages and was anchored off Berry Island.

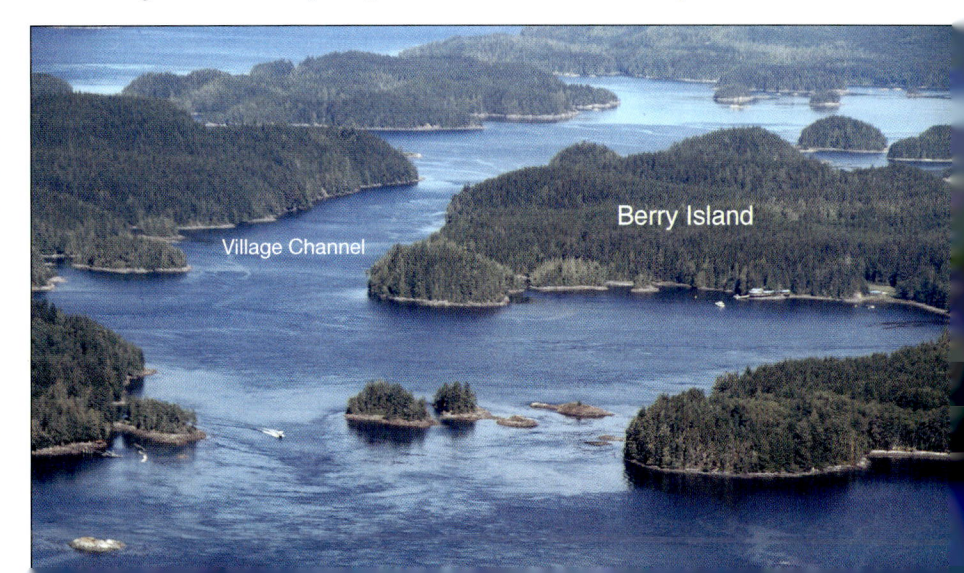

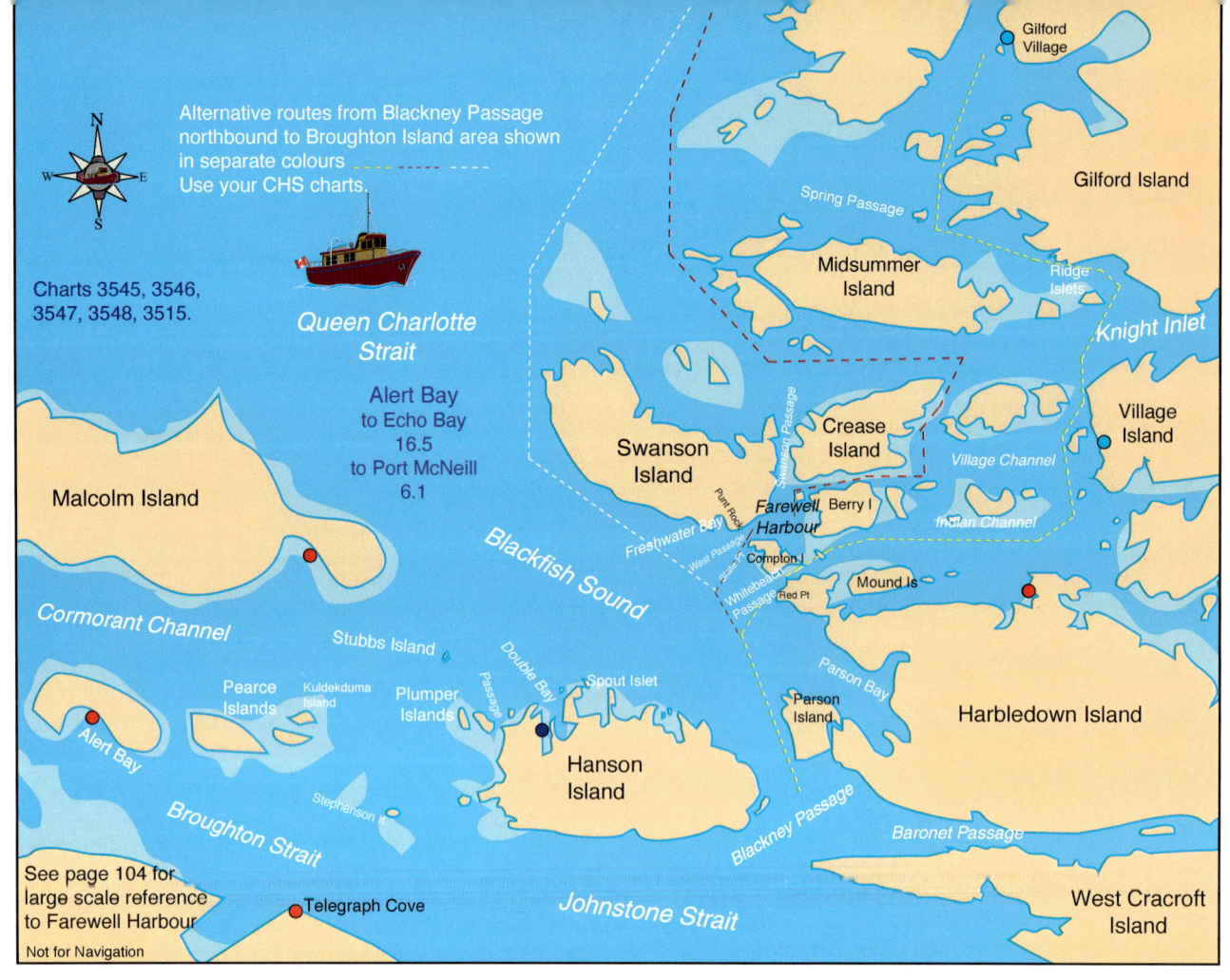

The north entrance to Farewell Harbour is through Swanson Passage which runs 2 to 3 knots and should be used with caution (see diagram on page 104). The same currents are present in Village and Indian Channels. Entering and leaving Farewell Harbour to the west is achieved by going carefully, preferably at slack, through West Passage winding north of Apple Islet and south or north of Punt Rock to skim by Slate Point on Compton Island or head straight out past Freshwater Bay. Mind Freshwater Rock on this entrance route. Use Whitebeach Passage on the other side of Compton Island. There is a shoal to be avoided on the south shore of Whitebeach Passage just past Red Point.

**Mound Island** appears to have a good anchorage off its south shore. This is not easily reached through the rocky passage off the west side of the island. The route into the anchorage is around the islands off the east side or between them, carefully avoiding a three-metre shallows in the middle, and possible fish farm structures beyond.

The anchorage is regarded with mixed feelings about the degree of shelter it provides. While it is protected from westerly winds it is subject to the swirling waters and currents from the adjacent Indian Channel. Mound Island was once occupied by the local First Nations people and traces of their residences can still be found in the undergrowth ashore.

We usually avoid dallying in the vicinity of the islands between Village and Indian Channels because of the constant currents and frequent wind in the area. However a slow cruise past the islands will produce a beautiful panorama.

A short distance across Blackfish Sound is Hanson Island with its rugged, almost inhospitable north shore. But it has two possible places to stop, **Double Bay** and an anchorage just to the east of **Spout Islet**.

---

**Freshwater Bay** on the south side of Swanson Island was the site of a fish buying camp run by Mrs Jae Proctor and her son Billy, now of Echo Bay (read *Heart of the Raincoast*–Horsdal and Shubart 1998). The name Freshwater Bay may come up in your travels and scouring of the charts. It once had a store, and the dock shown on some charts has long since been private. The bay can be used as an anchorage only for short durations in good weather. Parson Bay on Harbledown once had a village. Billy Proctor says there were some 75 native villages in the islands when he was a child.

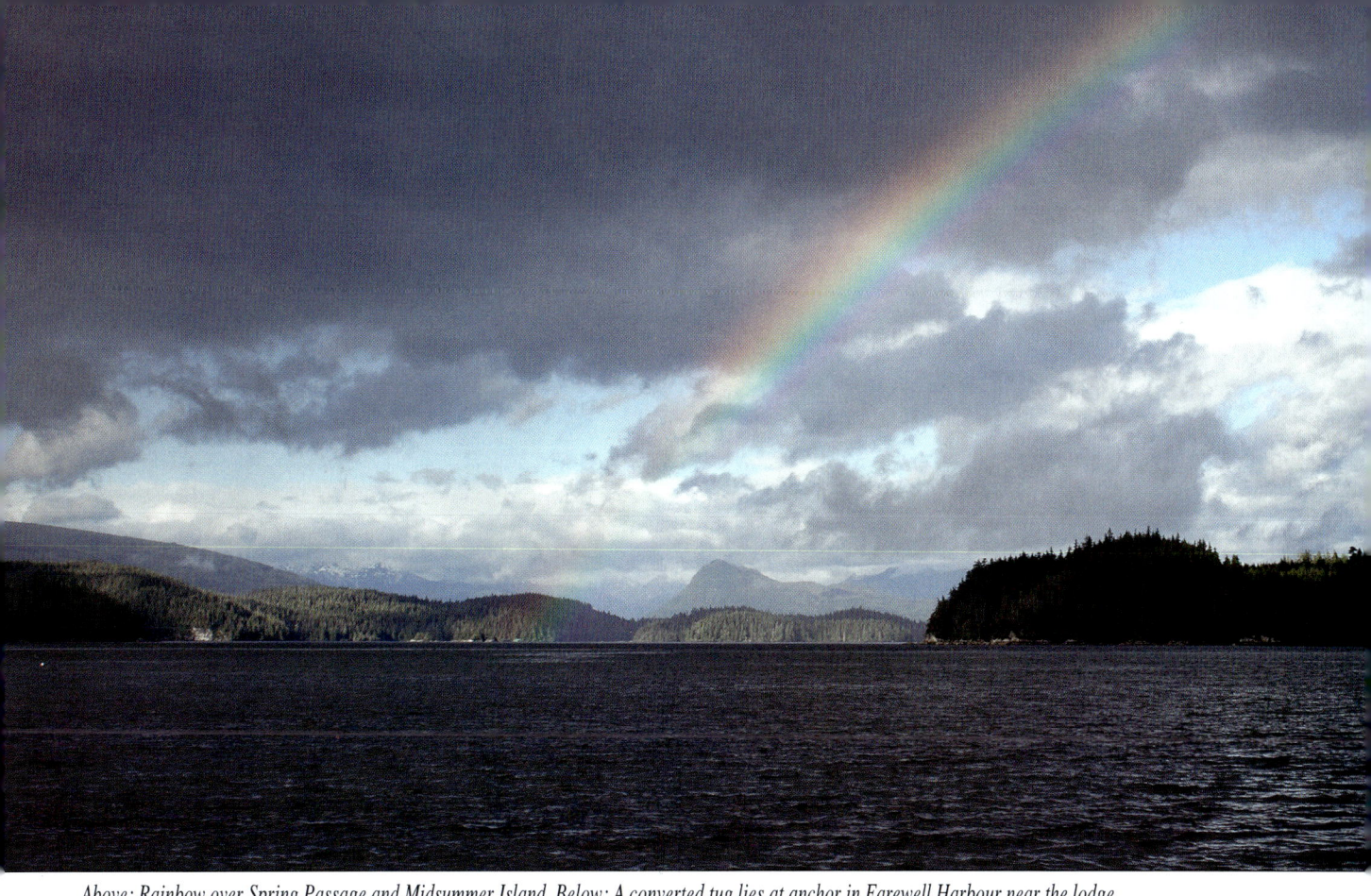

*Above: Rainbow over Spring Passage and Midsummer Island. Below: A converted tug lies at anchor in Farewell Harbour near the lodge.*

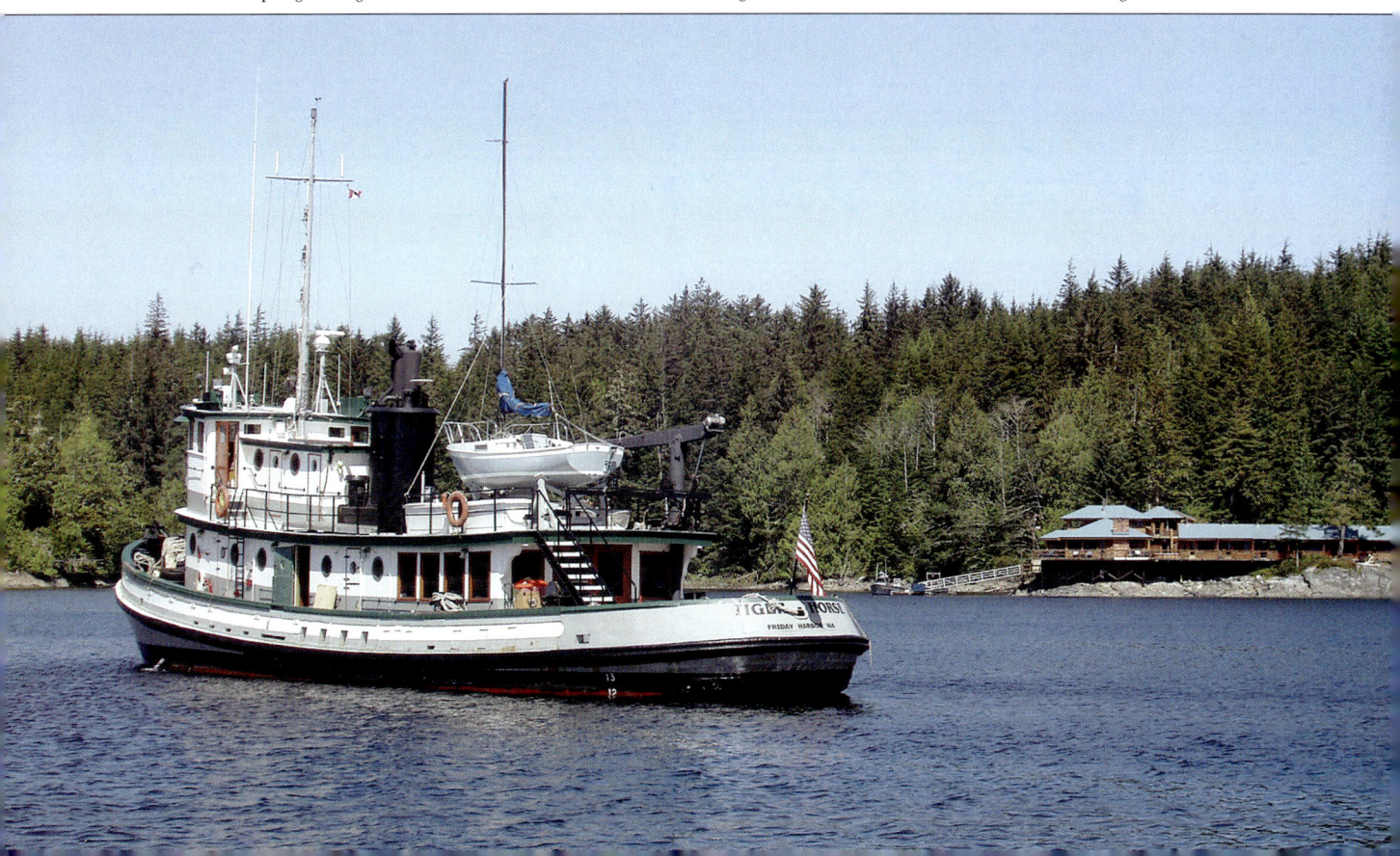

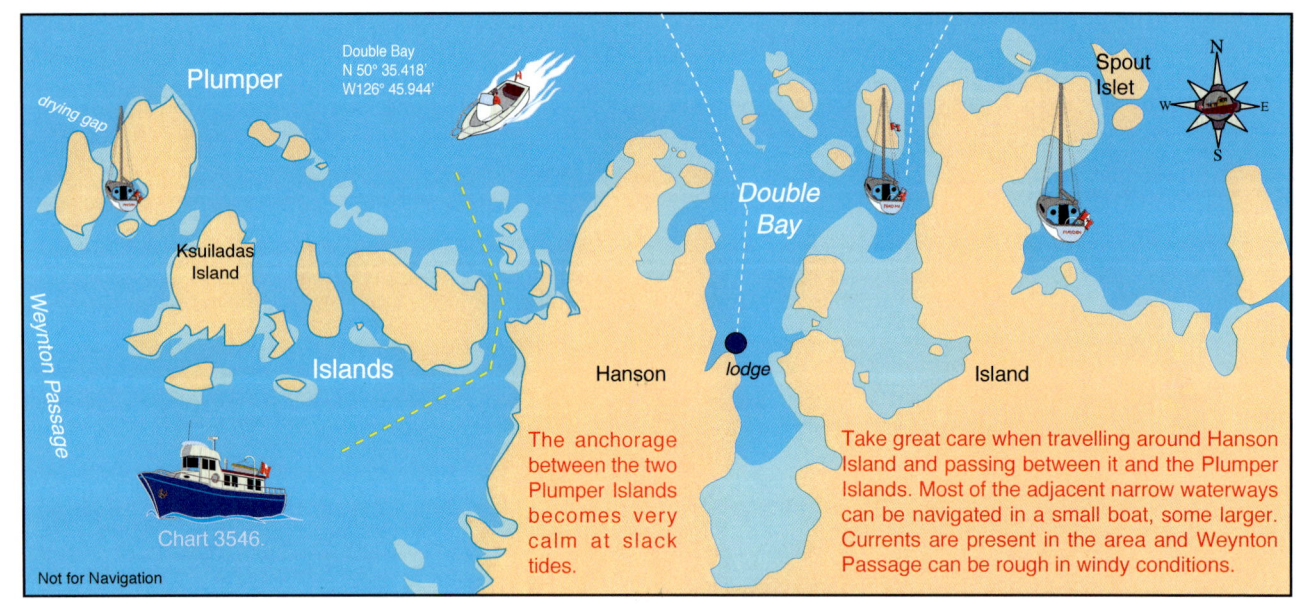

Map callouts:
- Plumper
- drying gap
- Double Bay N 50° 35.418' W126° 45.944'
- Spout Islet
- Ksuiladas Island
- Weynton Passage
- Islands
- Double Bay
- Hanson
- lodge
- Island
- Chart 3546.
- Not for Navigation

The anchorage between the two Plumper Islands becomes very calm at slack tides.

Take great care when travelling around Hanson Island and passing between it and the Plumper Islands. Most of the adjacent narrow waterways can be navigated in a small boat, some larger. Currents are present in the area and Weynton Passage can be rough in windy conditions.

We have taken passage through the above cut, indicated by a yellow dotted line, in a 39 metre, 10 knot cruiser near slack tide. Careful navigation or local knowledge is required (photo opposite).

## Hanson Island  chart 3546

There is shelter in Double Bay which makes for a good overnight stop. A lodge caters to fly-in guests June through September. This is a time when fishing and weather conditions are at their best. The large dock accommodates lodge boats for its fishing charters and sightseeing guests. The lodge haas been known to welcome transient morage customers at times and may well allow overnight moorage when not busy. The lodge may be reached on VHF channel 66A. Phone 250 949-1911. Anchorage may be found to the east of the entrance to the bay. Another reasonably good anchorage lies beyond **Spout Islet** east of Double Bay. Entrance is easy and the anchorage is generally good.

Double Bay is a fine place to view eagles, whales and dolphins. Safe entry into the bay requires careful but easy navigation down the west side keeping the rocks in the centre of the passage to port as you enter.

Nearby **Stubbs Island** is the centre of local tidal action. We went scuba diving on the east side of Stubbs Island once when it was slack, all five minutes of it, but the current was still running relatively strongly. As we surfaced and climbed into our pickup boat a tidal standing wave of about one foot formed alongside us and increased with the current. During that diving season, we were fortunate to have a large pod of killer whales come by barely 10 metres away.

Be mindful of the reefs between the **Pearse Islands** and the **Plumper Islands** when travelling back into Johnstone Strait. The Pearse Islands are covered later. See page 211.

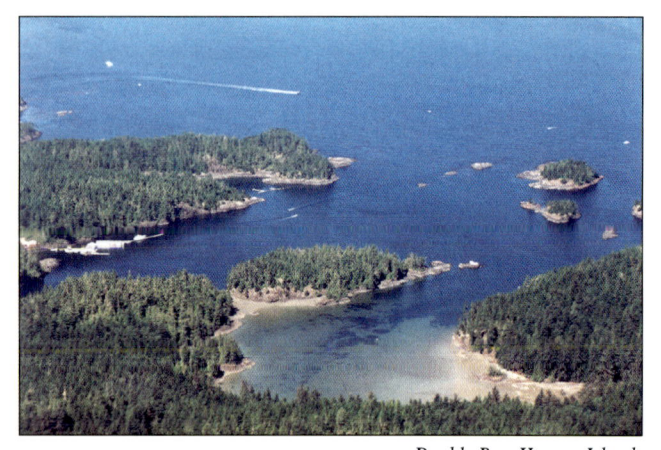

*Double Bay, Hanson Island.*

## Plumper Islands  chart 3546

Sheltered between the northwesterly islands of this group is a small anchorage good for perhaps three boats shore tied to the easterly island. We have anchored there in a 15 metre motor yacht quite easily, with comfortable room to spare for perhaps one or two more of similar size. The cove that is formed between the islands is a tranquil place with an outstanding view across Weynton Passage and Johnstone Strait towards Telegraph Cove. We have watched beautiful sunsets from this vantage point.

We have also sheltered among the Plumper Islands waiting out some fierce winds that kept us there for two days. During that time we discovered a strong current that runs through the cove at high tide when the water passes over the shallows of the narrow cut that divides the islands. A scuba diving club placed a float in the centre of the cove once and we were tied to the western side of the float but moved to the other side to escape the full force of the current.

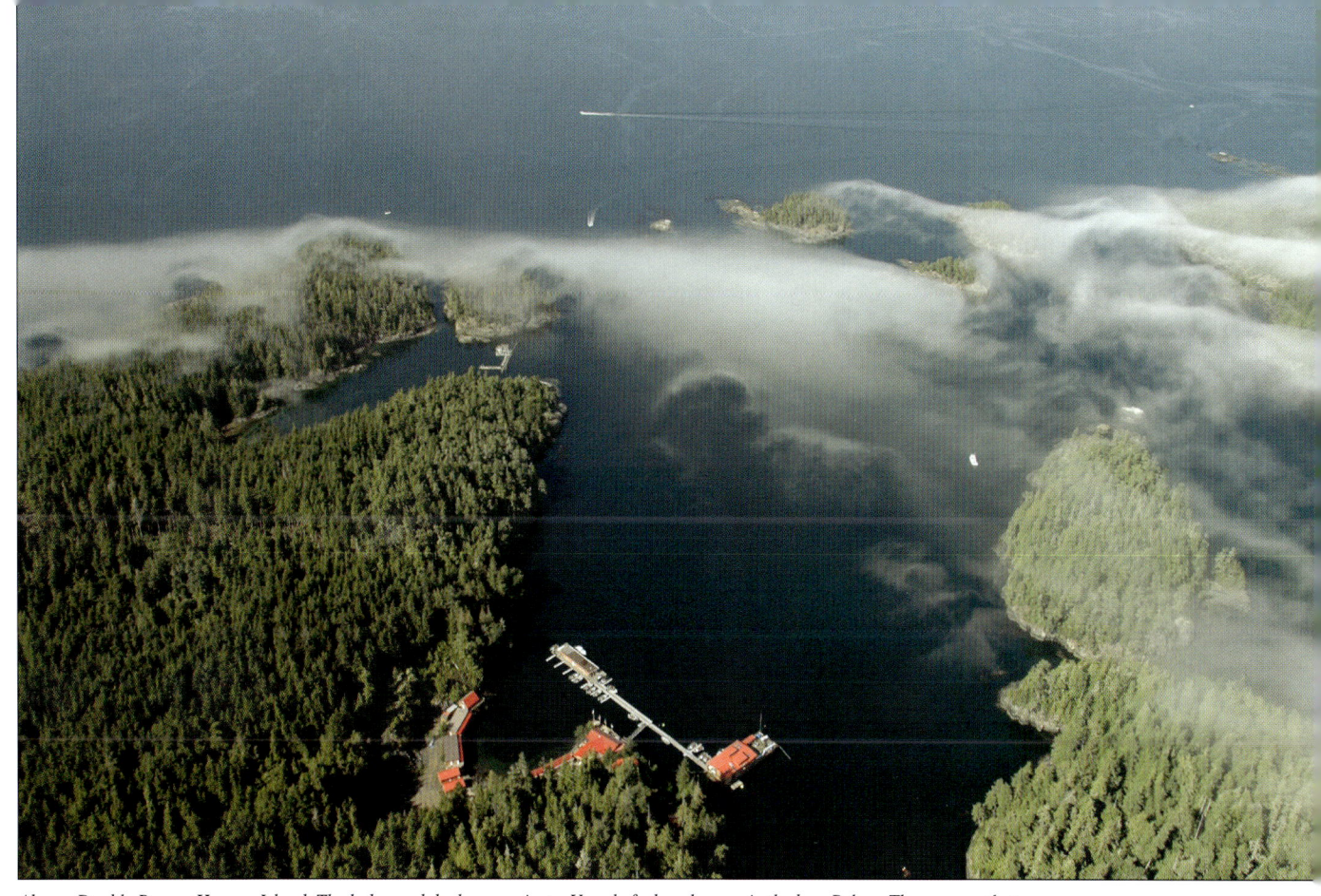

*Above: Double Bay on Hanson Island. The lodge and docks are private. Vessels find anchorage in the bay. Below: The passage that runs between the west side of Hanson Island and the Plumper Islands. It is used as a short cut between Blackfish Sound and Johnstone Strait.*

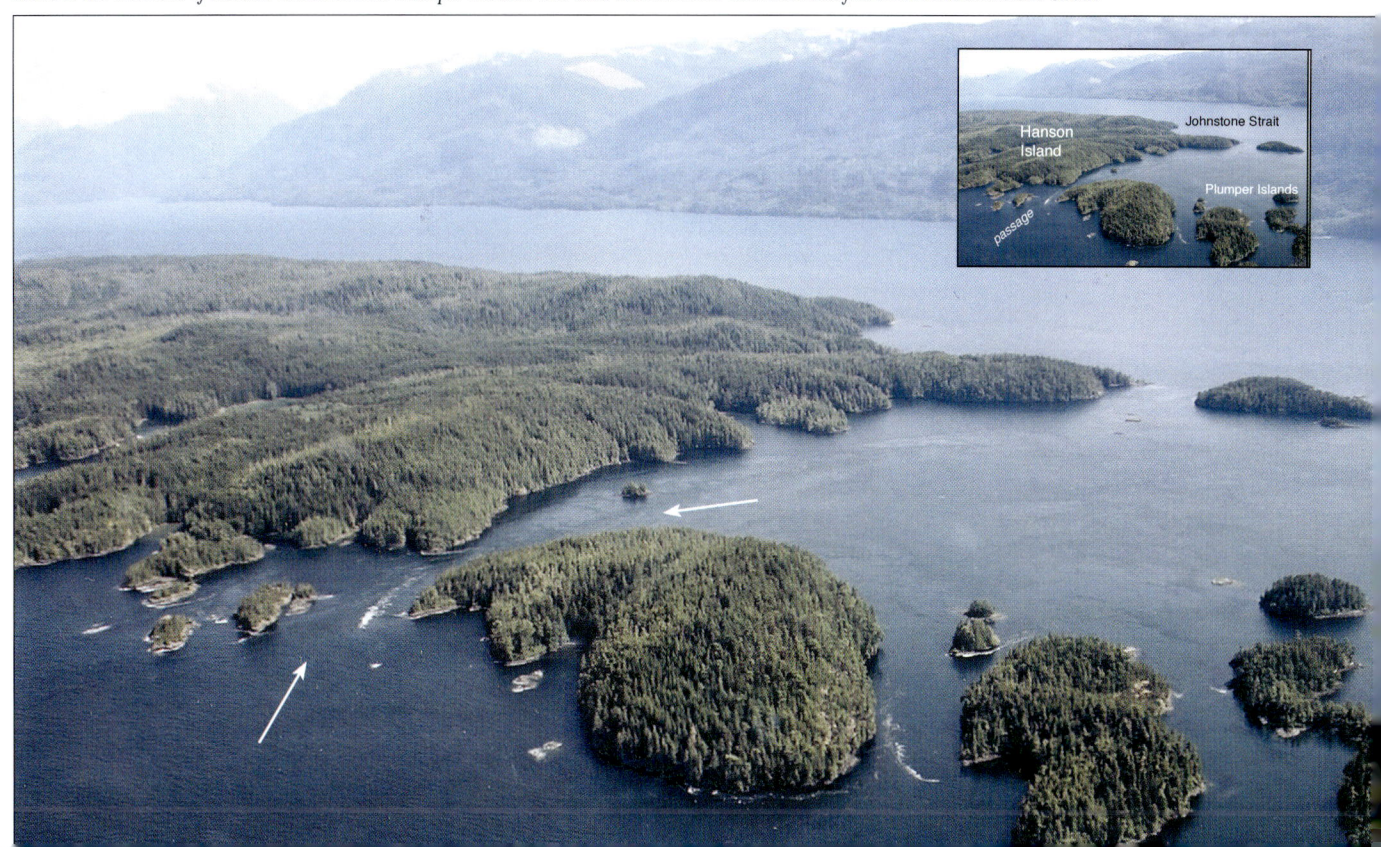

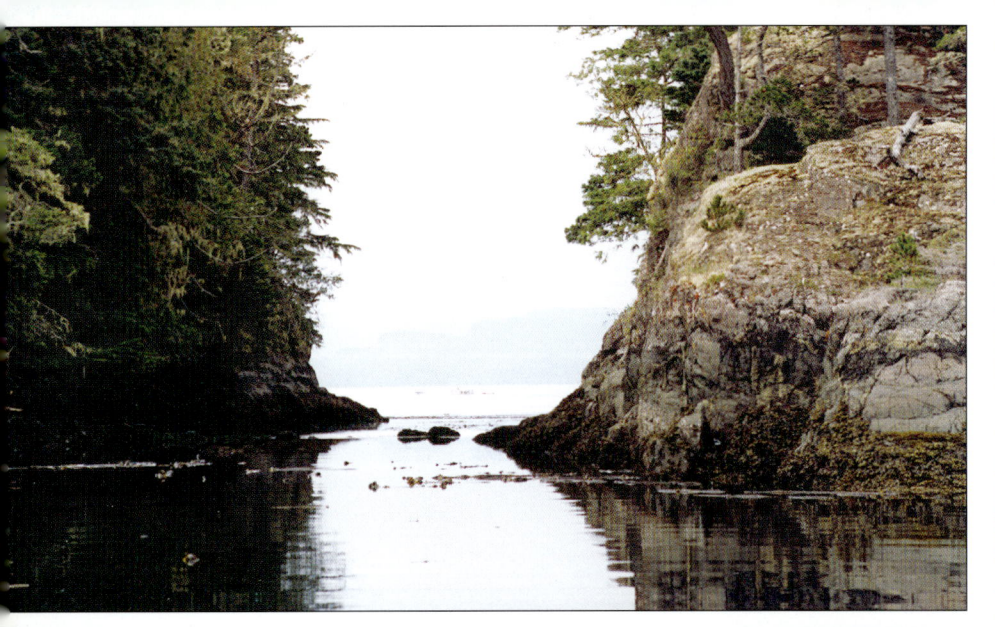

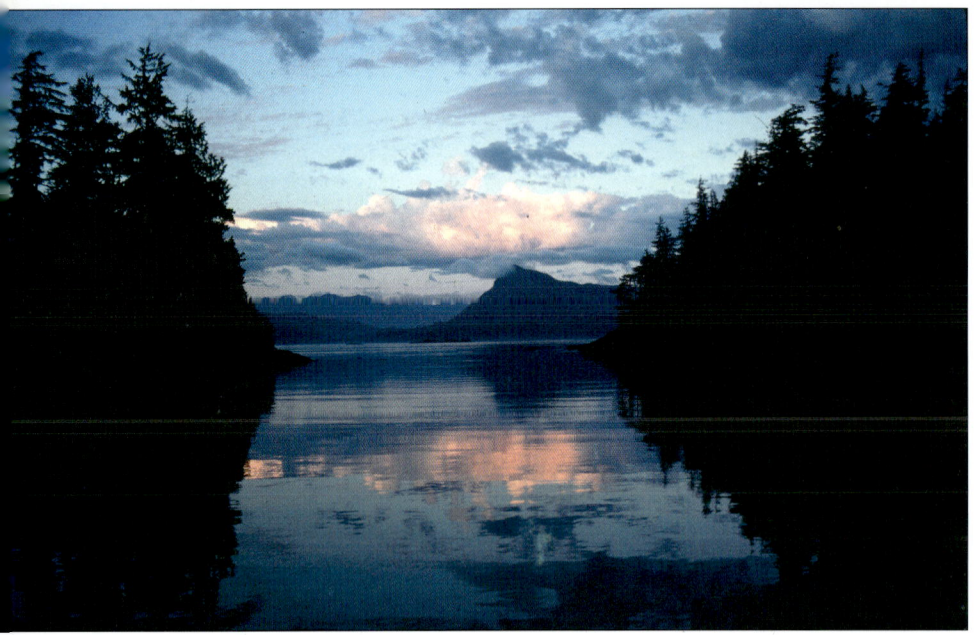

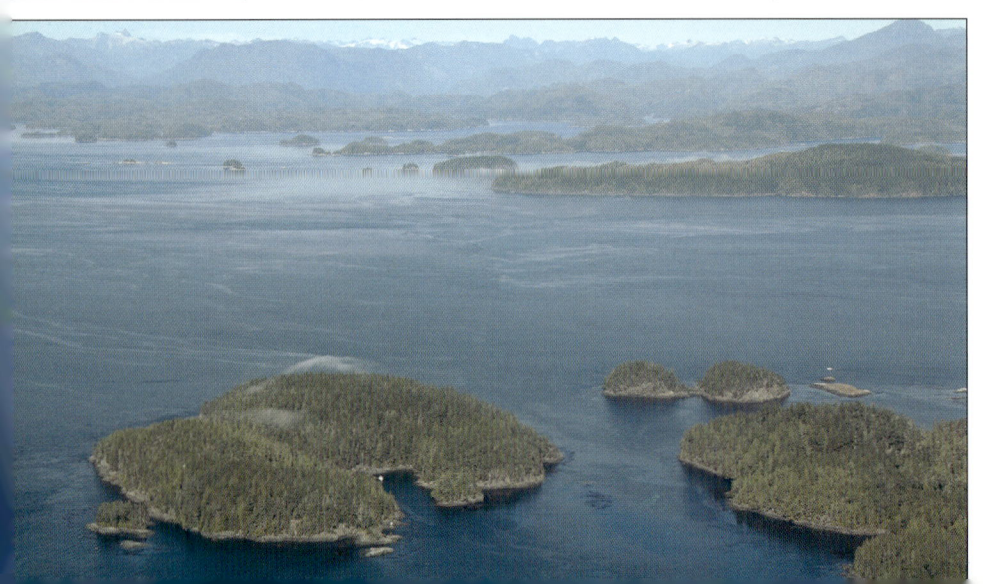

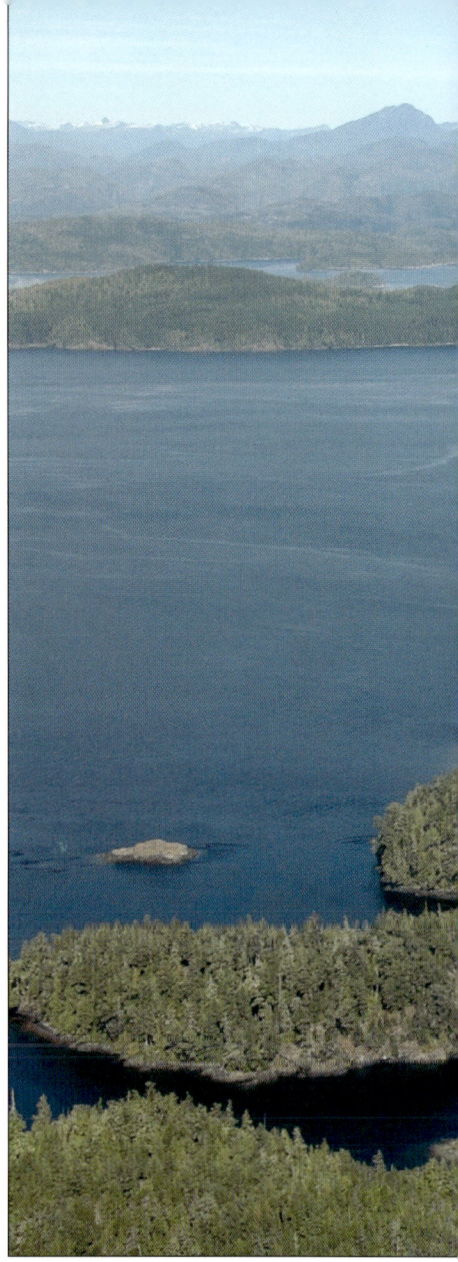

*Above: The inner Plumper Islands abutting Hanson Island with a light fog shrouding its north shore at the edge of Blackfish Sound. Note entrance to Farewell Harbour beyond. Left, top: Looking north through the non-navigable tidal passage from the anchorage between the outer two of the Plumper Islands. Left, centre: Looking towards Telegraph Cove at sunset from the anchorage in the gap between the outer Plumper Islands. Left, bottom: Anchored in the Plumper Islands. Right: Stubbs Island–the currents run fiercely around it. Far right: Scuba divers enter the water at Blackney Passage.*

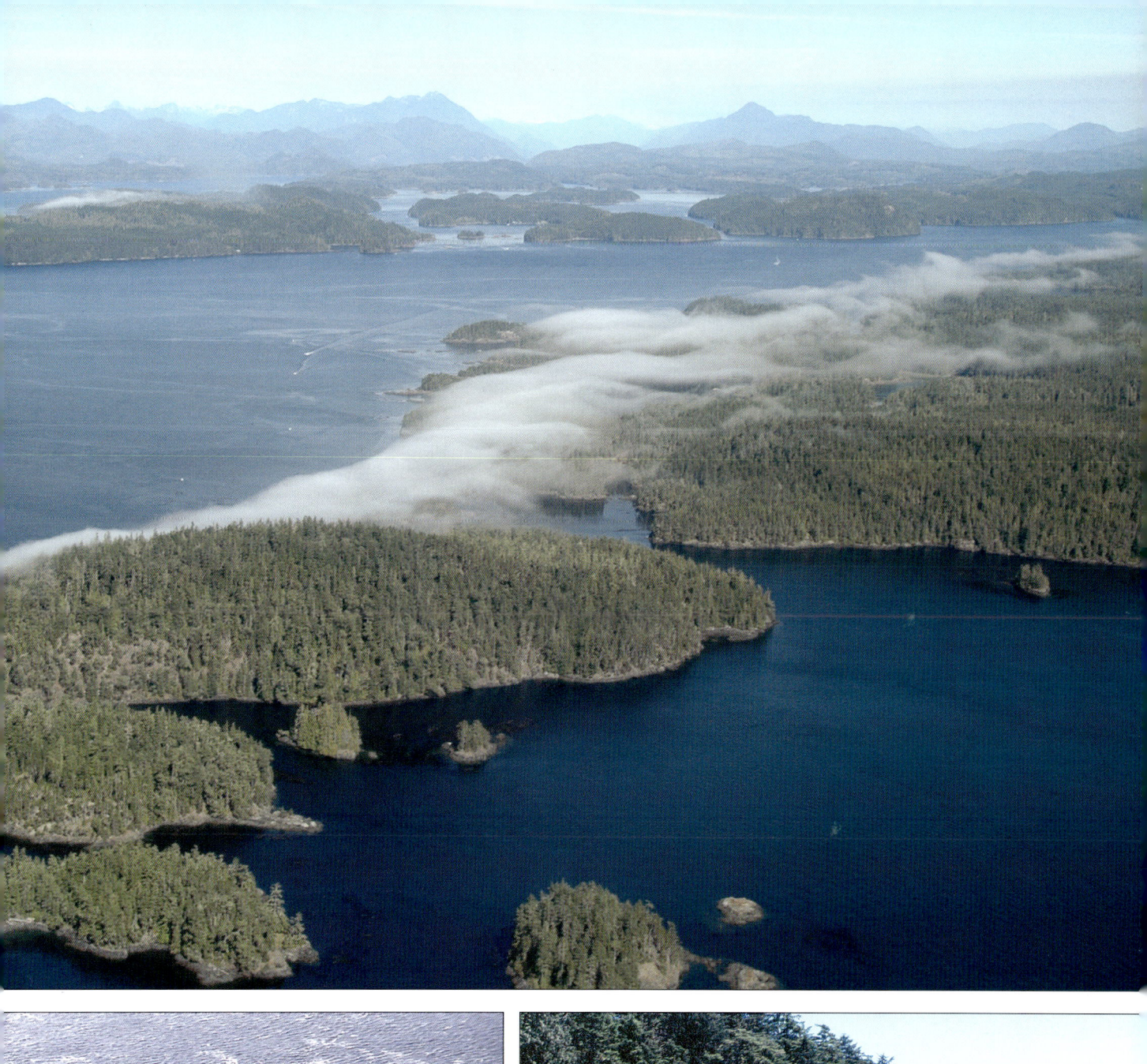

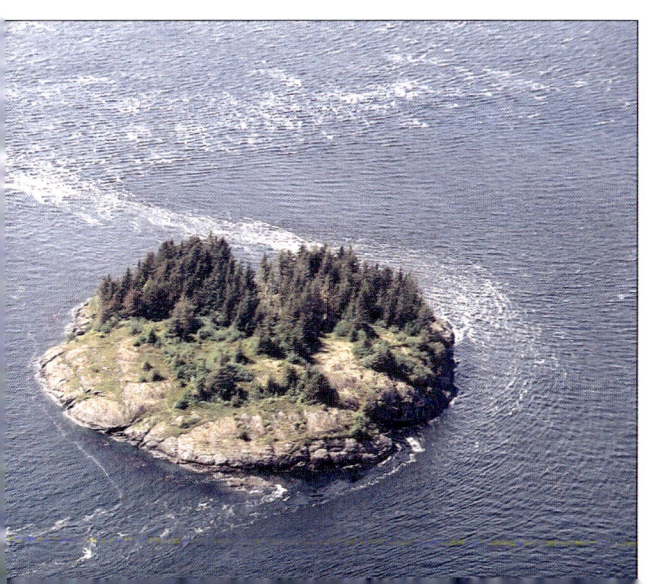

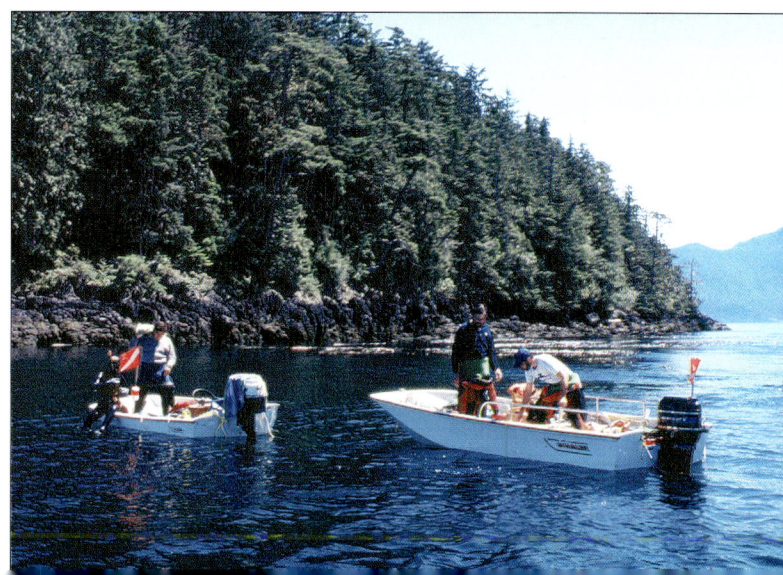

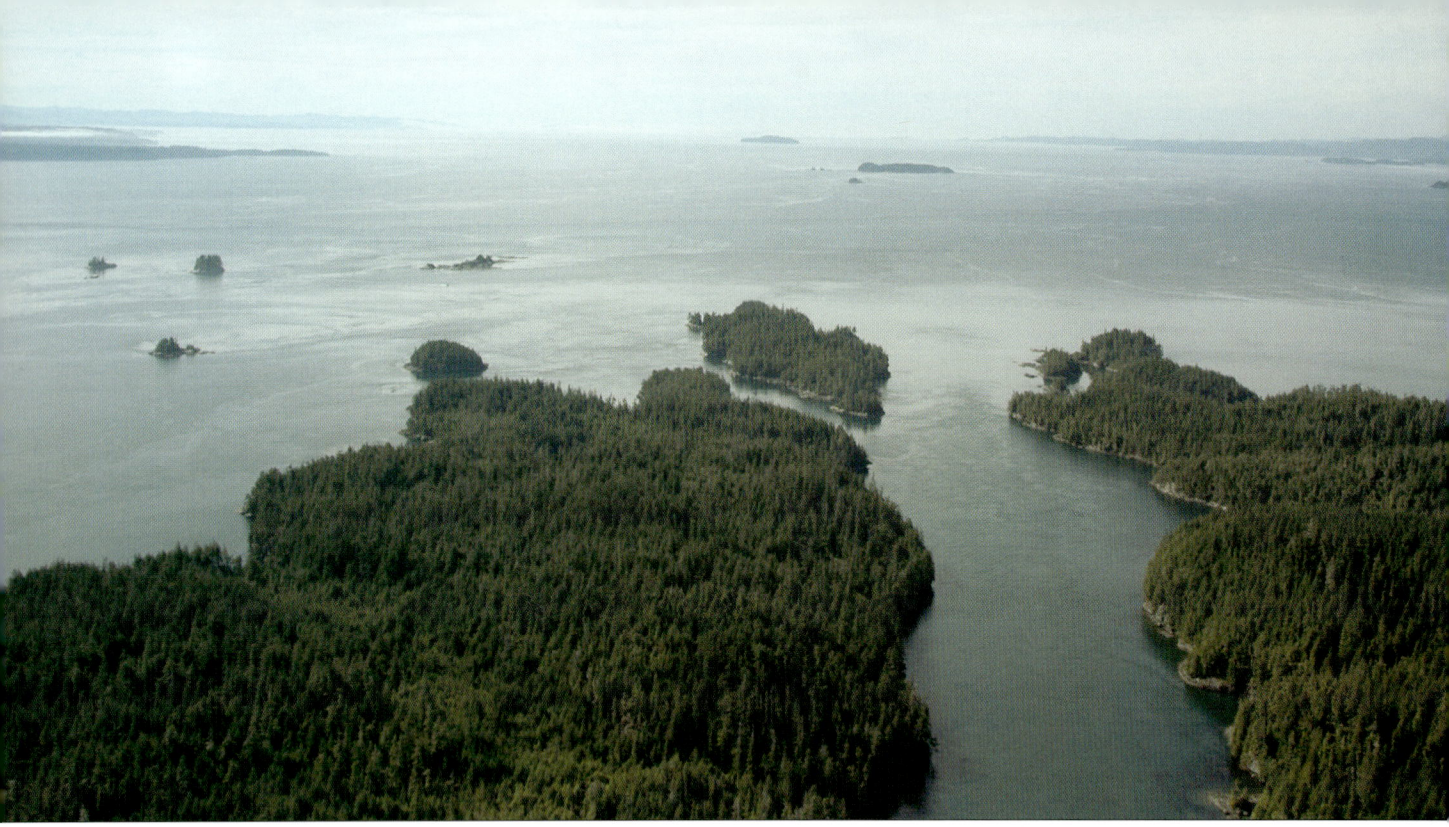

*Above: Midsummer Island, where Blackfish Sound meets Queen Charlotte Strait at the entrance to Knight Inlet. Below: Health Bay is also known as Gilford Village or 'Gwa yas dums'. The community welcomes visitors. A large gathering is held in June to commemmorate National Aboriginal Day.*

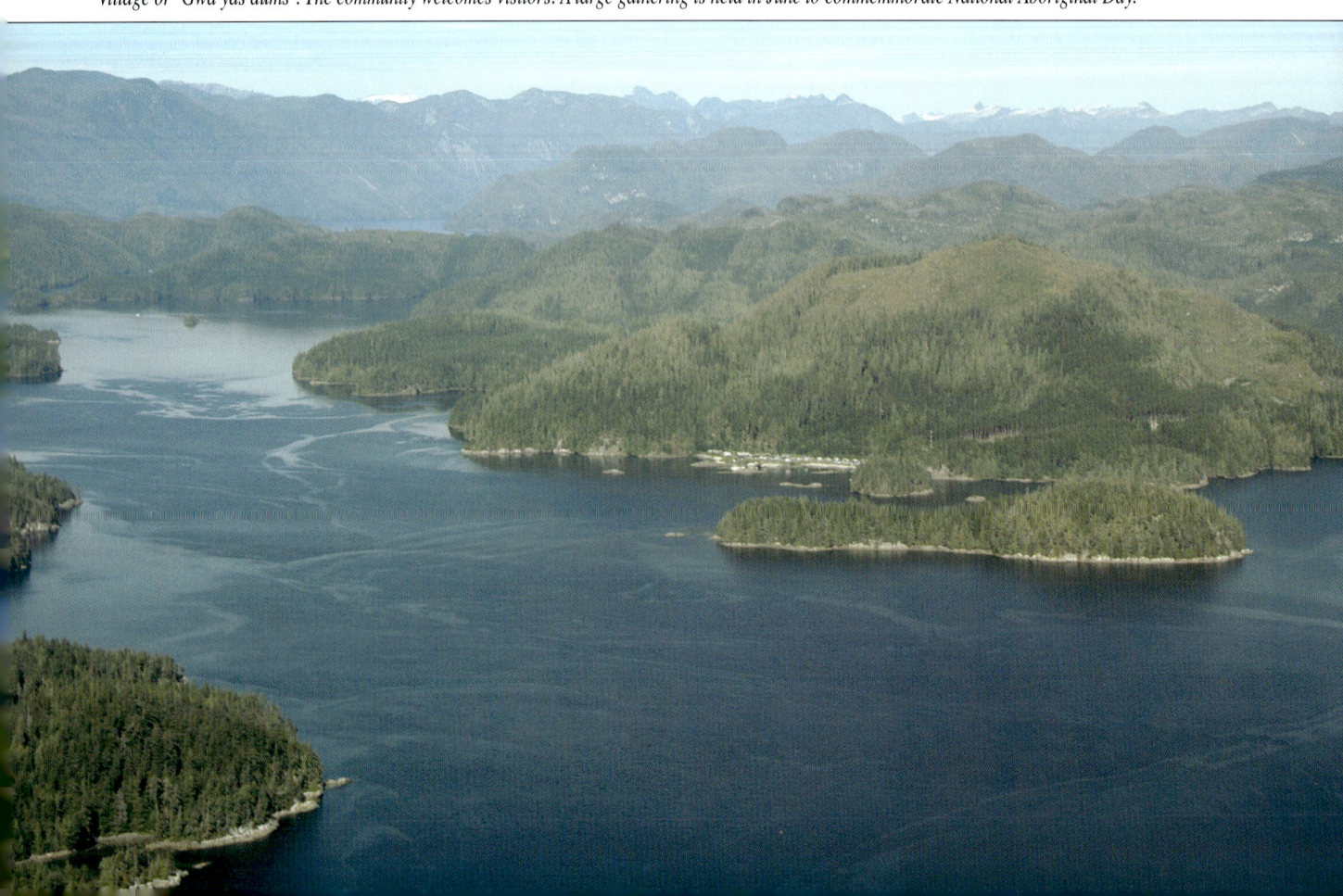

# Knight Inlet to Fife Sound
## Echo Bay via Gilford Village, Port Elizabeth and Retreat Passage

Charts 3515, 3545, 3546, 3547

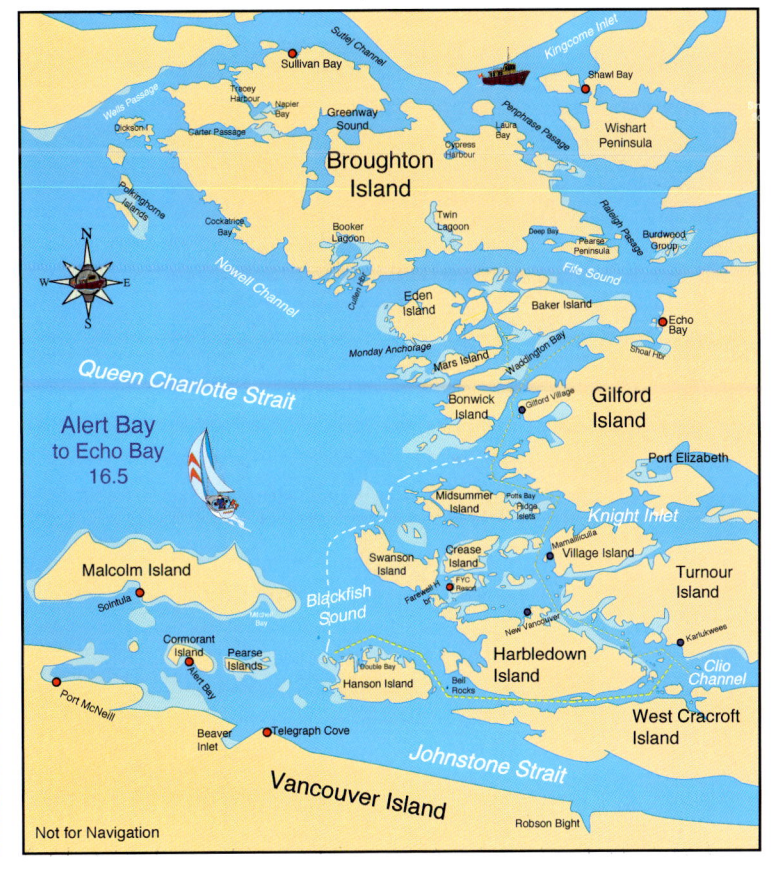

*If you wish to cruise directly to the Fife Sound area from Johnstone Strait, in calm weather make your way across Blackfish Sound from the Plumper Islands. Pass the western shore of Swanson Island to head up Retreat Passage on the way to more tranquil anchorages in the Broughtons or to the marina havens beyond. In inclement weather use the passages between the islands to reach your destination.*

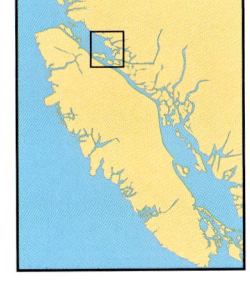

Travelling eastward into Knight Inlet mariners who know the area enjoy the majesty of the surrounding islands and mountains. Many stop in at Port Elizabeth while others venture beyond into the more remote reaches of the inlet, one of the longest on the coast. Spring Passage leads north from Knight Inlet as a major route for Mainlanders travelling between their homes and Johnstone Strait harbours.

(To differentiate from people who live in the north Vancouver Island area, such as at Telegraph Cove, those who live in the Broughton Islands and adjacent waterways refer to themselves as Mainlanders).

### Knight Inlet area  charts 3545, 3515

Old towboaters referred to the area as The Jungle, because of the profuse number of small independant logging operations, mostly around Knight and Kingcome Inlets. This was the centre of the float camp universe, with floating camp villages in Simoom Sound, Sullivan Bay, Claydon Bay and Minstrel Island, which at that time was its hub, the 'capital' of the region. The 1908 novel *Woodsmen of the West* by Martine Allerdale Grainger, had its setting at Minstrel Island.

Many yachtsmen have expounded on the marvels and beauty of the deep reaches of Knight Inlet with its lofty mountains. They are beautiful but most people prefer spending time among the group of islands, and in the small coastal communities where you can find comraderie among the permanent residents and the lore of the area. Anchorage in Knight Inlet is generally subject to weather, and there is plenty of wind and adverse conditions to make the experienced mariner either

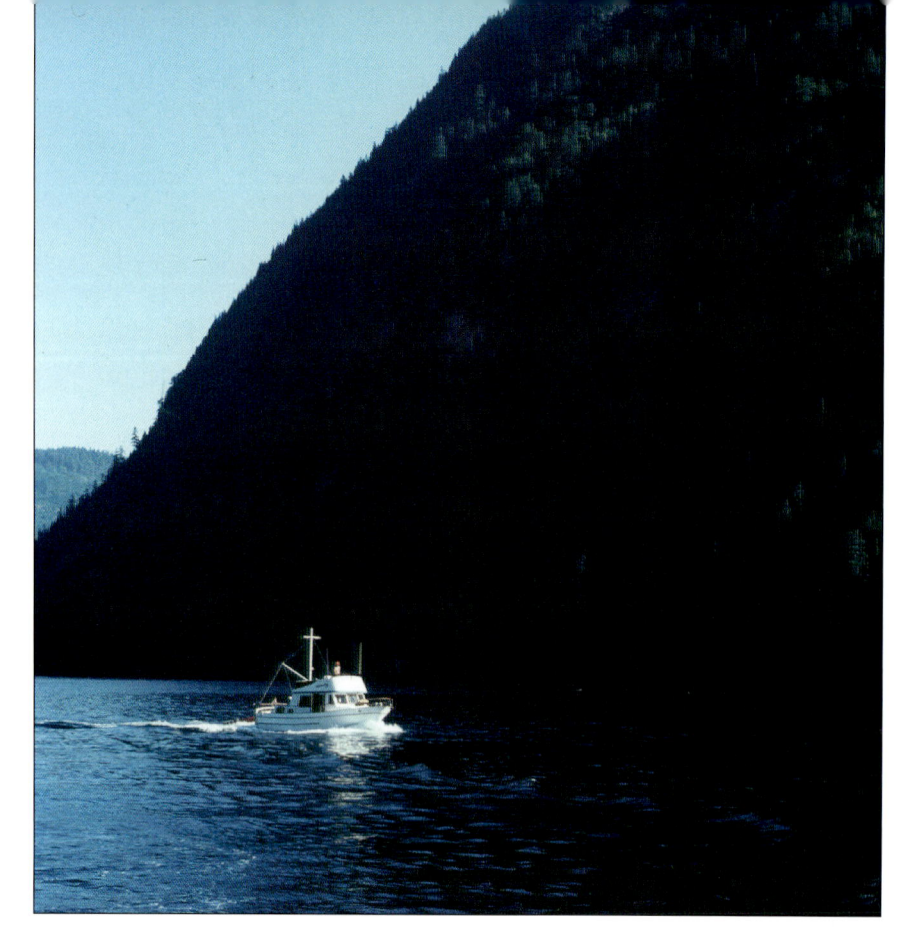

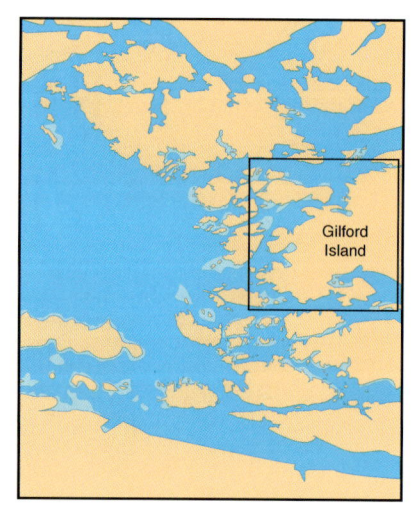

*How small a boat can look against the backdrop of even a relatively low mountain in the Broughton Islands area! This trawler is travelling west along Knight Inlet off Minstrel Island towards Village Island, thereby avoiding the navigational challenge of Beware Passage but missing out on the pristine anchorage at Potts Lagoon.*

stay out or go there knowing precisely what he or she is doing. An old settlement at **Glendale Cove** once attracted a fair amount of interest, and today while the remnants of industry are all but gone the activity in the cove has been replaced with a resort and whale and bear watching operation.

Most people going up Knight Inlet do so for the spectacular scenery and for the grizzly bear viewing at the head of the inlet or the whales that appear at times along the way. It is also renowned for its good fishing. But it's a long way up the inlet, and a long way back. About 70 nautical miles each way with frequent windy conditions and little shelter.

## Port Elizabeth   charts 3545, 3515

This large, mostly open port, lies near the mouth of Knight Inlet, about 10 nautical miles from Minstrel Island.

Travel down Knight Inlet from Minstrel Island in the direction of the delightful Village Island, for an easy, quick passage. Then enter the reef-strewn waters of the First Nations villages in the Village Group south of Knight Inlet where you may go ashore to look at the remnants of Mamalilaculla before continuing to Echo Bay. (See previous chapters.)

All too often we bypass Port Elizabeth in favour of smaller, cozier anchorages. Stop and check it out sometime.

Inside Port Elizabeth there are two anchorages that are readily accessible. **Duck Cove** at the west side of Port Elizabeth and **Maple Cove** at the entrance are the popular ones for small boats. Further anchorage can be found in the nook at the southeast corner of the bay near the end of the inlet. These anchorages are considered temporary so a careful watch should be kept in the event of winds. In an easterly blow favour the south shore. Maple Cove is suitable as an overnight stop only in ideal conditions. It's a fairly unprotected inlet due to the low-lying terrain surrounding it, particularly to the west. Best anchorage in Duck Cove is over mud, sand and gravel between the mainland and the small 47 metre high island shown on chart 3545. If you are a bird watcher you will find many of your favourite coastal species in Duck Cove.

## Midsummer Island   charts 3546, 3515

The islands at the entrance to Knight Inlet see a lot of open water action, making it best for the mariner to stay well inside during rough times in Queen Charlotte Strait. But when passage is calm there are all sorts of narrow channels and rock-lined short cuts between the larger passages. Knight Inlet to Bonwick Island and Waddington Bay offers the choice of following the larger Spring Passage into Retreat Passage, or taking the tighter but safer (from seas coming in off Queen Charlotte Strait) route skirting along the western shore of Gilford Island, passing on the east side of Henrietta Island and Seabreeze Island and then Sail Island taking in a view of or visiting Health Bay First Nations village. **Potts Bay** on Midsummer Island is protected by a chain of small islets and

114

## Map Labels (Top Map)

Tribune Channel
Fife Sound
Viner Sound
Davies Island
Baker Island
Blackney Pass to Cramer Pass Via Farewell Hbr, Knight Inlet, Retreat Passage 15.8
Scott Cove
Echo Bay
Cramer Passage
Gilford Island
Fox Group N 50°43.185' W126°34.975'
False Cove
Shoal Harbour
(Bootleg Bay)
Fox Group
Retreat Passage
Meade Bay
Bootleg Bay N 50°42.962' W126°34.2772'
Gilford Village (Gwa-yas-dums)
Sail I
Health Lagoon
Maple Cove
Health Bay
Gwa-yas-dums N 50°41.785' W126°35.892'
Duck Cove
Port Elizabeth
Henrietta I
There is a fish farm located in Potts Bay on Midsummer Island
Chop Bay
Tribune Pt
Gilford Point
Port Elizabeth N 50°39.092' W126°25.421'
Spring Passage
Potts Bay
Ridge Islets
Knight Inlet
Lady Is

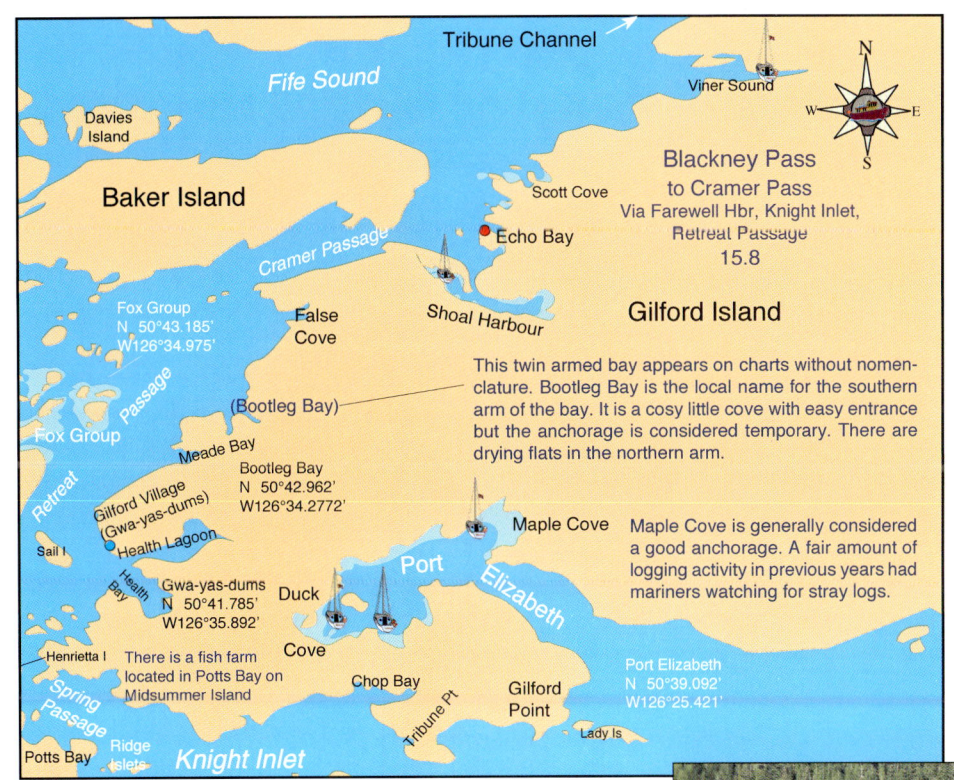

This twin armed bay appears on charts without nomenclature. Bootleg Bay is the local name for the southern arm of the bay. It is a cosy little cove with easy entrance but the anchorage is considered temporary. There are drying flats in the northern arm.

Maple Cove is generally considered a good anchorage. A fair amount of logging activity in previous years had mariners watching for stray logs.

**FOG CAUTION:** *"Coming out of Eliot Passage at Village Island where we had been in glorious sun, we were suddenly in dense fog, and had to take refuge in Potts Bay on the north side of Midsummer Island until it cleared"* —from the journal of fellow mariner, Chris Fraser.

*Below: Health Bay on Gilford Island is the location of an inhabited First Nations village called Gwa-yas-dums. It is also the name of the bay adjacent to Health Lagoon. Visiting these villages or the remains of abandoned ones should be done with consideration and care, and with the permission of those to whom they belong.*

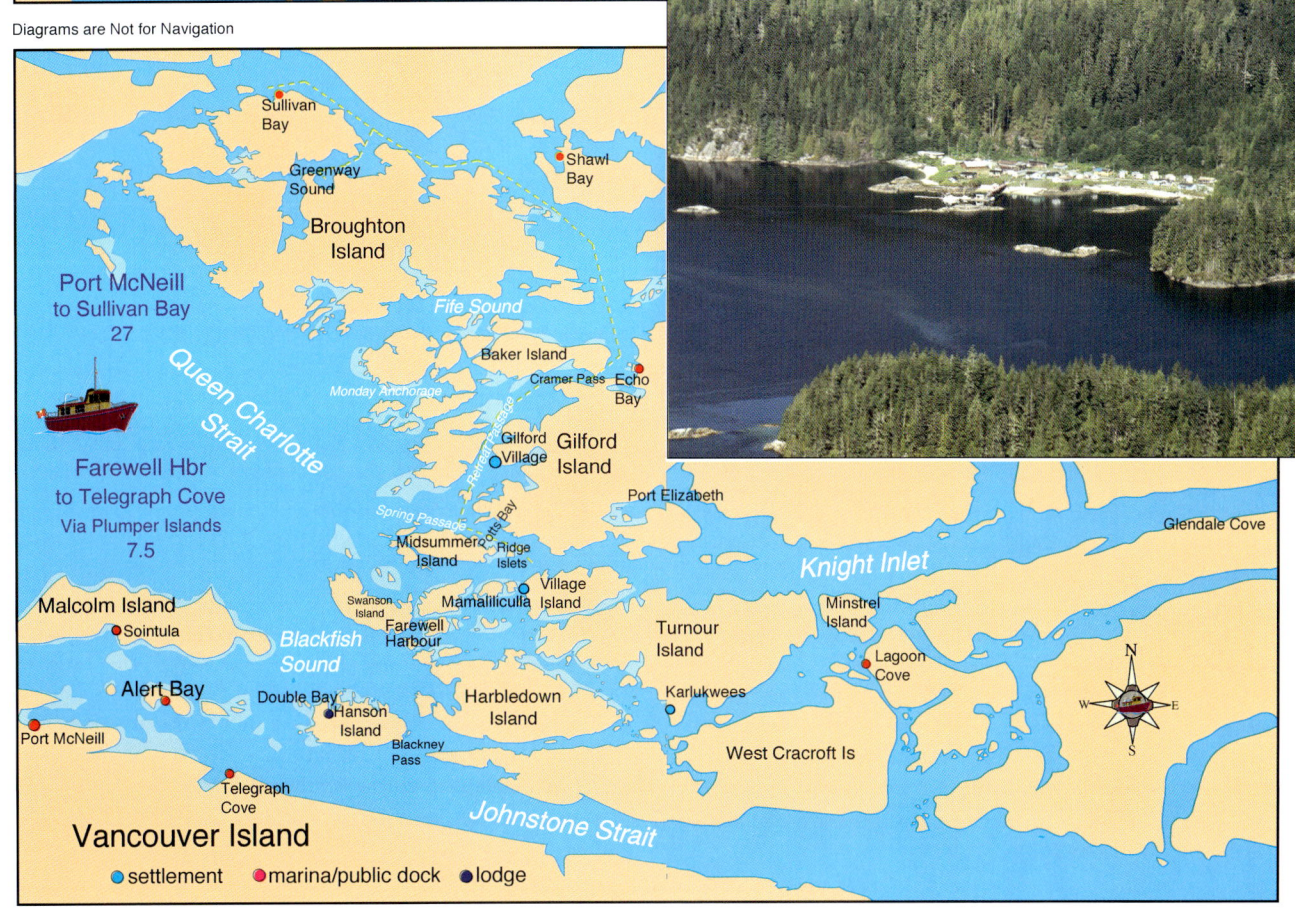

Diagrams are Not for Navigation

## Map Labels (Bottom Map)

Sullivan Bay
Shawl Bay
Greenway Sound
Broughton Island
Port McNeill to Sullivan Bay 27
Fife Sound
Baker Island
Monday Anchorage
Cramer Pass
Echo Bay
Queen Charlotte Strait
Gilford Village
Gilford Island
Farewell Hbr to Telegraph Cove Via Plumper Islands 7.5
Port Elizabeth
Glendale Cove
Spring Passage
Midsummer Island
Ridge Islets
Malcolm Island
Sointula
Swanson Island
Mamaliliculla
Village Island
Turnour Island
Knight Inlet
Minstrel Island
Blackfish Sound
Farewell Harbour
Lagoon Cove
Alert Bay
Double Bay
Hanson Island
Harbledown Island
Karlukwees
Port McNeill
Blackney Pass
West Cracroft Is
Telegraph Cove
Vancouver Island
Johnstone Strait

● settlement  ● marina/public dock  ● lodge

115

**Waddington Bay** Use charts 3515, 3546, 3547

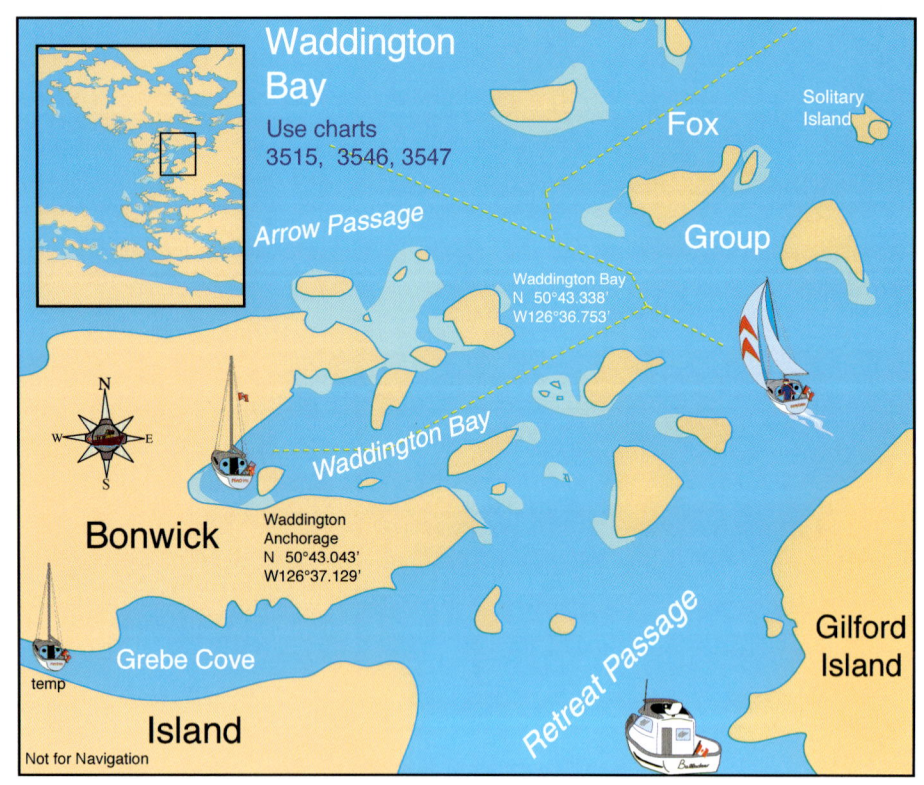

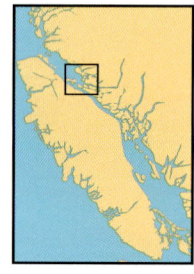

*Map labels: Arrow Passage, Fox Group, Solitary Island, Waddington Bay N 50°43.338' W126°36.753', Waddington Bay, Bonwick Island, Waddington Anchorage N 50°43.043' W126°37.129', Grebe Cove (temp), Retreat Passage, Gilford Island. Not for Navigation.*

*One of the most popular anchorages in the Broughton Archipelago is in Waddington Bay. Drop the hook in 5 to 8 metres over a muddy bottom. The favoured shore is north of the small island that dominates the inside cove. It is a good anchorage but northwest winds do blow in over the low hills at the head of the bay.*
*Photograph left top taken from the inner part of Waddington Bay.*
*Bottom: On an islet at the entrance to the bay. Nearby Grebe Cove is not ideal but has a good bottom. It would be wise to use a shore line if anchoring there.*

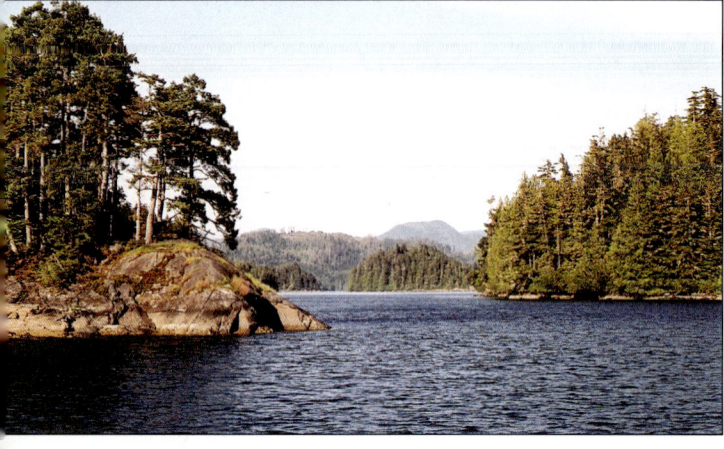

rocks but the flood and ebb wash the area with currents from the tide running through the bay. A fish farm lease is located there. The Ridge Islets are also subject to strong currents.

### Health Bay   charts 3546, 3545, 3515

On the west side of Gilford Island Health Bay will hold several boats in a protected anchorage, although an anchor watch should be maintained in the event of northwesterly winds. Health Lagoon is shallow and muddy and may be suitable only for excursions in a kayak at higher tides.

### Gilford Island Village   charts 3546, 3545, 3515

**Gwa-yas-dums**, also known as Health Bay or Gilford Island Village is a thriving settlement despite the relative abandonment of other First Nations villages in the area. New developments have been taking place there and we have seen a lot of activity as we passed by. Visitors are welcome and there are regular festivities in which to participate.

The passage on the east side of Sail Island is suitable for navigation. Watch for the rock that stands out far into the passage from the south shore of the reserve. This village celebrates National Aboriginal Day on the 21st of June each year when all comers are welcome.

The First Nations name for the village is Gwa-yas-dums. Traditional food, story telling and games for children are part of the day's events. The Big House is open to all and visitors get to wear traditional masks and regalia. Look for the Welcome Figure (totem) in front of the houses, at the top of the dock.

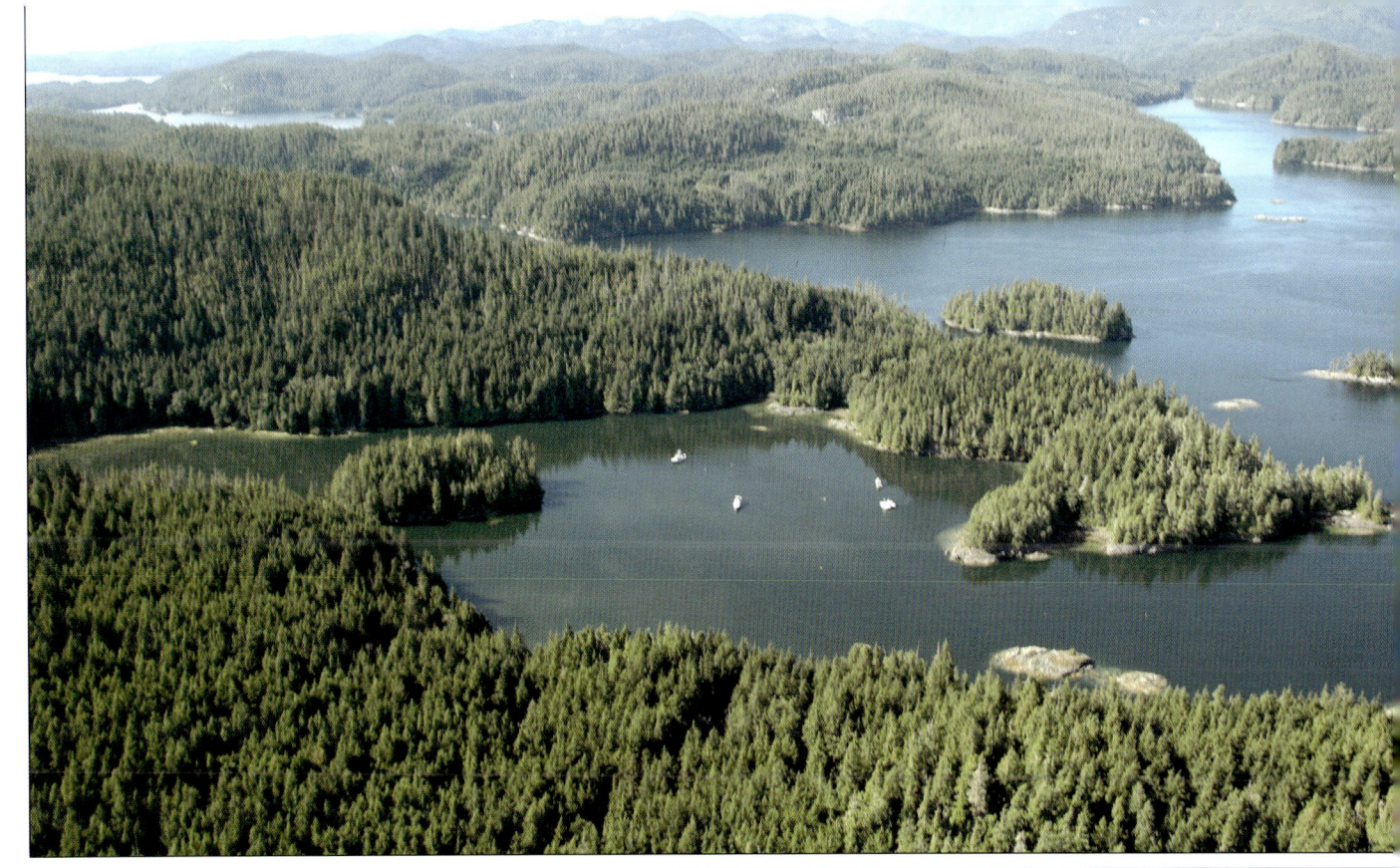

When crossing Knight Inlet and entering Spring Passage be mindful of Ridge Rock in mid channel and a cluster of submerged rocks around a small islet and exposed rock just beyond. To avoid this hazard we usually skim by the east end of Ridge Islets just off the east shore of Midsummer Island or between them and Midsummer Island with careful reference to the chart.

## Waddington Bay  charts 3515, 3546, 3547

After travelling past Gilford Village continue up Retreat Passage towards the Fox Group off the north end of Bonwick Island. Enter the east-west passage south of the Fox Group from either Arrow Pass or Retreat Pass and take the entrance southwestward into the bay.

It's easy to move into the bay's protected anchorage by following the fairly straight waterway with depths of 13 metres, quite constant, most of the way. Navigate carefully between the islands that hug the entrance. The bay opens up and anchorage can be taken anywhere around the island in the inner section of the bay. Waddington Bay has depths of 2 to 8 metres at low water in which to anchor. The bottom is muddy and you may have a job of washing down your anchor after sitting on the hook for a while.

In Retreat Passage **Carrie Bay, Grebe Cove** and **Meade Bay** are not ideal for anchorage and are best left to the locals who know what weather is suitable for using them. Those

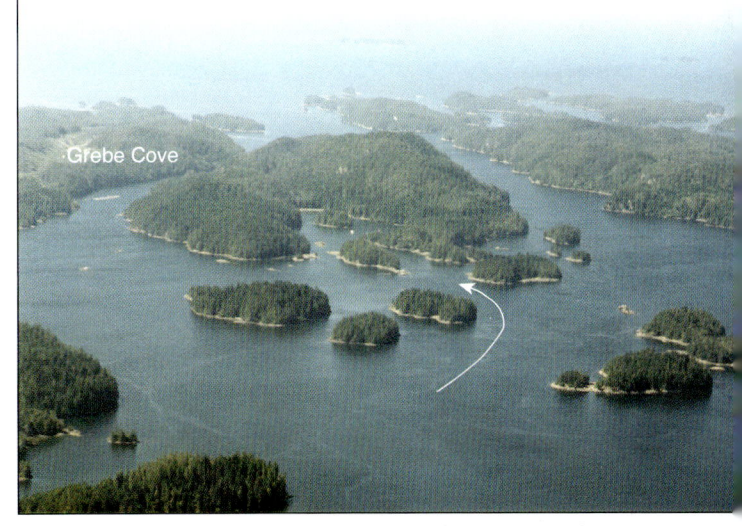

*Above: Waddington Bay can be seen in the centre of the top photograph. The lower photo shows islands at the entrance to the bay. Enter through the passages as shown in the diagram, opposite.*

who know the bays use them temporarily, and then only when the weather permits (diagrams page 116, 118, 119, 122). The southern portion of **Bootleg Bay**, (diagram page 118) is a cosy little cove. It has a narrow entrance but deep enough for passage at 6 to 13 metres. Some winds stir the anchorage at times. Anchor in 5 metres.

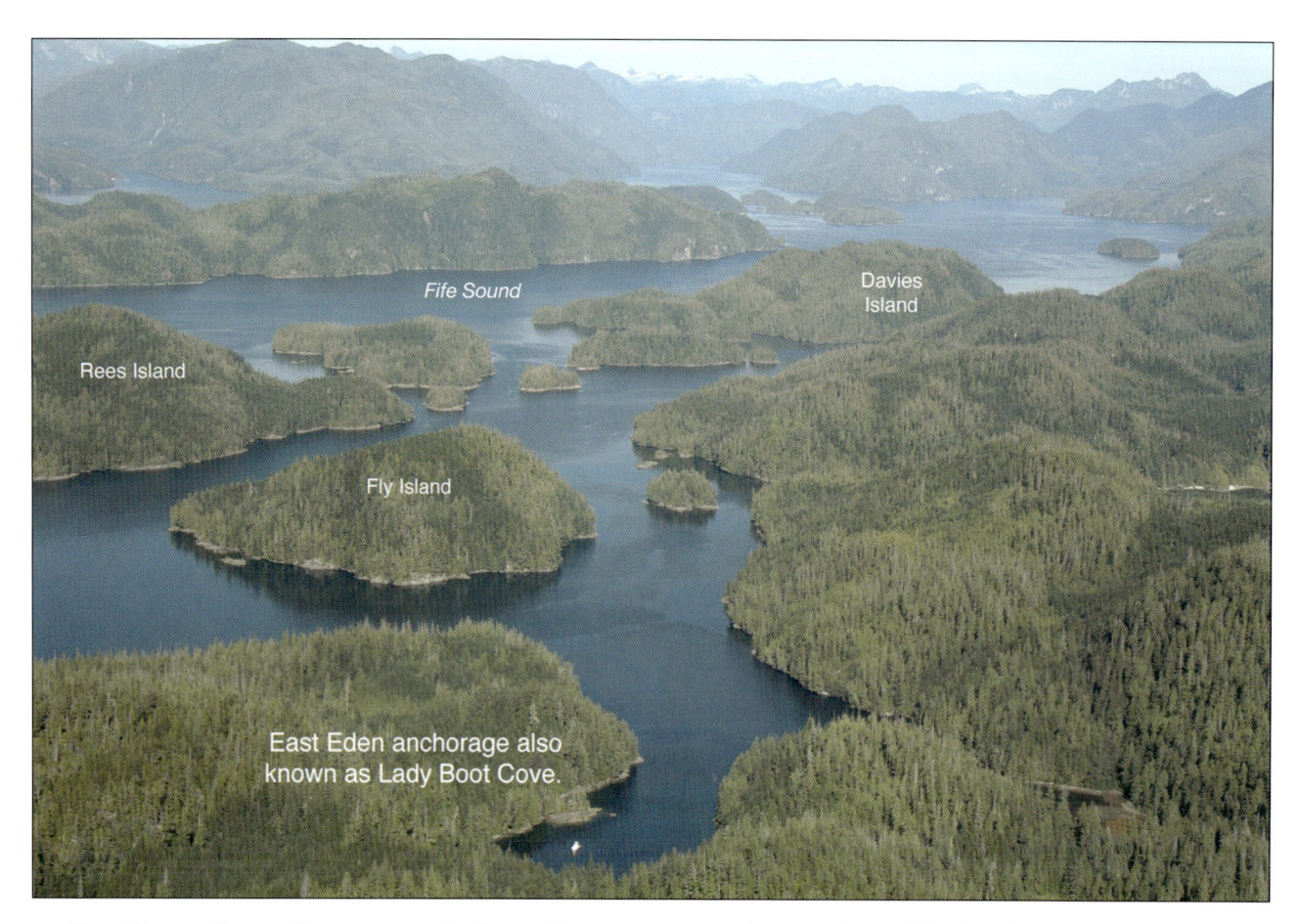

*Photo labels: Fife Sound; Davies Island; Rees Island; Fly Island; East Eden anchorage also known as Lady Boot Cove.*

Travelling up Retreat Passage towards Cramer Passage out of Waddington Bay you can cut through between the Fox Group and pass between Browne Rock to your starboard and the rocks and reef off Steep Islet to your port. Browne Rock can be a challenge. We have travelled past it without seeing any sign of it at times and at other times detected it by kelp on the surface. If you are uncomfortable with this passage, use Retreat Passage along the west shore of Gilford Island. Pass Solitary Islet either side and stay well to the right of Browne Rock taking a bearing on the tip of the islands off Isle Point. Curve around Browne Rock maintaining a course past False Cove close to those islets.

At the entrance to Cramer Passage you are also at the point where a turn to the west will take you to Monday Anchorage and the outer islands that are washed by the southeastern fetch of Queen Charlotte Strait. You could also travel up into this area around the outside from Spring Passage out of Knight Inlet. Do so only in calm conditions.

Pass the south side of Steep Islet and enter Blunden Passage to take you around Tracey Island into Monday Anchorage. The passages that lead to Fife Sound at George Point (diagram page 121) at the western tip of Baker Island make this excursion well worthwhile. Old Passage is a gorgeous, narrow "lane," wide and deep enough for most boats. The passage between Insect Island and Eden Island is also passable but not as well used as Old Passage. Mind the reefs at the north end. An anchorage opens into the north end of Eden Island, protected by Fly Island. This anchorage, **East Eden** is commonly referred to as **Lady Boot Cove** for its shape. Good anchorage can be found in the northern toe of the cove in about 5 metres. Misty Passage is wider than Old Passage but also very picturesque with a slight hint of ocean swells during relatively calm weather. The reward for a trip down Misty Passage is the anchorage at **Joe Cove.**

Using Queen Charlotte Strait from Spring Passage to these nooks and open, rather exposed Sunday Harbour and Monday Anchorage, you will pass the dubious anchorage at **Dusky Cove**. Travel on the west side of Bonwick Island by taking a rather tortuous route past High Island. It can be done easily enough with very careful navigation, in calm weather.

If you are looking for relaxation, use a route away from the dangers of the rocks and reefs off southwest Bonwick Island. If the weather is calm and you wish to go from Spring Passage to Arrow Passage then consider the waterway on the inside of the Sedge Islands south of High Island.

Crossing Arrow Passage you can enter Sunday Harbour or Monday Anchorage through Spiller Passage between Hudson and Mars islands.

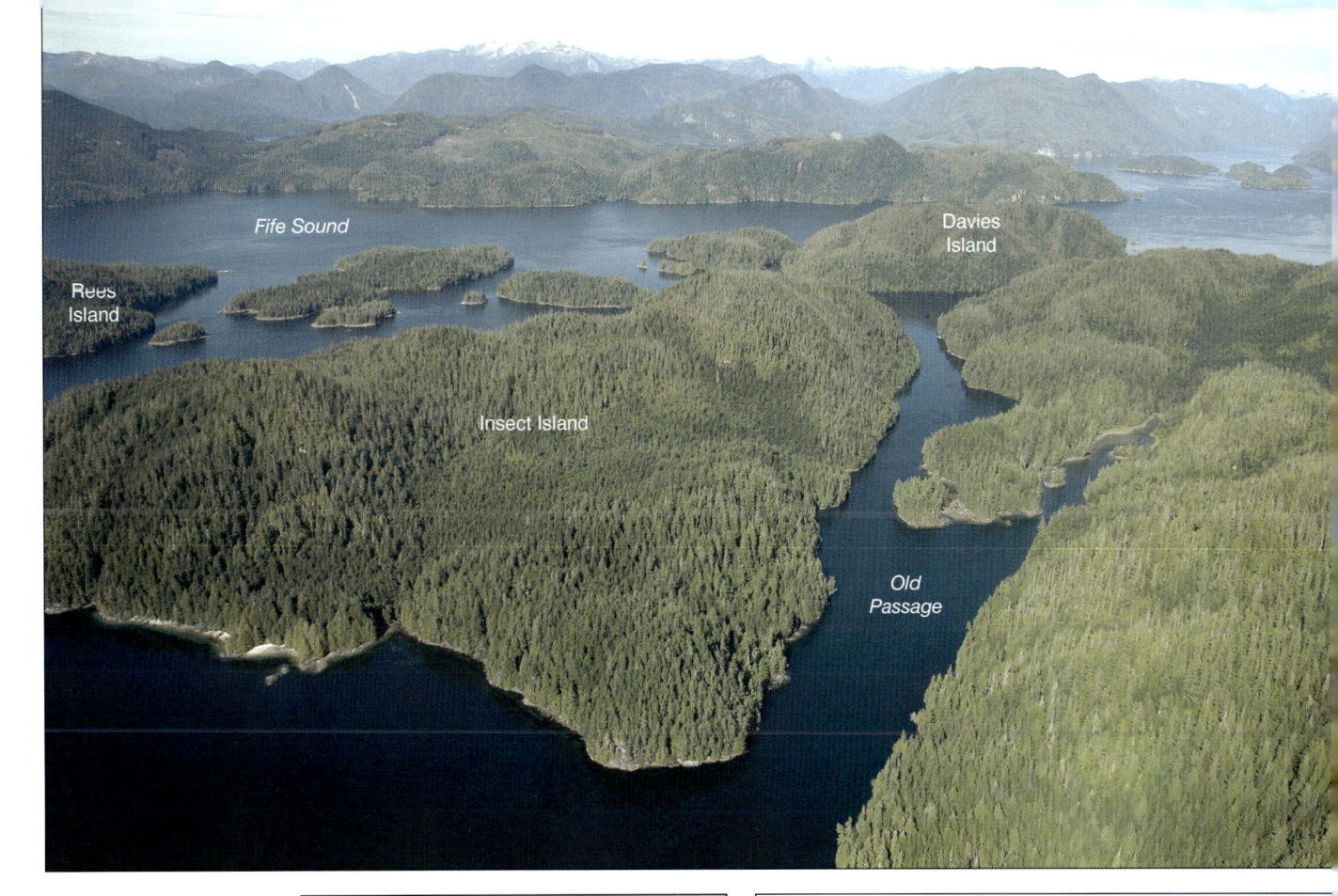

*Opposite: East Eden anchorage. Above: Old Passage with Fife Sound beyond. Right: Looking eastward into Monday Anchorage. Far right: Sunday Harbour and the entrance to Arrow Passage with references to the islands in the diagram below.*

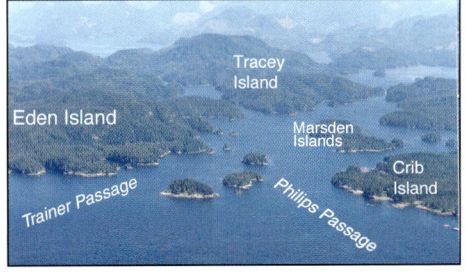

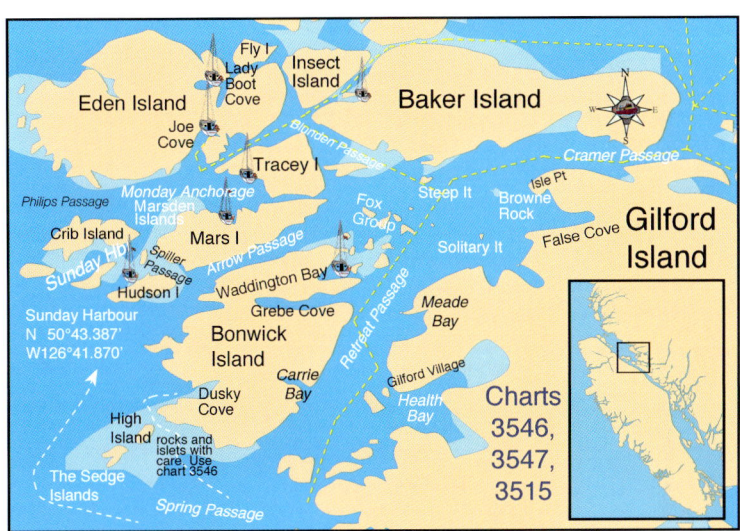

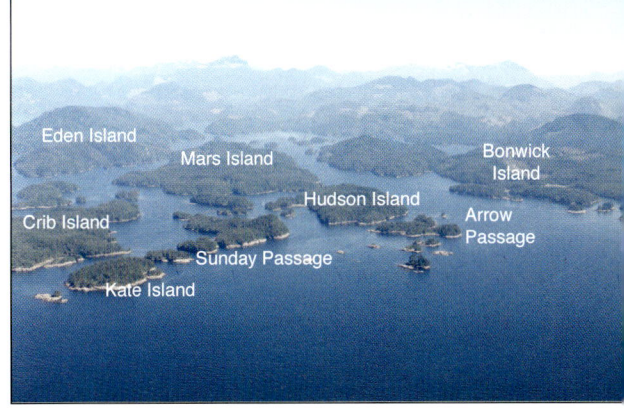

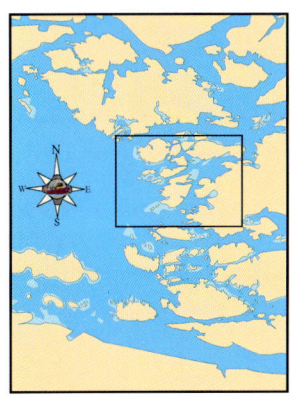

*Diagrams: Navigating northwards along the exposed west side of the Broughtons can take you past the Sedge Islands, Coach Islets and High Island, to Arrow Passage and Spiller Passage bound for Sunday Harbour.*

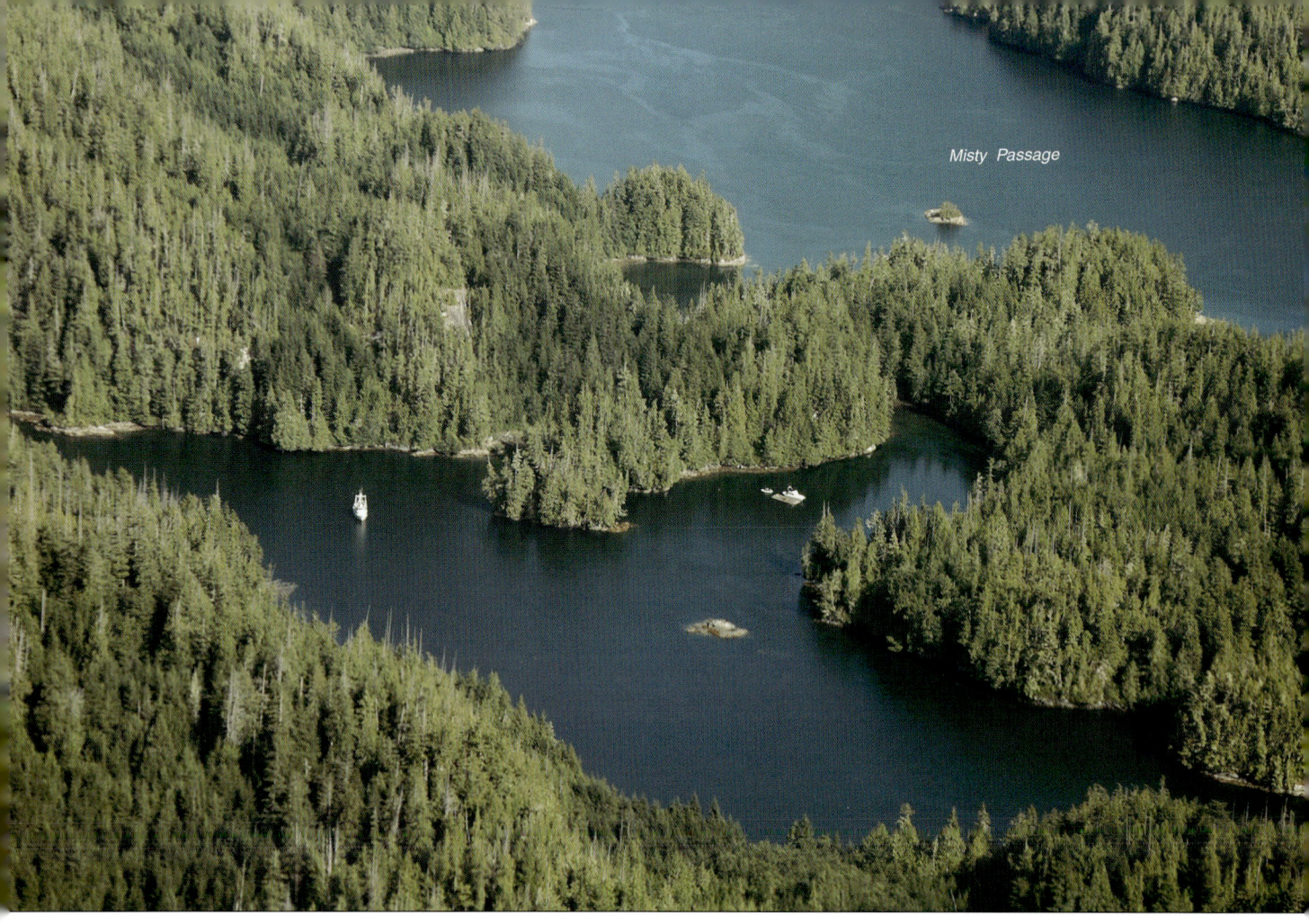

*Above: Misty Passage (and East Eden or Lady Boot Cove) almost connect with the anchorage in Joe Cove on Eden Island.*

## Eden Island
### Joe Cove chart 3547, 3515

This entire group of islands is a lovely area and well worth exploring. The most promising anchorage is in Joe Cove that opens into the south side of Eden Island. It is an easy entrance to the inlet. Deep inside the inlet the anchorage is good for half a dozen boats with the best spot in a small nook that opens off to the east.

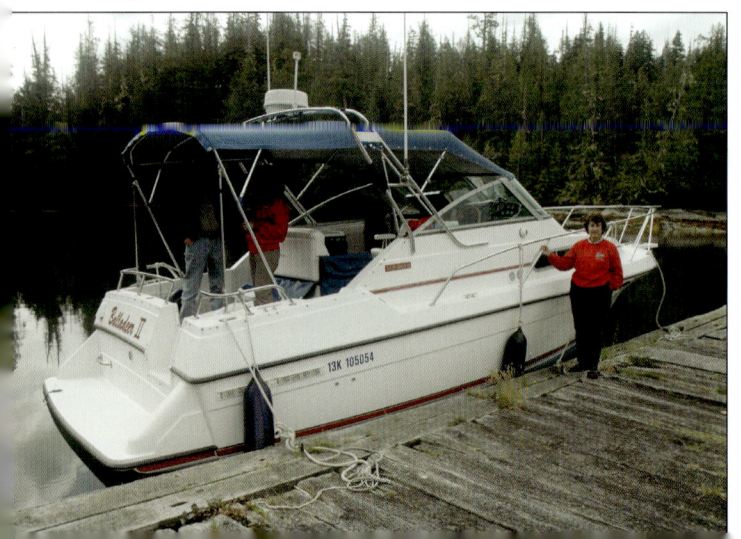

With care it is possible to easily enter this nook. Just be wary of the rocks protecting it. The anchorage is well sheltered from most winds but keep a watch during strong southwesterlies. Use large scale chart 3547. There is a raft anchored in the middle of the nook to which several boats could moor. Take your dinghy to the northern corner and walk the trail along the creek to a small lake half way between Joe Cove and Eden Island East (Lady Boot Cove).

### East Eden charts 3546, 3547, 3515

If you find yourself on the north side of Eden Island and in search of a place to anchor, try Eden East Cove, the inlet to the southwest of Fly Island. It reaches down and almost connects to Joe Cove. This anchorage is one of the better ones in the vicinity. Its far reaches are sheltered from practically all winds, even though getting through the entrance in windy conditions may leave you wondering. The large scale chart 3547 will help you wend your way out of Fife Sound or through the channels and passages around the Benjamin Group to reach this anchorage.

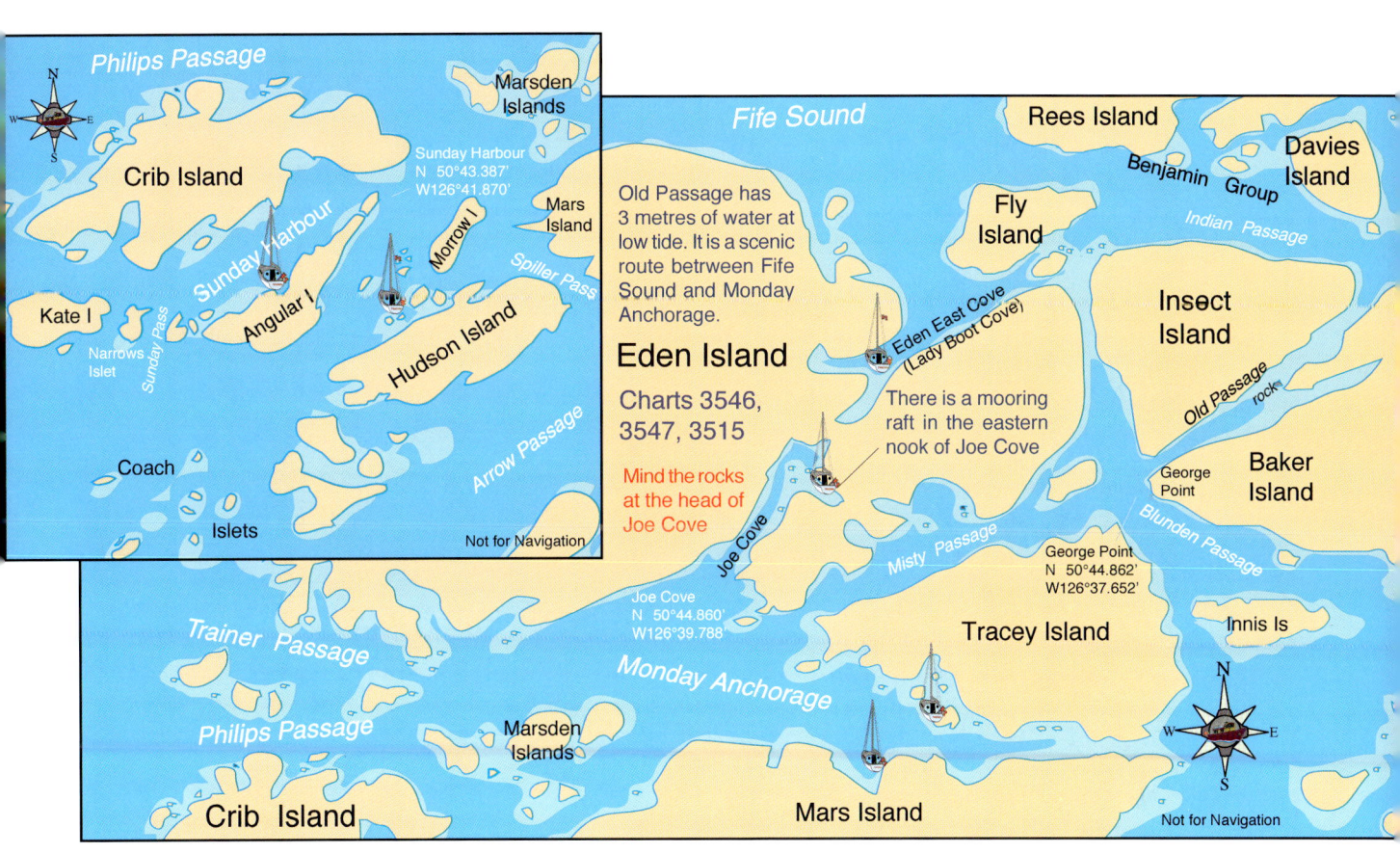

## Monday Anchorage   charts 3546, 3547, 3515

North of Mars Island is Monday Anchorage, a large open bay that affords some shelter in calm conditions. It is a large harbour capable of accommodating numerous pleasure craft, preferably in settled weather conditions because of its exposure to westerly winds.

Southeasterlies can be uncomfortable because of the way they sometimes are deflected off the slopes of Tracey Island into the anchorage.

The best, albeit temporary, anchorage is among the islets south of Tracey Island or the deep indent into Mars Island. This can be a busy, but seldom too crowded anchorage when lots of boats are about in mid summer. The nearest good shelter is at Joe Cove or Waddington Bay.

## Sunday Harbour   charts 3546, 3547, 3515

Some mariners choose to cruise the outer islands of Bonwick and Mars Islands. Here you will find myriad tricky passages, rocks and reefs combined with swell movement from Queen Charlotte Strait.

There are no anchorages in this area except a questionable temporary one in Sunday Harbour between Crib and Angular Islands.

*Right: Looking east over Joe Cove towards Fly Island and Rees Island in Fife Sound. Opposite: Tied up to a raft in the nook at Joe Cove.*

Some yachtsmen have taken shelter in the lee of **Hudson Island**, entering south of Morrow Island from Spiller Passage. Others choose Sunday Harbour. This is for the adventuresome type, those who don't mind sitting up all night on a dubious anchor watch. I would recommend anchoring in Waddington Bay and exploring the outer islands in a fast runabout during ideal conditions. An option is to cross Fife Sound and find anchorage in Cullen Harbour.

The best entrance to Sunday Harbour to ensure minimal affect of swells is from the east. Go around the rocks off the tip of Crib Island and then follow the centre of the harbour. Anchor in the nook on **Angular Island**. On a nice day the islands between Angular Island and Hudson Island look like a scene in the tropics.

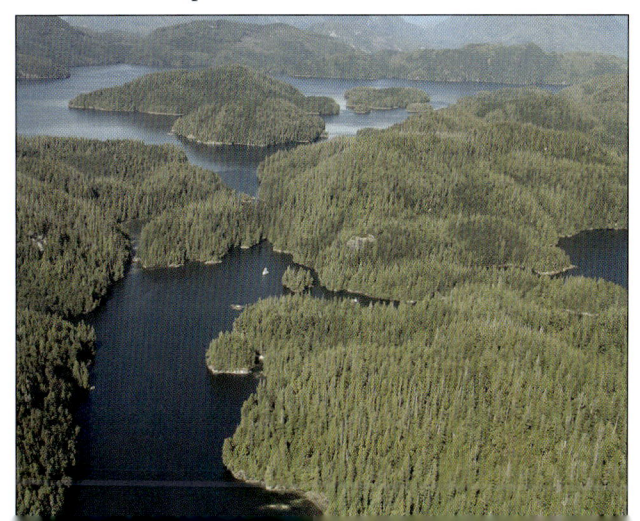

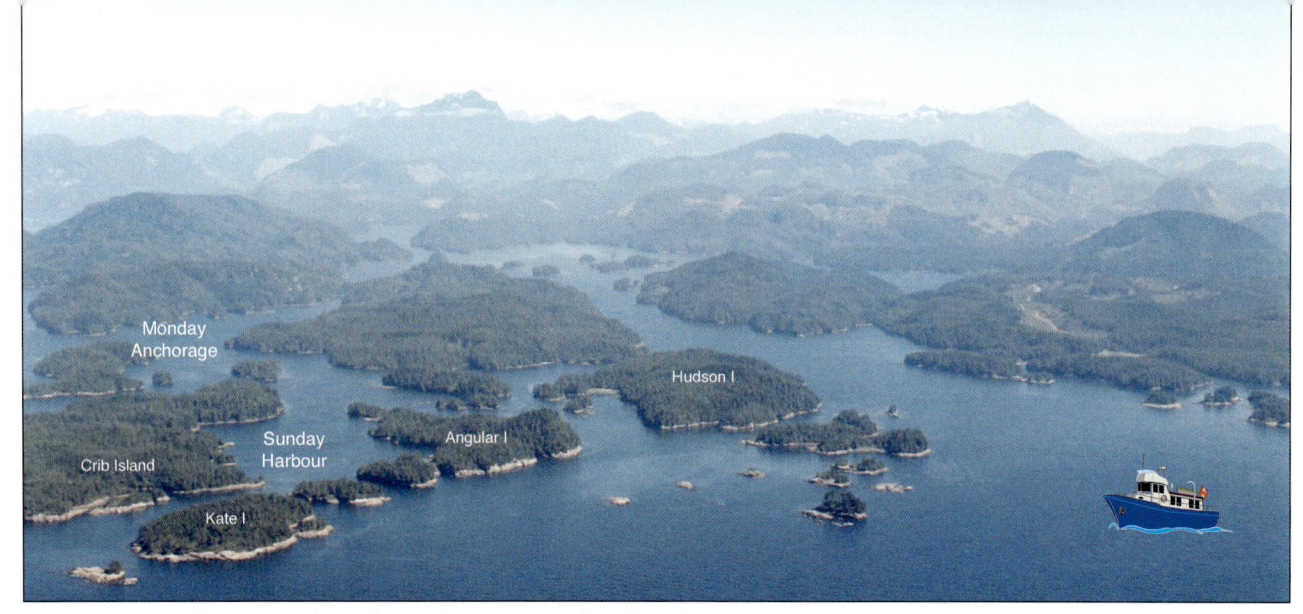

*Above: A view from the west of Sunday Harbour with Arrow Passage beyond. Sunday Harbour is not sheltered from strong winds. Hudson Island and Spiller Passage are in the centre of the picture, Kate Island is in the foreground. Angular Island, forming the south side of Sunday Harbour, lies between them. Sunday Pass is the second opening from Kate Island. A large drying rock obscures the entrance to the closer one. Opposite: The anchorage in Cullen Harbour is seen to the right of the islands. Entrance to Booker Lagoon is beyond the anchorage. See diagram at bottom of page and use chart 3547 to navigate.*

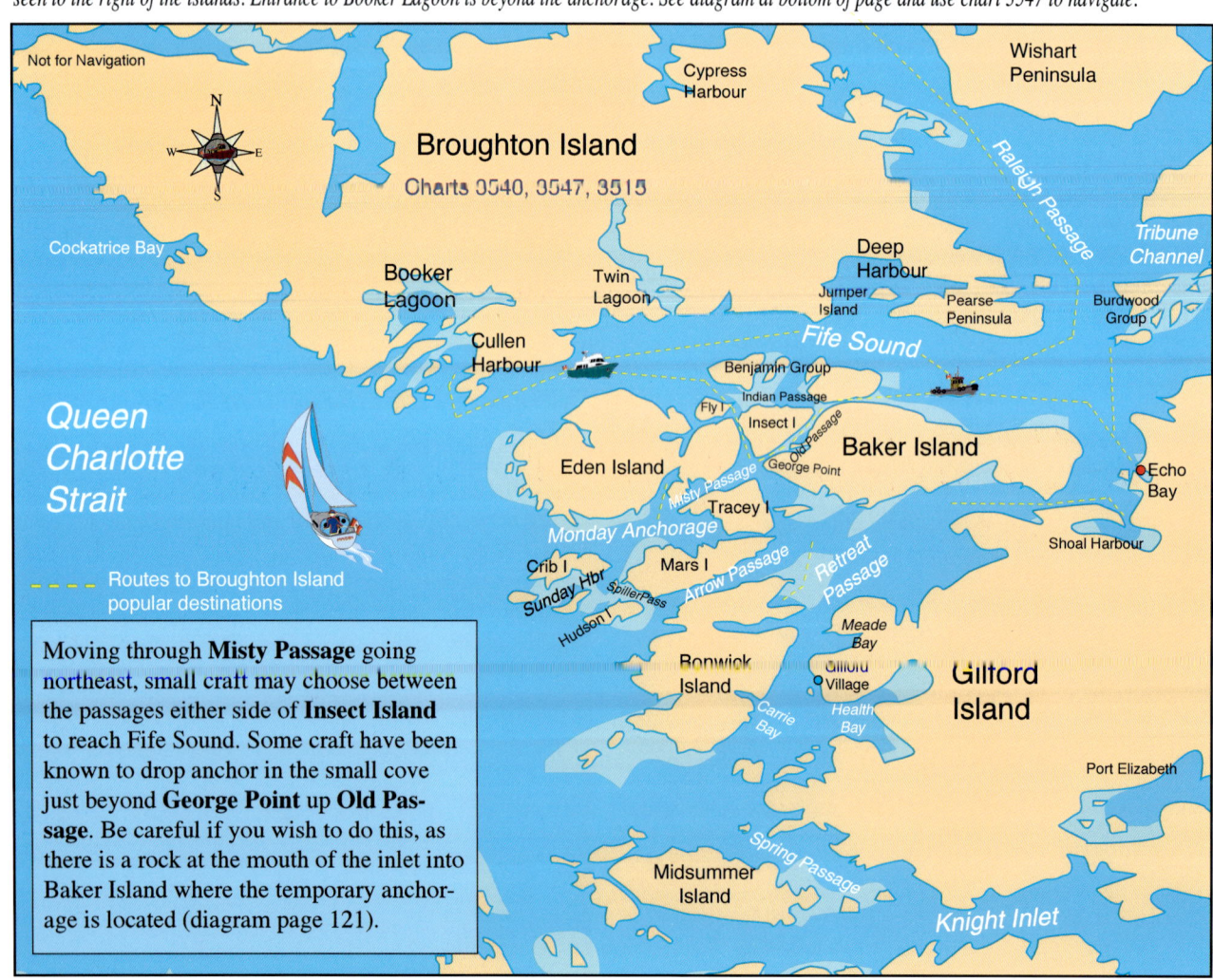

Moving through **Misty Passage** going northeast, small craft may choose between the passages either side of **Insect Island** to reach Fife Sound. Some craft have been known to drop anchor in the small cove just beyond **George Point** up **Old Passage**. Be careful if you wish to do this, as there is a rock at the mouth of the inlet into Baker Island where the temporary anchorage is located (diagram page 121).

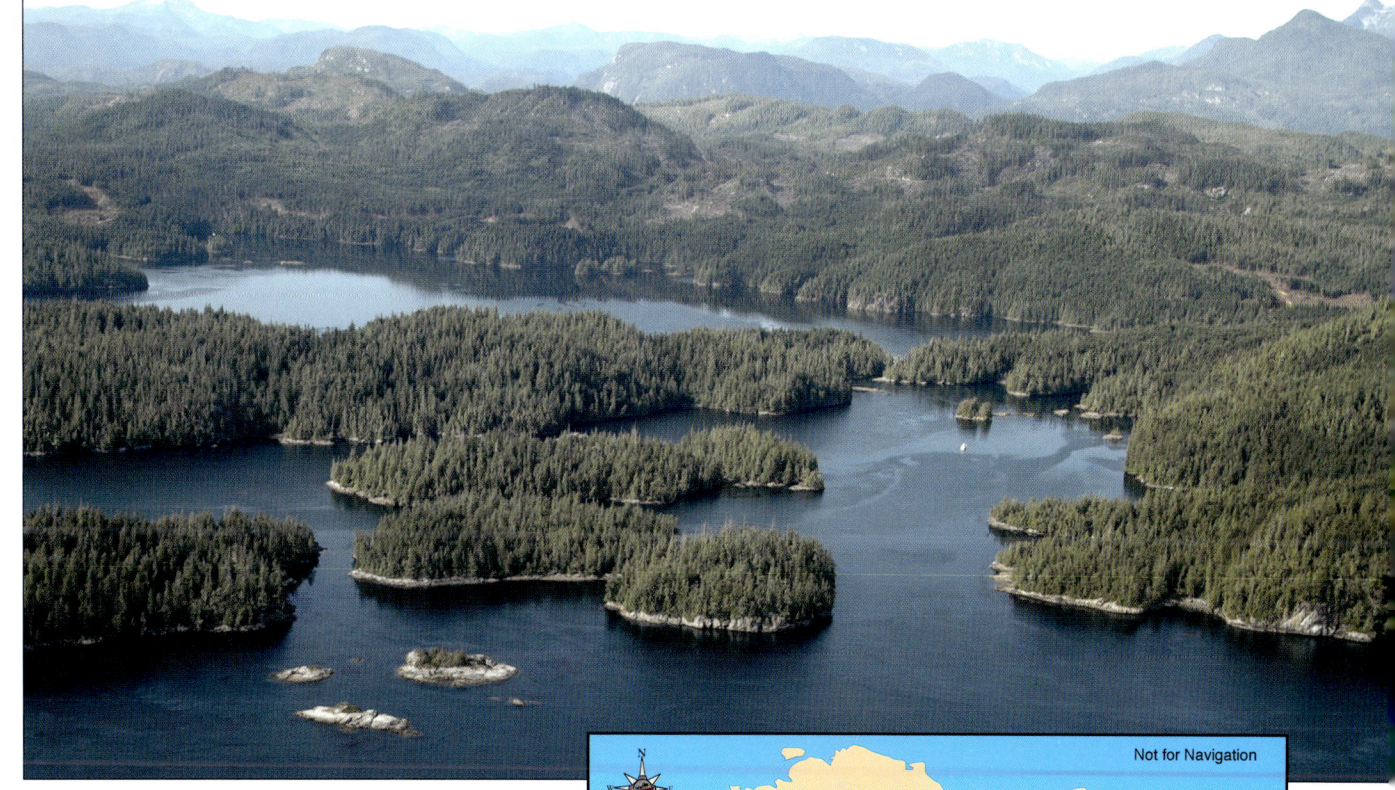

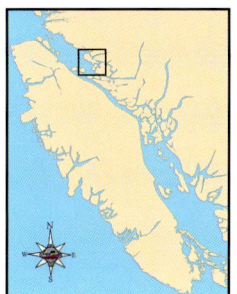

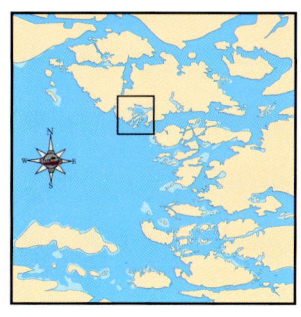

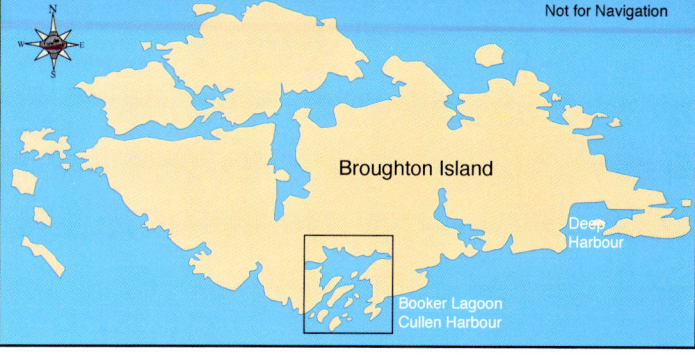

## Cullen Harbour  charts 3546, 3547

Leaving East Eden cove, cross Fife Sound from the Benjamin Group and find your way west to the south end of Broughton Island. Cullen Harbour lies at the entrance to Booker Lagoon, one of three lagoons on Broughton Island and the only one sounded by the Canadian Hydrographic Service. It is located to the east of the islands at the entrance to Booker Lagoon, which itself is not the best of anchorages. It can be entered only during slack tide.

The long fetch inside the lagoon allows a build-up of waves in a strong blow, which can cause the anchor to drag. The best anchorage is in Cullen Harbour.

Most mariners enter Cullen Harbour from the south and drop anchor in the centre over a muddy bottom. Enter west of Gordon Point. Some use a passage along the east side of Long Island, which is more of a challenge.

A good place to drop anchor is in the east side of the harbour in about 7 metres. The current flows strongly through the passage to Booker Lagoon and this should be taken into account when setting your anchor.

**The currents at the entrance to Booker Lagoon can be strong and dangerous if taken at the wrong times. Use the entrance only at slack or close to it. Slack has only about a ten minute duration.**

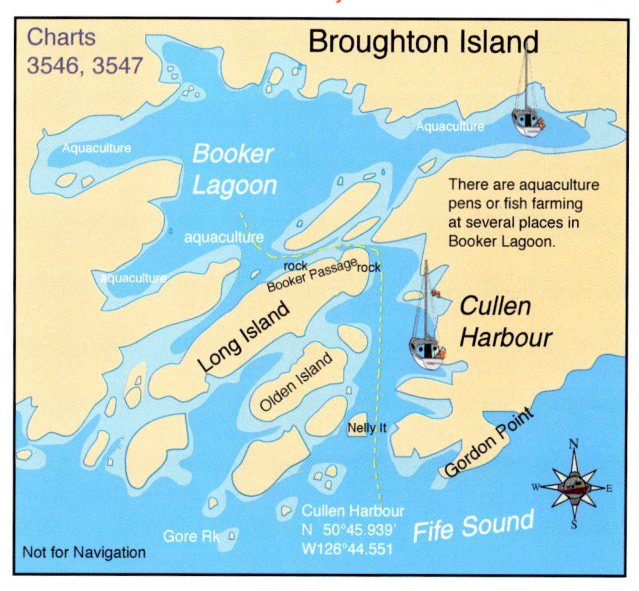

There are aquaculture pens or fish farming at several places in Booker Lagoon.

Cullen Harbour
N 50°45.939'
W126°44.551

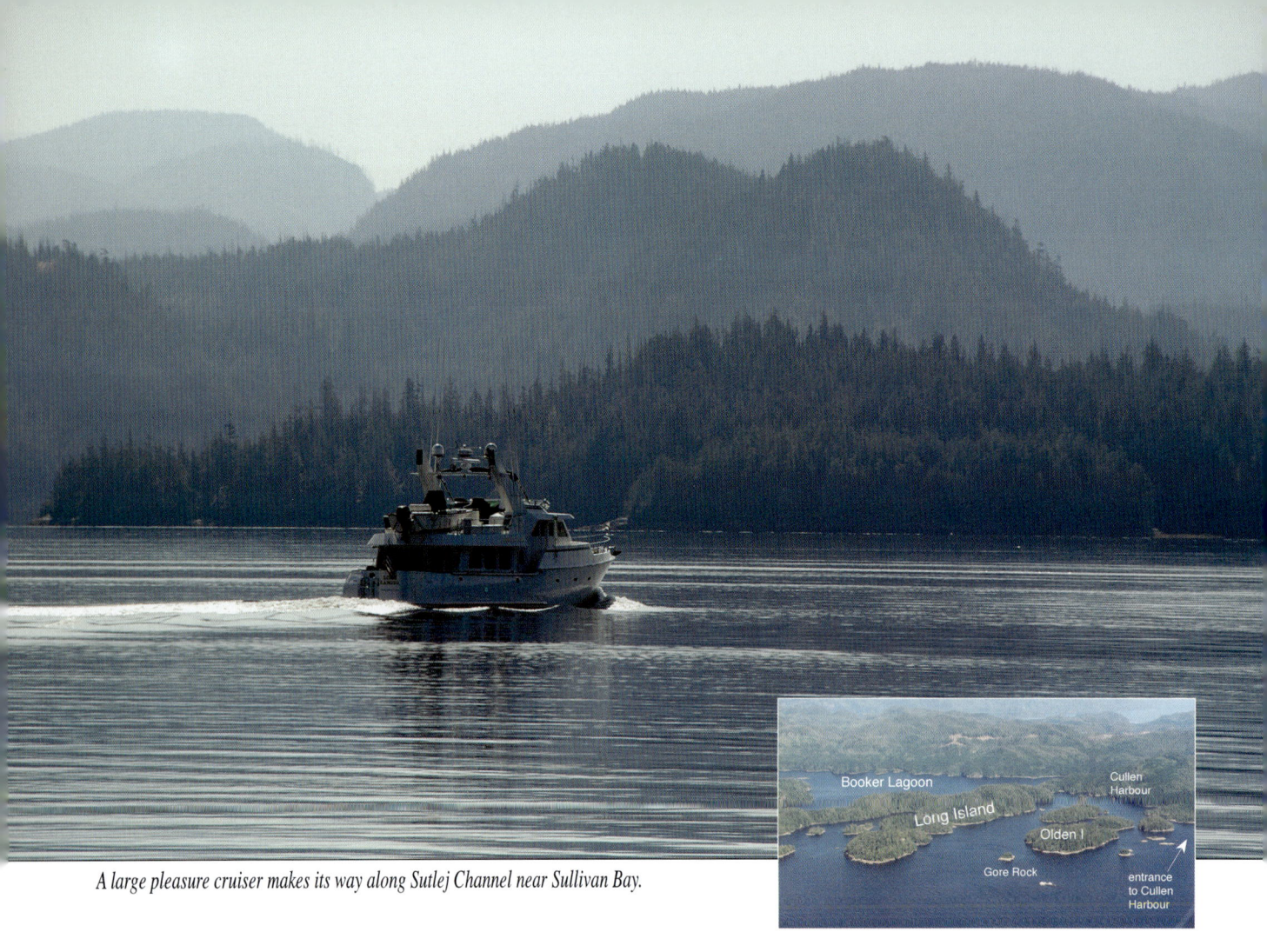

*A large pleasure cruiser makes its way along Sutlej Channel near Sullivan Bay.*

### Booker Lagoon  chart 3547

The entrance to Booker Lagoon is narrow and beset by currents. It can be accessed by small, preferably fast boats. However, one mariner said he had no difficulty entering the lagoon under power in his 8 metre, deep displacement sailboat, using a mark on a tree as a reference point. Use the entrance only at slack or close to it. Slack has about a ten minute duration.

From Cullen Harbour the entrance to Booker Lagoon is directly north with a sharp turn to port at the end of Long Island. Stay well clear as you round the reef that juts out at the tip of the island. The water here is about four metres deep at low tide and the passage is wide enough for easy transit, again, preferably during slack tides. The passage to the northwest of Long Island is also possible during slack tides, preferably high slack due to some shallower depths.

Inside, there is a fish farm near the entrance to the lagoon. Fish farming may preclude finding an ideal spot to drop the anchor for an overnight stay, both here and in other coves on the coast. Anchor in the vicinity of fish farms only if it is safe to do so, or find an alternative place to moor.

Booker Lagoon has been described as a remote wilderness, desolate and eerie with tall pines, black against the sky. It consists of four inlets, offering sheltered anchorage depending on the wind direction. Anchor deep in the bay over a muddy bottom immediately east of the entrance in 6 to 8 metres. This is the preferred, temporary anchorage for shelter from strong easterlies.

Passage to Echo Bay from Cullen Harbour and Booker Lagoon is eastbound along Fife Sound. Travelling westward to Wells Passage there is not much protection from the open seas of Queen Charlotte Strait, although in mild weather a stop at **Cockatrice Bay** may be appropriate (see page 189).

### Deep Harbour  charts 3547, 3515

The route to Echo Bay via Fife Sound will take you past Deep Harbour. If your objective is to remain in the area for a short while in fair weather try Deep Harbour as a temporary anchorage. The water is deep and a stern tie is recommended. Look for a sheltered spot beyond Jumper Island and the small island to the east of it.

# 'The Mainland'

## Vicinity of Echo Bay–Shoal Harbour to Sullivan Bay

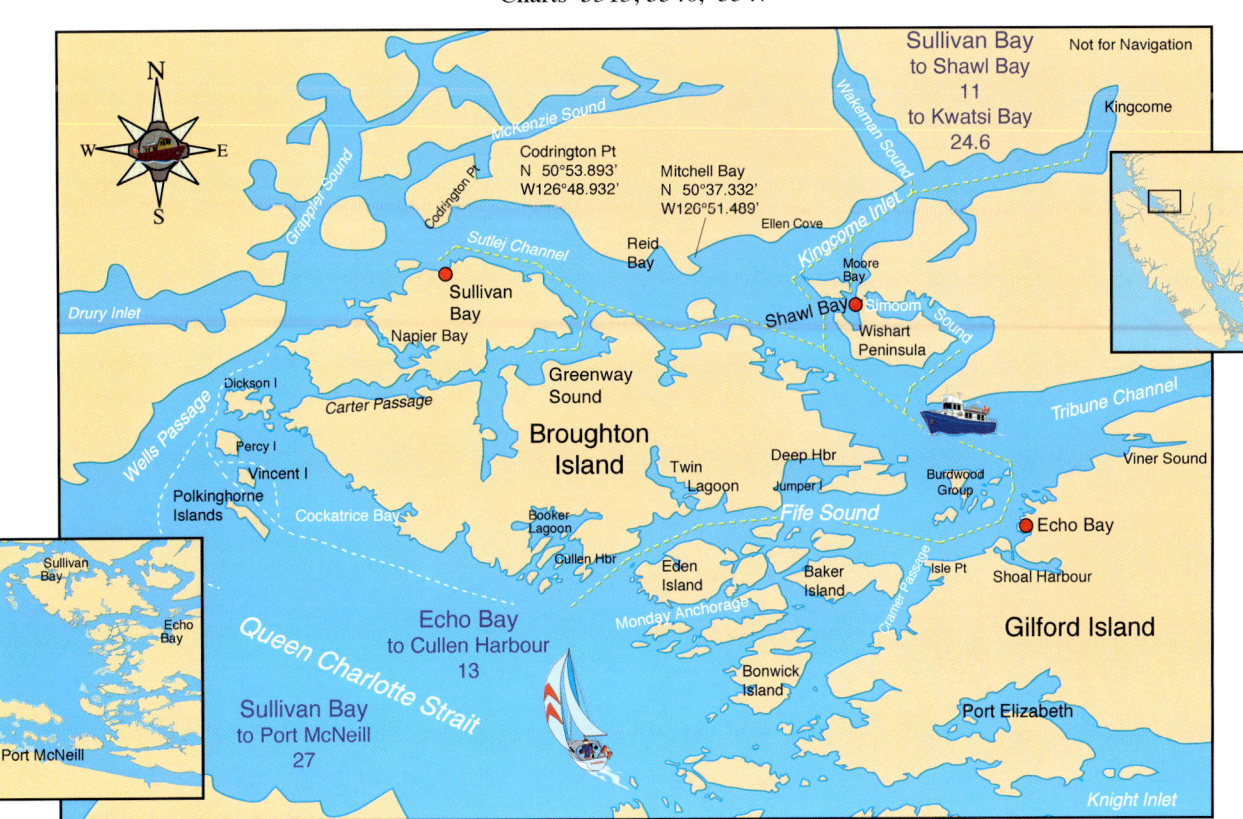

Charts 3515, 3546, 3547

Note: the mileages given are always from the first named place.

If you are travelling the outside route to Wells Passage it is easiest to navigate north of the Polkinghorne Islands, especially if the seas are building in Queen Charlotte Strait. Alternatively go south or north of Vincent Island, remaining clear of Percy Island on the approaches to Wells Passage. Stop along the way and explore the Polkinghornes by dropping a day hook in the lagoon on the north side of the larger island, but only if weather permits. Use **Dickson Island** as an anchorage or temporary stop if you plan continuing up the mainland coast towards Blunden Harbour (see page 187 and 190).

Use the alternative route via Fife Sound around the north of Broughton Island to Wells Passage if the weather is unfavourable. This takes you to the settlements from Echo Bay to Sullivan Bay with many interesting stops between.

### Shoal Harbour   chart 3515

The most secure anchorage in Shoal Harbour is in the west arm in about three or four metres. There is also an anchorage behind the island just inside the entrance.

This latter spot is usually considered a temporary anchorage although we have seen boats anchored there for overnight stays on many occasions. The west winds are of little concern when anchored in Shoal Harbour but be alert when easterlies are in the weather forecast.

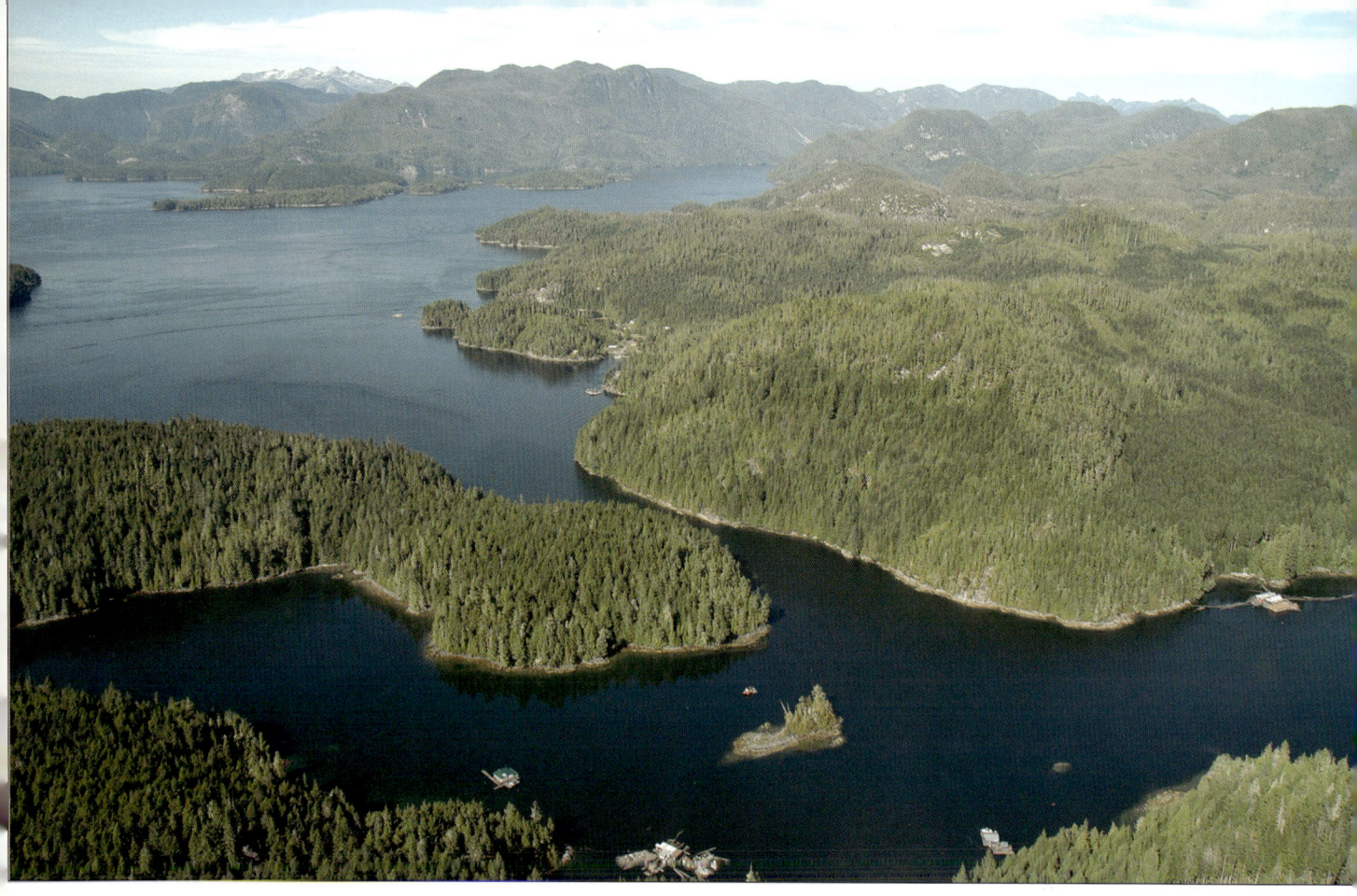

*Shoal Harbour. Best anchorage is in the bight at lower left in the photo.*

Shoal Harbour has long been a hub of logging activity and related residential settlement. Private mooring, booms, crab traps and a logging camp greeted us over the years when we dropped anchor in the mud shallows.

For secure moorage we usually find our way into Echo Bay where tying up at a dock for the night ensures secure shelter from any weather. Echo Bay has served mariners and local communities as a hub and safe haven since the earliest logging and settlement in the area.

## Echo Bay  chart 3515

Be mindful of the rock just off the entrance to Echo Bay. Inside the bay you will find a wide variety of services and provisions. Pierre's Echo Bay Resort offers internet connection, all marina facilities, fuel, a post office and accommodations. The marina and resort have a long history of ownership with Bob and Nancy Richter having passed the reins in recent years to Pierre and Tove Landry and Jerome and Lucy Rose.

Echo Bay has welcomed guests for many years and its various owners have built the resort from a rambling, rustic facility and single float to its present status as lodge and fully equipped marina. The Richters took advantage of the sale in Washington State some years ago of part of the old floating bridge across Lake Washington. The large concrete section of the old structure now resides anchored at the entrance to the bay and serves as the base for the store and post office as well as other utility buildings for the marina and lodge operation, and for special events.

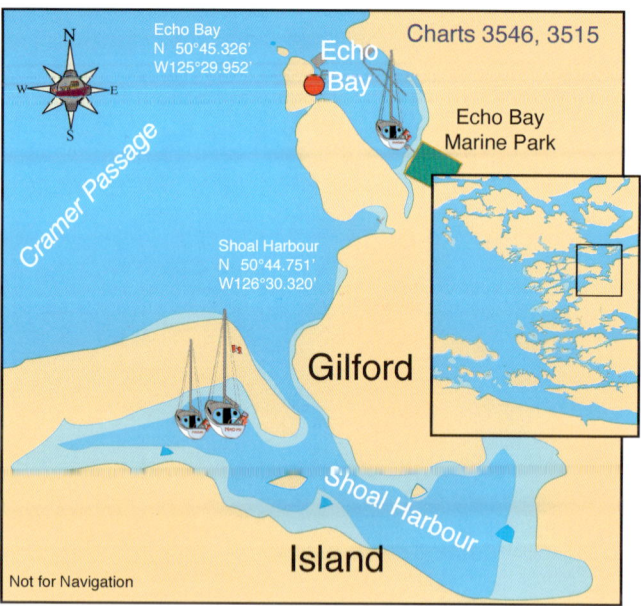

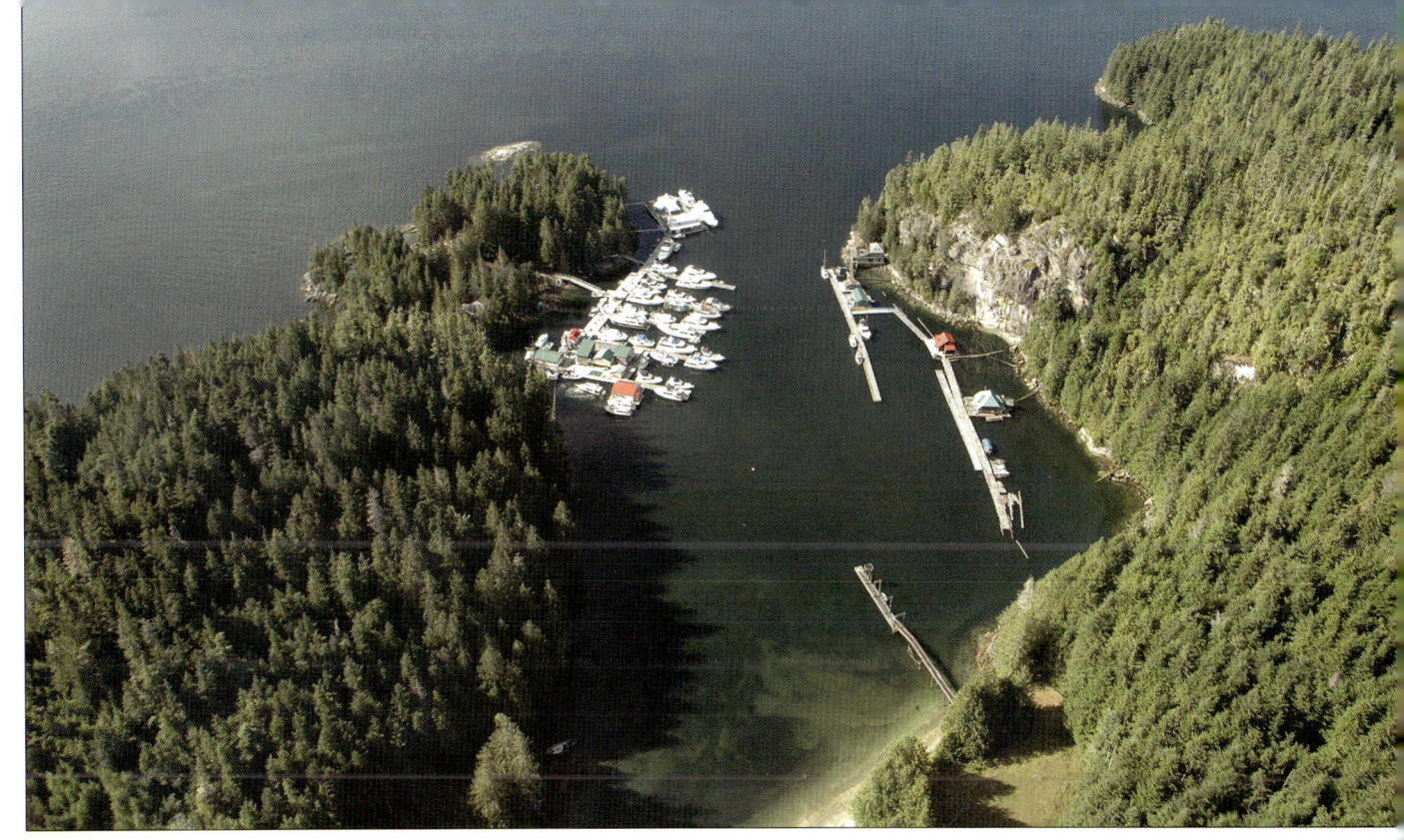

*Above:* The settlement at Echo Bay includes Pierre's Echo Bay Resort located in the lee of the island. There are docks on the opposite shore. A public float extends from a sandy beach, for dinghy use only, giving access to the marine park lands adjacent to the bay.
*Right:* The peninsula and island giving shelter to Echo Bay, located at the north end of Cramer Passage and opposite Fife Sound. Billy Proctor's residence and museum are in the cove in the foreground, lower right.
*Bottom:* Echo Bay with the marine park at its head. At one time a school house served the outlying and local communities. Now the area is cleared and designated marine park.

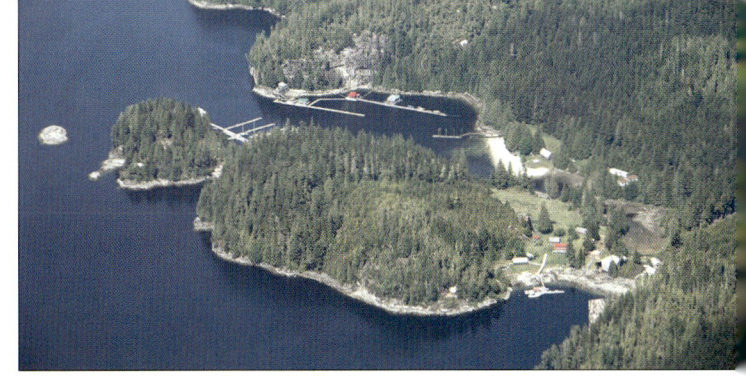

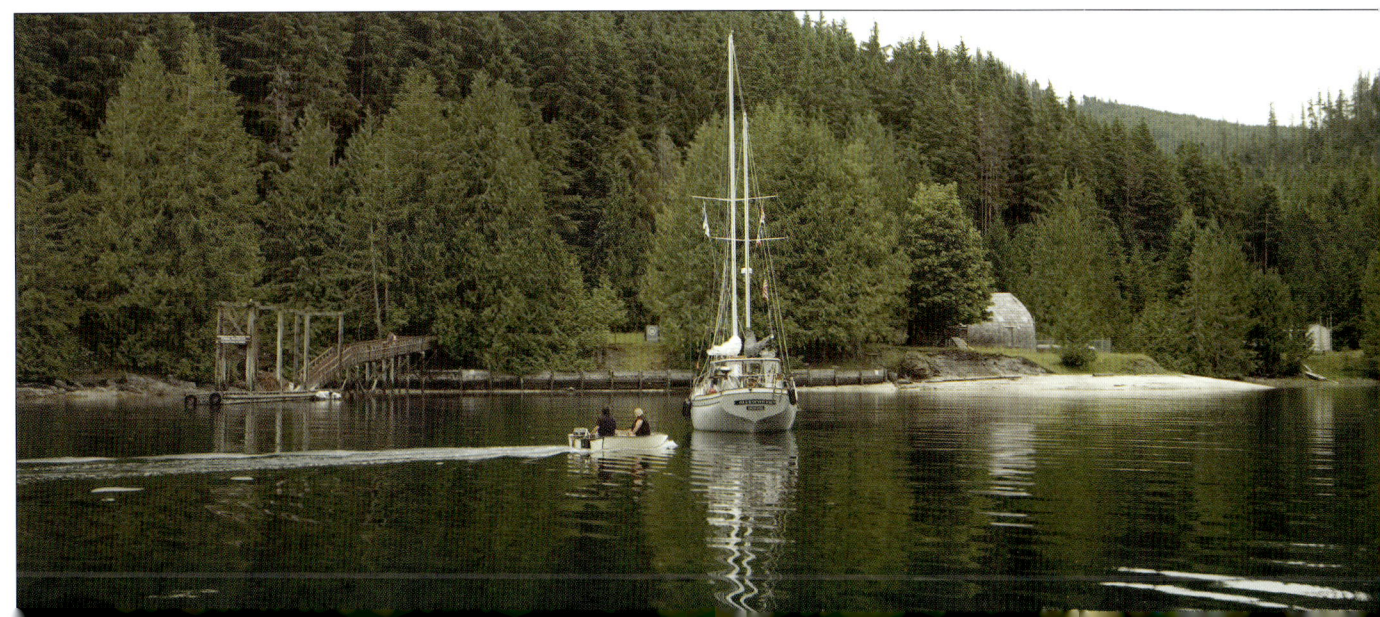

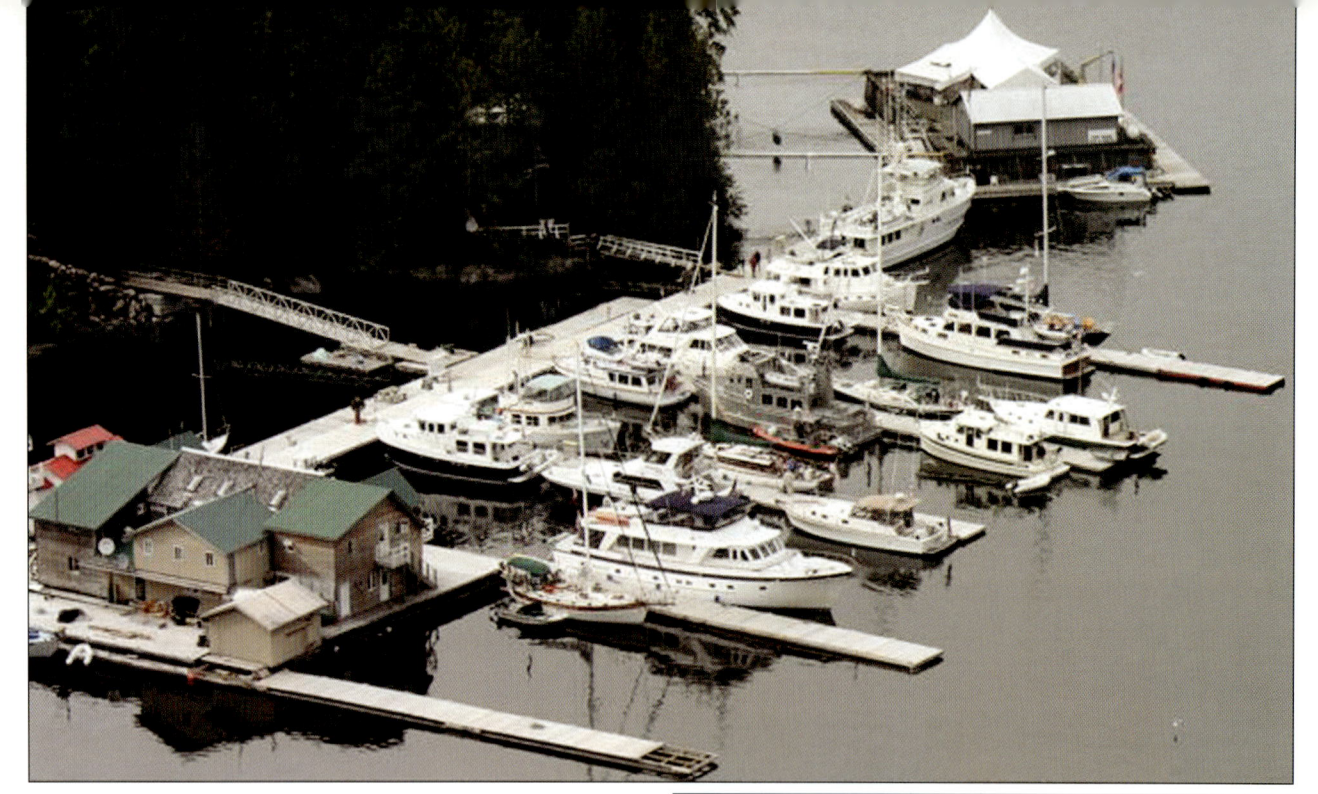

## Pierre's Echo Bay

128 GD Simoom Sound BC V0P 1S0
Phone 250-713-6415
email: info@pierresbay.com
www.pierresbay.com

Pierre's Echo Bay Resort is a popular place. It has a daily happy hour and regular theme nights featuring pig roasts, rib roasts and Italian nights. For details visit their website.
The marina offers power hook-ups—15, 30 and 50 amps, and there is water at the dock (limited in summer). Rental suites are available. Fuel services are available for gas, diesel and propane. There are laundry facilities, showers and washrooms. A store and post office are on the main float. Block and party ice, fresh and frozen produce, groceries, books and charts are available. There is cell phone service and the marina offers wireless internet. For the hardy, there is a rustic path to Billy Proctor's Museum, or use the public dock nearby.

Caution: Keep well clear of the rock at the entrance off Echo Bay. Locals take passage inside of it, but visitors should exercise caution by passing around the outside.

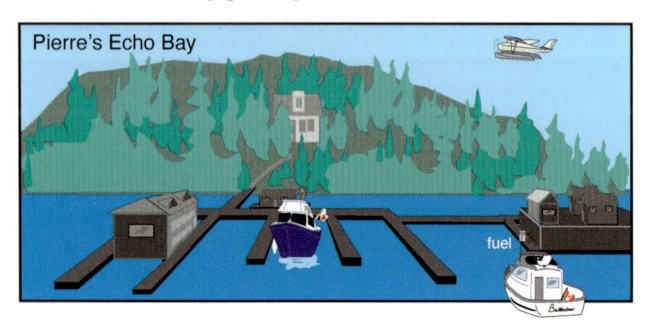

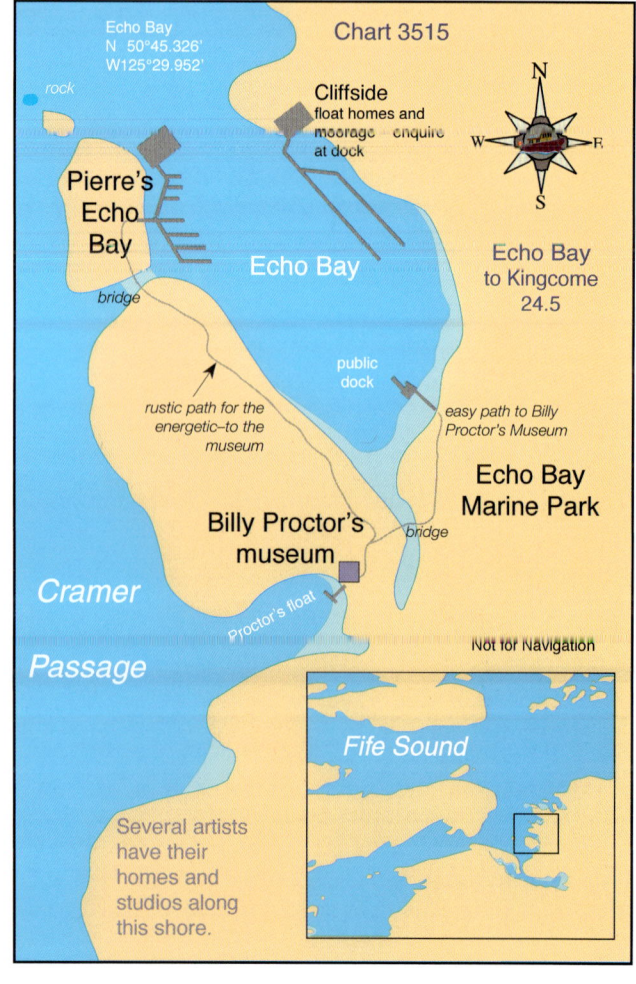

128

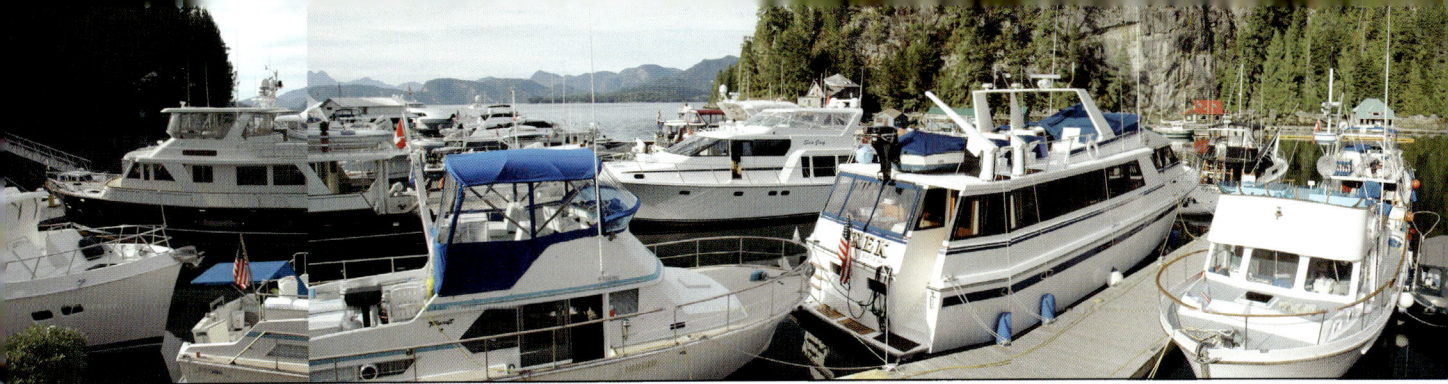

*Above: Vessels docked at Pierre's Echo Bay for a mid summer weekend. Right: Approaching Echo Bay from Cramer Passage. The view in the background is Fife Sound and the Burdwood Group. Opposite: The structures at top include the marina office and barbecue tent with dining area. The docks include the large building that has accommodations for overnight guests. Settlements and communities on "The Mainland", as the area that includes the adjacent groups of islands is known, depend on one another for help. It is not unusual to learn that many of the local residents have come together to help build a home or move one by float to another nearby location.*

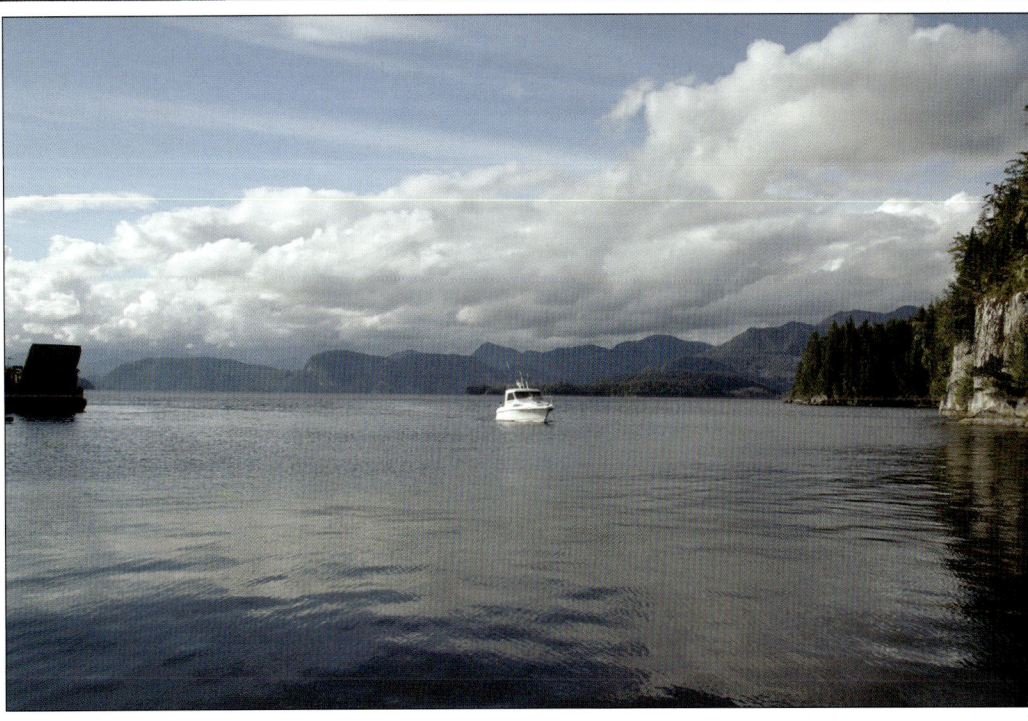

Some mariners visiting the bay may remember the former owners of Echo Bay Marina and Lodge, Ray Rosback, who for many years since has provided marine services at Alert Bay and Port McNeill. During his tenure he provided supplies and services to a large community in nearby Simoom Sound, Scott Cove and other logging camps dotting the nearby waterways.

The original lodge was built by Lena Laviolette as a hotel in the 1920s. She and her husband lived on the property. Their location and the number of transient visitors in the area at that time inspired them to build the hotel. After Lena sold the hotel she continued to live in the vicinity in a floating home.

There is a pathway to the scenic view above the bay. Former marina operators gave directions to access the trail. "Take a lunch and a hand held VHF," they said, "and walk at a 'legal limit', which means not in a hurry, to the parkground up from the public dock at the head of Echo Bay. Behind the site of the former school there are water lines that run up the hill. Follow these until you arrive at a dam. Continue almost to the top of the path, where there are four small trees, two on each side, with fluorescent flags attached. Turn left between the flags and follow a series of flags going up the hill until you reach the logging road. This is edged by a stoned slope which you will have to climb over to access the logging road. Turn left and follow the road up another hill to the end of the road. The lookout is at the end of the road where you can see from Cramer Pass to the Burdwood Group including Fife Sound and Penphrase Passage."

Opposite Echo Bay Marina and Resort is Cliffside Moorage, formerly known as Windsong Sea Village, which may be able to provide overflow moorage for visitors. Enquire at the dock. It offers no electrical hook-ups or overnight amenitites. The facility belongs to the owners of Sullivan Bay.

Echo Bay is a hub for communications and socializing in the area. Regular flights stop in the bay with float planes from Kenmore Air and Pacific Coastal. Grizzly Helicopters also will be seen frequently flying in and out or overhead en route to other nearby locations. A small public float serves as access to the park and provides a landing for boat owners going ashore in their dinghies while anchored off the white

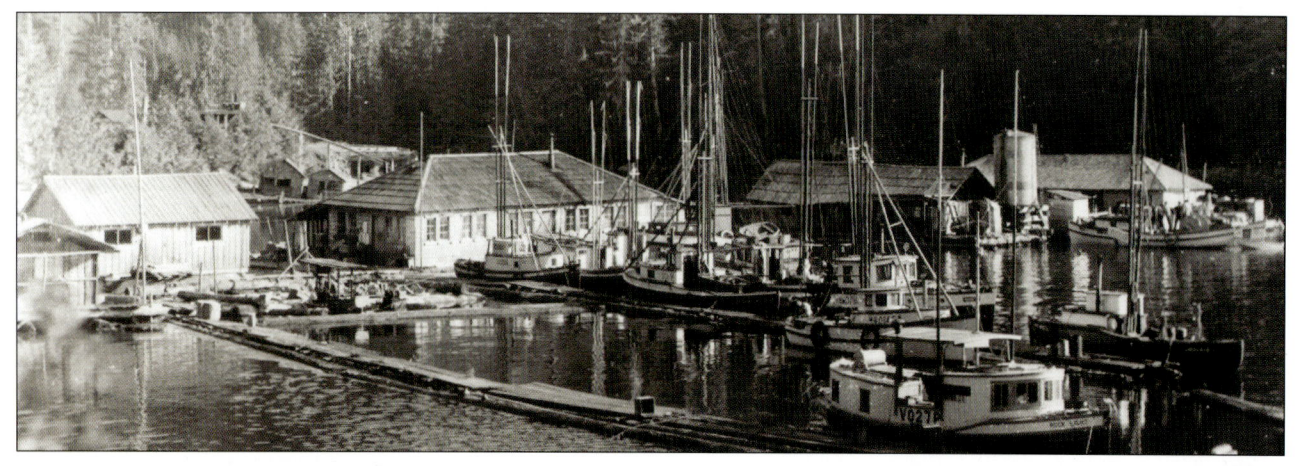

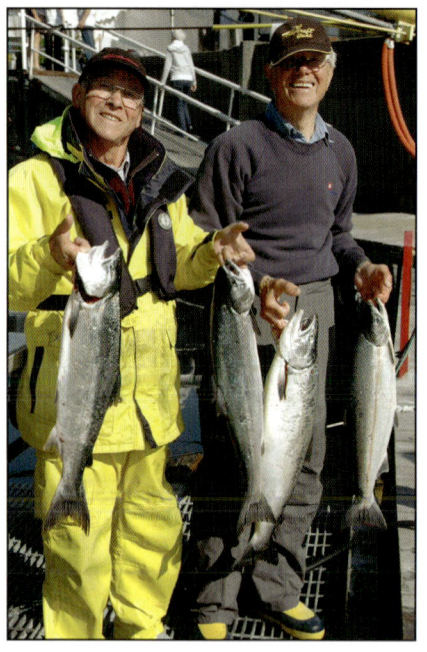

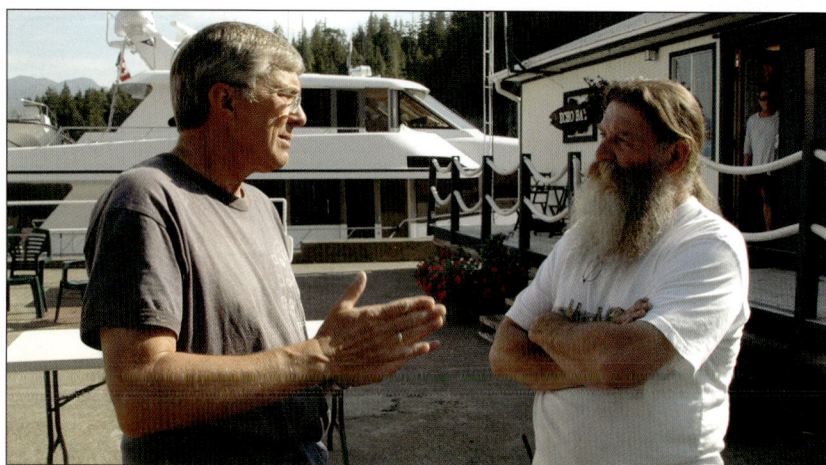

*Top: The early days at Echo Bay. It has long been a busy hub of "The Mainland." Above: Visitor Bruce Jackman (of Port McNeill Fuel Dock) and Echo Bay's Pierre Landry. Left: Fishing attracts many boaters to the area and catches can be rewarding. Right: Whale spy hopping off Echo Bay.*

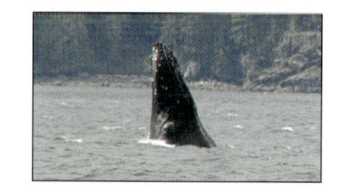

sandy beach. One year we noticed strange sounds coming from the woods behind the school building. It was the noise of many herons in their rookery. We heard it for the first time in 2002 and again a year later. There were about 15 pairs of herons and we were told they return to the rookery from time to time.

From the park, a short walk along a winding trail leads to the other side of the isthmus where Billy Proctor has his home and museum. Cross a stream, and walk along the trail, passing over a small bridge to Billy Proctor's property. The optional rustic path from the marina is longer and best for those who are fit.

You can also go there by boat. Follow the shoreline out of Echo Bay keeping a short distance offshore around the island, minding the rock on the outside. Continue to the south side of the isthmus, where his dock is located in the cove between Echo Bay and Shoal Harbour.

Billy Proctor will gladly show you his collection of artifacts and bottles from the early years on the coast. His museum is becoming well known far and wide and he welcomes you to tie up briefly at his dock while visiting him. His collection includes Chinese and Japanese bottles, a mimeograph machine dated 1910 that came from Minstrel Island, stone arrowheads, and a Simoom Sound post office scale, among the many items representing the history of the area in the early part of the 20th century.

For interesting information about the area read *Full Moon, Flood Tide* by Billy Proctor and Yvonne Maximchuk, and *Heart of the Raincoast*, which Proctor coauthored with his former neighbour Alexandra Morton, well-known whale researcher, photographer, artist and writer. Yvonne Maximchuk is a local artist whose studio is near Proctor's museum. She invites mariners to call her at 250-974-8134 and view her work or sign up for some of her painting classes.

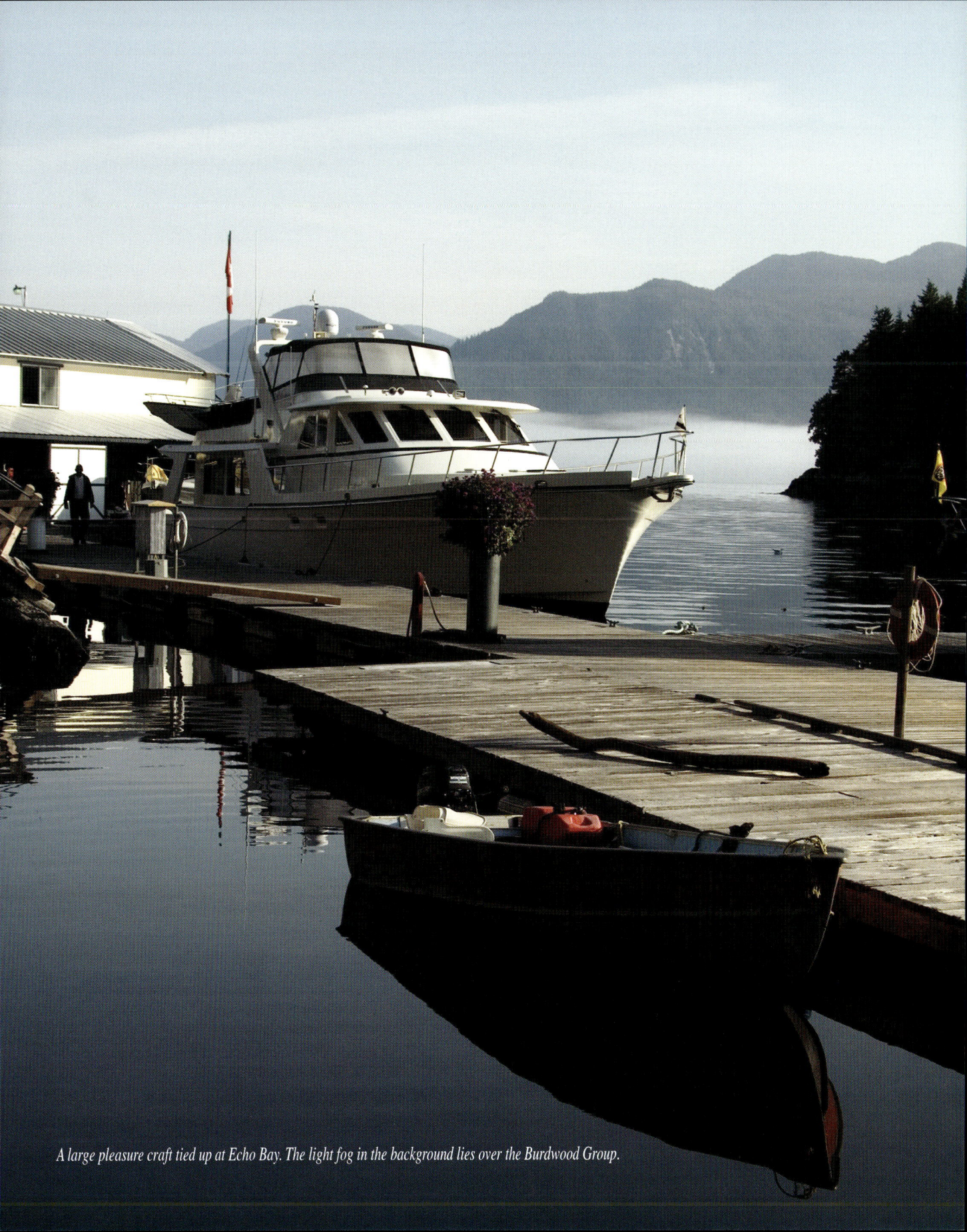

*A large pleasure craft tied up at Echo Bay. The light fog in the background lies over the Burdwood Group.*

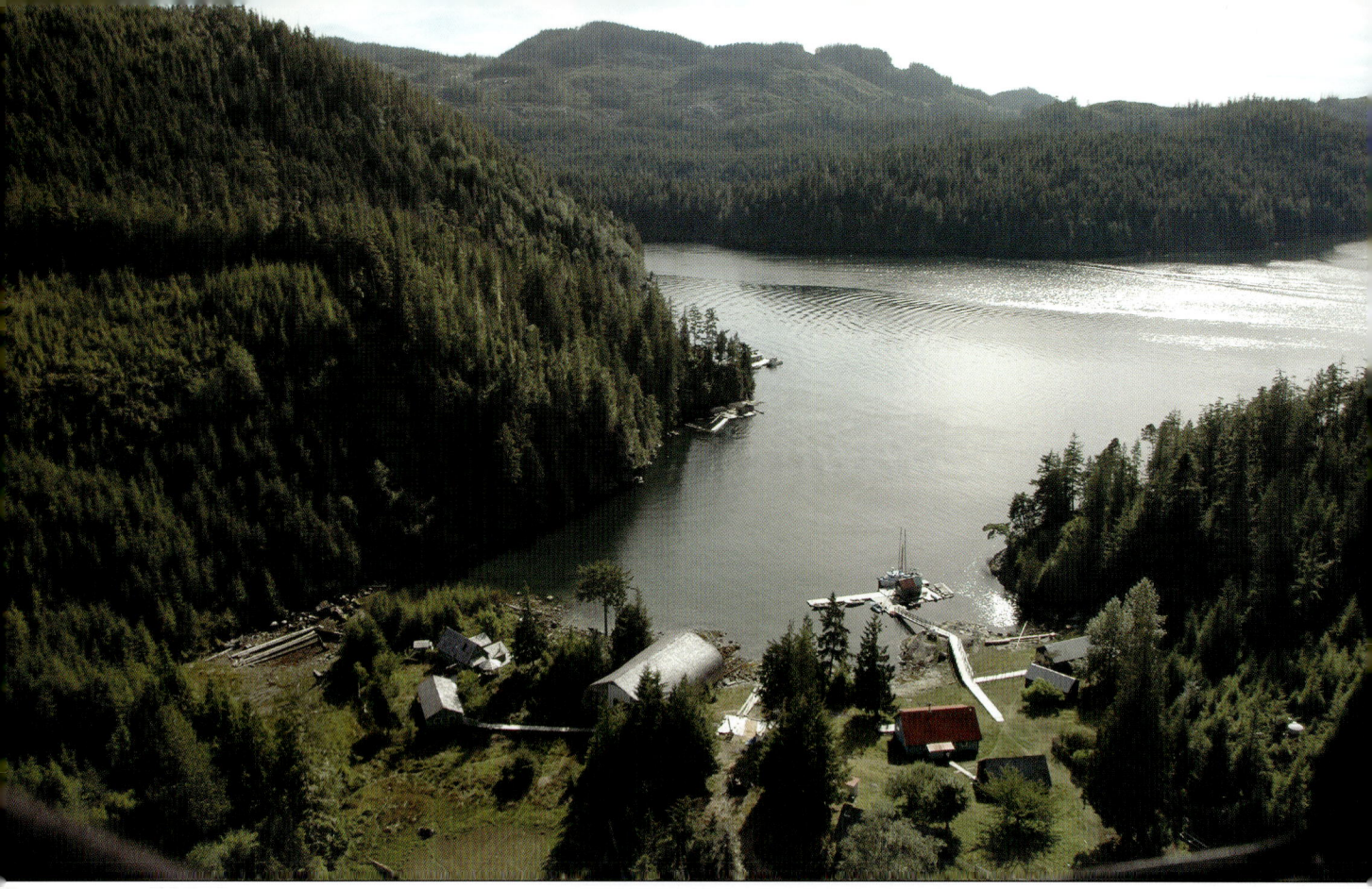

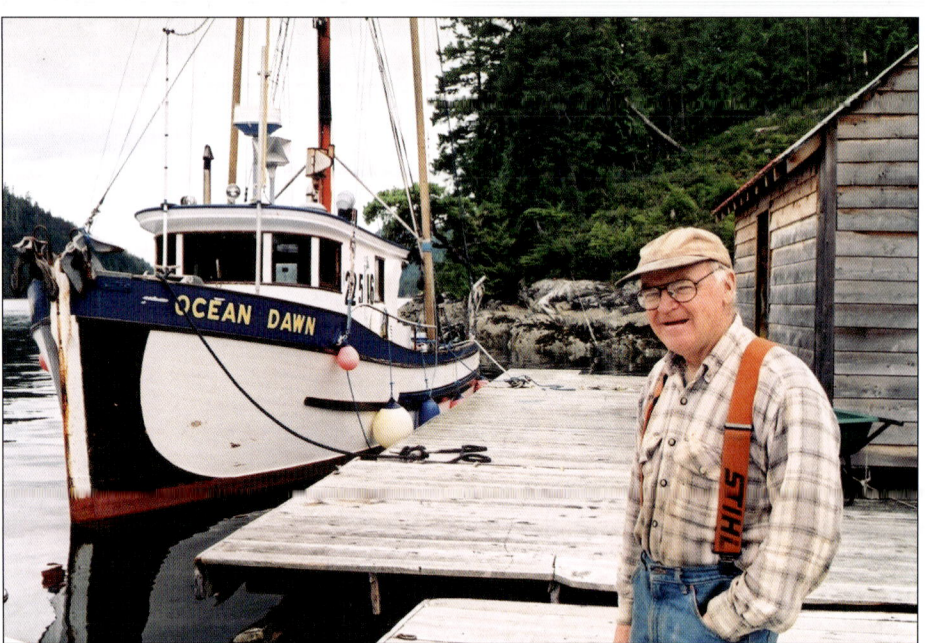

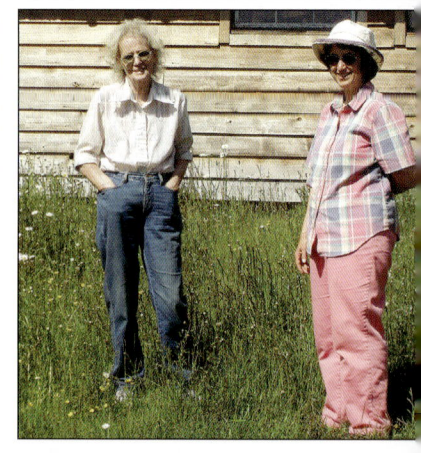

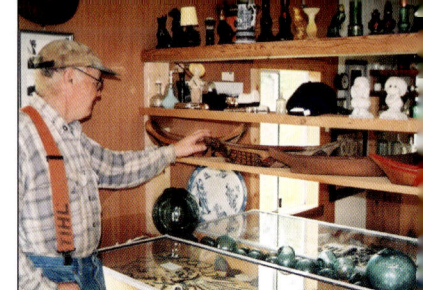

Top: Billy Proctor's homestead and dock. Above right: His late wife Yvonne talking to the author's wife, Carla, in the late 1990s. Above: Billy Proctor on his dock.
Right: Proctor in his museum (which depicts much of the history of the area by way of the Chinese and Japanese bottles and artifacts he has collected over the years.

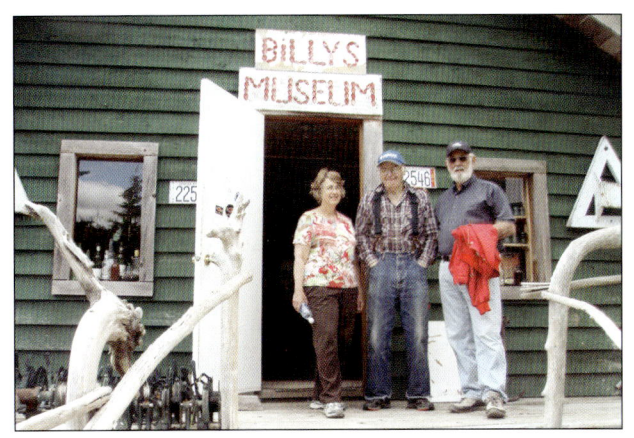

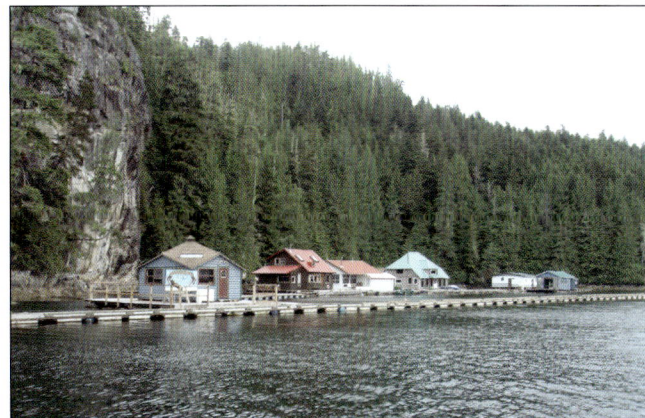

*Above left: The author and his wife with Billy Proctor at his museum.*
*Above right: The docks at Cliffside (formerly Windsong Sea Village) belongs to owners of Sullivan Bay. Overnight moorage is available on enquiring at the dock.*
*Right: Scott Cove, location of the former post office that served the loggers of Simoom Sound at the entrance to Tribune Channel. The post office is now located at Echo Bay.*
*Below: A boat cruises up Cramer Pass towards the Burdwood Group. Scott Cove and Echo Bay are to the right.*

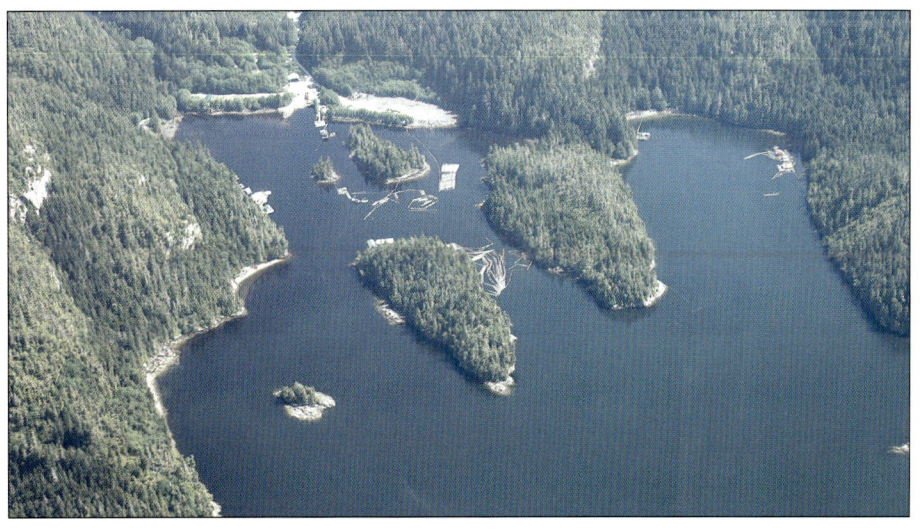

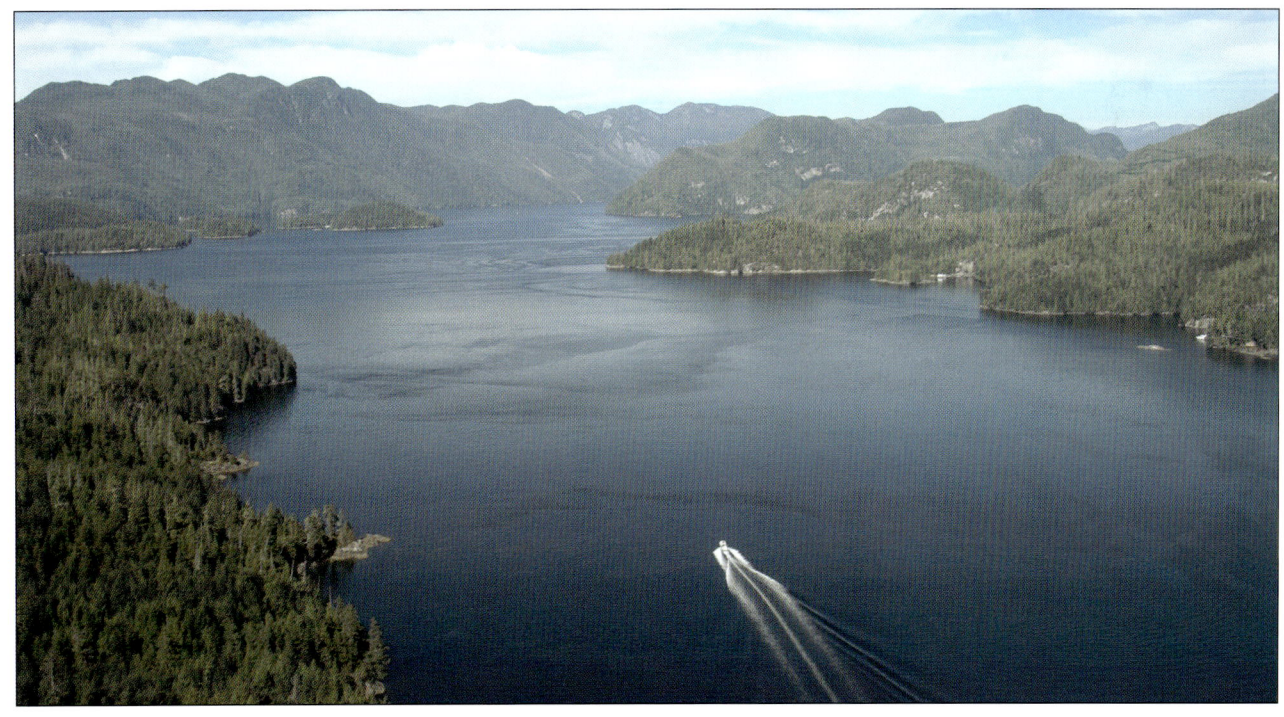

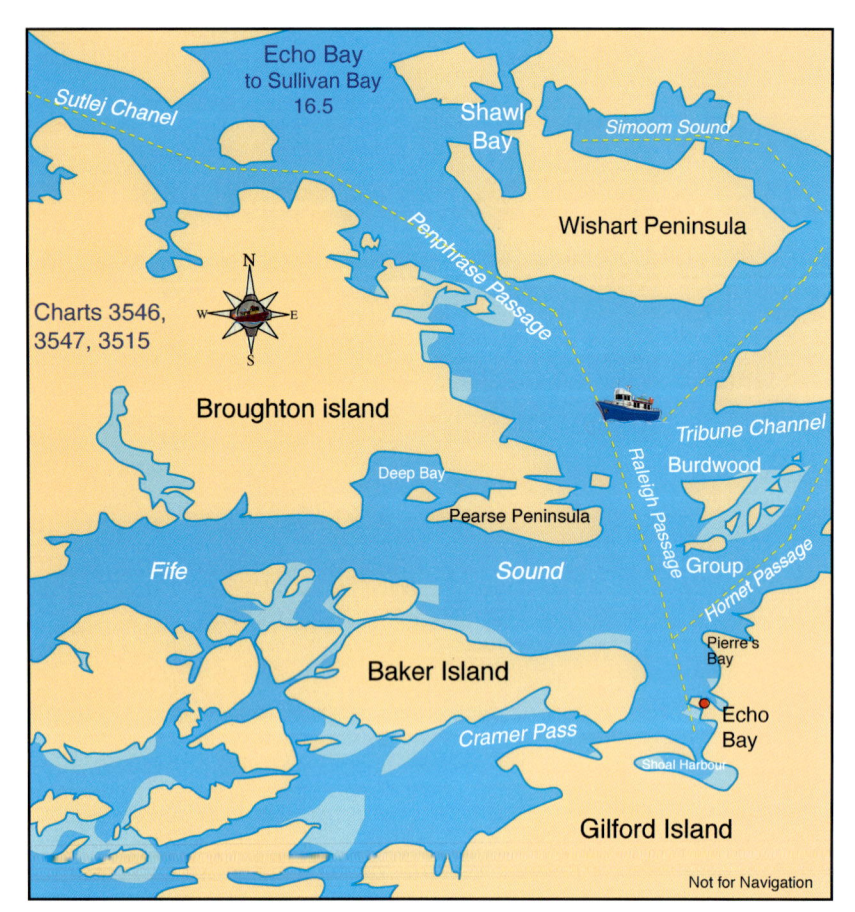

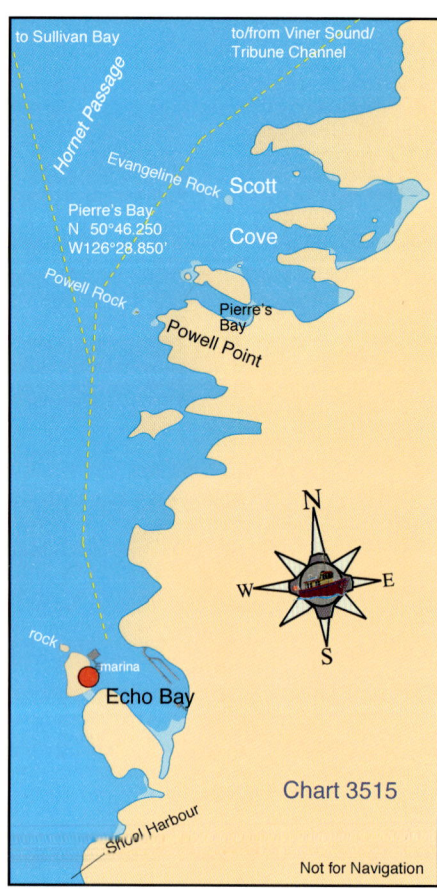

## Scott Cove  chart 3515

Scott Cove near Echo Bay was the home of Pierre and Tove Landry who have since moved to Echo Bay. Scott Cove was once a very populated place. Until as recently as the 1970s and into the '80s there was an active logging camp with residential float houses strung along its west side. Then the Landrys set up their lodge, an imposing building that appeared prominently at the entrance to the tiny cove that became known as Pierre's Bay. Since the move to Echo Bay, residential floating homes remain in the tiny nook, sheltered from most weather conditions.

Several years ago members of the Des Moines Yacht Club presented Pierre and Tove with a very large barbecue which, along with all the other structures, was transferred to Echo Bay where visitors have been enjoying a variety of barbecues during the season. The lodge that once stood in the entrance of Pierre's Bay, is now a fixture of the docks at Echo Bay and provides comfortable accommodations for guests who arrive by boat or fly in to visit the facility.

There is a network of logging roads that can be used to link various trails to and from the current and once-inhabited places on the island. One of these logging roads can be reached by a trail out of Scott Cove that links the many others on Gilford Island.

## Cramer Pass to Shawl Bay  chart 3515

If you hug the shoreline on the east side of Cramer Pass, travelling towards Scott Cove, it would be wise to give Powell Point a wide berth (diagram above). Powell Rock is a nasty hazard not always marked by kelp. At low tide it can be seen just above the surface. A short way beyond is the entrance to Pierre's Bay in the south corner of Scott Cove. Your passage to Shawl Bay takes you past the Burdwood Group, along Penphrase Passage and on to Kingcome, Greenway Sound and Sullivan Bay.

## The Burdwood Group  chart 3515

This is where you arrive at the west end of Tribune Channel after travelling that route from Minstrel Island towards the Fife Sound area. See Route 1 on page 8.

The Burdwood group of islands and the surrounding waters are somewhat like the hub of a large turnstyle, with channels and inlets leading off in several directions. Tribune Channel enters from the east, Fife Sound from the west, Cramer Passage from the south and Penphrase Passage from the north. Simoom Sound and Viner Sound get in on the act with their openings abutting the circle where Tribune Channel's north and south shores flare apart. The islands are popular among cruising yachtsmen for their beautiful vistas

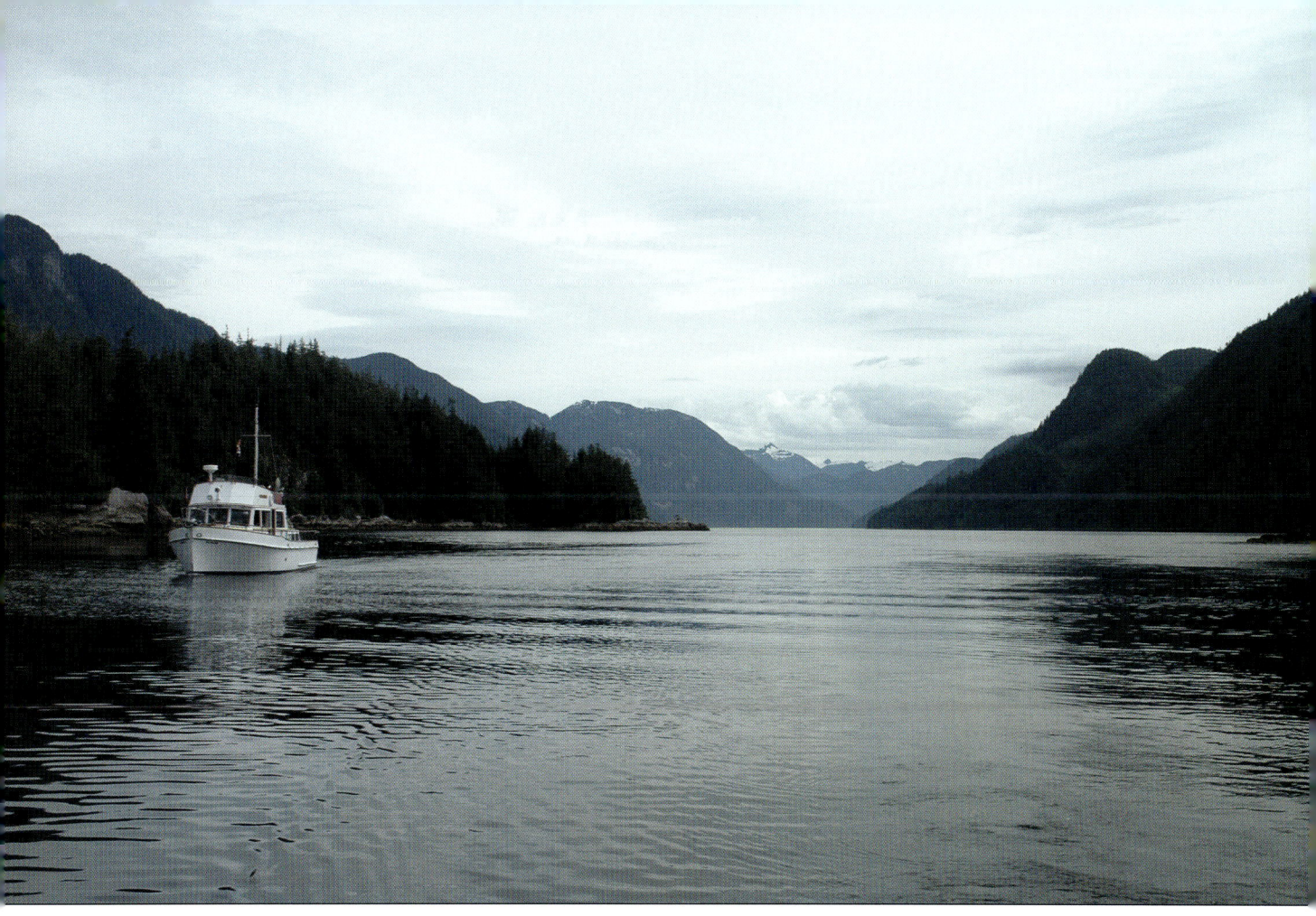

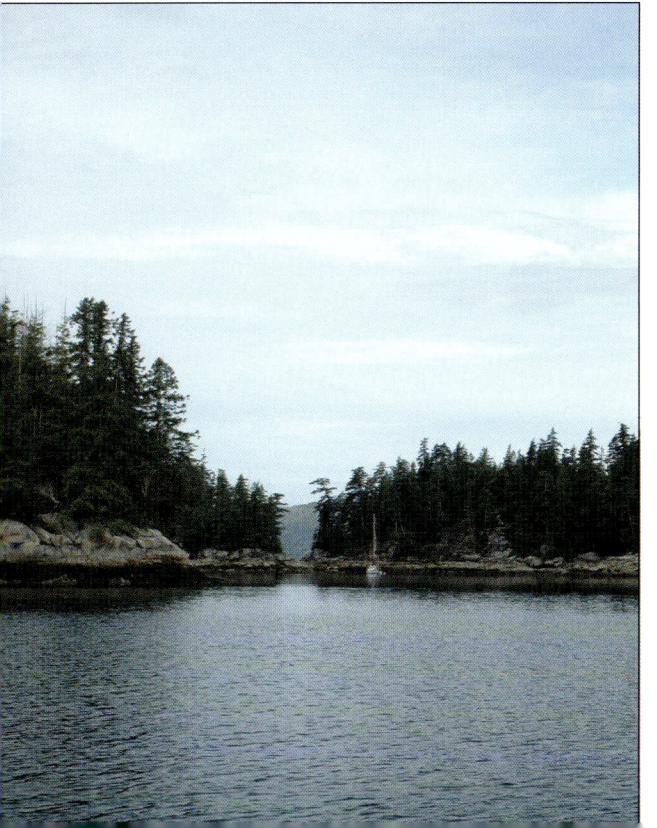

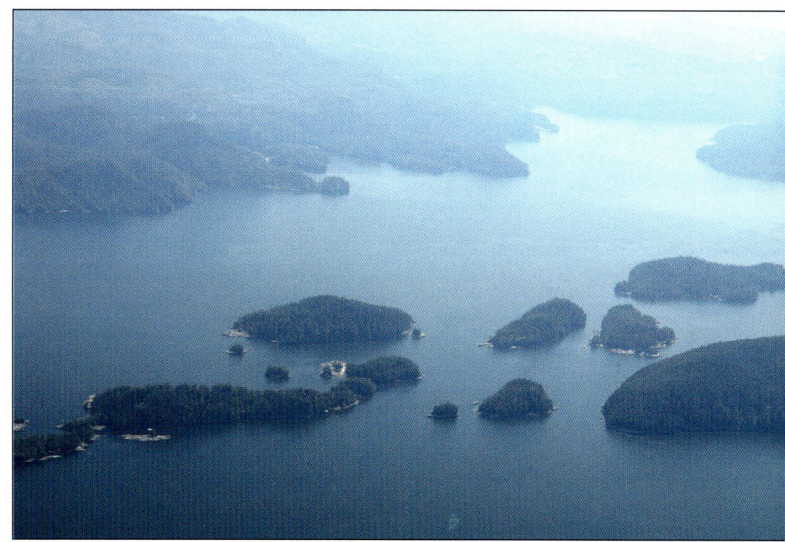

*Top: A boat slowly idles through the Burdwood Group heading for a quiet spot to drop anchor. In the distance is Tribune Channel. The view above shows the Group and Cramer Passage leading off to the south with Echo Bay at left. The image on the left is of an anchorage in the Burdwood Group of islands.*

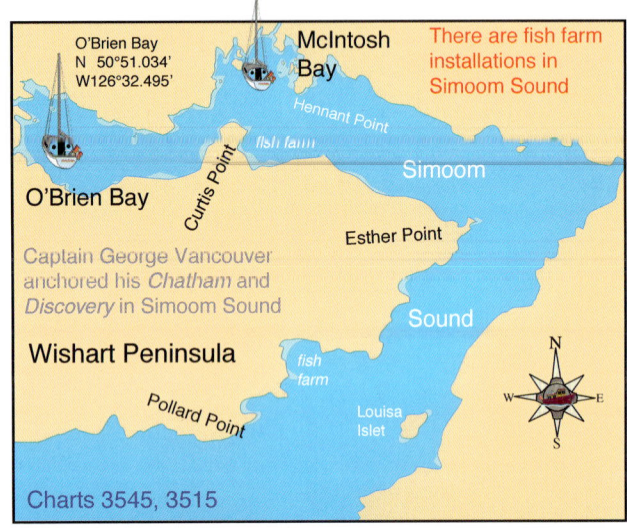

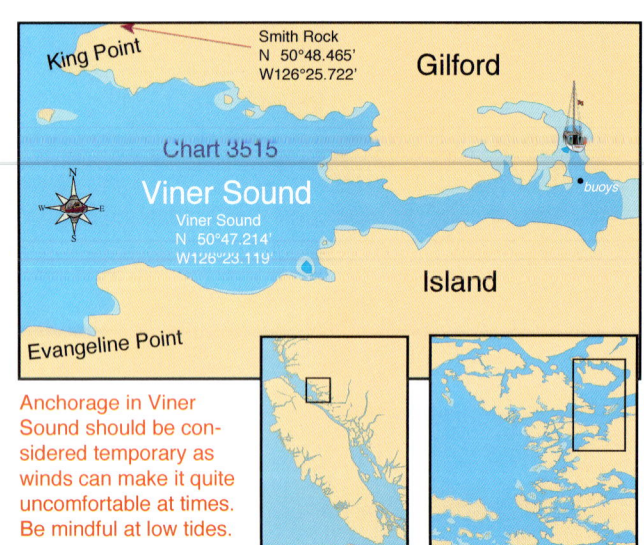

## Map labels (left upper map)

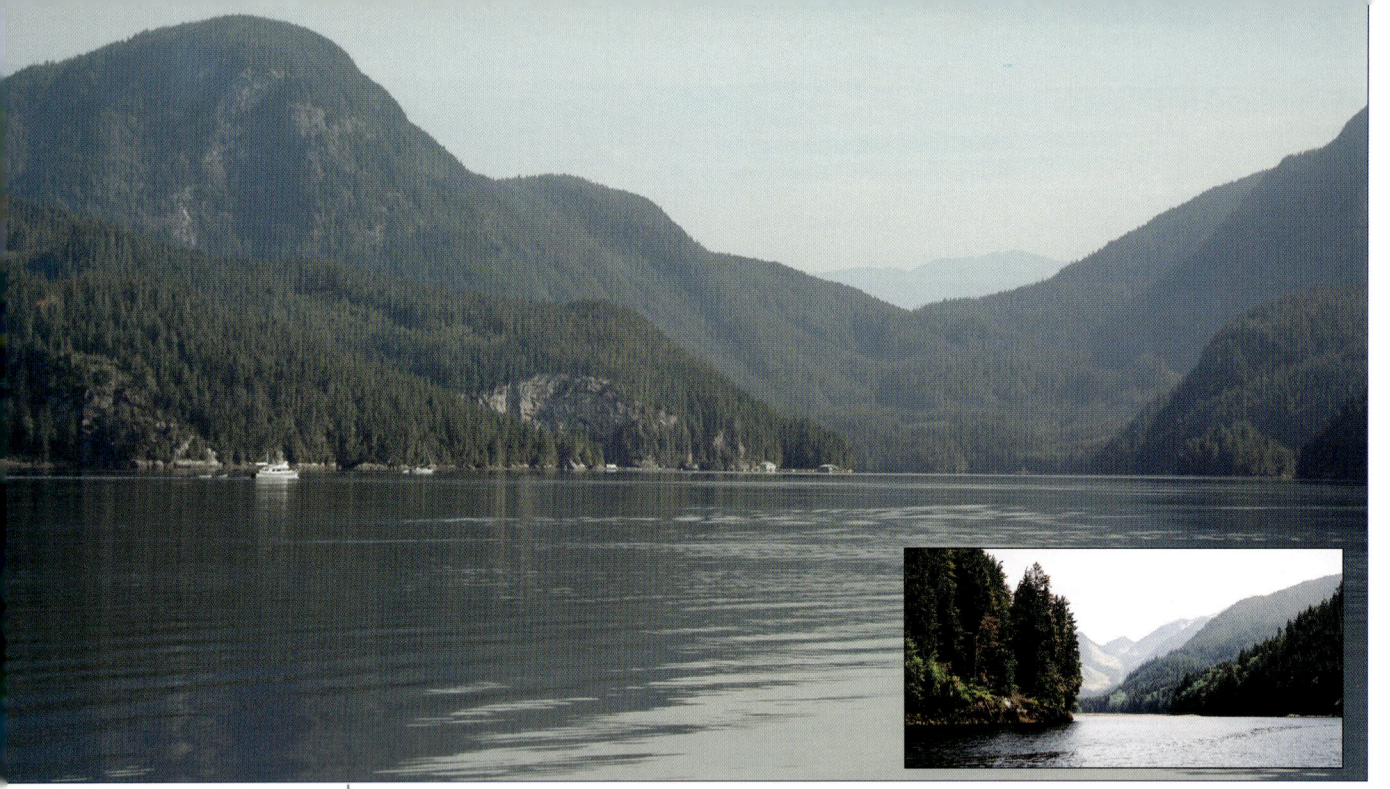

O'Brien Bay
N 50°51.034'
W 126°32.495'

McIntosh Bay

There are fish farm installations in Simoom Sound

Hennant Point
fish farm
Curtis Point
O'Brien Bay
Simoom
Esther Point

Captain George Vancouver anchored his *Chatham* and *Discovery* in Simoom Sound

Wishart Peninsula
Sound
fish farm
Pollard Point
Louisa Islet

Charts 3545, 3515

## Map labels (right upper map)

King Point
Smith Rock
N 50°48.465'
W 126°25.722'
Gilford

Chart 3515
Viner Sound
Viner Sound
N 50°47.214'
W 126°23.119'
Island
buoys

Evangeline Point

Anchorage in Viner Sound should be considered temporary as winds can make it quite uncomfortable at times. Be mindful at low tides.

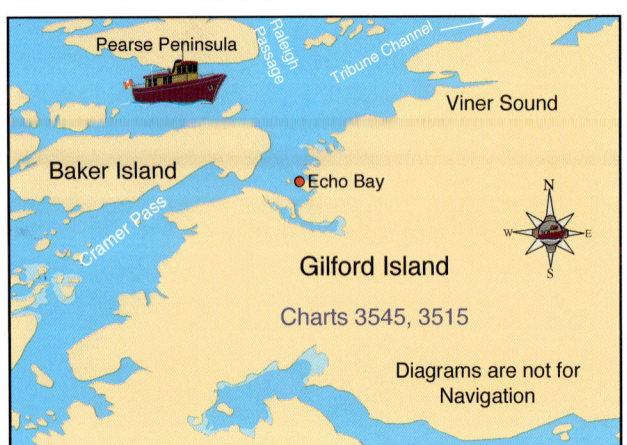

## Map labels (lower map)

Pearse Peninsula
Raleigh Passage
Tribune Channel
Viner Sound
Baker Island
Echo Bay
Cramer Pass
Gilford Island
Charts 3545, 3515

Diagrams are not for Navigation

---

and white beaches, with some nooks suitable mostly for daytime anchorage. They are surrounded by rocks and reefs and although several passages are possible, the best entrance to the middle of the group is from Hornet Passage to the east or the two passes from the north. Raleigh Passage and Hornet Passage lie on either side of the Burdwood Group.

When arriving from Tribune Channel you have the option of continuing south past Viner Sound to Echo Bay, Shoal Harbour, and beyond to the lower Broughtons, or northwest towards Shawl Bay and Sullivan Bay.

The direction to Sullivan Bay takes you into or past Simoom Sound, to Laura Bay and Shawl Bay then on to Kingcome Inlet or Wells Passage via Sutlej Channel.

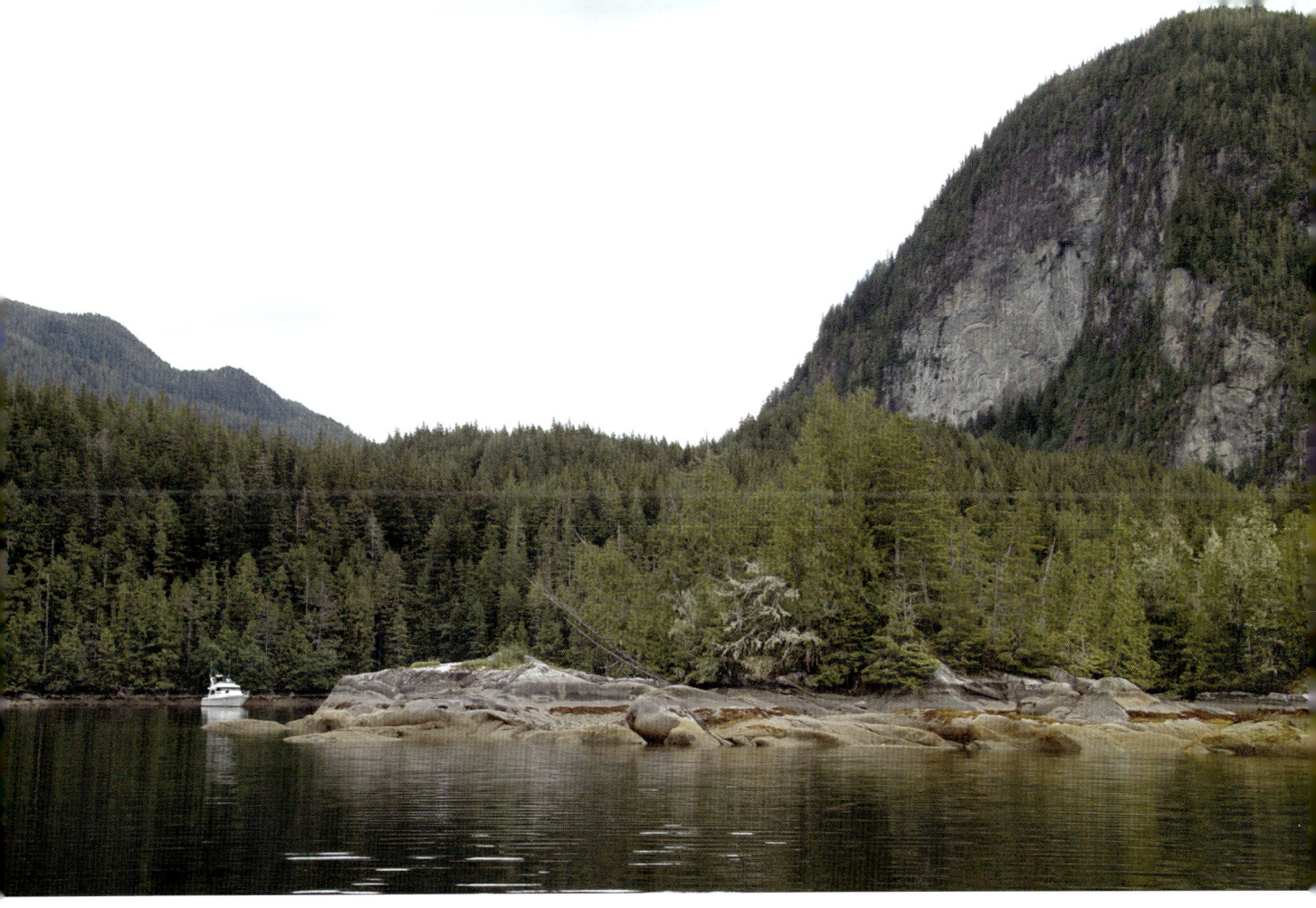

*Above: Calm waters and a tranquil anchorage in McIntosh Bay, Simoom Sound. Opposite page: Approaching the entrance to Simoom Sound. Inset: Viner Sound on the northwest side of Gilford Island. A small basin affords anchorage for two or three boats and several mooring buoys are available at the head of the sound.*

Sea conditions around the Burdwood Group may help you decide on your further plans, or to alter those already in place. Sometimes windy conditions can make it uncomfortable around the islands themselves. Westerlies bear watching closely south of the islands, and easterlies north of them.

## Viner Sound chart 3515

Viner Sound lies beyond Hornet Passage. By all means look for shelter inside if the wind is favourable. You have about 3 miles to go into the sound to find reasonably protected anchorage in a delightful cove with a depth of 4 metres. There are four mooring buoys at the entrance to the nook and space for a few boats to anchor. Small craft drop the hook here or well inside the inlet in the shallows west of the drying portion. It's the type of slightly out of the way place you would explore when you have the time. Day anchorage is good in settled weather. Check the tide tables carefully before anchoring. The currents in this area and the tidal exchanges are strong and large enough to cause you problems as the tide falls.

## Simoom Sound chart 3545, 3546

If you have arrived at the western end of Tribune Channel from Kwatsi Bay (page 77) enter Cramer Passage from Hornet Passage east of the Burdwood Group to reach Echo Bay. Or continue west along Penphrase Passage if Shawl Bay is your objective.

If you have just left Echo Bay pass the Burdwood Group via Raleigh Passage to reach Simoom Sound or to continue to Shawl Bay. Simoom Sound lies beyond Deep Sea Bluff in the lee of the Wishart Peninsula. It was once the location of much logging activity and today it is possible to see helicopter logging at times on the steep hillsides nearby.

Simoom Sound is known historically as being one of the extended anchorages used by Captain Vancouver in HMS *Discovery* and *Chatham* during his voyages of exploration in the summer of 1792. Best anchorage in the sound can be found at **O'Brien Bay** or in **McIntosh Bay**. It is possible to take shelter in some conditions and in emergency in the lee of Louisa Islet near the mouth of Simoom Sound, or adjacent to the fish farm on the opposite shore. Another fish farm lies farther up in the sound.

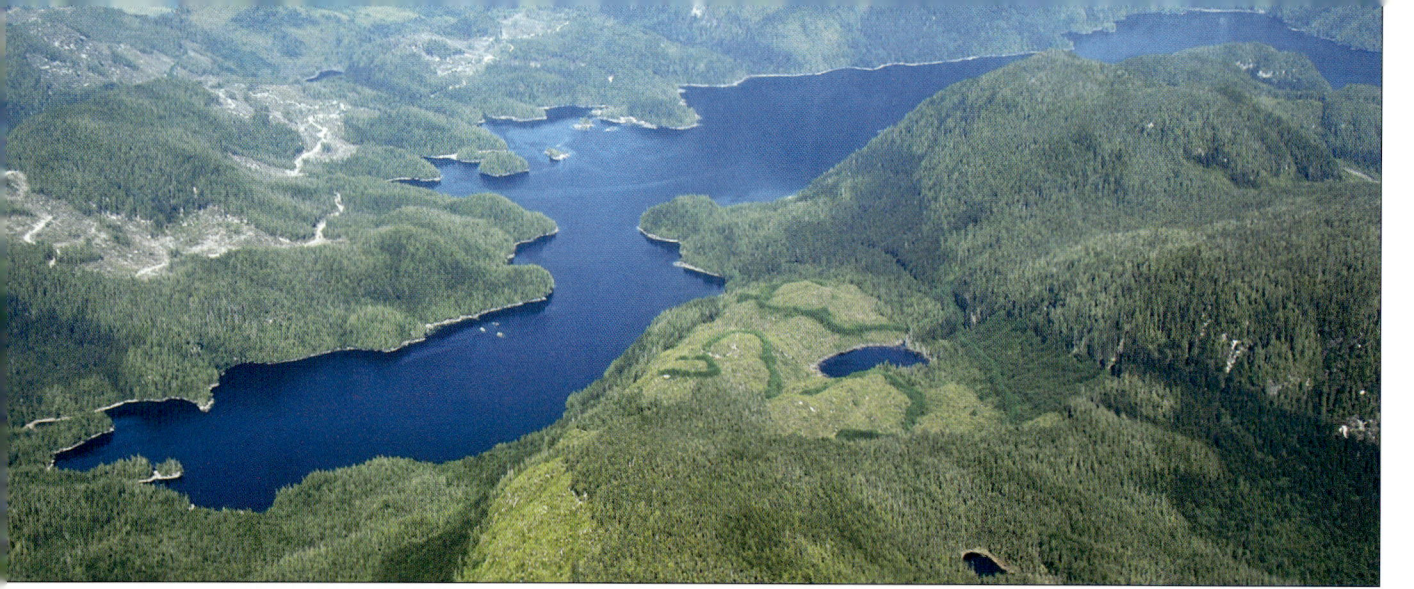

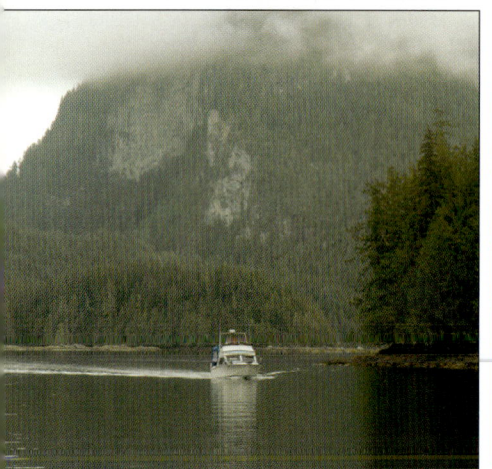

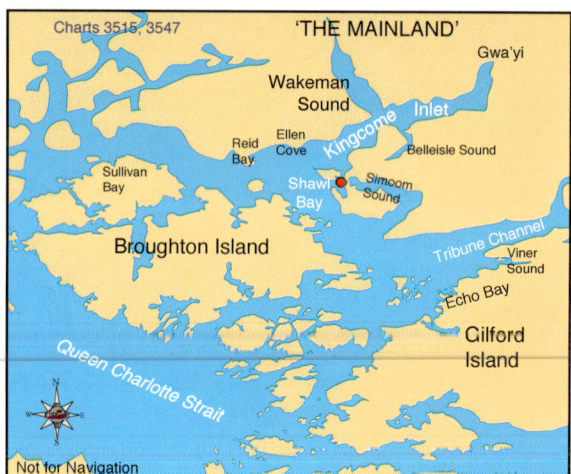

*Above: The head of Simoom Sound with O'Brien Bay in the foreground and McIntosh Bay at top centre. Bottom: Simoom Sound, where Captain Vancouver anchored in 1792. Left: Slipping into the innermost reaches of Simoom Sound. Bald Mountain forms a backdrop to the view from inside O'Brien Bay. Opposite page: Relaxing and enjoying the ambiance of Shawl Bay. This floating resort and the well-known family who owns it have a long history on 'The Mainland' coast.*

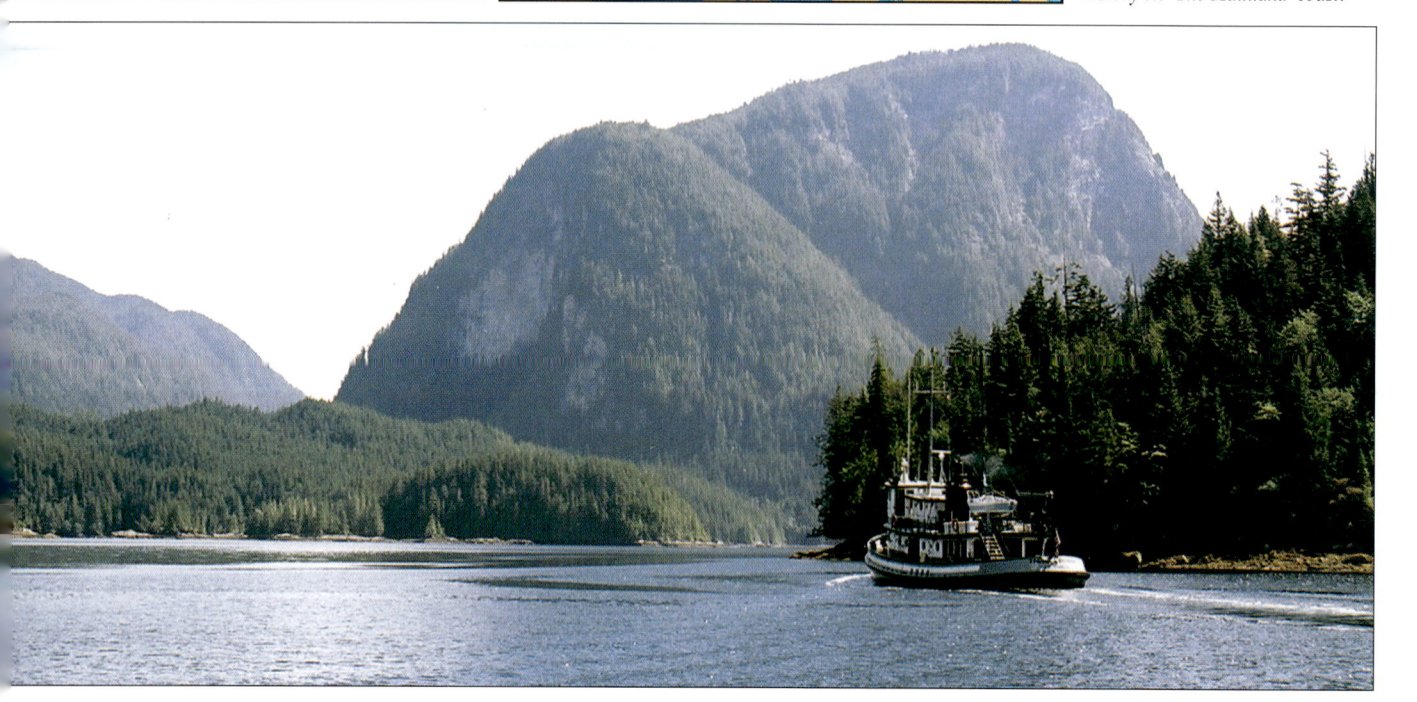

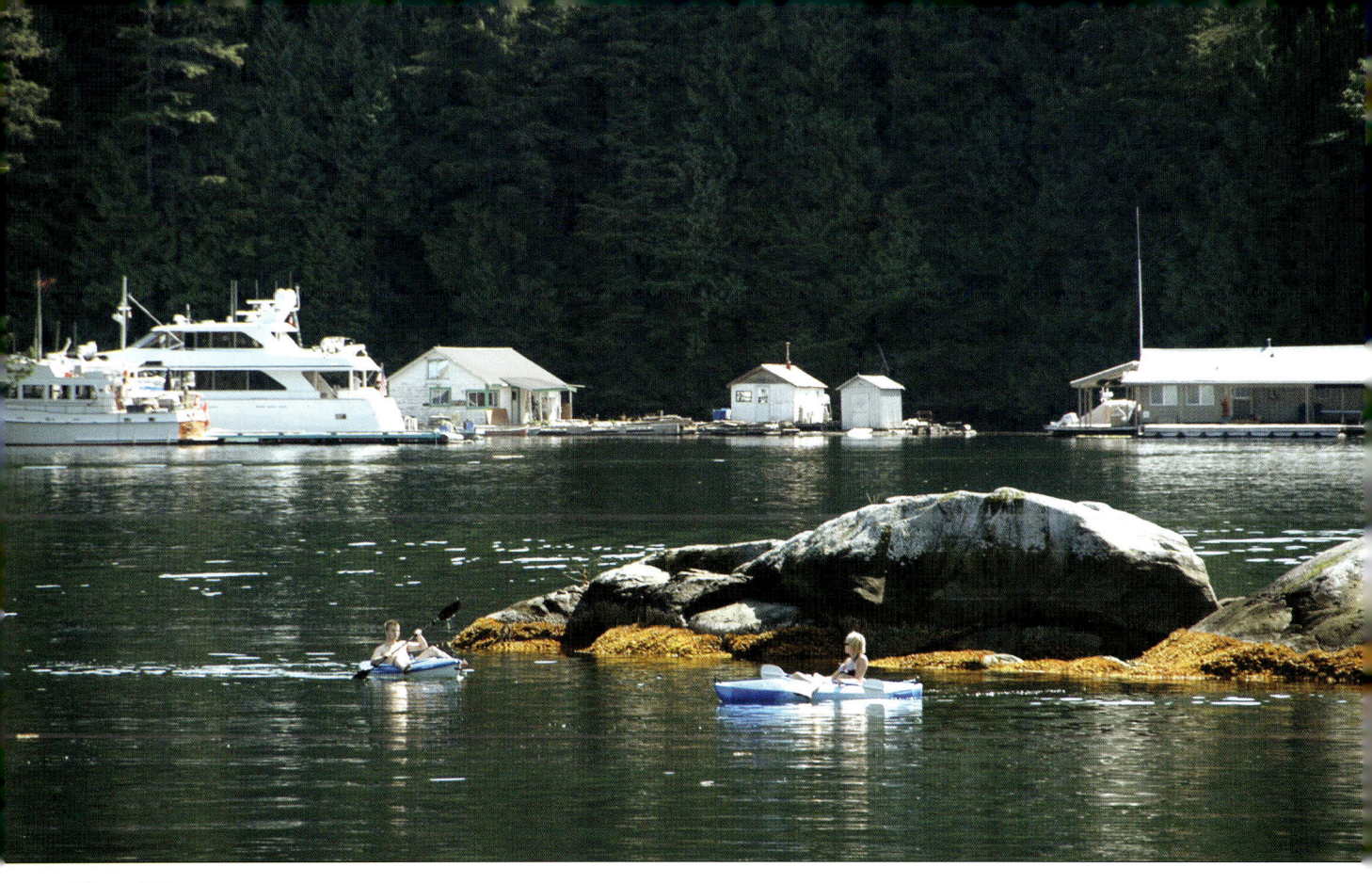

## Shawl Bay  chart 3515

Breakfast at Shawl Bay is legendary. Introduced in the mid to late 1990s and carried on through the years, it has been a delightful fare of pancakes and coffee and other treats, but the gesture on the part of the owners Lorne and Shawn Brown has made it very special. Lorne's parents and their family were the former owners of the floats and store in the bay. The docks were there in the early days to serve the needs of local logging camps. They were part of the original Viner Logging Company located in adjacent Moore Bay. When Lorne's father, Allan, died, the facility was maintained by his mother, Edna. She and her sister Jo Didrikson ran the marina for some years, before Edna passed away in the mid 1990s leaving the marina to be run by her son Gary, Lorne's brother, and then eventually by Lorne and his wife Shawn with the assistance of their son Robert. Aunty Jo continued to collect the moorage fees from overnight guests until her recent death. She also took care of the business side of rental cabins, small, tidy units usually occupied by fly-in guests or those who arrive aboard small boats that do not have adequate onboard accommodations. The flights that bring guests to the bay usually come out of Port McNeill or Campbell River.

The marina is quite extensively endowed with floats and several small buildings that accommodate, among other things, a laundry and a gift shop. Regular visitors know to look for the popular sticky buns and bread baked fresh by Shawn. The pancake breakfast with coffee is a morning ritual, provided complimentary by the family to overnight guests. Other special dinner evenings include alternating seafood chowder and turkey.

Shawl Bay Marina has two generators to provide electrical power to the cottages and docks. These, along with a water supply line, were brought in during a renovation undertaking when Lorne took over the facility. Other upgrades to the marina included redecking of the docks and the addition of a large, covered social area with picnic tables.

For the use of overnight guests who have canine commitments, the marina has a doggy walk, or what the family refers to as the K-9 Yacht Club, with a real grass lawn and plastic fire hydrants.

## Moore Bay  chart 3515

When the tide is on the rise and beyond the half way mark, it is possible for some boats to navigate through the narrow pass at the north side of Shawl Bay into Moore Bay. Mind the ledge off Gregory Island. Locals use this waterway as a means of travelling between Shawl Bay and Kingcome Inlet. Some slip through to anchor in the shelter of Gregory Island in the lee of Thief Island. Mind Thief Rocks which can be difficult to locate at some tides. There are two mooring buoys in the eastern corner of Moore Bay. Use these with discretion.

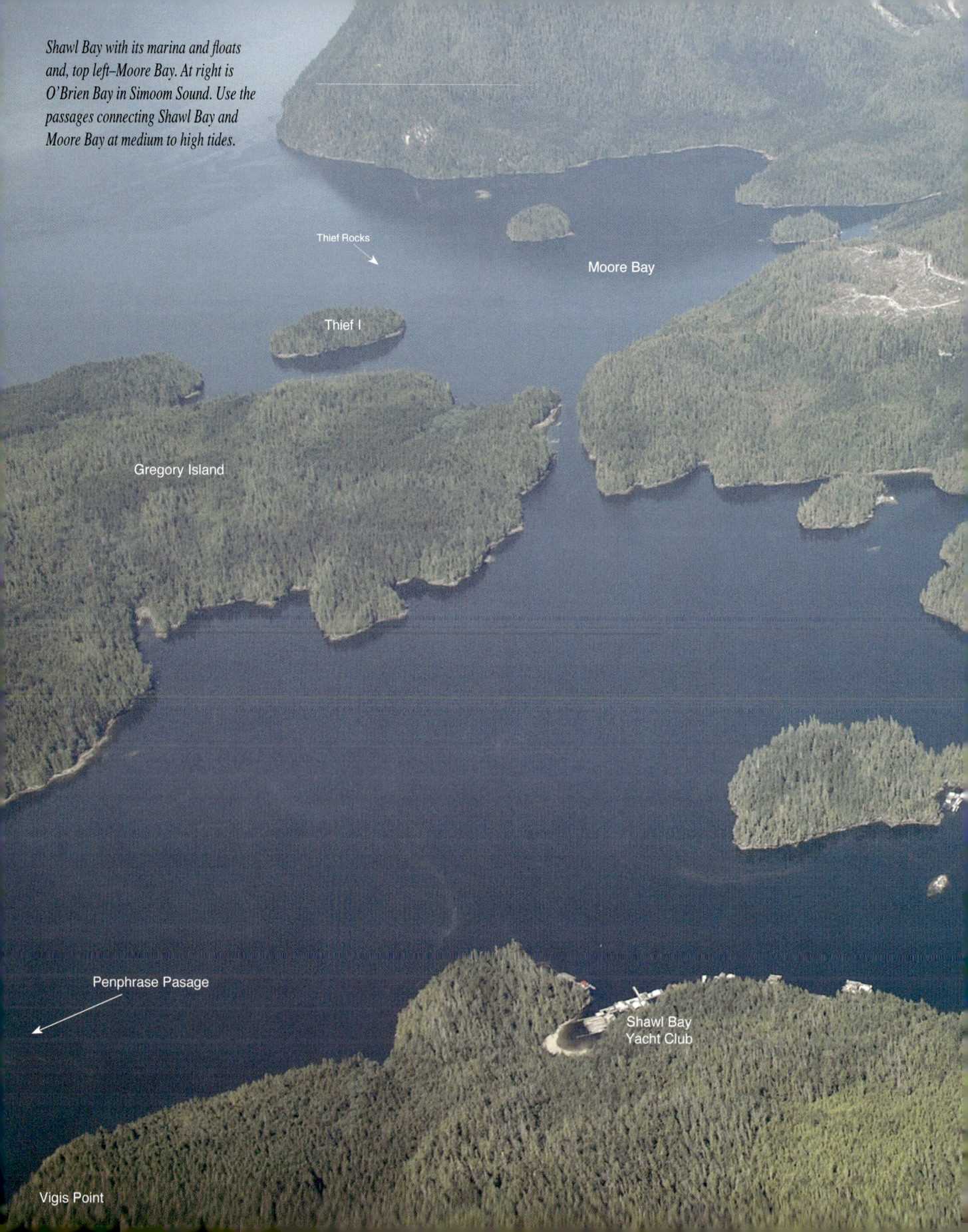

*Shawl Bay with its marina and floats and, top left–Moore Bay. At right is O'Brien Bay in Simoom Sound. Use the passages connecting Shawl Bay and Moore Bay at medium to high tides.*

anchorages in McIntosh Bay

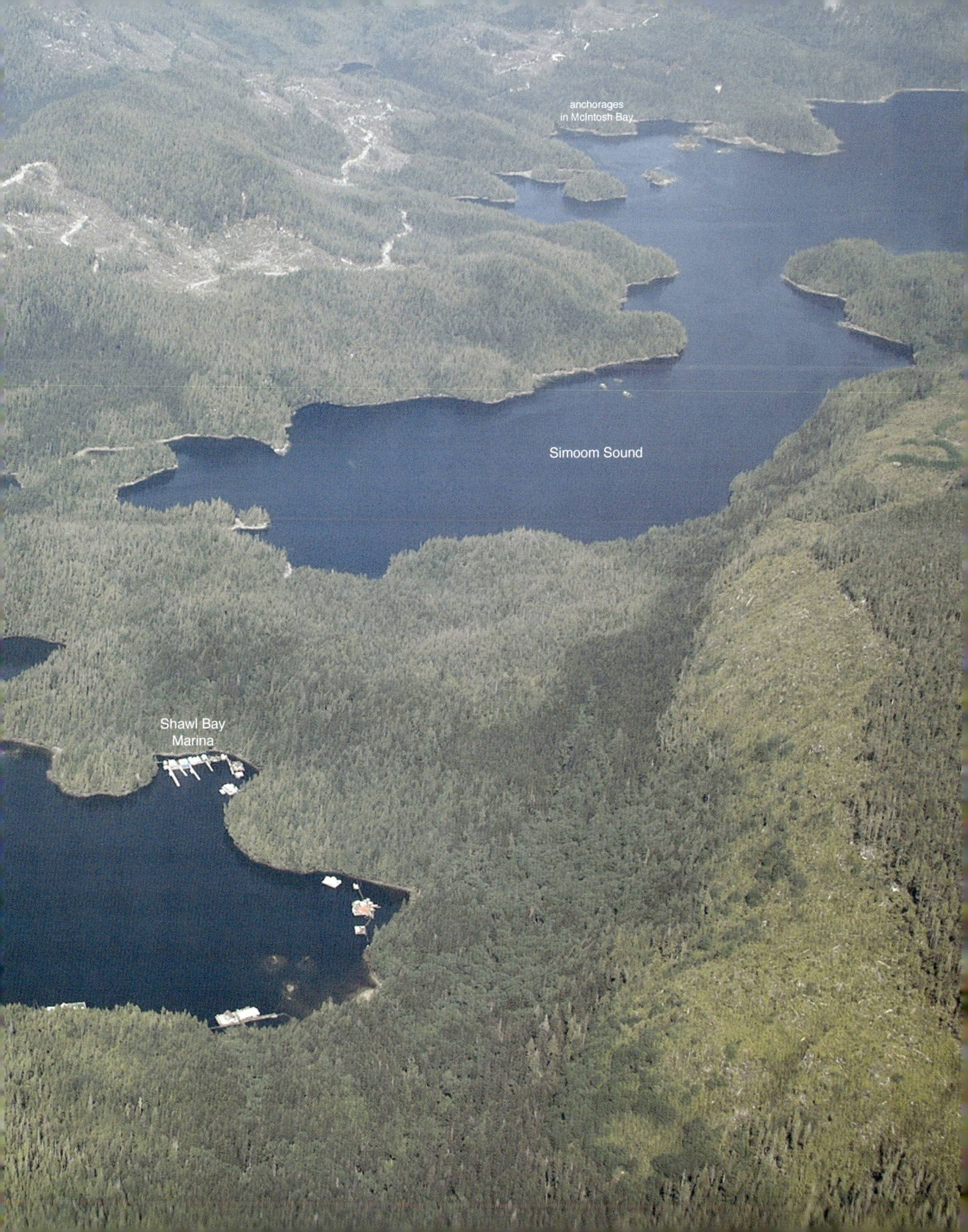

Simoom Sound

Shawl Bay Marina

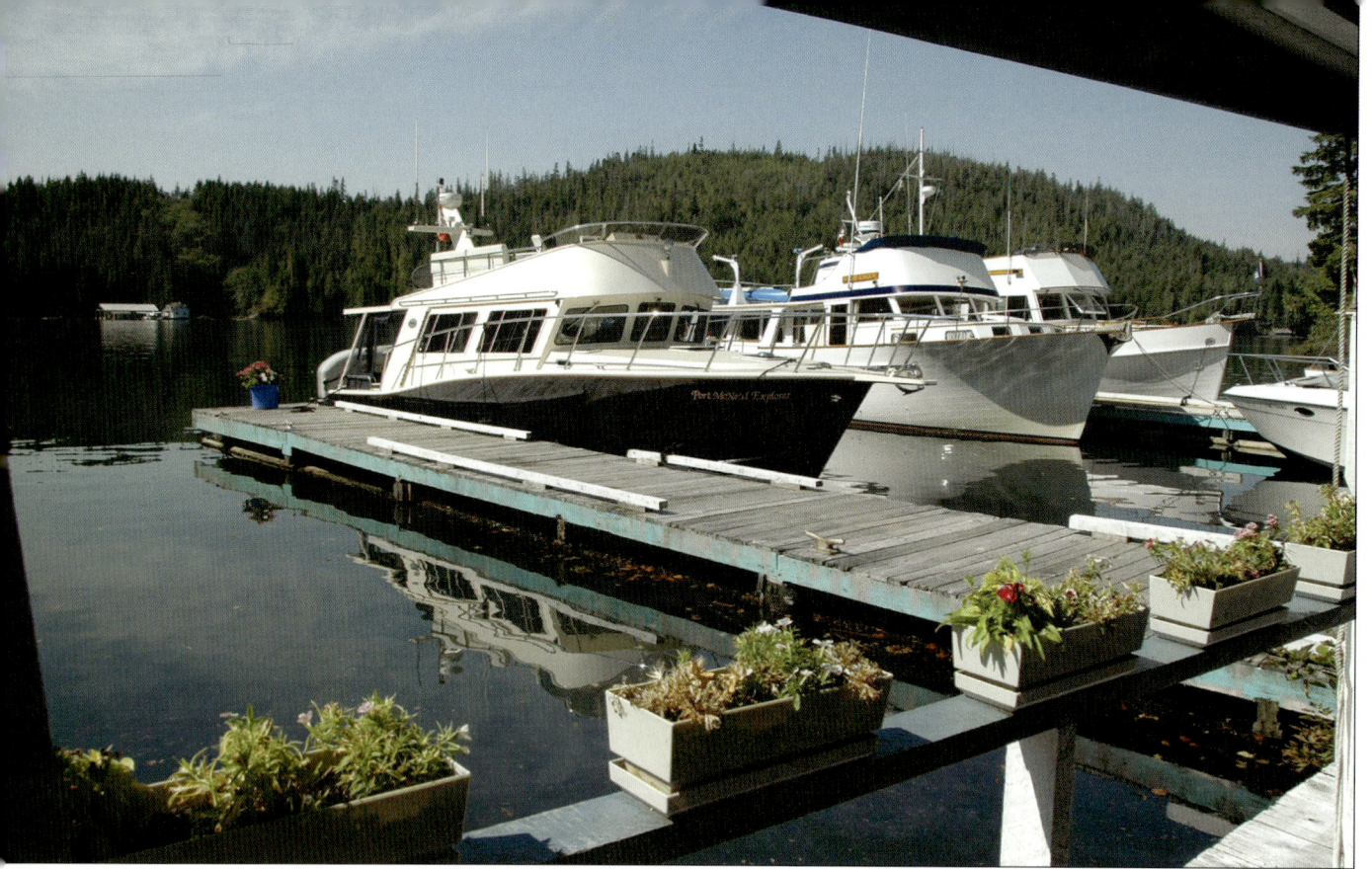

*Visiting boats at Shawl Bay. Each year the boats arriving at the Broughton Islands seem to become larger than before. Docks and amenities have been upgraded at this and other marinas to cater to the bigger vessels and the needs of their crews. Below: There is a covered patio float at Shawl Bay where visitors gather for evening social times and for pancake breakfasts. The buildings accommodate the owners, a gift shop, laundry and other facilities for mooring guests. A comfortable cabin is available for overnight visitors who fly in or arrive as guests aboard a boat.*

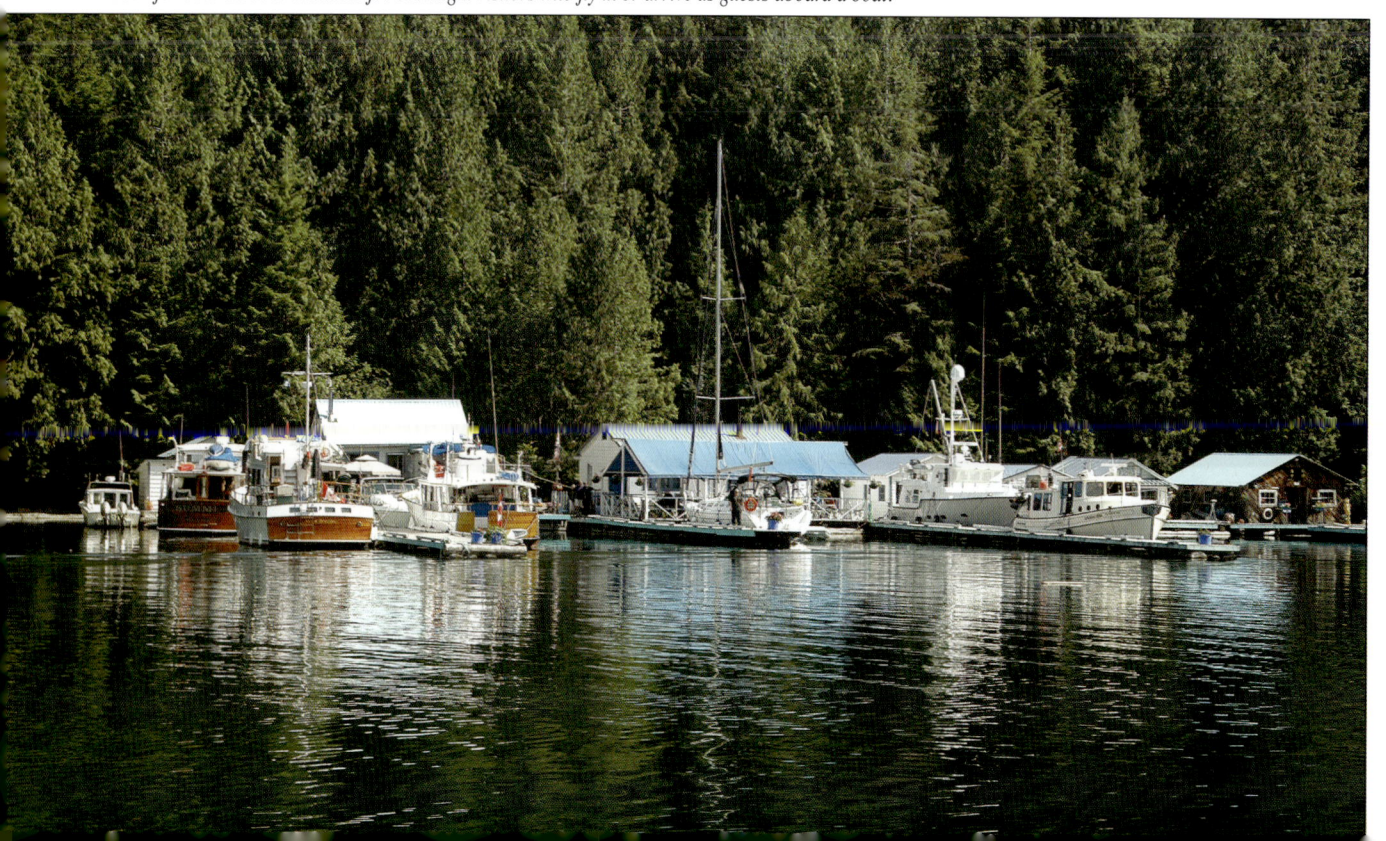

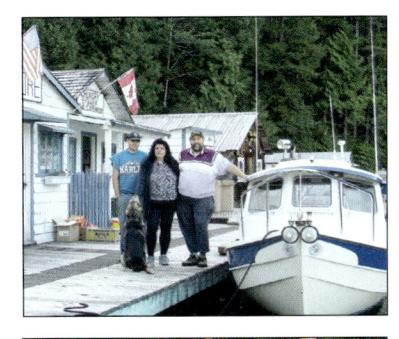

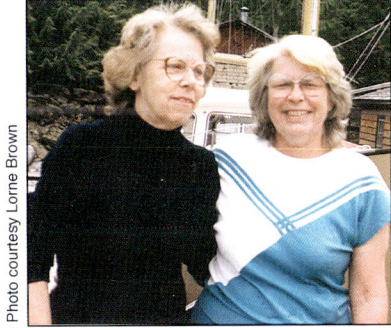

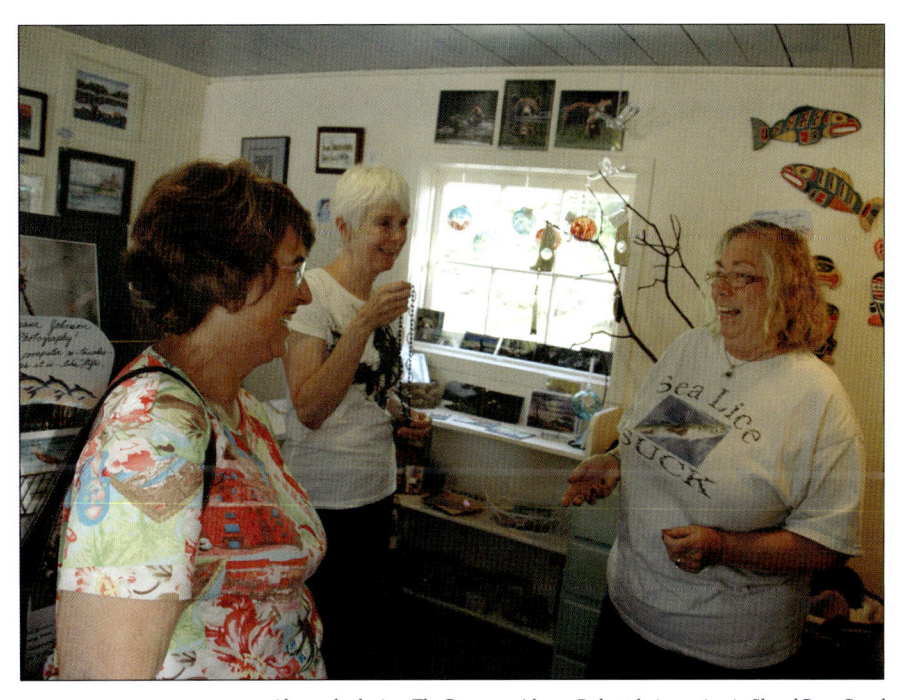

## Shawl Bay Marina
General Delivery
Simoom Sound  BC  V0P 1S0
Phone  250-483-4169  VHF 66A
email:  shawlbaymarina@hughes.net
www.shawlbaymarina.com

The marina has 1,000 ft of dock space, some reserved for yacht clubs, a small store with some provisions and a gift shop. A pancake breakfast is included with overnight moorage courtesy of Lorne and Shawn Brown. The marina also provides water, laundry, covered picnic tables, showers, fresh bread, pies and cinnamon rolls. This is the nearest marina to Kingcome Inlet (and the village of Gwa'yi).
When entering Shawl Bay from Penphrase Passage, pass Vigis Point and, at no wake speeds, slip by the Shawl Bay Yacht Club floating homes immediately inside the bay. Follow the curve of the bay around the island in the centre and proceed slowly towards the turquoise docks and white cabins with wedgewood trim, against the far shore.
Anchorage in nearby Moore Bay. Use the passage between Shawl Bay and Moore Bay only at medium to high tides.

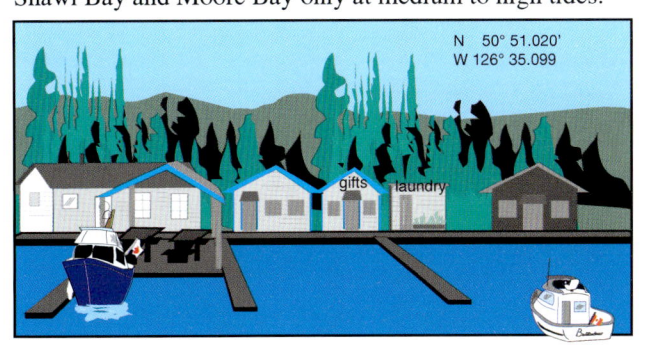

*Above clockwise: The Browns with son Rob at their marina in Shawl Bay. Carol "the Bead Lady" shows guests Carla Vassilopoulos and Nancy Jackman some of her gift selections. Sisters the late Jo Didriksen and Edna Brown, former family owners of the facilty. Bottom: Rustic building on the docks at Shawl Bay and the "K-9 yacht club" adjacent to the USA and Canadian flags.*

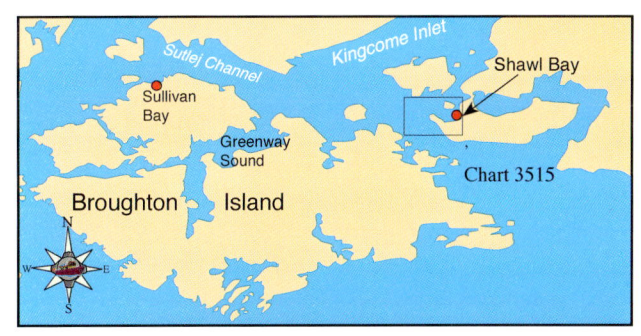

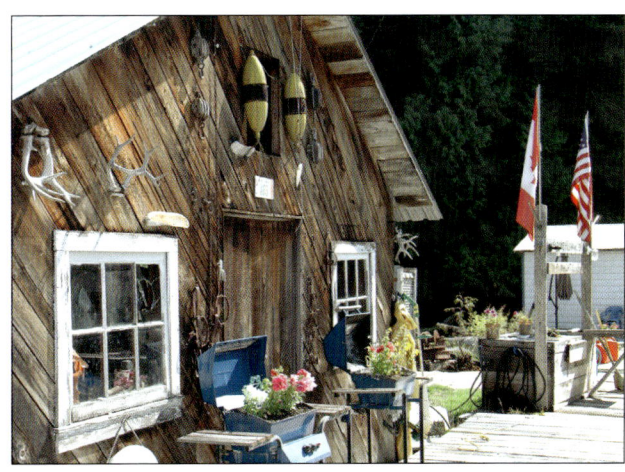

N  50° 51.020'
W 126° 35.099

**Shawl Bay**
to Sullivan Bay 11
to Echo Bay 5.5
to Kingcome 13.5

Note: the mileages given are always from the first named place.

to Kingcome Inlet

Kingcome Inlet

rock
mooring buoys
dinghy dock
Thief Rocks
Thief Island
Moore Bay

to Greenway Sound and Sullivan Bay

Bradley Point
Chart 3515
**Gregory Island**

This passage is navigable only at half tides plus and frequently used by local boats to about 40'. Check with marina.

Simoom Sound
O'Brien Bay

Shawl Bay
N 50°51.020'
W126°35.099'

Vigis Point

Penphrase Passage

Shawl Bay Yacht Club

Shawl Bay

Shawl Bay Marina

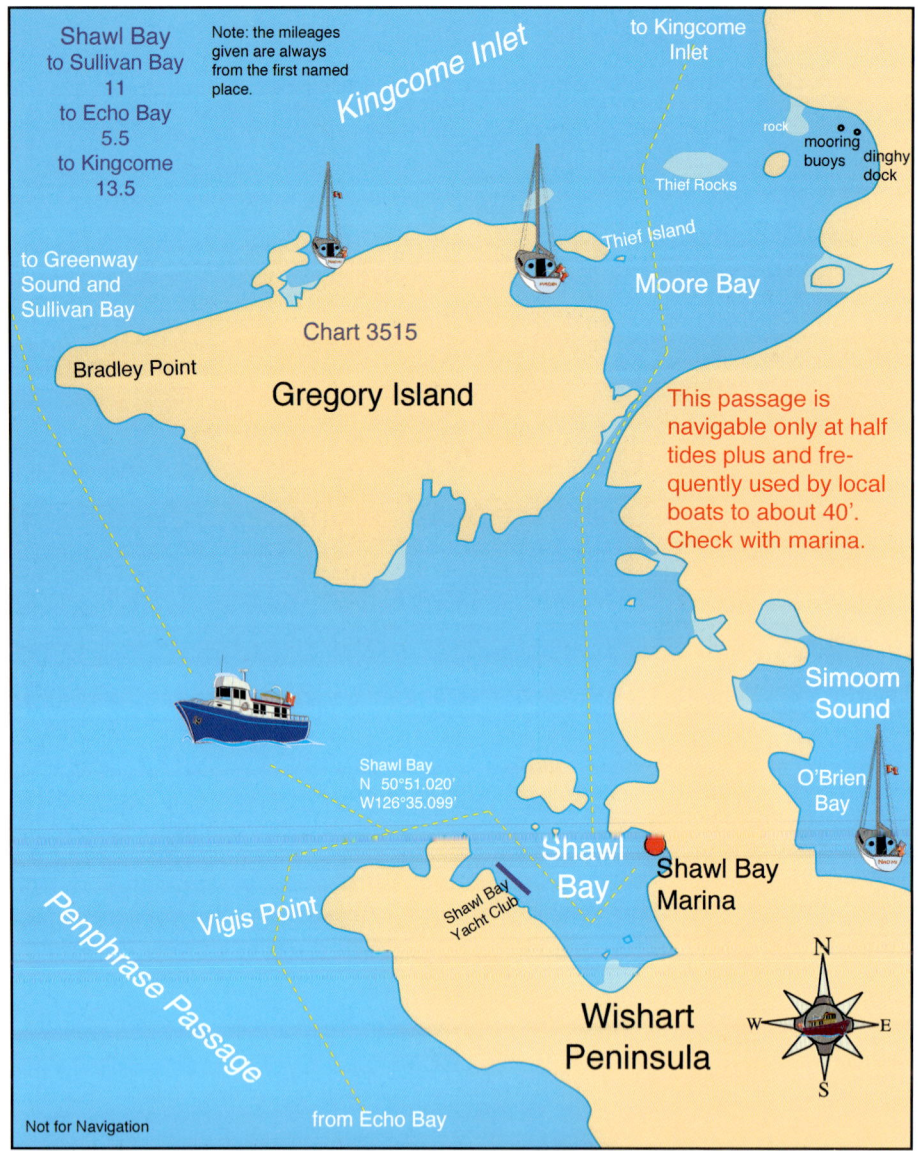

**Wishart Peninsula**

from Echo Bay

Not for Navigation

*Opposite: Looking east up Kingcome Inlet towards its confluence with Wakeman Sound. Bottom: The logging camp at Wakeman Sound, and Kingcome Inlet from above the mountains overlooking the village of Gwa'yi (Kingcome).*

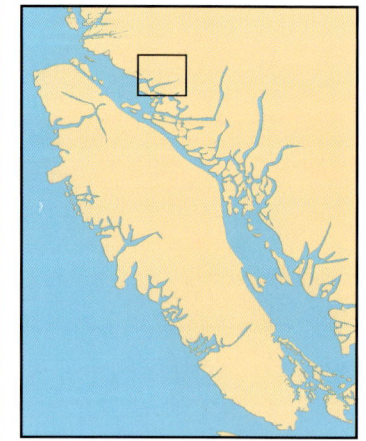

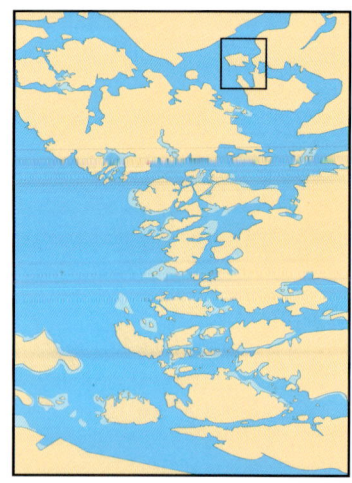

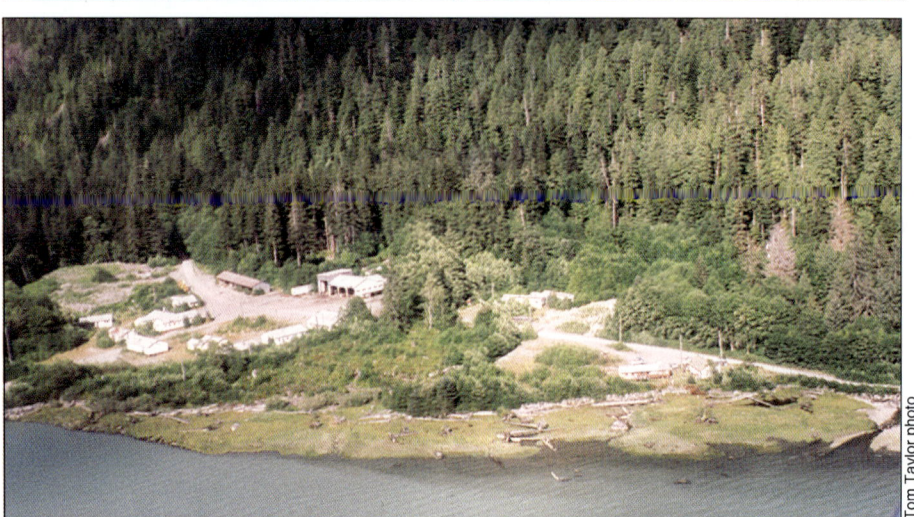

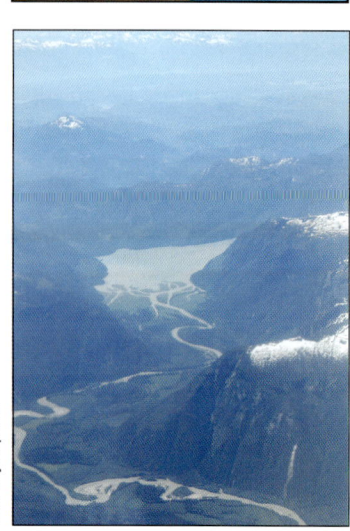

Tom Taylor photo

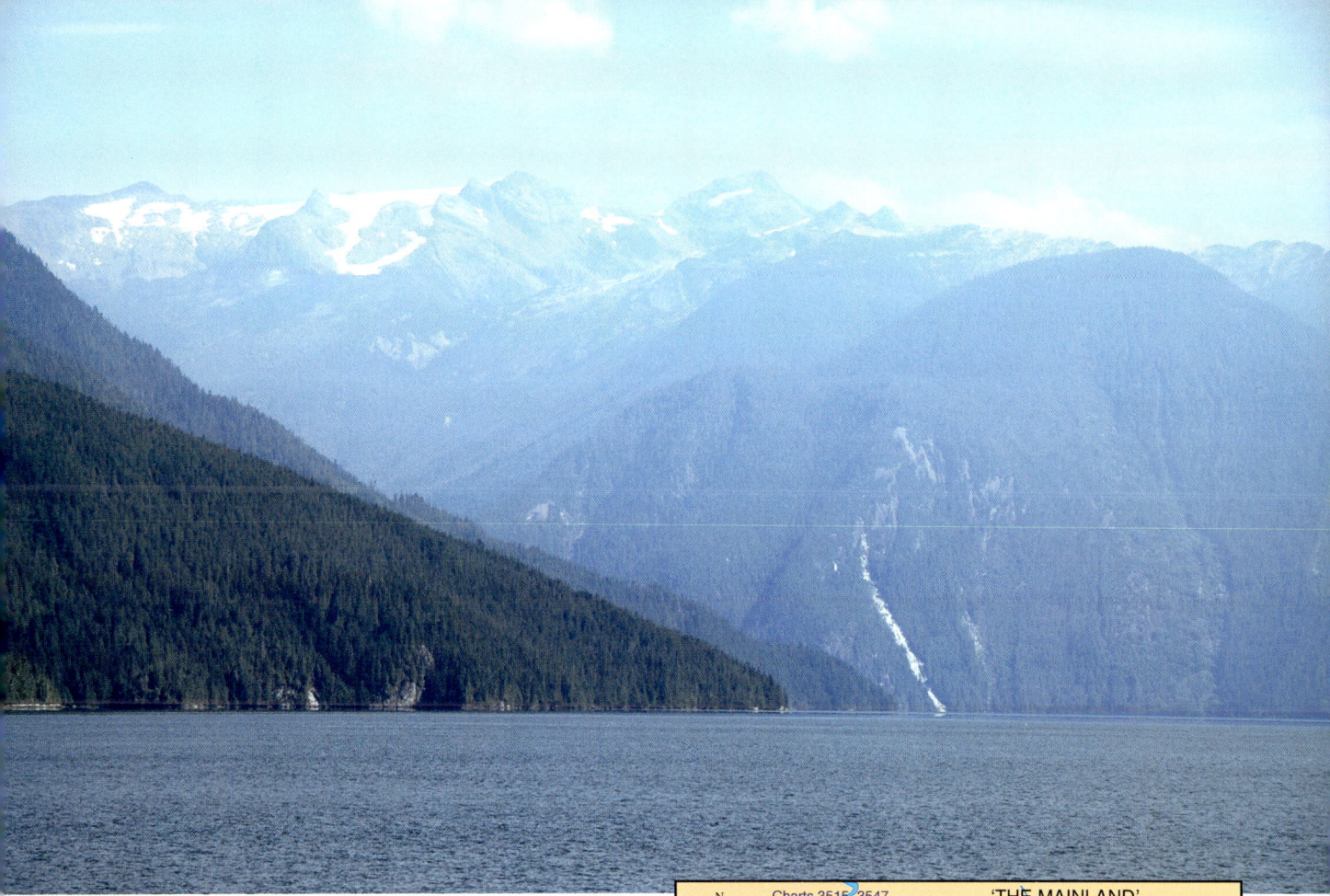

### Kingcome Inlet  chart 3515

From Shawl Bay, passage into Kingcome Inlet can be taken via Moore Bay or around Gregory Island. There is not much by way of shelter along the 17 miles of Kingcome Inlet. Beyond Magin Islets, **Reid Bay** opens on the west shore of the entrance to Kingcome Inlet but is not considered a reliable anchorage. Rather, if you need to find a temporary place of shelter try the small bay to the south of it. This bay offers protection from easterlies. Anchor in about 10 metres, but watch for rocks if you enter from the south. As you travel farther up Kingcome Inlet along the northern shore you can take shelter from rising westerly winds in **Ellen Cove**. **Wakeman Sound** is a wide, scenic sound that opens to the north off Kingcome Inlet, part way to its head. Individuals cruising into the sound may see bears on shore and possibly whales along the way.

Steve and Retta Vesely, the former owners, were well known in the area for three decades. Their Gypsey II Fishing Camp catered to people flying in to fish, watch bears, bird and wild life. More recently other owners and managers running the operation at Wakeman Wilderness Camp added other eco-tourism elements to the experience and visitors came to watch salmon spawning and perhaps do some river rafting and paddling in the lower delta of the river. While the Interfor company dock serves the coming and going of small crew boats it can be used temporarily by a small to medium sized boat. Otherwise it is necessary to anchor in a bight nearby. It is advisable not to tie up to the large buoy near the dock due to its exposed position.

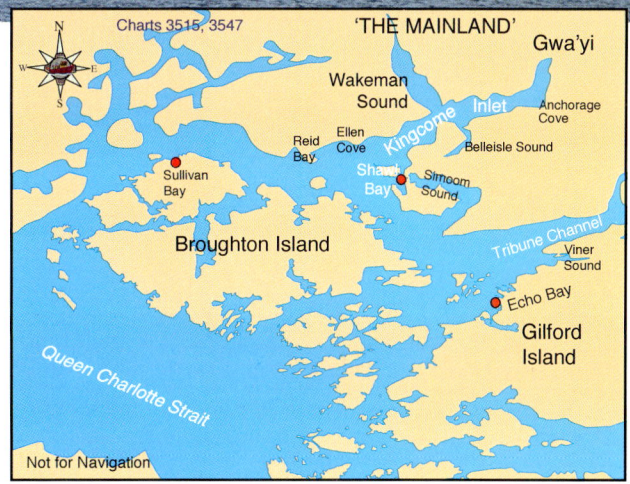

It was fascinating to watch helicopter logging in Wakeman Sound. We were fascinated as we cruised by the tall mountains and long narrow waterfalls taking in the magnificent views.

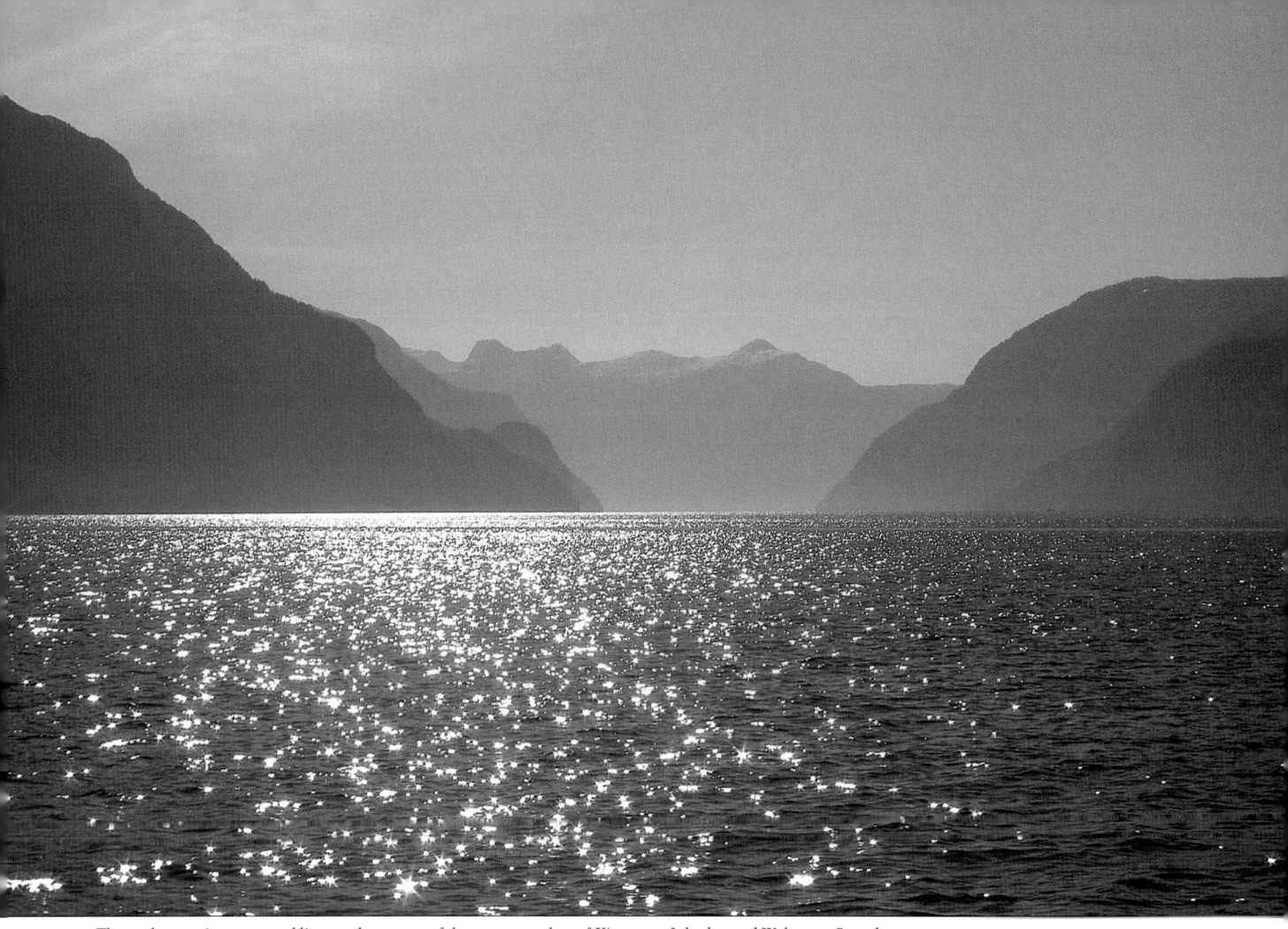

*The early morning sun sparkling on the waters of the upper reaches of Kingcome Inlet beyond Wakeman Sound.*

Equally grand are the views up Kingcome Inlet. Logging is a big industry but it has its disadvantages for mariners looking for peace and quiet. Cypress Harbour, for example, may not be the best place to anchor overnight if you wish to escape the sounds of industry.

**Belleisle Sound** opens off to the south of Kingcome Inlet but is deep throughout with the exception of a small beach off a piece of First Nations land, located beyond a small islet on the east shore a short distance beyond the narrow entrance. There is a reef off the south end of the beach and any anchoring in this area should be in the lee of the island and only for a short period, preferably during daylight and while the winds are calm. Robert Hale, founder of *Waggoner Cruising Guide* says he and his wife Marilyn spent the night at anchor here once, in calm conditions. But be warned of possible strong westerly winds.

Near the head of Kingcome Inlet you are not only in the land of the First Nations of Gwa'yi, but also at the site of large rock paintings on the cliff overlooking the deep inlet. Nearby is the former home of the Halliday family. This is a landmark in Kingcome Inlet. The old ranch was home to the Hallidays since being established in 1895 by William and Ernest Halliday. Their farm became a focal point on the coast with steamships calling, logging and of course, farming. The Hallidays farmed cattle and produced hay and fresh greens.

At the head of Kingcome Inlet you can tie alongside a public float and work your way up the river in a small, shallow draft boat. Nearby is **Anchorage Cove** where you can drop anchor in settled weather. This is the land of *I Heard the Owl Call My Name*, a book by Margaret Craven that told of the life of the Gwa'yi people, and of a missionary at the village. To visit Kingcome Village, Gwa'yi, it is best to make arrangements first. Ask for information at Shawl Bay Resort or at Port McNeill. Trips into Kingcome Inlet or the Wakeman Sound wilderness can be arranged.

The Kingcome Inlet village of Gwa'yi has been well maintained and the people living there sometimes welcome visitors. The missionary John Antle established a mission station at this most famous of all First Nations historic villages. The church building was erected by the local population in the 1930s and has been well maintained in its anomalous place among the totem poles and First Nations homes.

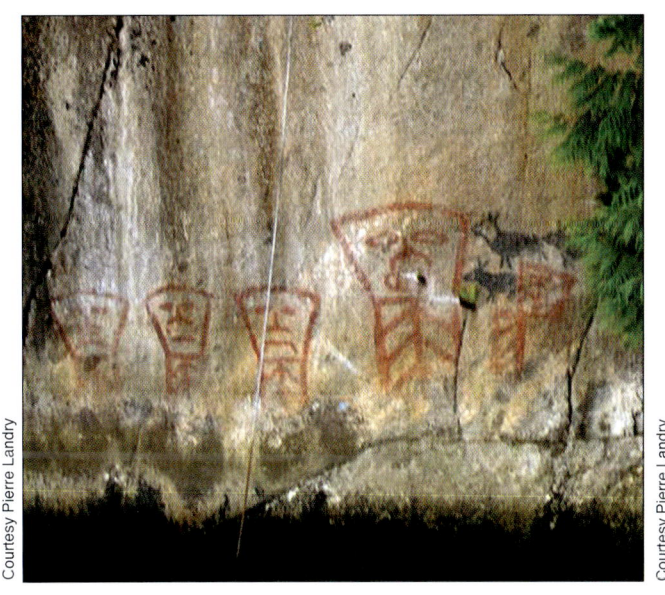

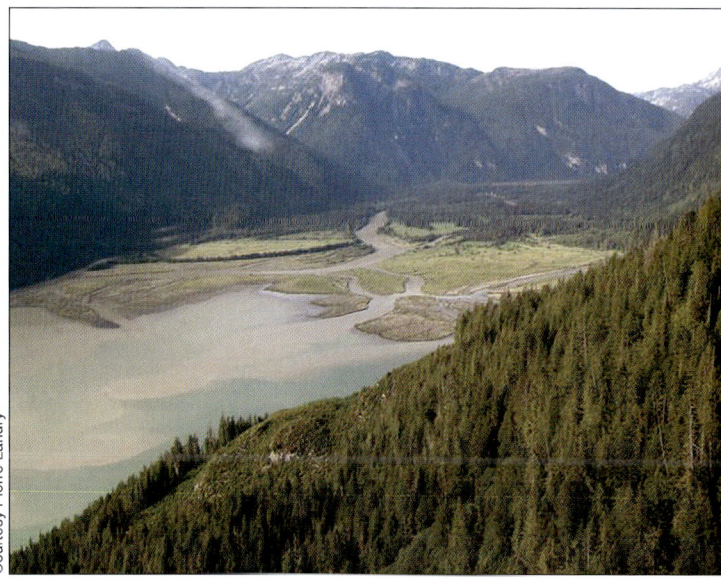

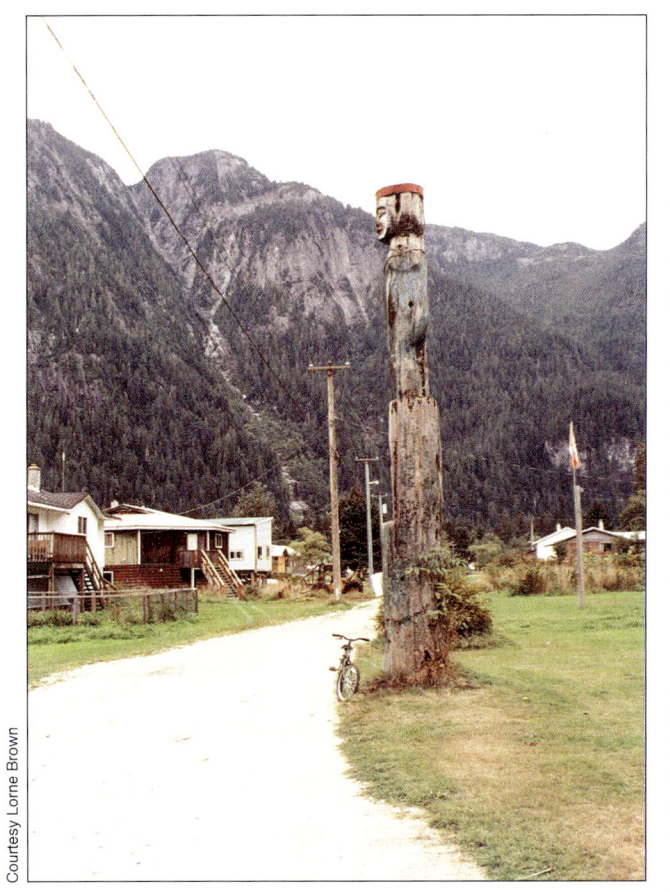

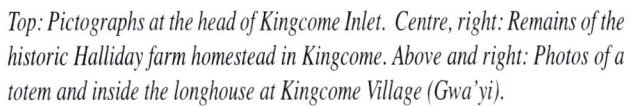

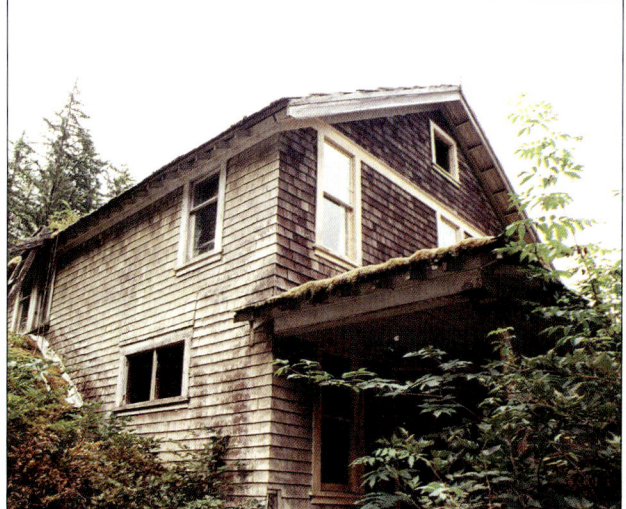

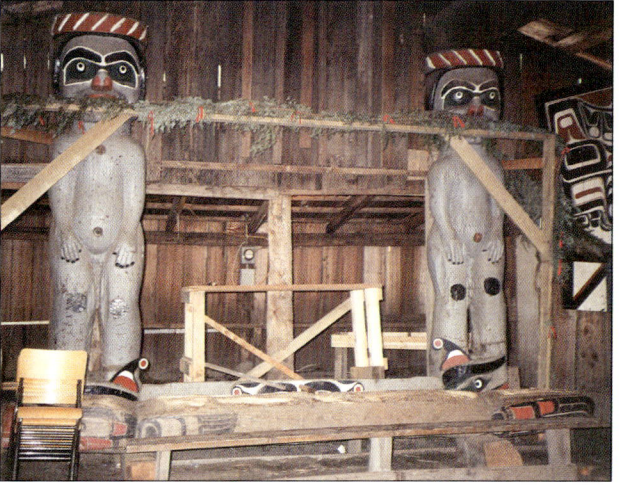

*Top: Pictographs at the head of Kingcome Inlet. Centre, right: Remains of the historic Halliday farm homestead in Kingcome. Above and right: Photos of a totem and inside the longhouse at Kingcome Village (Gwa'yi).*

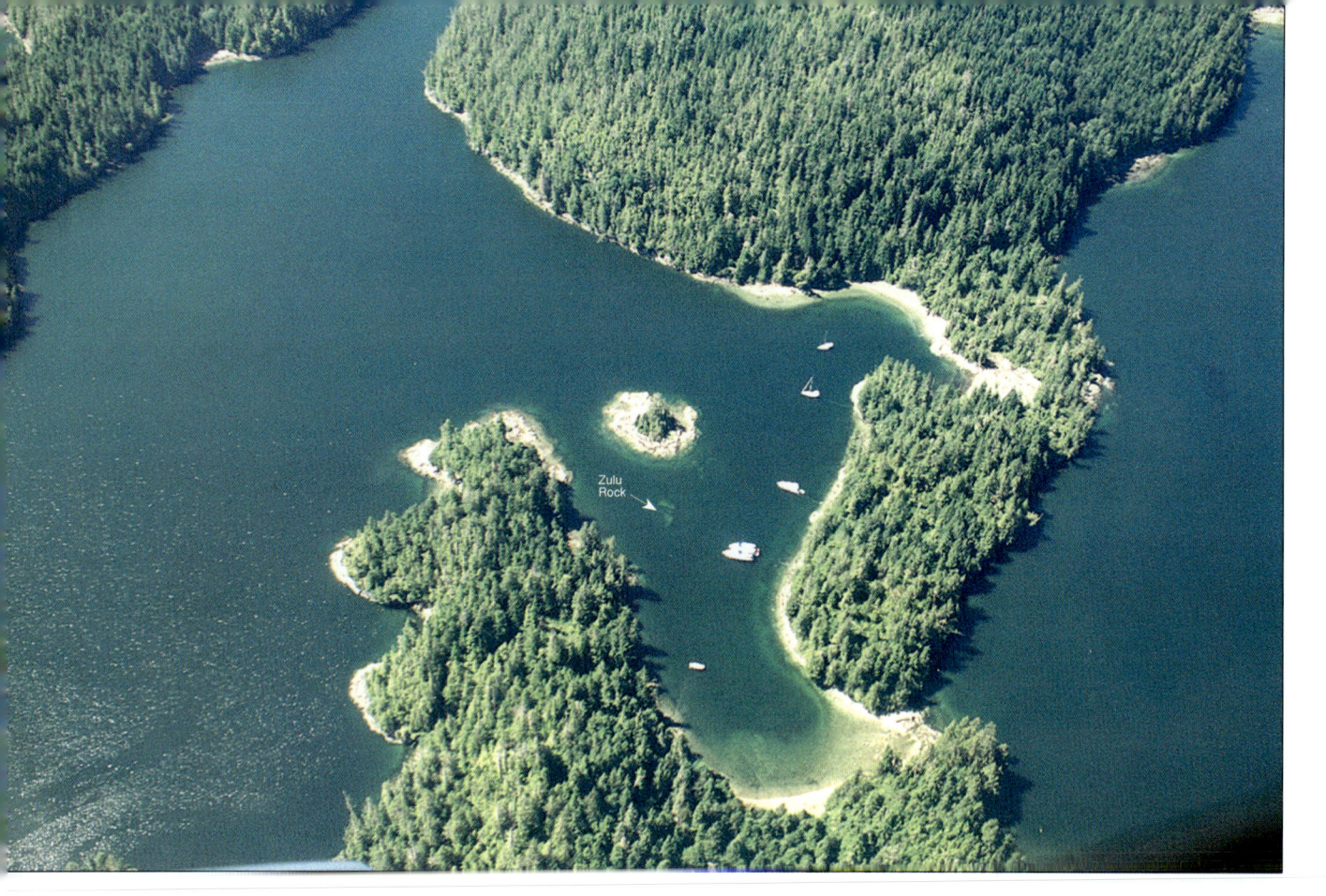

## Fife Sound to Sullivan Bay  chart 3515, 3547

Travelling along the north side of Broughton Island you may want to spend a while stopped at anchor. Bermingham Island on the Pearse Peninsula abutting Raleigh Passage, protects a small unnamed cove guarded by rocks at the northern entrance, and a reef in the middle of the eastern entrance. But this latter passage can be navigated carefully either side of the reef, clearly marked on the chart. Boats have been known to anchor in this cove but it is deeper than most people like to trust their anchoring. It is best used as a temporary stop in good weather.

## Laura Cove  chart 3515

The cove in Laura Bay is the preferred anchorage. It lies about three miles west of Slmoom Sound and has proven to be a favourite anchorage for us over the years. Find a spot to drop anchor between Trivett Island and the hook of Broughton Island that pokes into Penphrase Passage. The islet in the middle of Laura Cove provides good shelter for several small craft. Mind the rock just east of it and check the set of your anchor as some seaweed is reported on the seabed.

Hayle Bay is too open and unprotected for safe anchorage overnight. Fishing in this area is generally very good. Carla once caught a 10 kilogram salmon in Hayle Bay just to the south of Hayle Point that forms the southern breakwater for Laura Bay. In recent times fish stocks have been under close scrutiny in the midst of a dispute over the harmful effects of fish farming. Sports fishing is still enjoying good catches in the area, however.

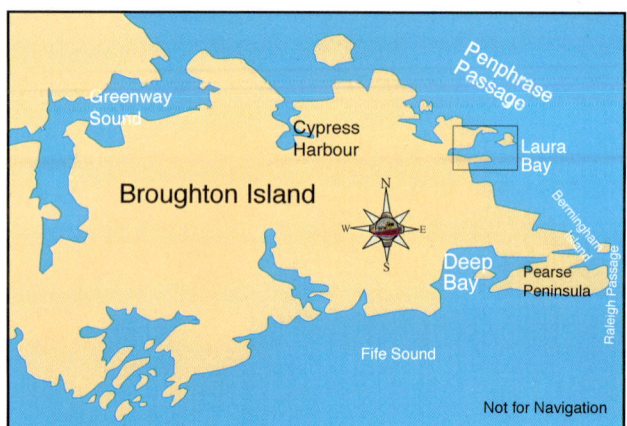

On your approach to Laura Bay, if you are rounding the east side of Trivett Island be aware of a shallow ledge off its south shore. Watch also for Trivett Rock which is indicated on the chart as more than two metres below the surface at low tide. It is of little concern to small boats but was the nemesis for a Union Steamships vessel, the *Cassiar*, in 1917.

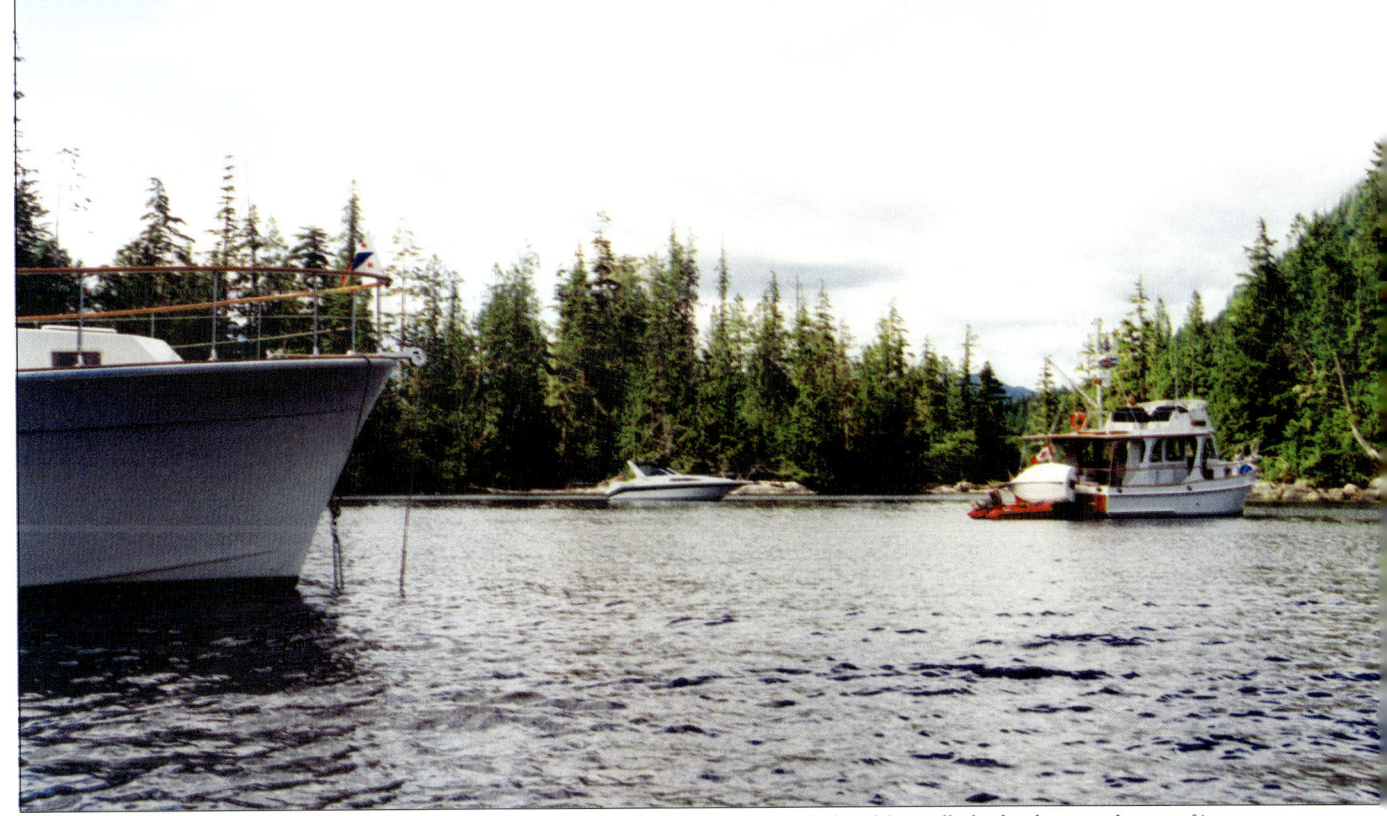

*Laura Cove is a popular anchorage off Penphrase Passage. It can accommodate several boats in the lee of the small island and more to the west of it. Always check the set of your anchor. Some reports state kelp has been found on the seabed in Laura Cove causing anchors to slip.*

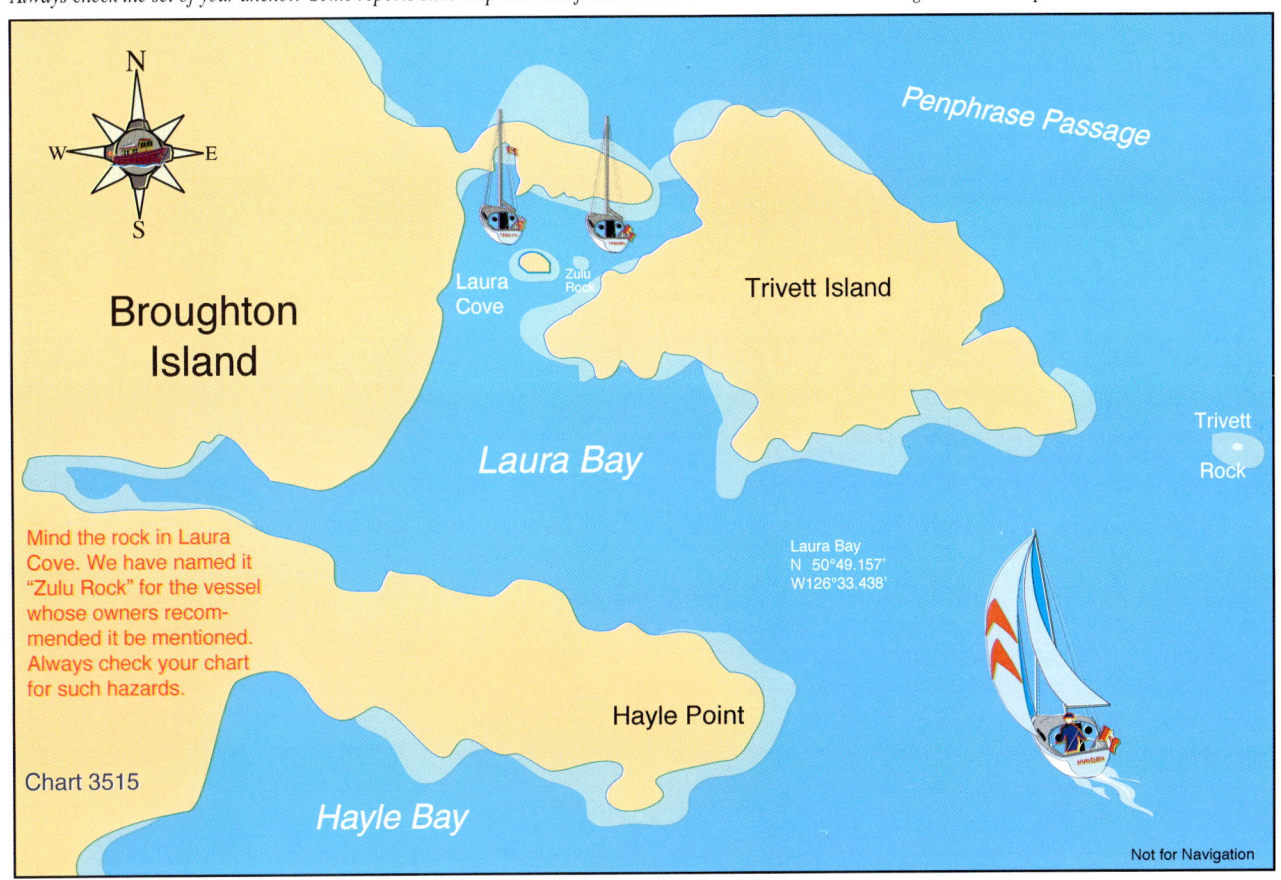

Mind the rock in Laura Cove. We have named it "Zulu Rock" for the vessel whose owners recommended it be mentioned. Always check your chart for such hazards.

Chart 3515

Laura Bay
N 50°49.157'
W126°33.438'

Not for Navigation

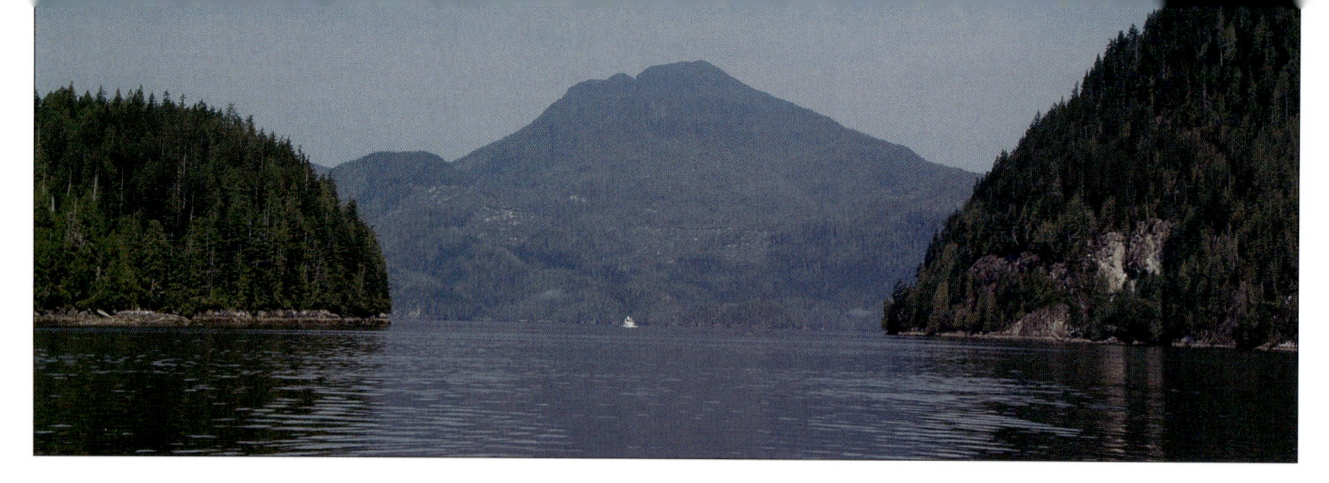

## Sir Edmund Bay  charts 3547, 3515

Sir Edmund Head is a prominent hill that is the main feature of a peninsula protruding into Penphrase Passage. Easily identified by its rounded shape, it is an indicator to mariners of the location of Laura Bay to its south and Sir Edmund Bay to the west of it. Sir Edmund was governor of the Hudson's Bay Company for a five year tenure in the 1860s. The bay is the site of a former logging operation and old cables and machinery ended up on the bottom when the camp was abandoned. Care should be taken when anchoring in the bay. Avoid westerly winds and occasional strong easterlies from the direction of Laura Bay. Laura Cove, opening off this exposed bay, is the favoured anchorage in the area (diagram page 149).

*Cruising on beyond Shawl Bay and the entrance to Kingcome Inlet, Penphrase Passage, Sharp Passage and Sutlej Channel take you to Cypress Harbour, Greenway Sound and Sullivan Bay and also to the entrance of Drury Inlet. The passage above shows the east end of Sutlej Channel north of Broughton Island. Stop along the way at Laura Cove or visit Grappler Sound.*

## Cypress Harbour  charts 3547, 3515

Enter Cypress Harbour through the east side of its mouth. Fox Rock, protruding from the opposite shore extends farther into the entrance than most people realise.

We once sat at anchor in **Miller Bay** in about 4 metres, while it rained hard and long. There were logging activities in the harbour and we watched the coming and going of commercial boats throughout the day. Then the rain lifted and we went fishing and hooked the biggest salmon we had ever had on a line. Too heavy for our line, it snapped the nylon and took off after our brief attempt to play it and reel it in.

Deeper in Cypress Harbour are shallows with kelp and mud that could cause difficulty when trying to weigh anchor. An alternative anchorage to Miller Bay is **Berry Cove**, which is not as sheltered as the former, but good in most conditions except for easterly winds. Anchor in about 6 metres. Continuing to Greenway Sound, travel along Sutlej Channel going either side of Stackhouse Island to Walker Point then turn south into the sound.

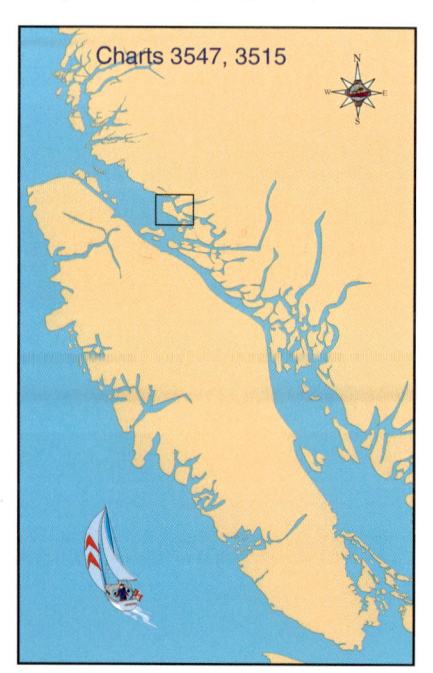

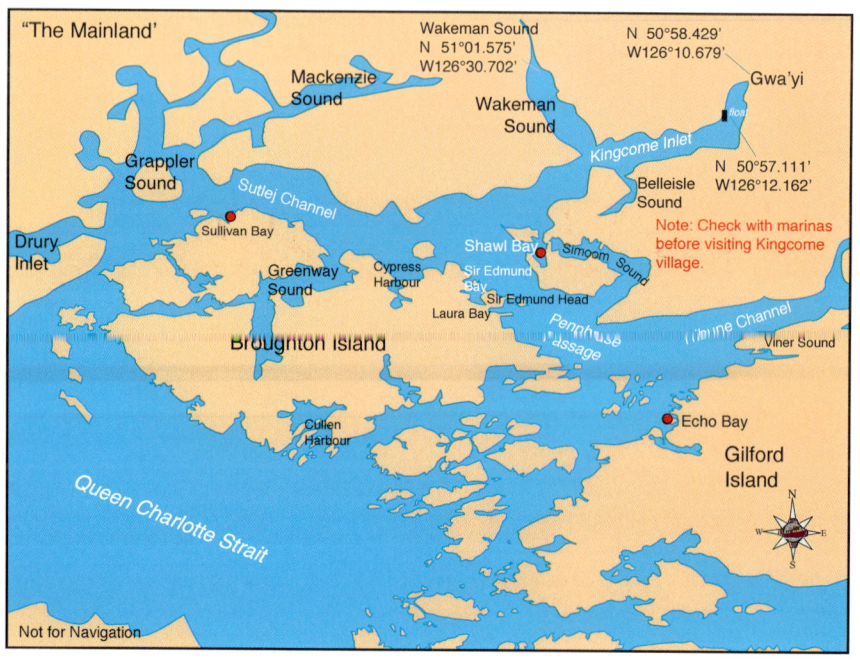

**Map callouts:**

Greenway Entrance
N 50°51.889'
W126°43.954'

Sutlej Channel • Stackhouse Island • Walker Point • Sharp Pass • Greenway Sound • Maude It • Moore Pt • Cecil I • Woods Point • Donald Head • Fish farm • Berry Cove • Miller Bay • Broughton • Cypress Harbour • 100' • 65' • Lagoon 38' • rock • Broughton Island • rocks/islets • 28'

Our route into and inside the lagoon, including our depth readings in feet

It is not wise to try to enter Broughton Lagoon unless you have some experience at doing so. It is possible in a small boat and then just after the tide turns at high slack. Use only the north entrance and be prepared to leave soon or stay until the following high slack. The lagoon is not charted. Watch for a rock off the point on the lower west side.

Not for Navigation    Charts 3547, 3515

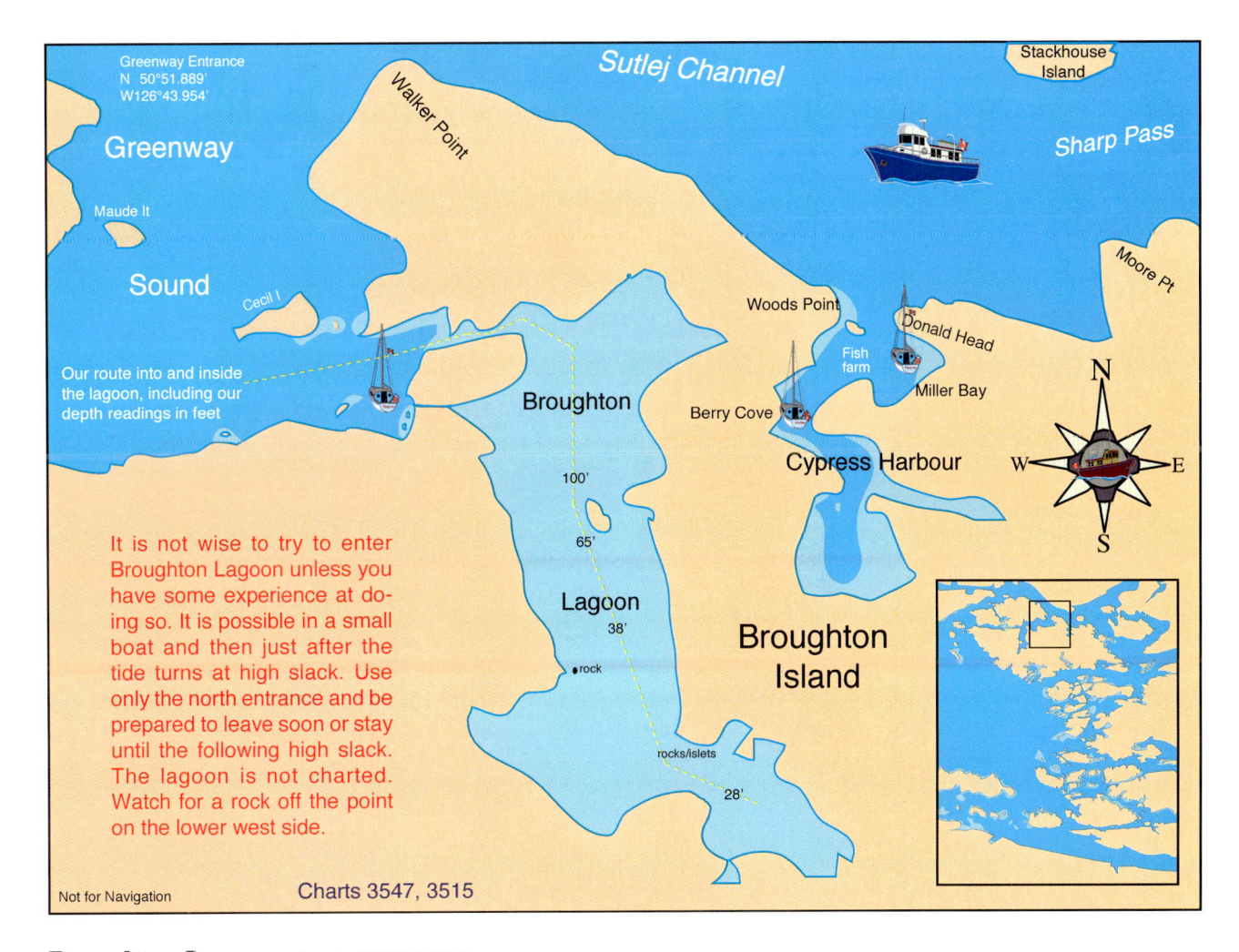

## Broughton Lagoon  charts 3547, 3515

Broughton Lagoon can be accessed at high tide, but only after the tide turns, using the tide tables for Alert Bay and adding one hour and 20 minutes to it. The entrance, just beyond Cecil Island, cannot be taken at high tide when the water is still flowing in. Tom Taylor, founder of Greenway Sound Resort says "the currents all chase the tide. It always takes a while for the water flow following a tide change to actually turn, so wait until after the tide has reached its peak before using any fast flowing waterway."

There are two passageways into the lagoon but only the northerly one is navigable. The other one dries. It is too narrow, too shallow and too dangerous. Once inside, Tom Taylor told us, it has a beautiful charisma. It has a magnificent setting, a grand view of a mountain peak and overall scenery. Inside the lagoon there is one rock off the point on the central lower west side, otherwise depths seem adequate. The water in Broughton Lagoon is partially salty and brackish. It is possible to linger inside the lagoon for about half an hour on the same tide before returning. If you want to remain longer and explore it, then wait and leave on the next high tide.

Tom Taylor once accompanied the *Inlet Transporter* to move a logging camp in the lagoon and was aboard when it navigated through the entrance. This vessel is 105' by 31' beam, and 15' draft. It touched sides as it went through.

The passage is adequately deep and the width about 10 metres with a sharp dogleg in the middle to the right and then to the left, going in. We entered it accompanied by Tom, at the prescribed one hour twenty minutes after high slack on Alert Bay plus one hour for daylight savings time. There was still a notable flood of water going through with us.

With care we slipped through the narrow passage. Then returned to a similar condition in reverse after about half an hour inside the lagoon.

The sunlight late in the day (it was 7.30 pm when we were inside the lagoon) hit us right in the eyes as we found our way back out, making it very difficult to see the sides of the passage. With all these challenges, we do not recommend trying to enter Broughton Lagoon. However, if you must, then do it first in a small, fast runabout and only at the times suggested, or with an experienced guide.

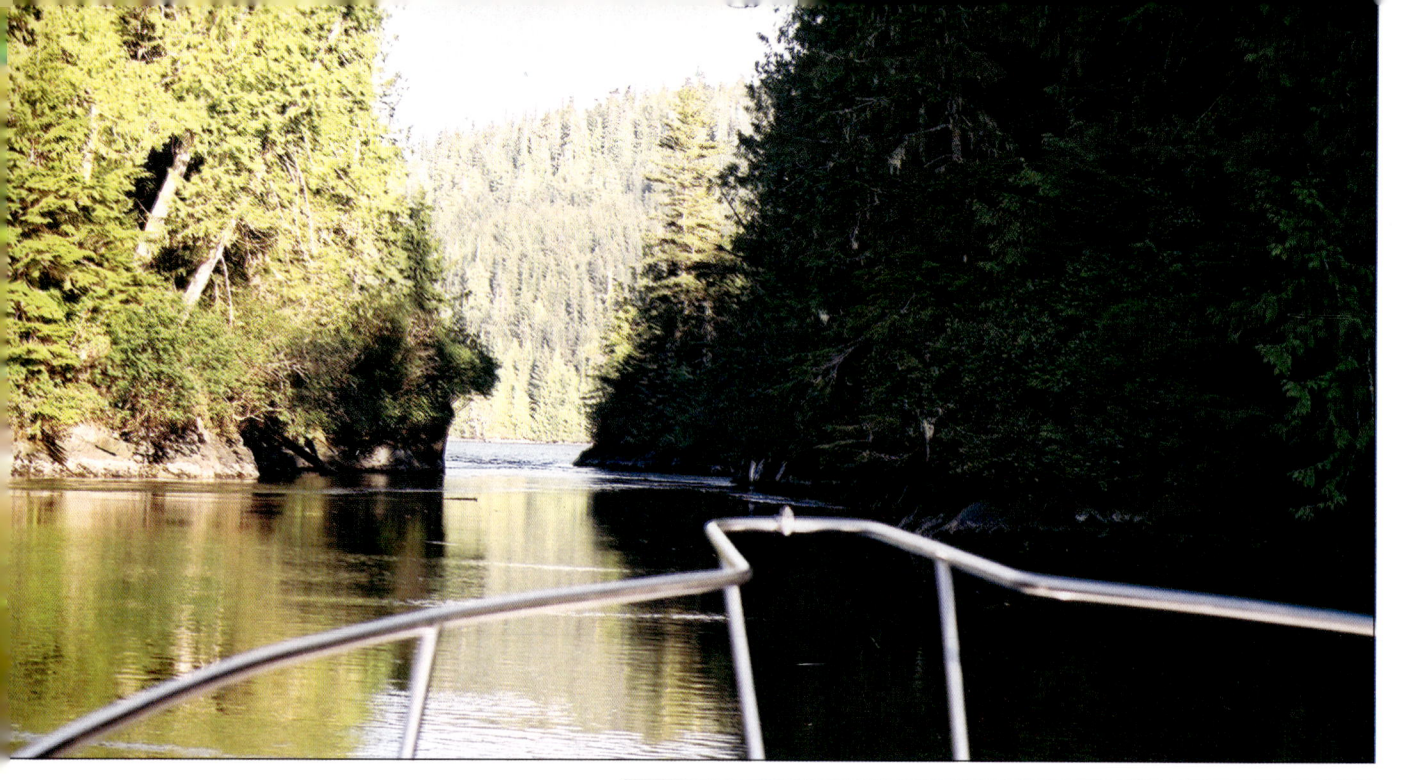

Photos top and centre show the entrance to Broughton Lagoon. It is narrow and difficult to locate when leaving the lagoon. When leaving do not mistake the larger opening on the inside seen in the photo opposite. Bottom left: Another view of the exit from the lagoon.

> "The currents all chase the tide. It always takes a while for the water following a tide change to actually turn, so wait until after the tide has reached its peak before using any fast flowing waterway."
> –Tom Taylor

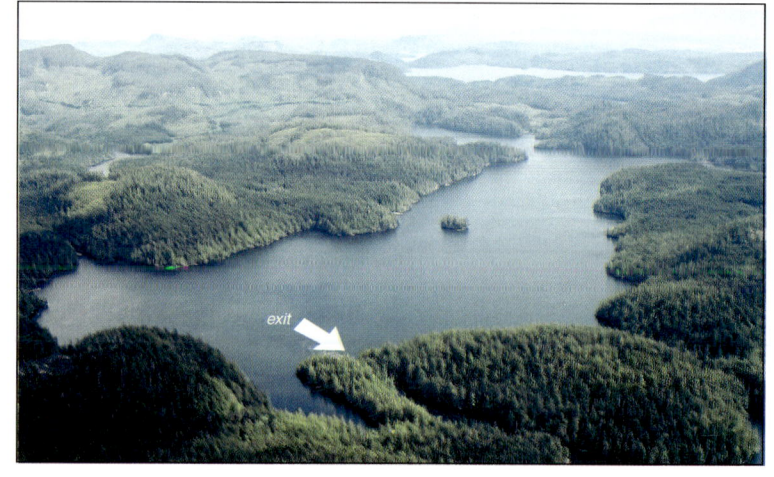

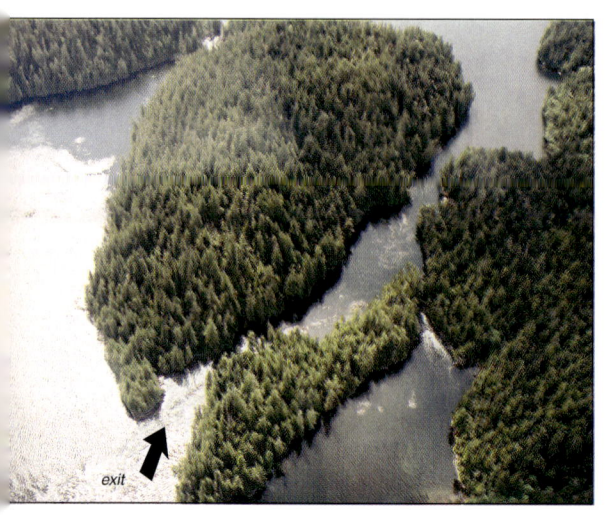

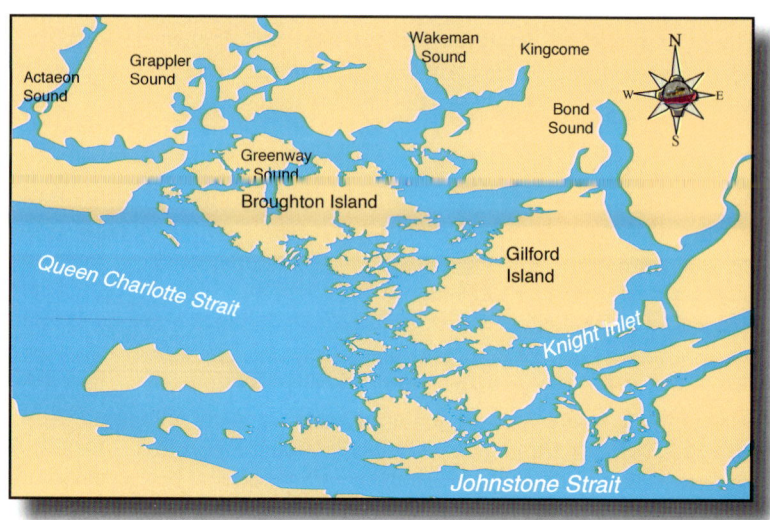

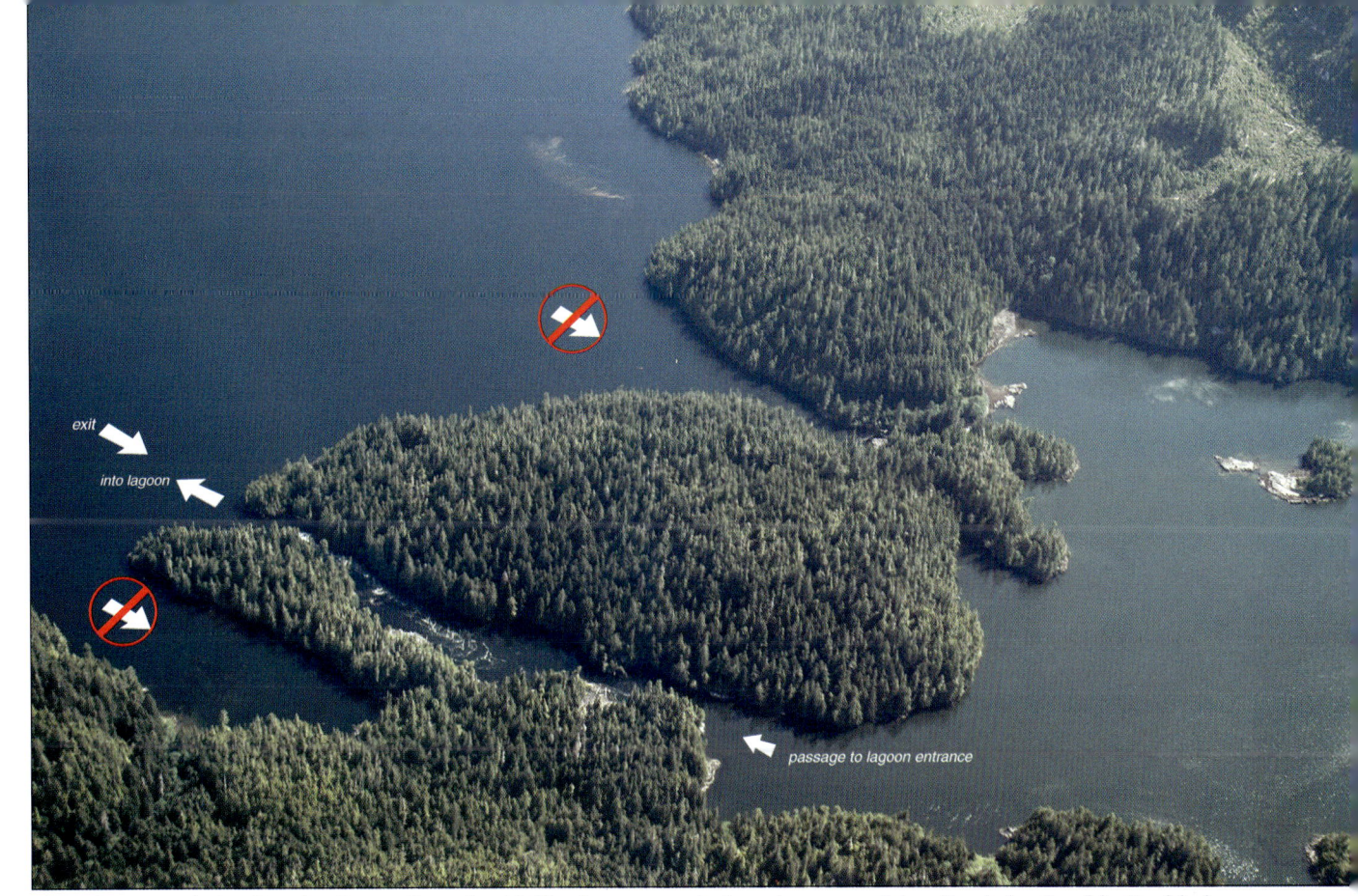

*Above: Entrance and exit at Broughton Lagoon. Do not be misled by what appears to be the easier passages. Below: Note the location of the site of the former Greenway Sound Resort and the BC Forestry Service dock with the trail up the mountainside to Broughton Lake.*

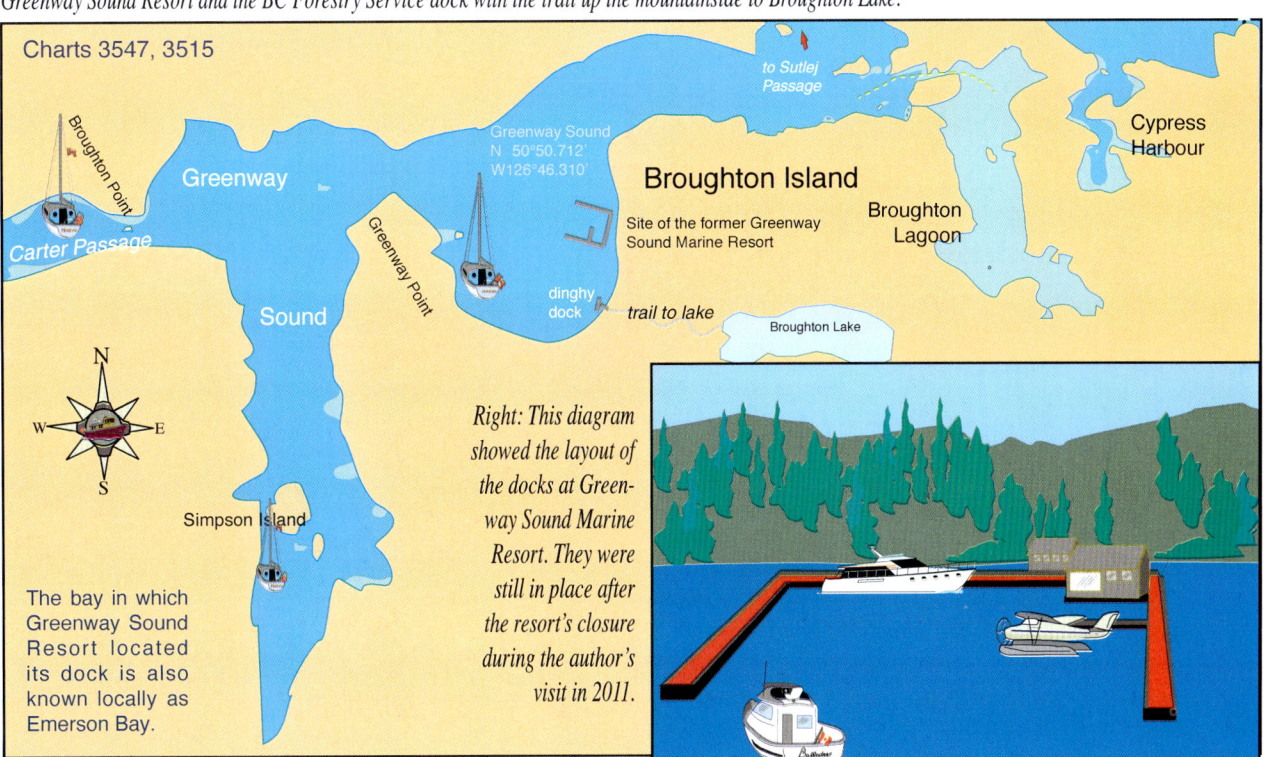

Charts 3547, 3515

Broughton Point — Carter Passage — Greenway Sound — Greenway Point — Simpson Island — to Sutlej Passage — Greenway Sound N. 50°50.712' W126°46.310' — Broughton Island — Site of the former Greenway Sound Marine Resort — dinghy dock — trail to lake — Broughton Lake — Broughton Lagoon — Cypress Harbour

The bay in which Greenway Sound Resort located its dock is also known locally as Emerson Bay.

*Right: This diagram showed the layout of the docks at Greenway Sound Marine Resort. They were still in place after the resort's closure during the author's visit in 2011.*

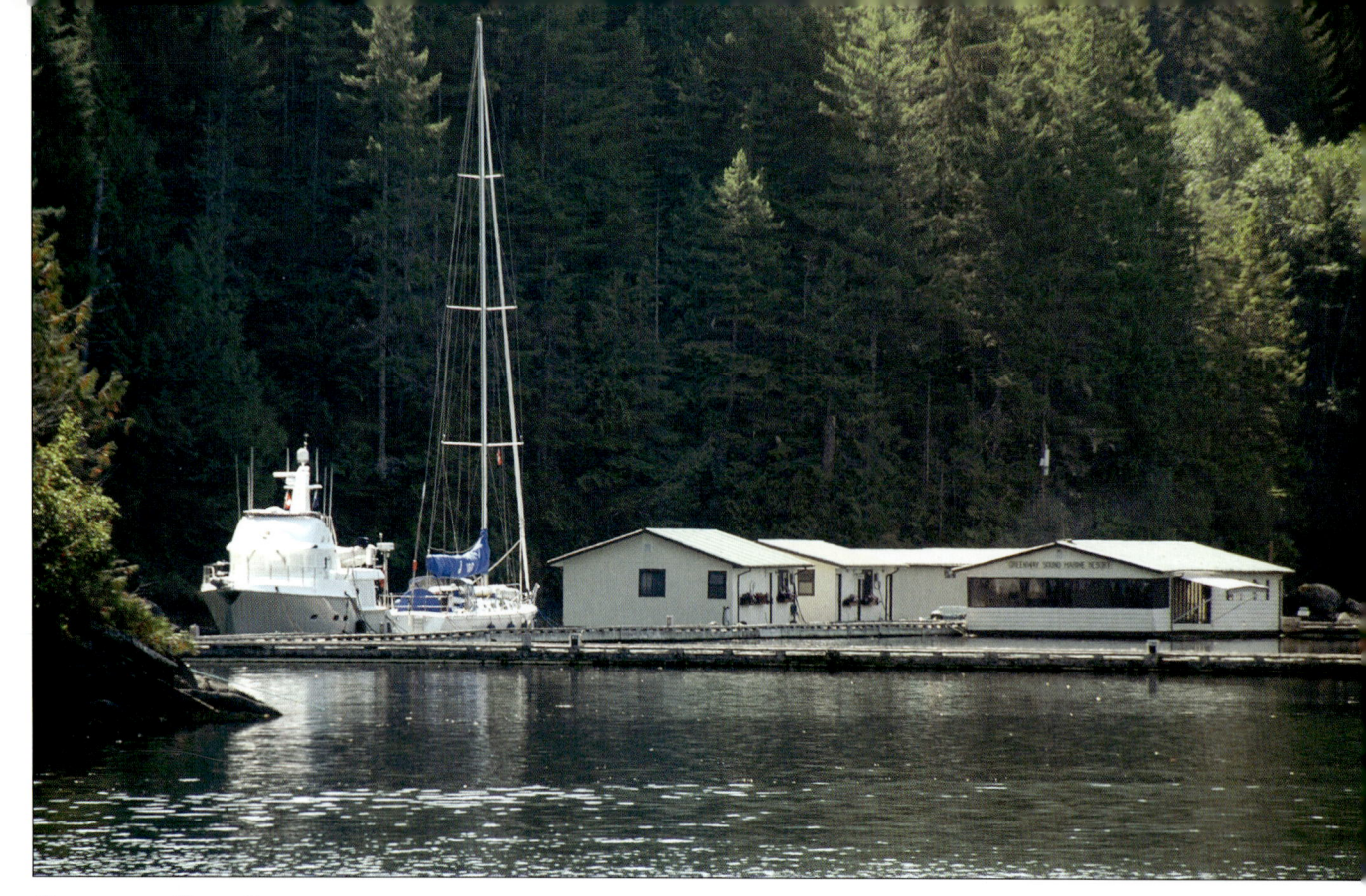

## Greenway Sound  charts 3547, 3515

Greenway Sound is a large body of water that separates Broughton Island from North Broughton Island and forms a deep inlet that almost splits the larger island in two. This area has been a favourite destination for cruising mariners, especially during the tenure of Tom and Ann Taylor at Greenway Sound Marine Resort. This open, alluring establishment in the sound was established by the Taylors in 1984 as a haven for boats, large and small, seeking a place to call home away from home during summer. The Taylors arrived in the sound looking for an alternative location for a marina after trying to establish the old cannery harbour at Butedale. That attempt became futile when it was found that the cost of maintenance was far beyond potential revenues. Furthermore, with the increase in cruise ship traffic to Alaska the wash from the passing massive vessels was causing havoc at the rather exposed docks. So the Taylors moved and established the resort at Greenway Sound instead.

The marina at Greenway Sound saw many years frequented by large and small vessels from BC and the United States on their way to Rivers Inlet, Hakai Pass or Alaska. Some mariners used the location as a base where they met up with friends flying in to join them for a cruise in local waters.

The facility in Greenway Sound soon became known for its long stretch of carpet-covered dock, its restaurant and store, and the many amenities to make guests comfortable. It was not unusual to see boat crews walking the docks for their daily exercise. The docks were laid out in a wide square 'U' with a float plane-docking finger pointing into the square near the far corner where the facilities were located.

In conjunction with their marina facility the Taylors worked with the BC Forest Service to establish and maintain a trail and float nearby for hiking access on the island to the large Broughton Lake that sits alongside Mount Ick. Realizing the value of the trail to visitors the Taylors collaborated with the Forestry Service to ensure its maintenance. Visitors enjoy the three-kilometre walk to the lake where swimming is popular. There is a float and ramp adjacent to the shore at the base of the trail and visitors can tie up their dinghies there while hiking to the lake.

The marine resort site is located an easy run from the north side of the island part way down the sound. Beyond that and well before the end of the sound, Carter Passage branches westward along the south side of North Broughton Island. This passage is not an easily navigated passage, other than by canoe or kayak or by a very shallow draft boat. Mariners willing to negotiate its tricky rocks, shoals and shallows should do so only at high tide. There is a drying bar at the narrows at the east end and a tidal rapids at the narrows at the western side of the passage. I have always considered the two islands as one, leaving Carter Passage to the more adventuresome types. Both ends of Carter Passage are used regularly as sheltered anchorages.

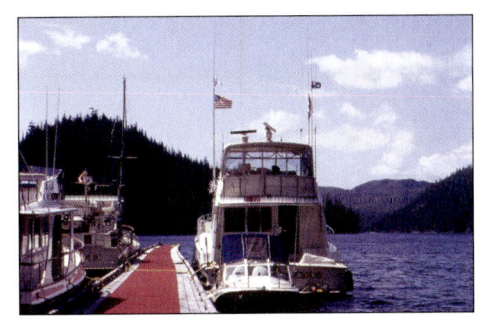

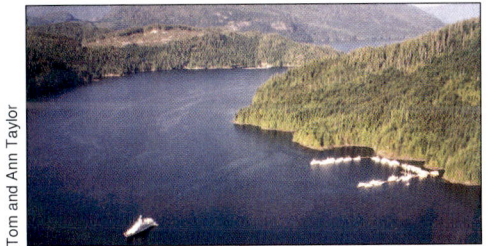

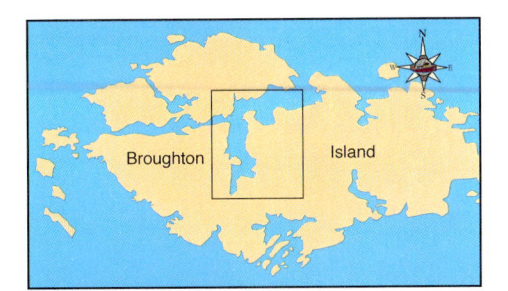

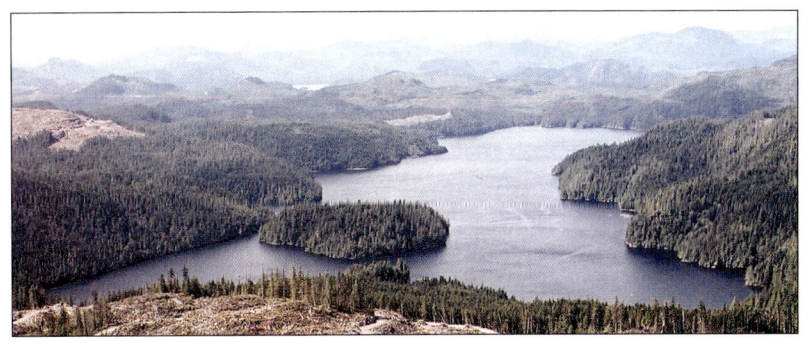

*Above left and left: Greenway Sound Resort. The red carpet treatment was what the marina offered to all guests. The entire dock was carpeted, all half a mile of it. Guests would use the carpeted dock as a place to exercise, taking in the distance as a morning or evening stroll or run. Above: South end of Greenway Sound showing Simpson Island anchorage. Right: Tom and Ann Taylor, who founded the resort, retired in 2010 and closed the resort. Below: The dinghy dock near the site of Greenway Sound Resort's location, gives access to the trail that leads to the lake.*

*Opposite page: Early season at Greenway Sound Marine Resort in its heyday.*

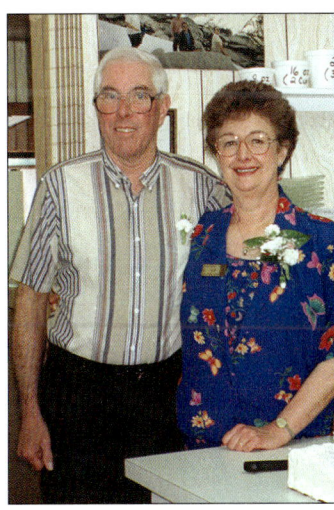

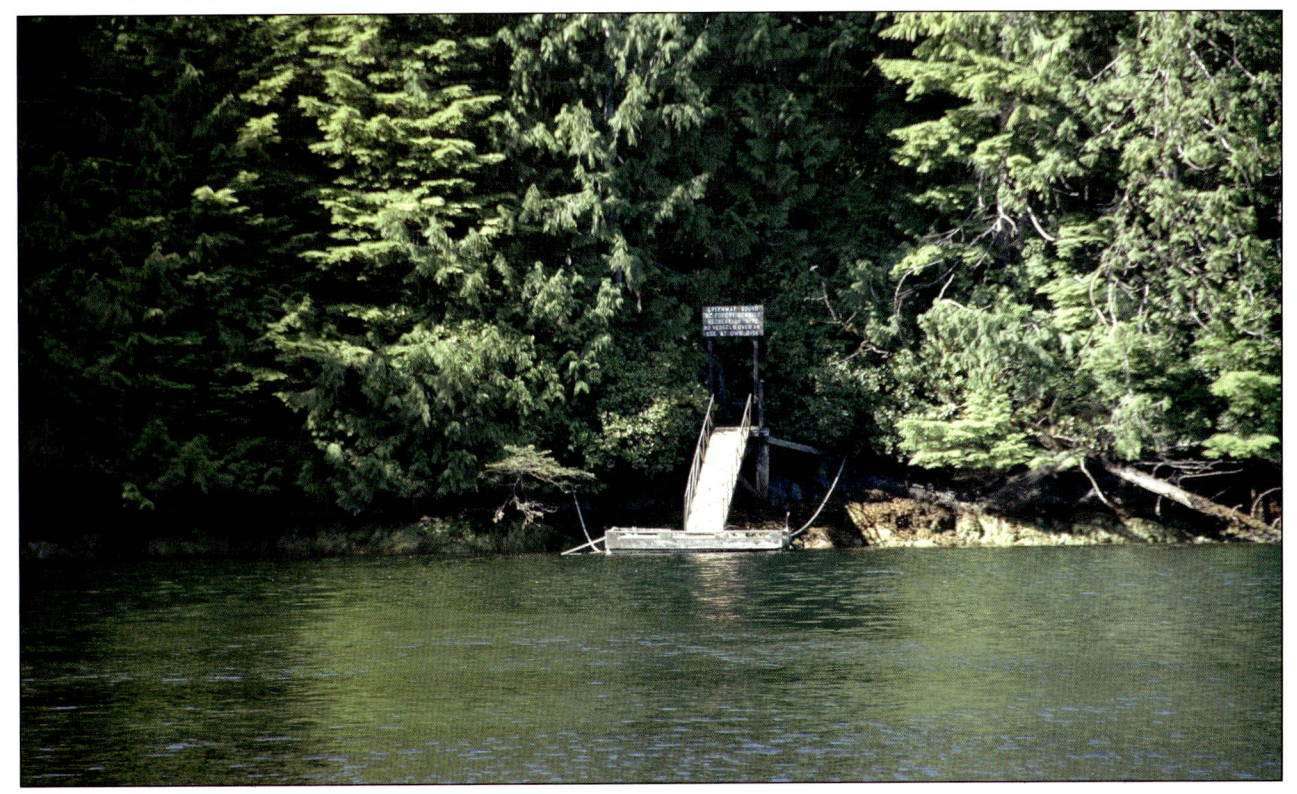

155

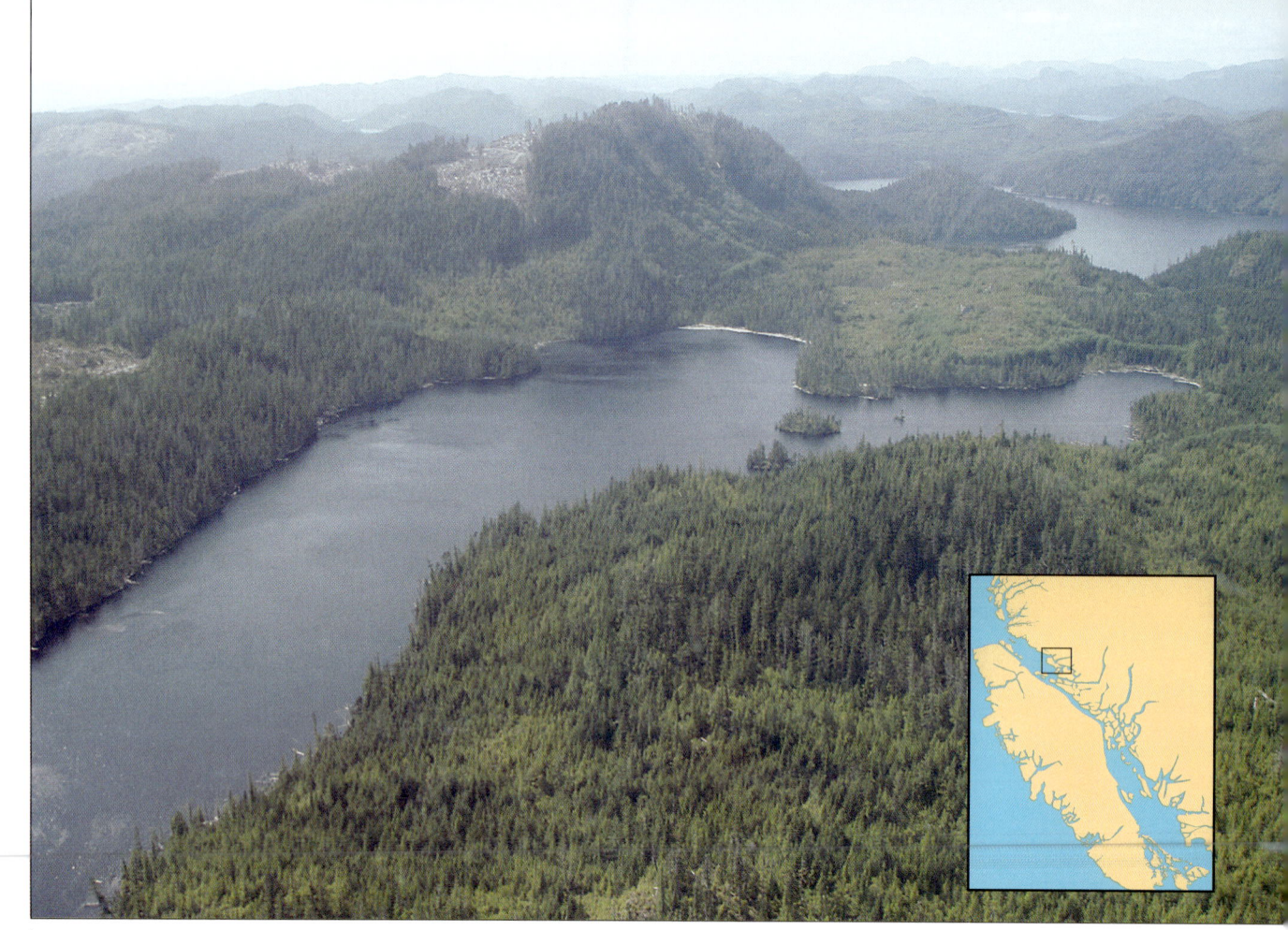

## Trails and lagoons

Mariners love to find trails to hike, paths to follow and lakes to swim in. The Broughton area has no shortage of such available resources. Where lakes are not easily accessible, warm, shallow lagoons suffice. Some marinas and the Forestry Service have established trails to hike, and landings to serve eco tourists and pleasure boaters. Some trails have been left behind by former loggers, miners, fishermen and woodsmen who settled the coast during the heyday of those industries in the area. The trails are sometimes connected to lakes, streams and waterfalls where bathing in refreshing or surprisingly warm lake water can be the reward for a vigorous hike, or a casual stroll. A good start is Broughton Lake.

## Hiking Trails

A great deal of logging takes place in the vicinity of Greenway Sound, on the mainland and in the islands. This can be seen readily from the air. The logging roads serve as hiking trails and can be accessed in some cases by trails leading from the shore. Some of these exist on Broughton Island and other islands in the group. Parklands can be found also at Turnbull Cove and Moore Bay, all with walking trails, some of which link up with lakes, cross the islands and return to the shore elsewhere. Scott Cove and Echo Bay have trails. Minstrel Island, Lagoon Cove and Shawl Bay have trails or nearby access to trails. Go and walk them, but be mindful at all times of the presence of bears. Grizzlies are seen frequently on the mainland.

## Carter Passage chart 3547

Tom Taylor reports that it is possible but not recommended to go through Carter Passage. He says if you want to explore by dinghy use the passage only at high tide and only in a small boat. We recommend that anyone using Carter Passage for gunkholing in a small boat carry with them a hand held VHF radio and stay in touch with their mother vessel. Boats may use the wide opening at the east end of the passage as an anchorage.

*Above: Broughton Lake is accessed by trail from Greenway Sound–partially seen beyond the ridge of the mountain. Anchor opposite the site of the former resort and dinghy to the Forestry Service dock at the foot of the trail.*
*Note: There are no expectations at the former marina, but there is always a possibility of a new resort or availability of a dock for visitors.*

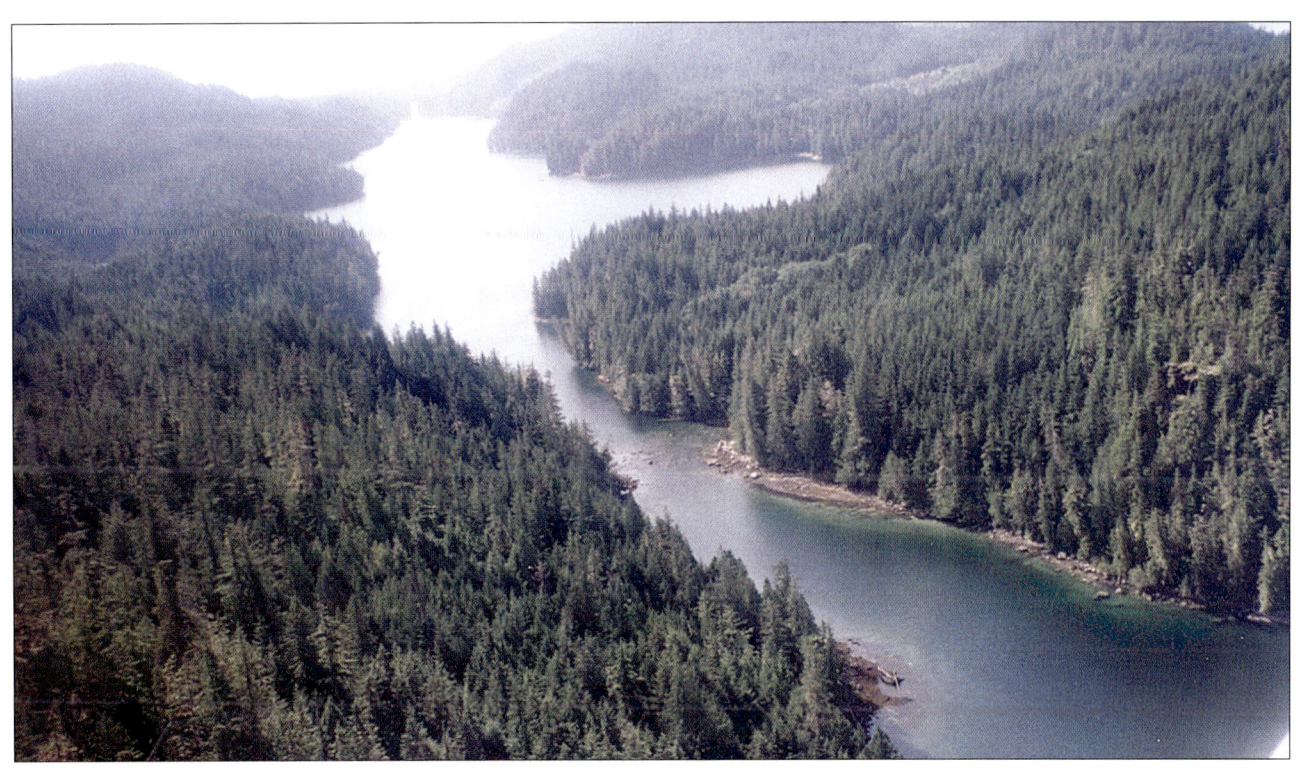

*Above: Carter Passage looking west. It provides some sheltered anchorage a short way in on either side of the passage but a drying ledge near the east entrance restricts passage to small boats only at high tide; Right: Entering the east side anchorage in Carter Pass. The diagram below shows how Carter Passage and Greenway Sound split North Broughton Island from Broughton Island.*

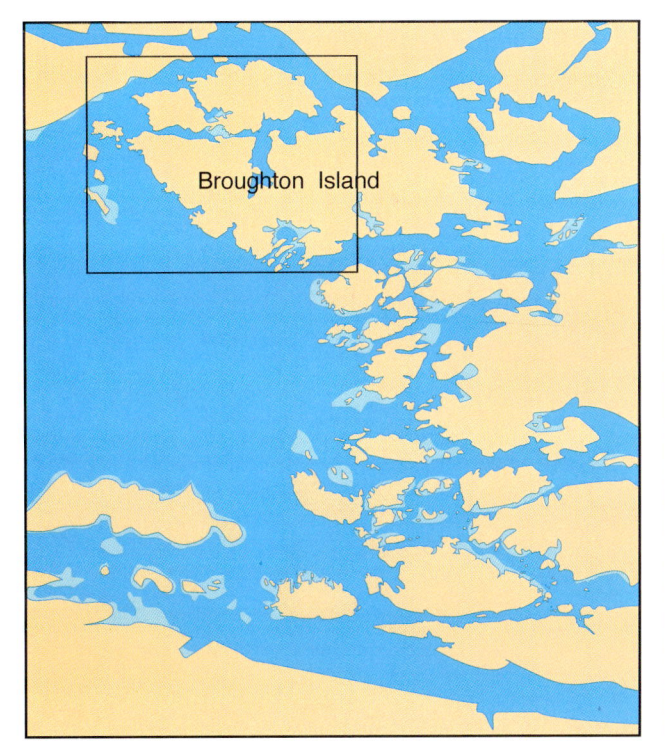

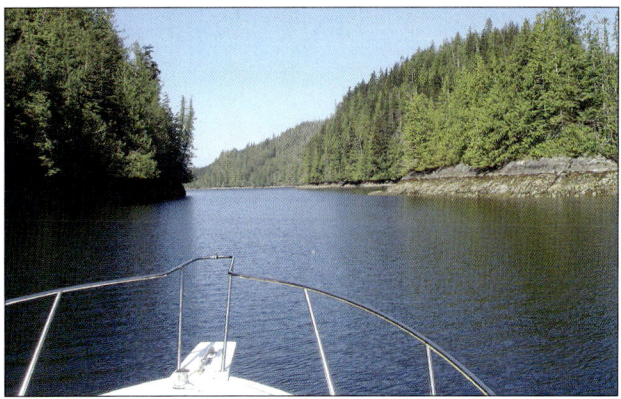

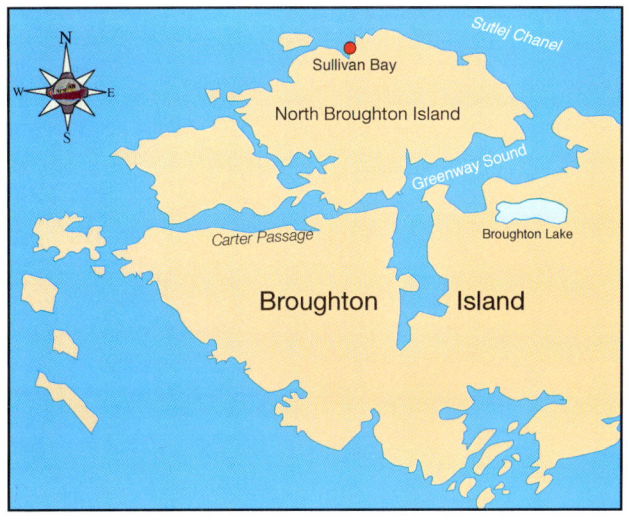

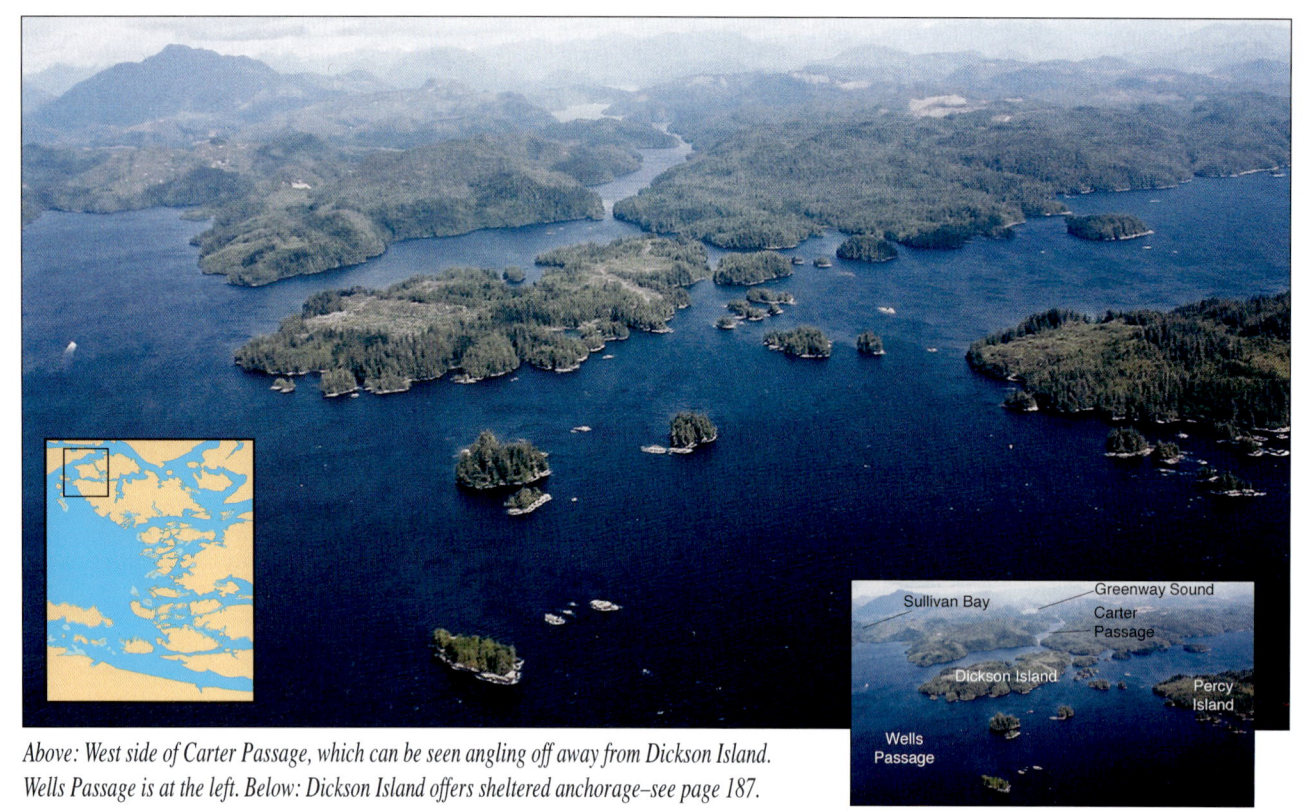

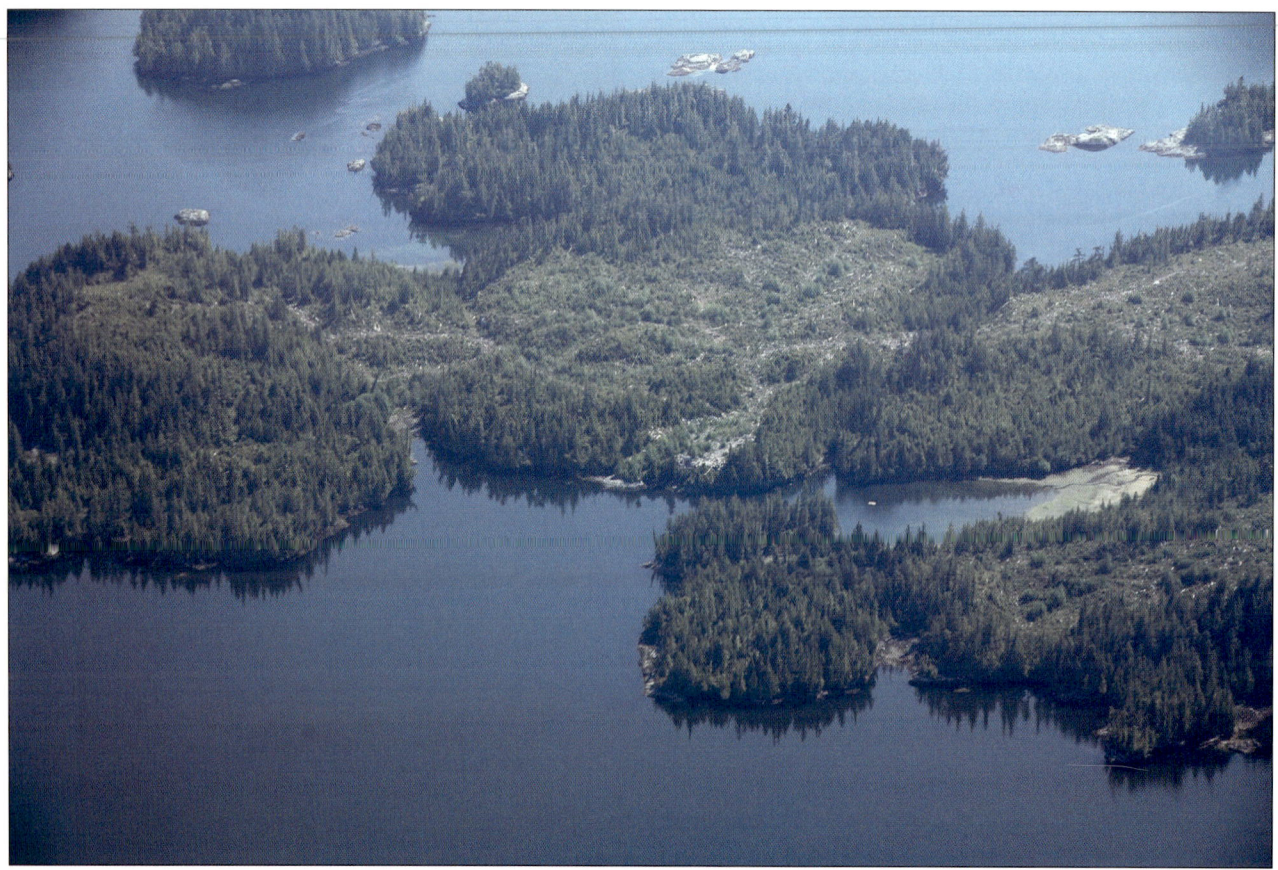

*Above: West side of Carter Passage, which can be seen angling off away from Dickson Island. Wells Passage is at the left. Below: Dickson Island offers sheltered anchorage–see page 187.*

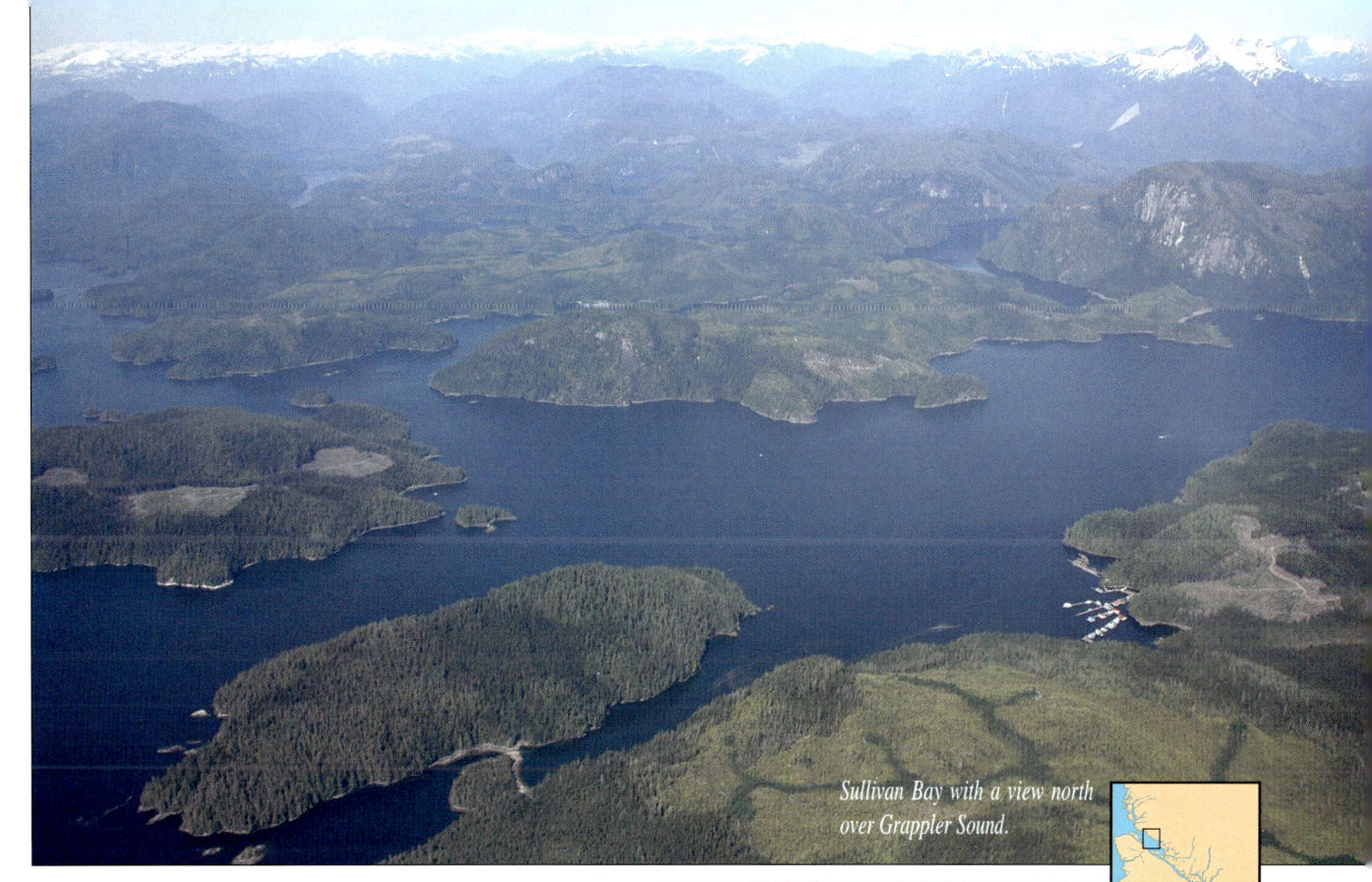

*Sullivan Bay with a view north over Grappler Sound.*

## Sullivan Bay Marine Resort
Sullivan Bay BC V0N 3H0
Phone 250-629-9900
VHF 66A   chart 3547
www.sullivanbay.com

This marina is a well-known fuel stop. It has diesel, gas and oils. It offers 15, 30 and 50 amp 110 and 220 volt shore power. The marina comprises 4,000 feet of dock. The outer fingers of the dock are for visiting boats to 300 feet, while float home owners have the docks closer to shore.

Note the large, modern homes on floats. Visitors are reminded to respect their privacy.

Facilities and amenities include a restaurant and a store with groceries, produce, ice, tackle, souvenirs, books, gifts, charts and video rentals. There is a liquor store, a mail drop and a library. It also has a one-hole links. In past decades it also became known for its "street signs."

The marina offers specialized boat sitting.

Scheduled and charter float plane service is available to Seattle, Campbell River, Port McNeill and Vancouver.

The marina is busy in summer with the coming and going of regular visiting yachts. It is the gateway to Drury Inlet, Actaeon Sound, Grappler Sound and Mackenzie Sound in addition to Wells Passage and the open waters of Queen Charlotte Strait. Prawn boats operate extensively through the area, in Drury Inlet and Mackenzie Sound.

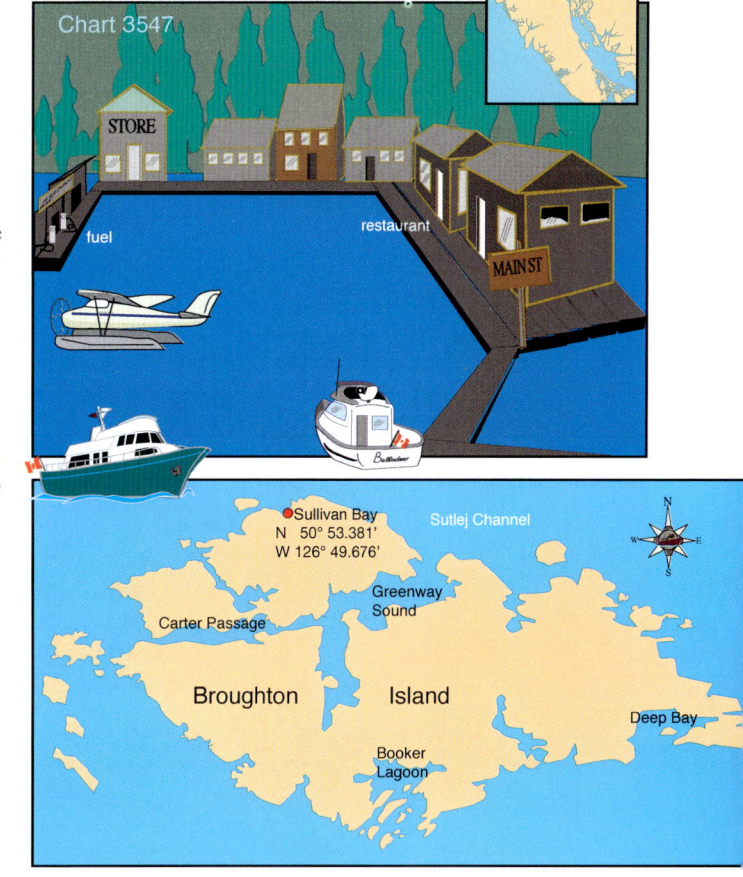

Chart 3547

Sullivan Bay
N  50° 53.381'
W 126° 49.676'
Sutlej Channel
Carter Passage
Greenway Sound
Broughton Island
Booker Lagoon
Deep Bay

159

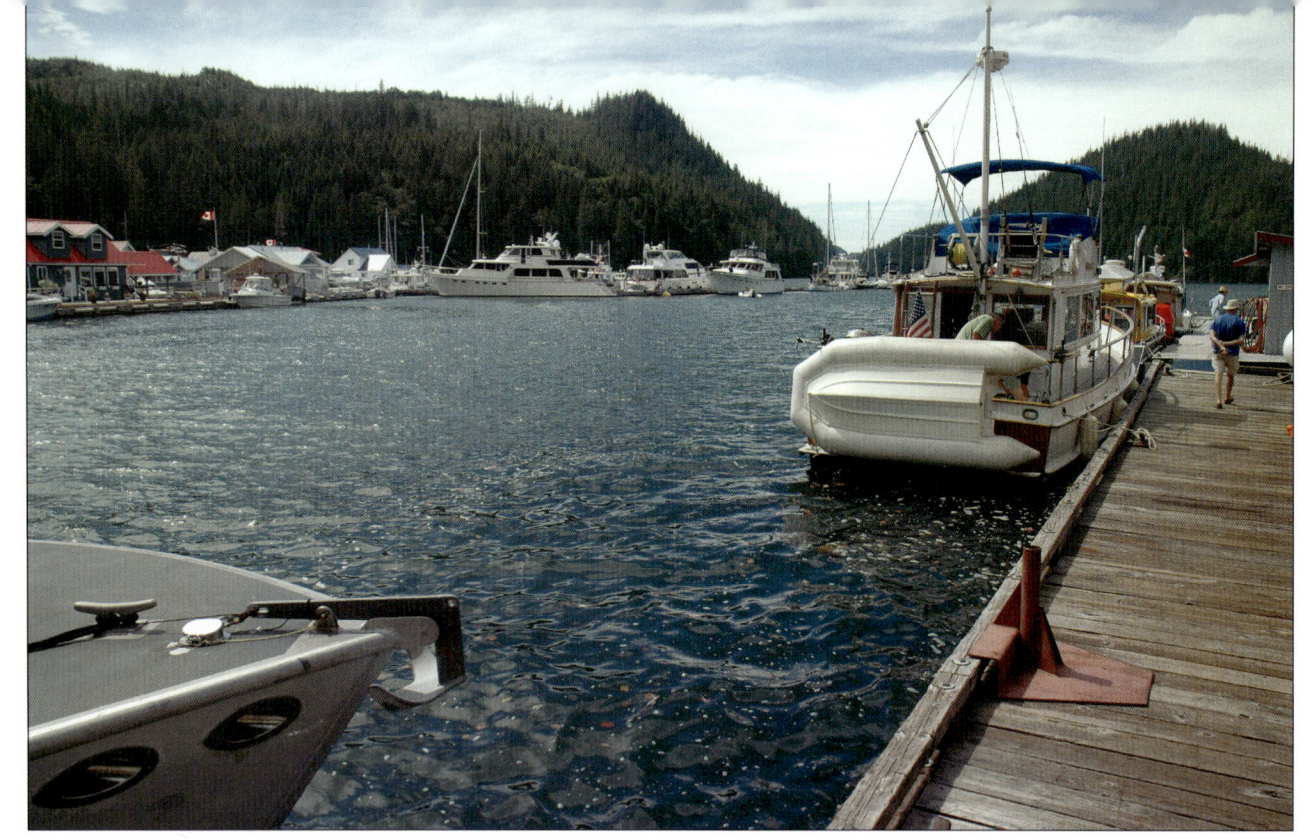

*Above: Sullivan Bay marina, busy in summer, from the fuel dock and store access float. The private floats are to the west of the main docks (top left in photo). The fuel dock, opposite page, has seen the coming and going of all types of craft over a long history of serving the boating and aviation communities. The bay lies in the lee of a point of land protecting it from east winds in Sutlej Channel while Atkinson Island protects it from westerlies out of Wells Passage.*

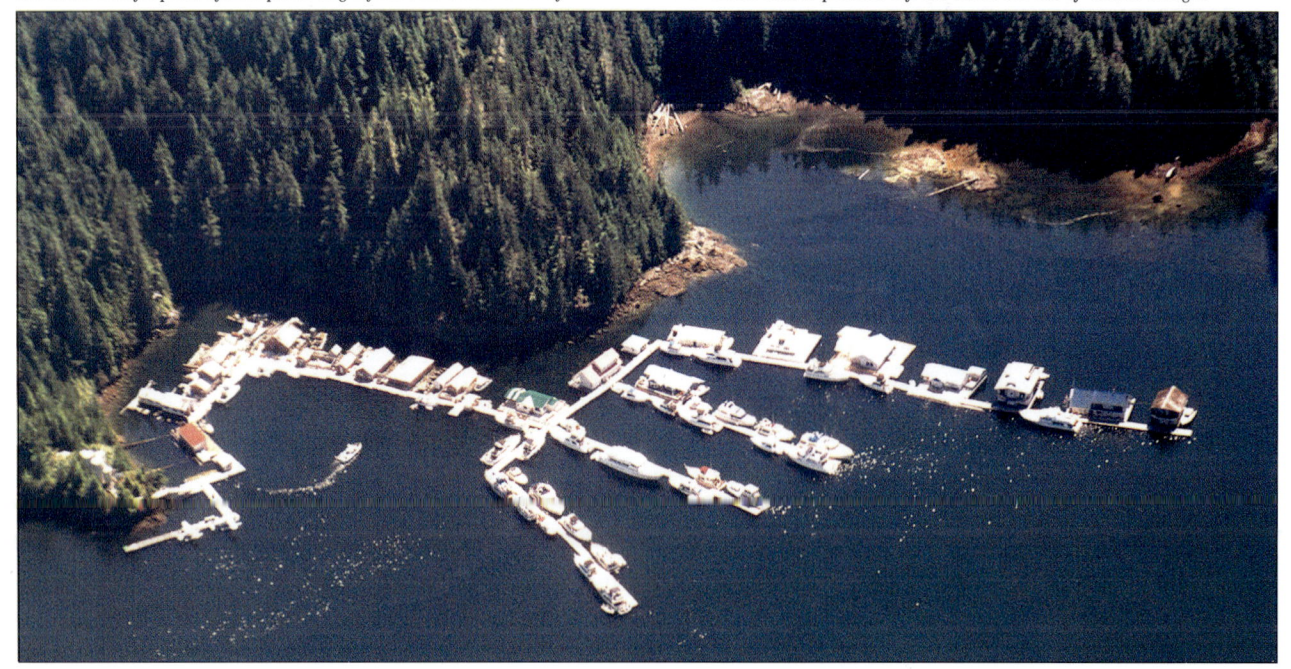

*Above: This aerial photograph shows the layout of the docks. The newer buildings are mostly on the inner fingers branching off the main dock with visitor moorage available on the outer floats (foreground). The buildings on the main floats of Sullivan Bay Marina include the store (opposite page), laundry and washrooms, restaurant and other character cabins around the 'Sullivan Bay Square,' to the left of the fingers occupied by visiting boats and floating homes.*

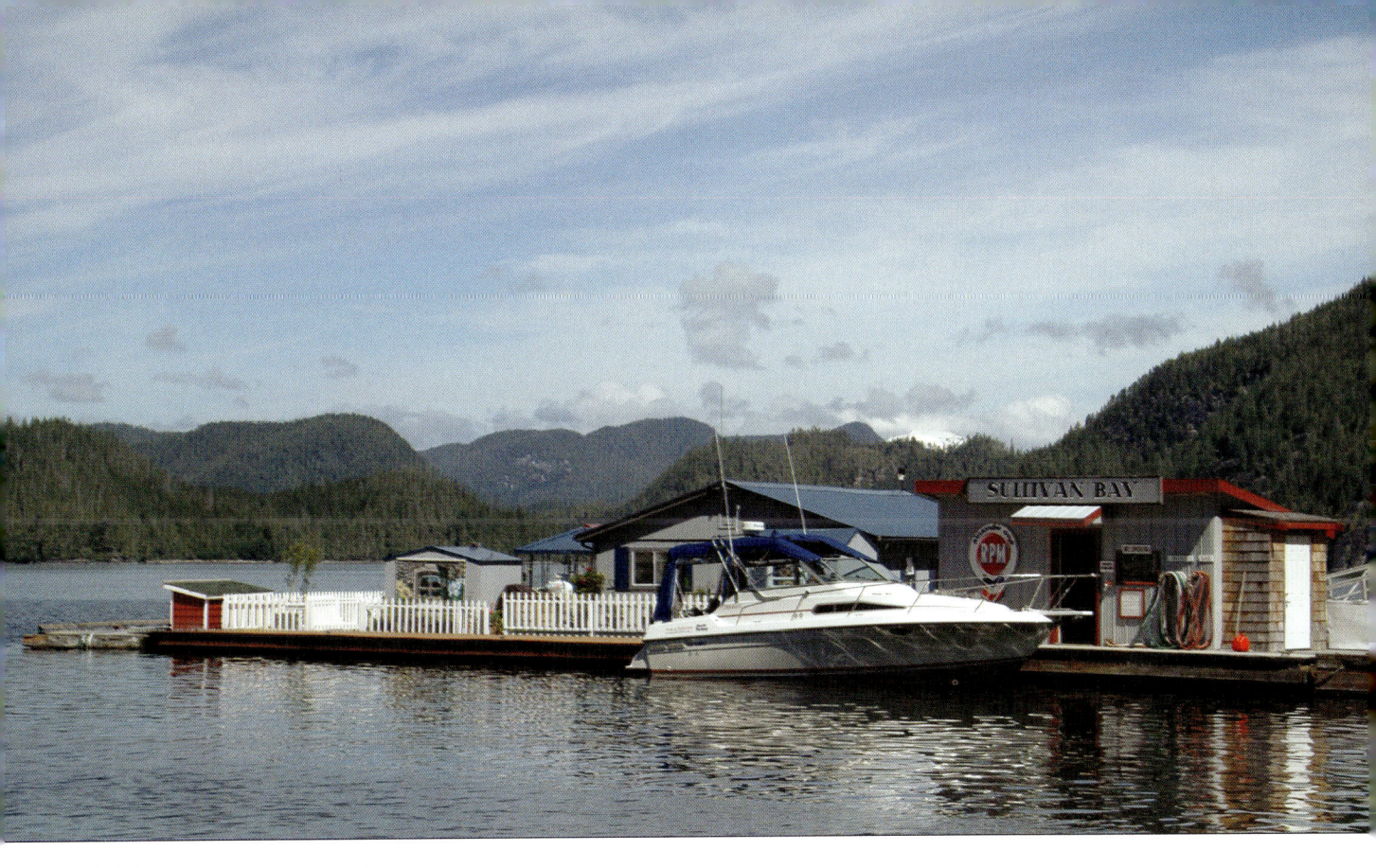

## Sullivan Bay  chart 3547

The history of Sullivan Bay is a story in itself, best left to be expanded on by historians. It was established in 1945 by Bruce and Myrtle Collinson. Since that time the settlement has seen the coming and going of vessels of all types over its checkered past. Mission boats stopped in for fuel and supplies and to conduct services for the community. Fisheries and Forestry boats made Sullivan Bay their focal point in the area. Seaplanes used it as a major fuelling stop. It served as such for Queen Charlotte Airlines which belonged to the late Jim Spilsbury (read his book *Accidental Airline*).

A characteristic of Sullivan Bay Marina is its quaint village charm, with street signs, names on buildings and directional sign posts. Property owners have established some fine floating homes along the dock, occupied by families and guests during summer and dutifully maintained by a skeleton staff in the winter. A small but comprehensively stocked store supplies a large resident and transient community all year round. Fuel is available at Sullivan Bay Marina, not only for mariners but also for aviators who use regular gasoline. In 2011 managers Chris Scheevers and Debbie Holt pointed out the 'Sullivan Bay Square' for happy hour, and various new structures and modernized conveniences. Take your favourite putter and try your luck for a night's moorage on Sullivan Bay Marina's one-hole golfing links.

Pat Finnerty and Lynn Whitehead became the joint managers of the marina shortly after the death of Lynn's husband Michael in the late 1970s, in an aircraft accident. After the tragedy Pat Finnerty bought into Sullivan Bay and ran it with Lynn until about 2008. Some of the owners of the large yachts seen at the bay each summer are shareholders in the operating company and the facility has the look and feel of that kind of involvement, with the presence of large floating homes, some with decks for small aircraft or helicopters.

The camp that became the present day Sullivan Bay Marina was once located in the lee of one of the islands on the other side of Patrick Pass, probably Kinnaird Island.

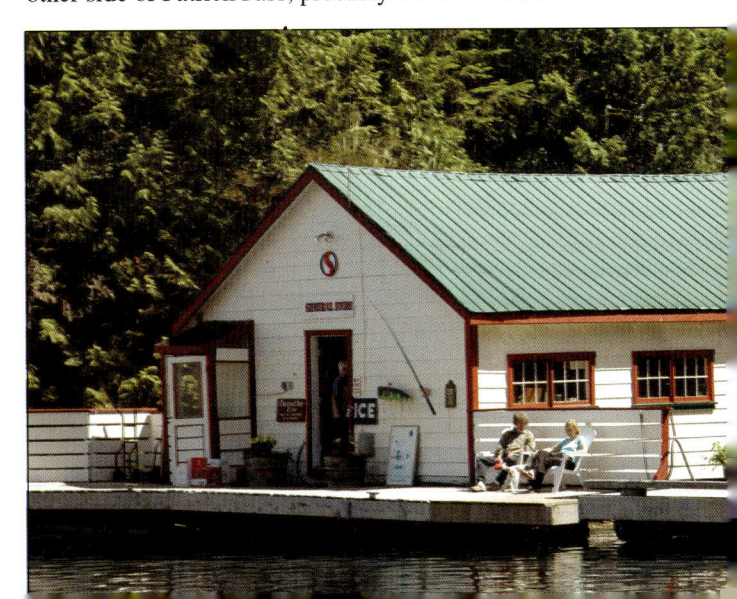

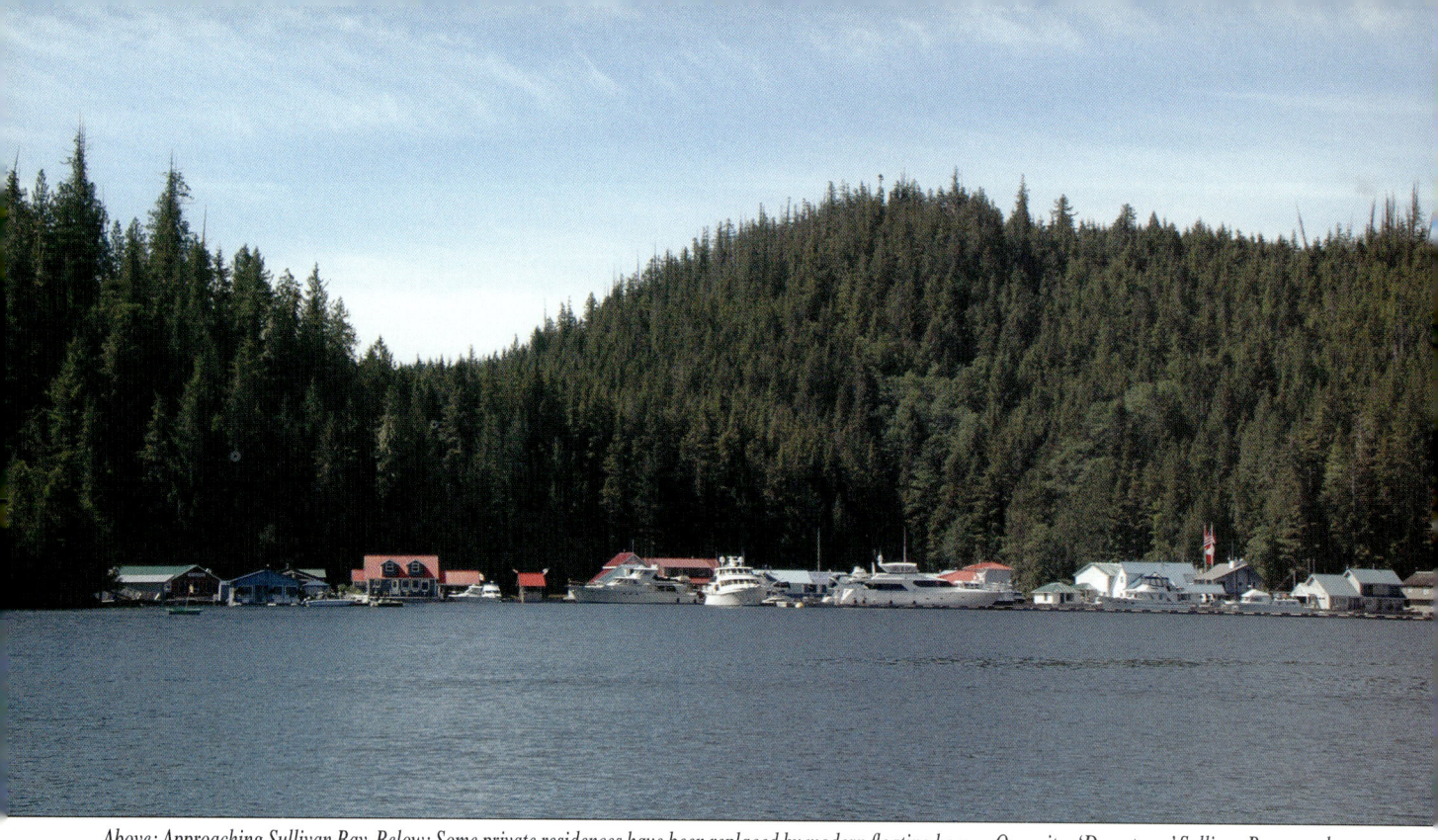

*Above: Approaching Sullivan Bay. Below: Some private residences have been replaced by modern floating homes. Opposite: 'Downtown' Sullivan Bay complete with grocery store, restaurant and quaint historic buildings. Playfully the owners have established a jail (the Sullivan Bay Brig). Don't forget to let your crew out after you've taken their picture. Note the black and white photos from a collection of old photographs that were on display at Sullivan Bay Marina. The floating settlement was always busy with visiting aircraft and ships, summer and winter. Inset: Inside the well-provisioned grocery store at Sullivan Bay.*

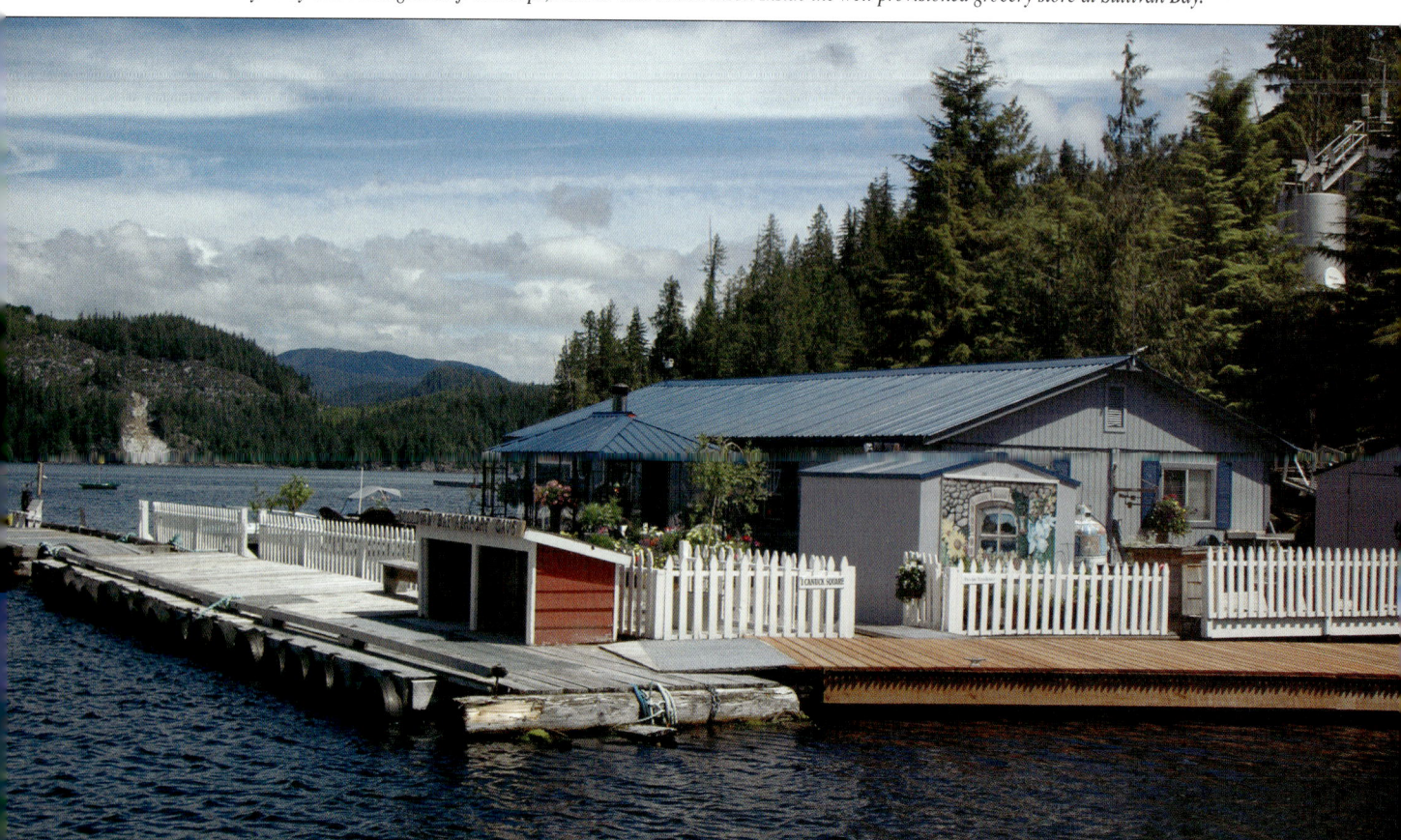

163

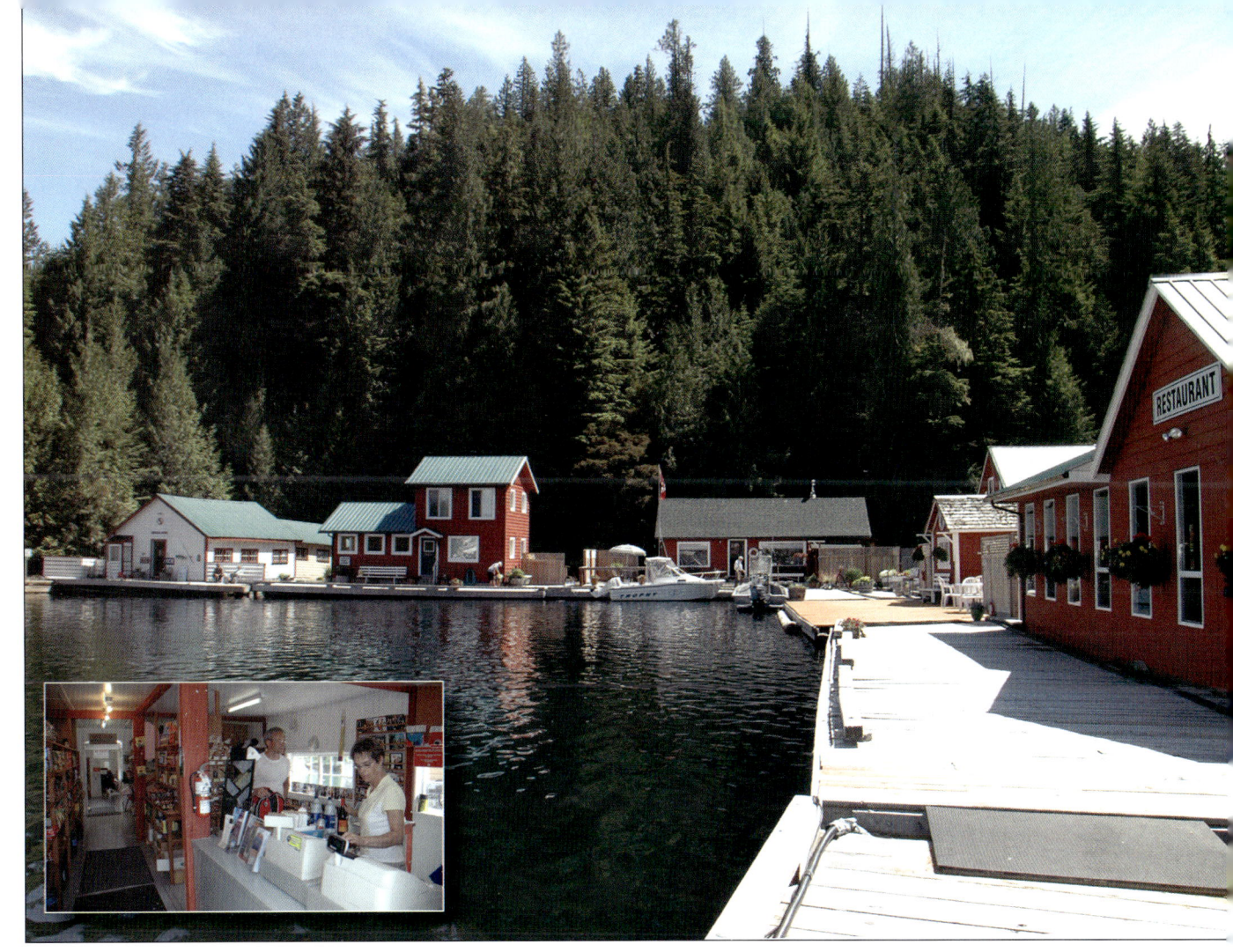

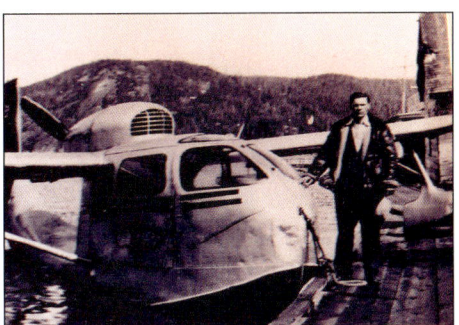

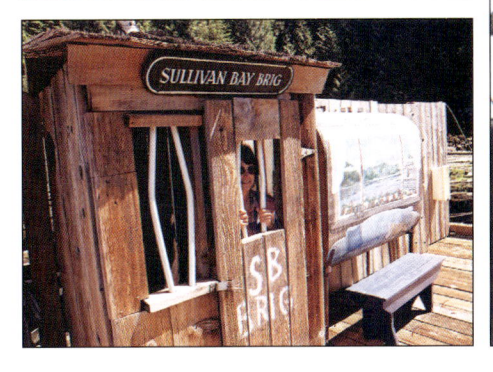

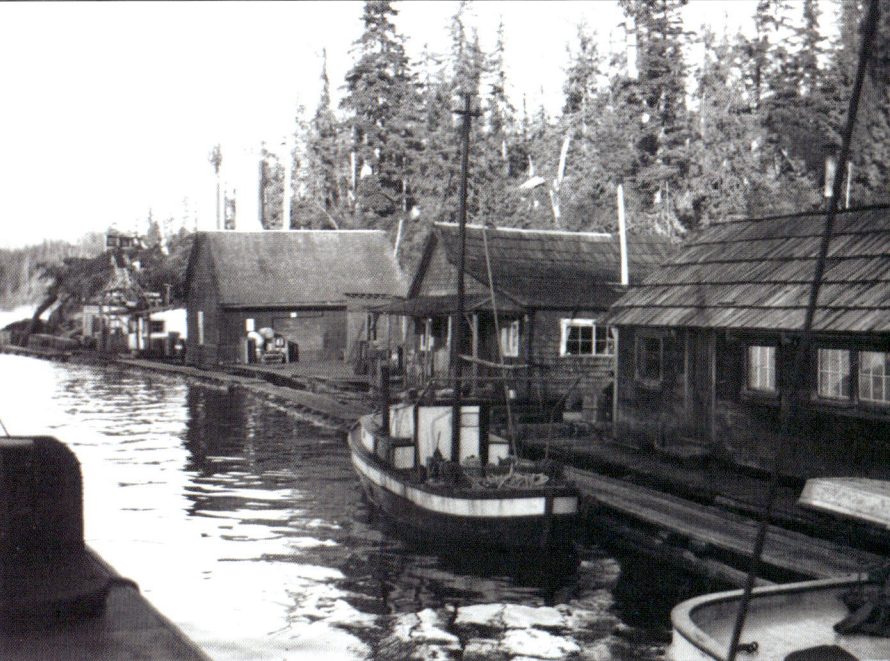

# Grappler Sound and Mackenzie Sound

From Watson Island to Nepah Lagoon and Nimmo Bay

Chart 3547

## Watson Island  chart 3547

In the vicinity of Sullivan Bay there are several anchorages popular among cruising mariners who know the area. Grappler Sound lies to the west of Watson Island and is the hub for access to Drury Inlet, Hopetown Passage, Kenneth Passage and Mackenzie Sound. And there are numerous anchorages in the area such as at **Claydon Bay**, **Hoy Bay** or **Turnbull Cove.**

Travel across Sutlej Channel northwest through Dunsany Passage and turn north at Cunning Point to enter Hopetown Passage. This is not a passage in the true sense of the word as it is only passable in very small boats at high tide. However, the anchorage in Hoy Bay on the north side accommodates several boats in about 12 metres of water. Easterlies blow into the anchorage but it is protected from the west. If it blows from the east chances are the wind will be strong, funnelling through the narrows of the passage from Mackenzie Sound. These winds can be rather intimidating as they have been known to form small but scary looking twisters.

Mackenzie Sound lies to the east of the island. It is obscured by the narrow Hopetown Passage at the south end of Watson Island and by Kenneth Passage at the north end, but access through this latter passage is quite straight forward.

## Claydon Bay  chart 3547

West of Watson Island, across Grappler Sound, look for shelter in Claydon Bay on the mainland side. Claydon Bay is a good anchorage in all weather provided you use the lee shore in the winds you are trying to avoid. Anchor at the north end for best protection from most winds–westerlies in particular, and in the south bay for protection from easterlies.

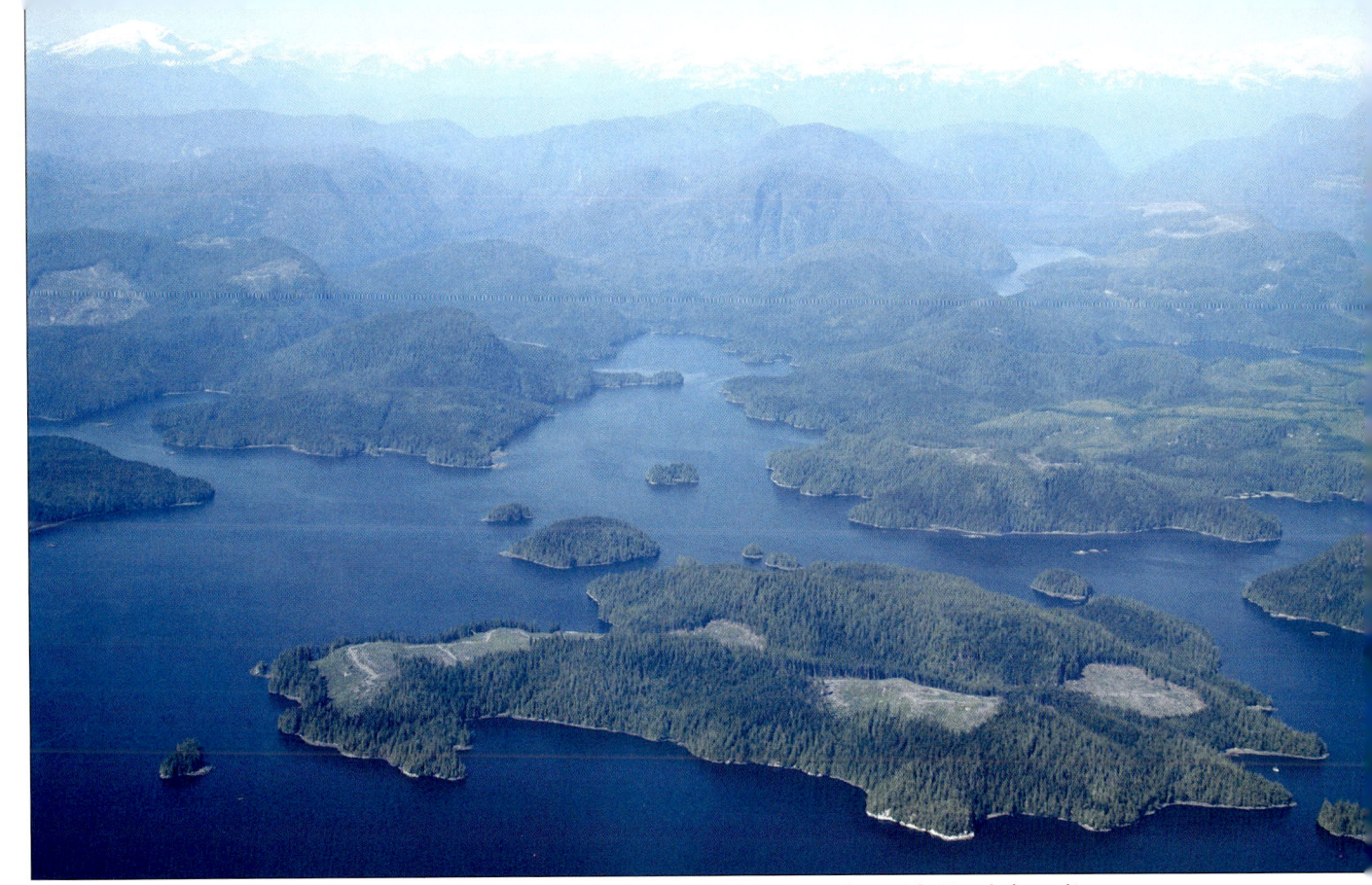

*A view up Grappler Sound showing Claydon Bay opening to the left and Hopetown Passage entrance at lower right. Note the boat taking temporary anchorage off the eastern tip of Kinnaird Island in the foreground. Beyond Watson Island lies Nepah Lagoon angling off towards the mountains.*

Chart 3547 shows easy passage into the bay clear of the rock and reefs to your starboard as you enter. Keep the small islet to your starboard too, as you proceed to the north bay. Between Claydon Bay and Turnbull Cove it is an easy passage along the west side of Watson Island, watching for the pinnacle just south of Watson Point. Going south down Grappler Channel you may be tempted by the appearance of Carriden Bay. Avoid it. It is too unpredictable when winds are forecast.

Nearby **Embley Lagoon** is not a recommended anchorage. It shallows out almost immediately inside the entrance. The tidal currents through the entrance are also restricting, limiting passage to slack tide. See diagram page 167.

### Turnbull Cove  chart 3547

This is a good, but sometimes windy, anchorage at the north end of Kenneth Passage. A narrow but easy entrance provides access to this favoured spot. Anchor over a flat, muddy bottom. Take your dinghy to explore from there.

Back in the 1970s we had the pleasure of meeting Owen and Clara Lane who owned a large logging camp on a nearby lake and made Turnbull Cove their home. The Lanes lived aboard a large pleasure cruiser, *Invader* and spent six months of the year at Turnbull Cove or Sullivan Bay, and the other six months moored at the Bayshore Inn in Vancouver. Their boat eventually became part of the charter fleet providing dinner and sight-seeing cruises in Vancouver harbour.

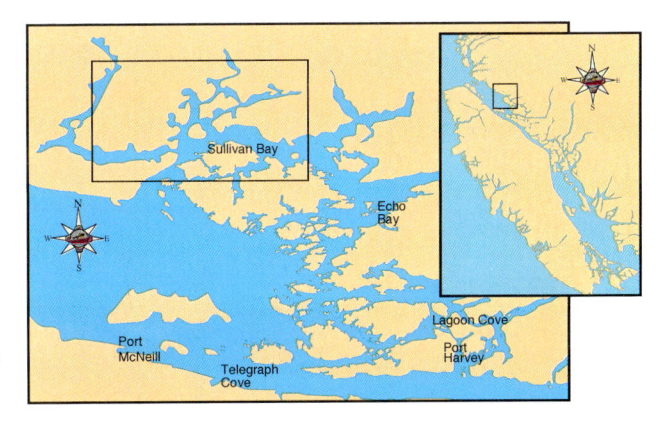

You may choose to avoid nearby **Nepah Lagoon**, or explore it only in a fast runabout. Enter and leave quickly during the very brief slack tide. It pays to observe the performance of the **Roaringhole Rapids** from outside the entrance for one or more tidal exchanges before attempting it (see pages 167 and 171). Or be prepared to remain inside the lagoon until the following slack tide. If you do find yourself trapped inside the lagoon between tides anchor temporarily in **Yuki Bay** a short distance from the entrance on the east side.

165

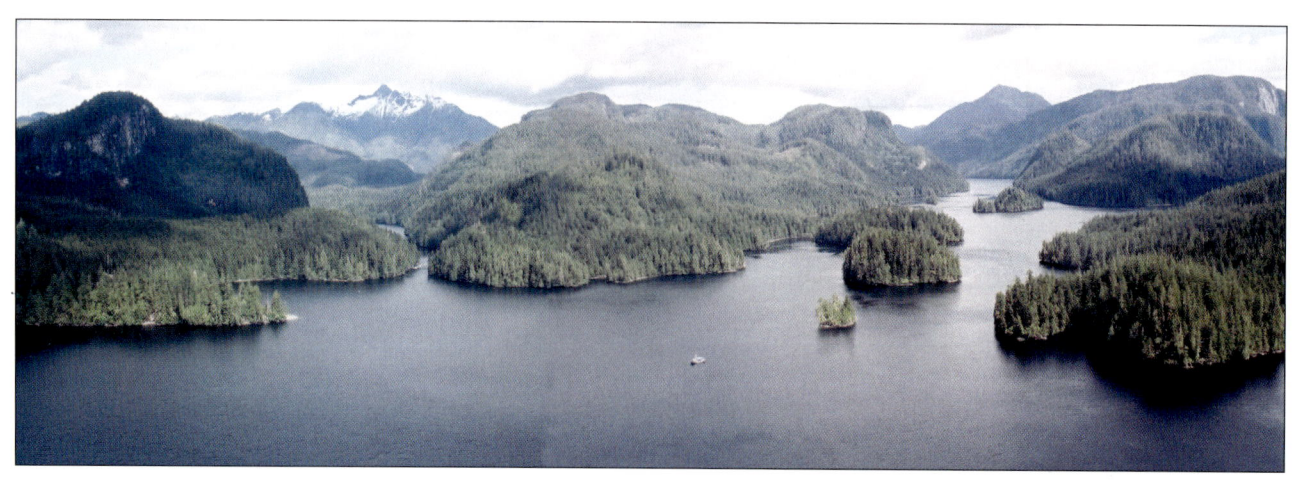

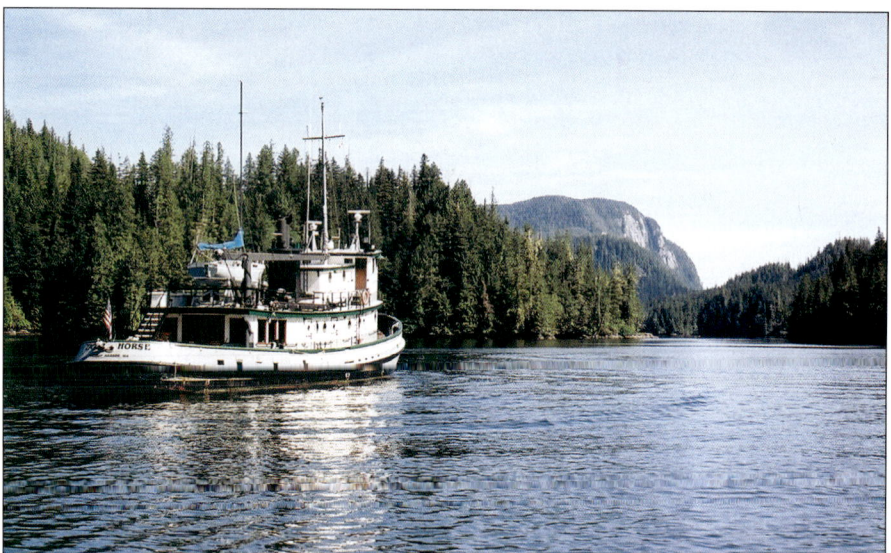

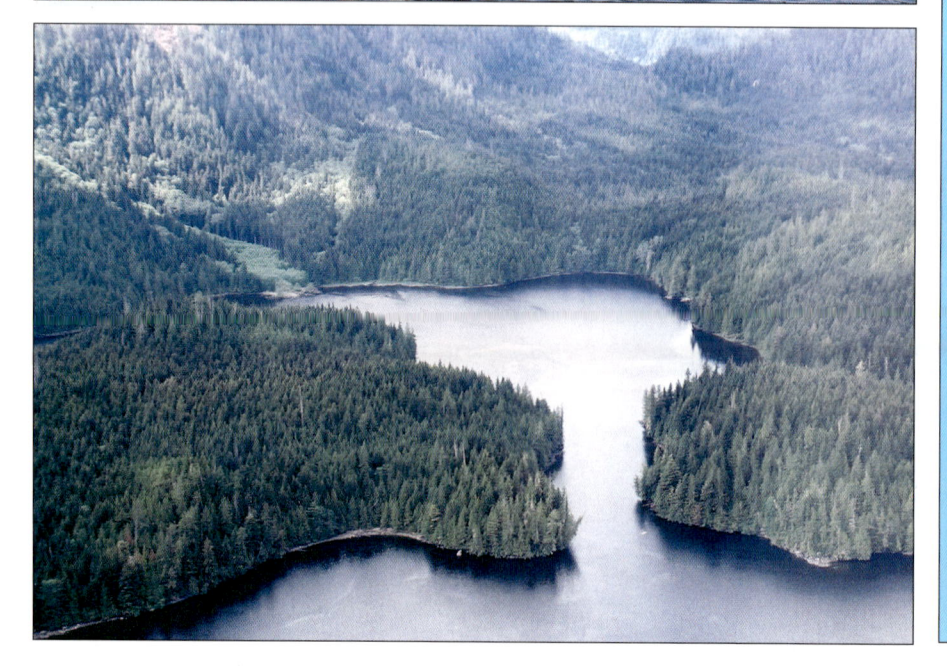

*Above: The head of Grappler Sound showing the entrance to Nepah Lagoon directly in front of Mount Stephens, with Kenneth Passage to the right.*

*Left: This large tug was anchored inside Turnbull Cove. It is a mostly sheltered place to drop the hook for large and small boats.*

*Bottom: Turnbull Cove with its narrow entrance is shown from the air.*

### Homesteaders

The entire Broughtons area was dotted at one time with homesteaders and a number of industrial enterprises, which included logging camps. Some remained only a short while. As logging moved on very few homesteaders stayed for any great length of time and today there are more vague signs of former settlement than there are remaining settlers.

Most coves and bays where settlers set up their homesteads are now either occupied by recently established holiday homes or simply returned to the dense underbrush of the forests.

There are still some signs of former industry, such as where a roadway was built for the logging industry. Some remnants of an elevated roadway can be seen in the shallows of Claydon Bay (opposite page).

## Chart 3547

**Turnbull Cove** N 50°57.301' W126°49.688'

**Jessie Point** N 50°57.105' W126°49.146'

**Kenneth Passage** N 50°56.788' W126°50.885'

**Claypole Point** N 50°55.930' W126°46.695'

**Claydon Bay** N 50°55.552' W126°53.098'

**Hoy Bay** N 50°55.337' W126°49.535'

**Burly Bay** N 50°55.553' W126°47.063'

**Dunsany Passage** N 50°54.846' W126°50.370'

Locations on map: Turnbull Cove, Overflow Basin (tidal falls), Embley Lagoon, Nepah Lagoon, Yuki Bay, Roaringhole Rapids, Jessie Point, Kenneth Passage, Watson Point, Watson Island, Steamboat Bay, Claypole Point, Mackenzie Sound, Claydon Bay, Woods Bay, Hoy Bay, Hopetown Point, Hopetown Passage, Burly Bay (temporary), Grappler Sound, Morton Point, Buckingham Island, Dunsany Passage, Cunning Point, Linlithgow Pt, Carriden Bay, Pandora Head, Kinnaird Island, to Sullivan Bay

Anchorage in Hoy Bay east of Hopetown Point.

Travel through Hopetown Passage only at very high tides and in very shallow draft boats.

Watch for strong curents off Cunning Point.

*Not for Navigation*

---

## Claydon Bay — Chart 3547

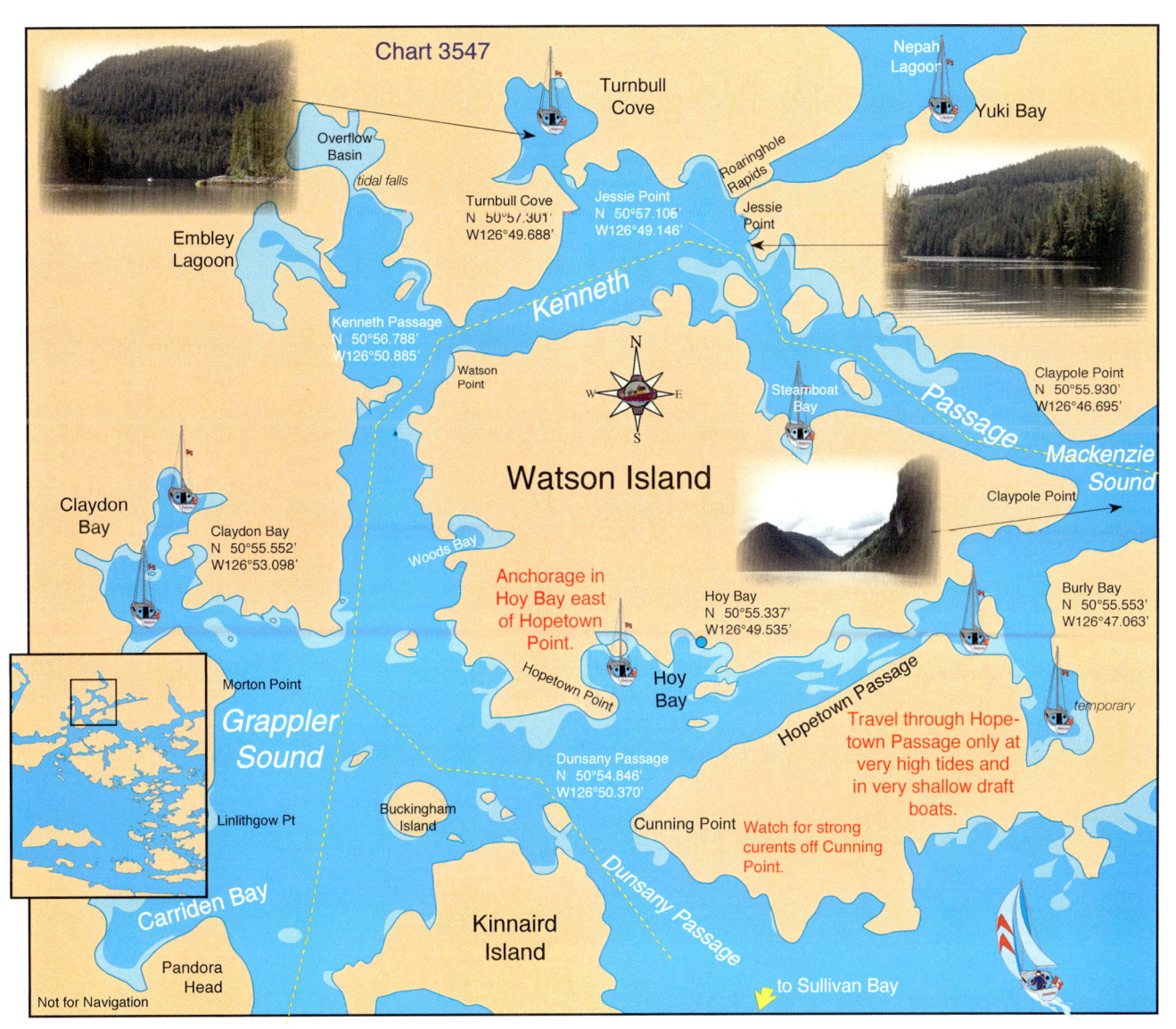

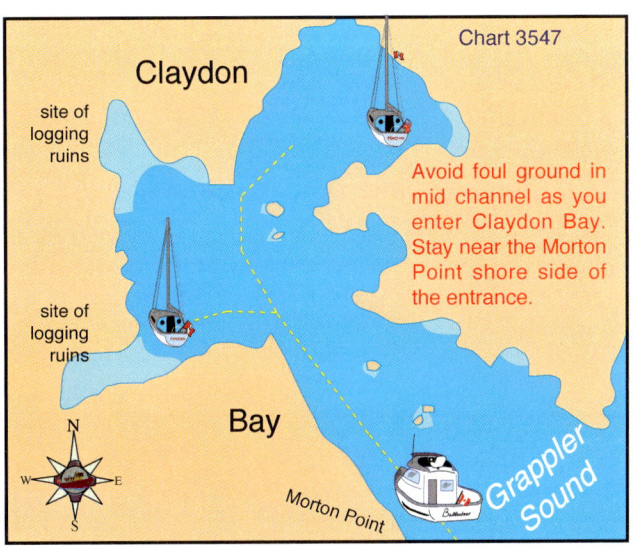

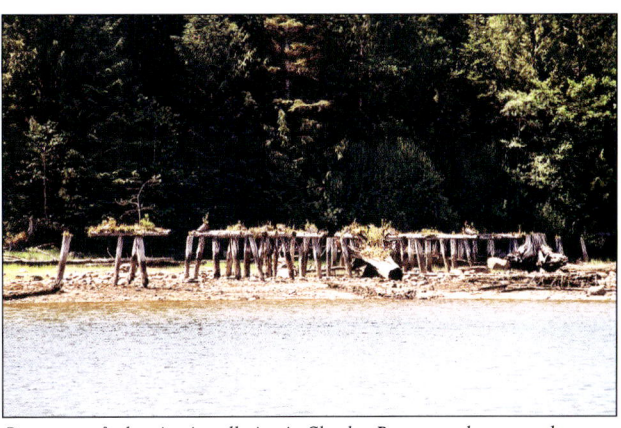

site of logging ruins (×2)

Morton Point, Grappler Sound

Avoid foul ground in mid channel as you enter Claydon Bay. Stay near the Morton Point shore side of the entrance.

*Remnants of a logging installation in Claydon Bay–a trestle-mounted roadway at one time used by logging trucks.*

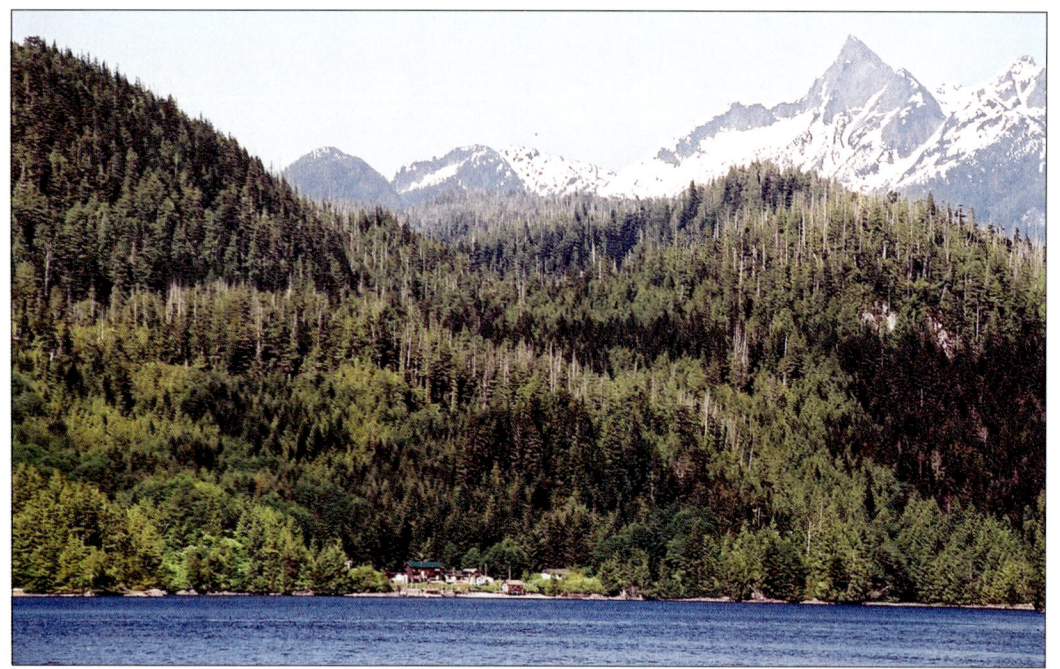

*Left: Hoy Bay, nestled deep in Hopetown Passage is dwarfed by the towering peaks of the Colville Range on the mainland. The private residences in the bay are on First Nations land.
Centre: Hopetown Passage from the west shows Buckingham Island in the foreground left with Kinnaird Island's northern shore in the right corner. A bay in the northwest side of Kinnaird Island (to the right in the photo) was once the location of the floating camp that was moved to Sullivan Bay to become the busy centre it is today.
Left: The eastern entrance to Hopetown Passage. It should be taken in small boats (dinghies, kayaks) at high tide only. The passage is blocked at low tide by rocks that dry over three metres. Strong winds funnel through the passage at times. Anchorage in Hoy Bay (centre right in the photograph) is generally quite good.*

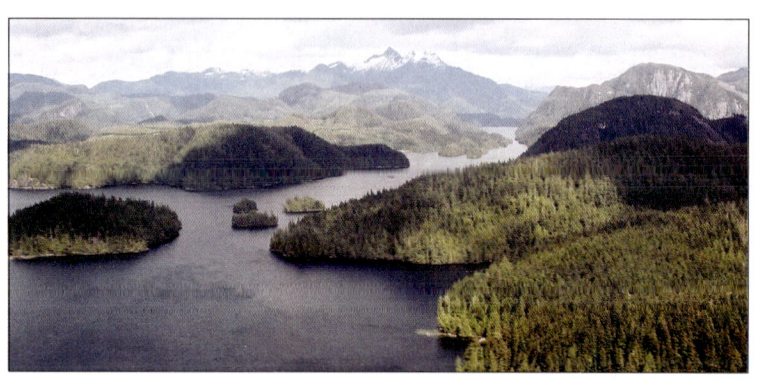

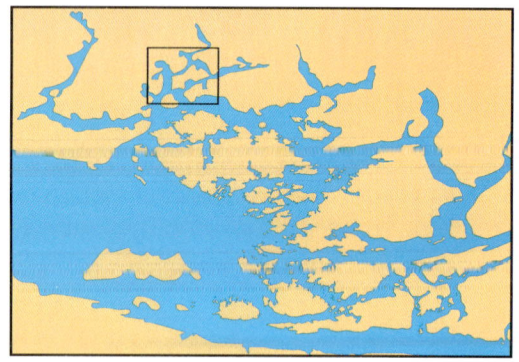

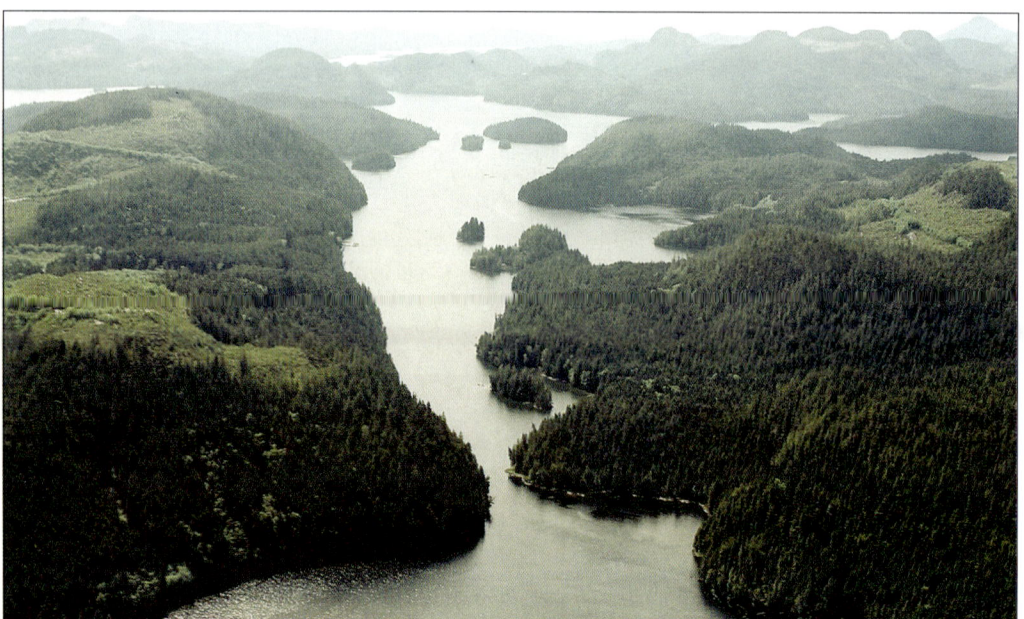

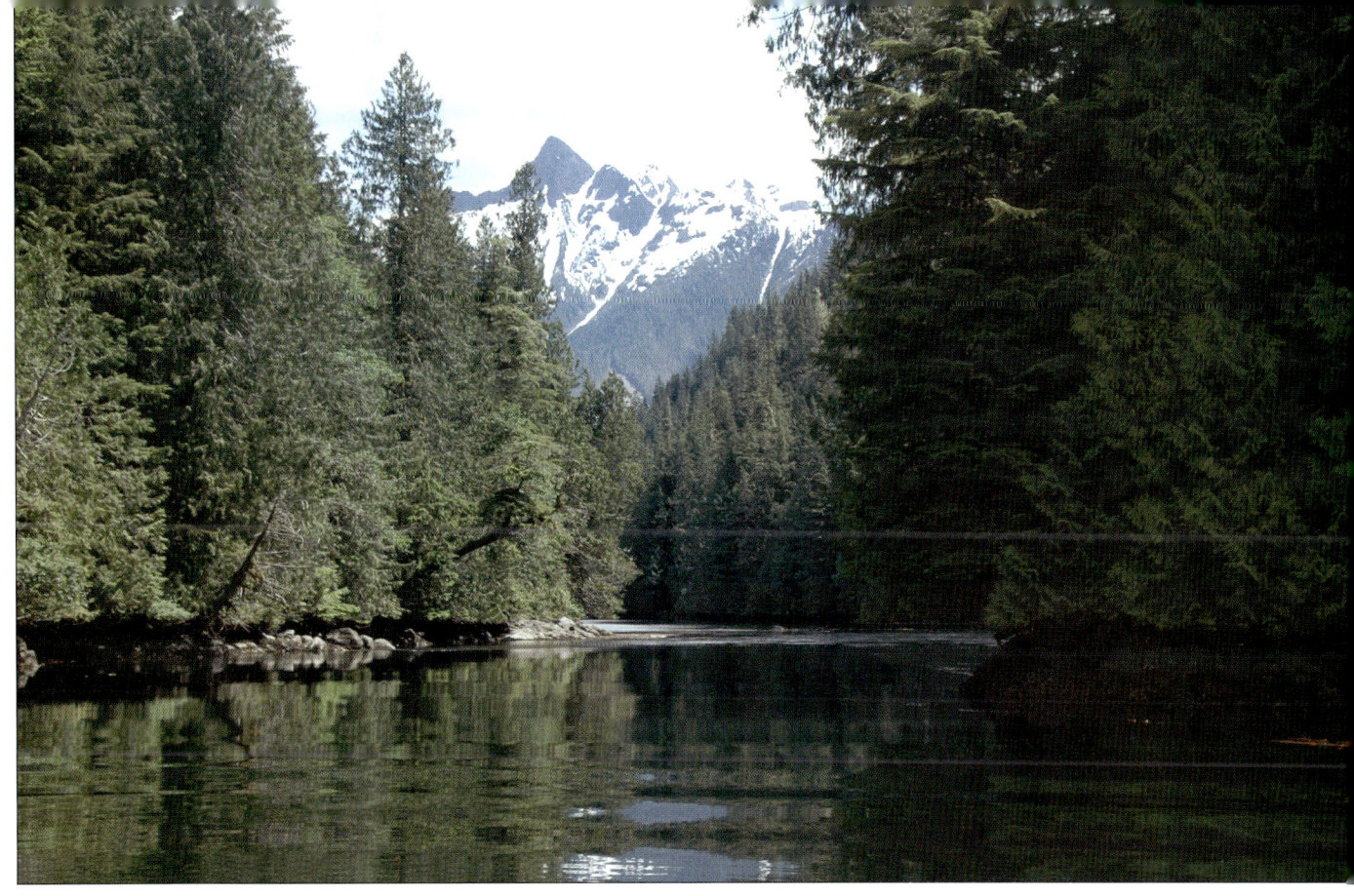

*Above: The Roaringhole Rapids limits entrance to Nepah Lagoon to slack tides. Once inside anchor at Yuki Bay and check the tides and times for leaving.*
*Below: The entrance to Mackenzie Sound from Kenneth Passage provides an exquisite view of Mount Stephens as it does from almost anywhere in Grappler Sound and Mackenzie Sound. This photograph was taken in Mackenzie Sound near the south entrance to Kenneth Passage.*

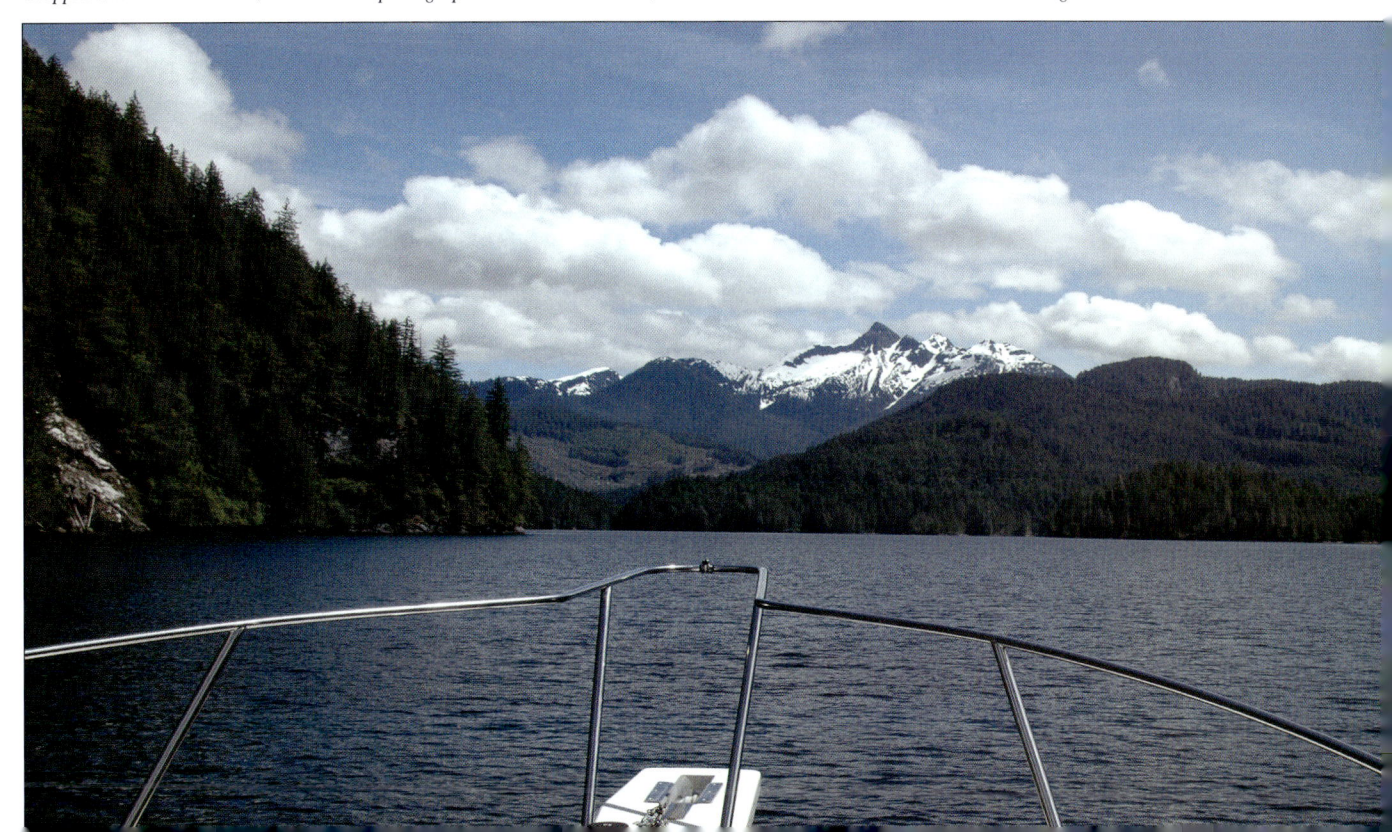

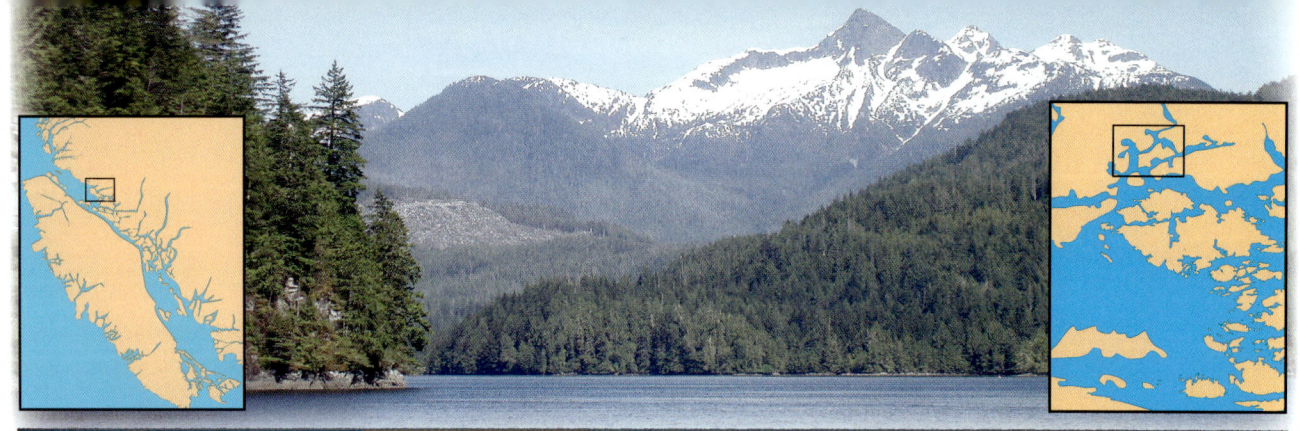

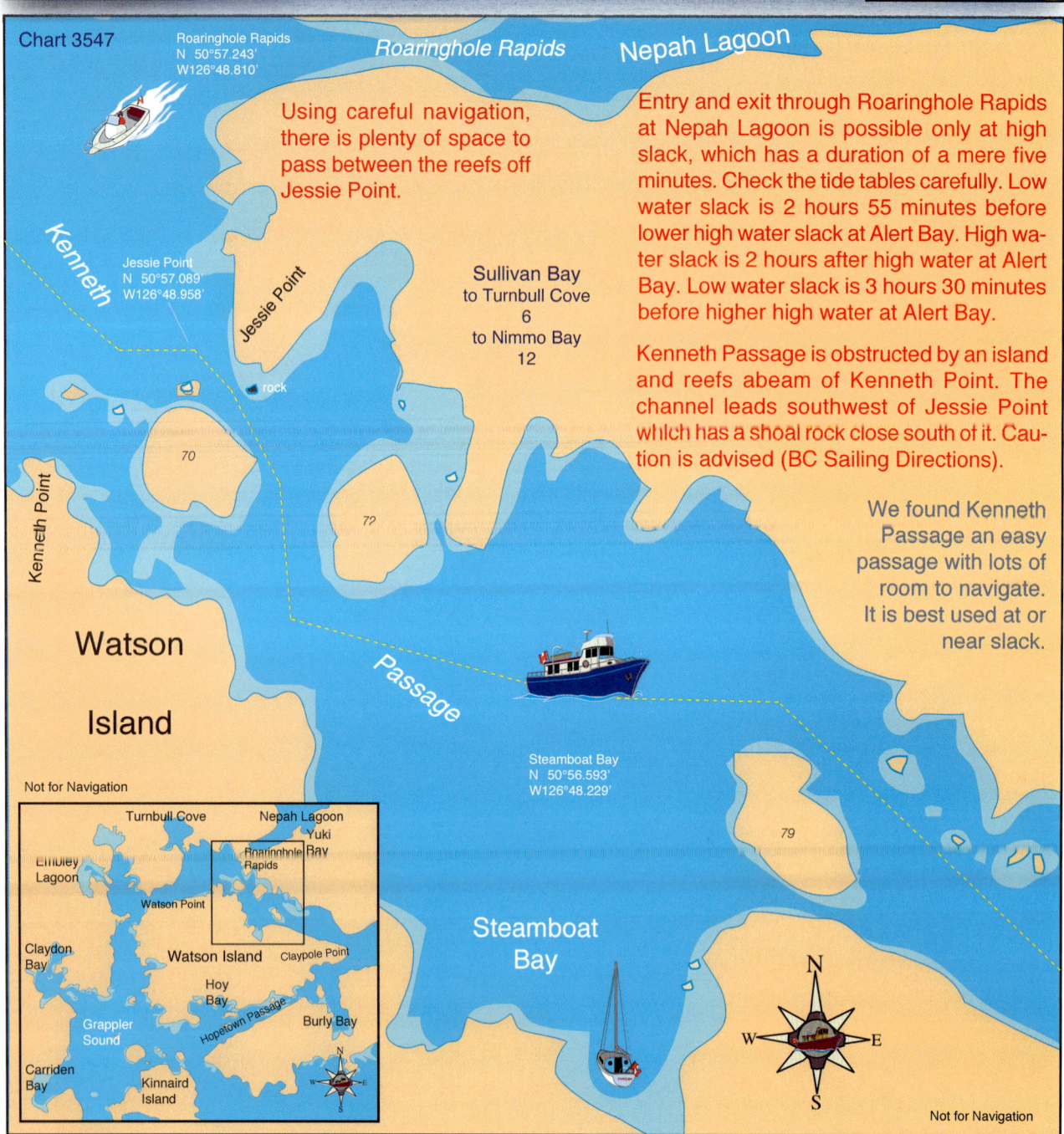

## Chart 3547

**Roaringhole Rapids** — N 50°57.243' W126°48.810'

### Roaringhole Rapids — Nepah Lagoon

Using careful navigation, there is plenty of space to pass between the reefs off Jessie Point.

**Jessie Point** — N 50°57.089' W126°48.958'

Sullivan Bay to Turnbull Cove 6 to Nimmo Bay 12

Entry and exit through Roaringhole Rapids at Nepah Lagoon is possible only at high slack, which has a duration of a mere five minutes. Check the tide tables carefully. Low water slack is 2 hours 55 minutes before lower high water slack at Alert Bay. High water slack is 2 hours after high water at Alert Bay. Low water slack is 3 hours 30 minutes before higher high water at Alert Bay.

Kenneth Passage is obstructed by an island and reefs abeam of Kenneth Point. The channel leads southwest of Jessie Point which has a shoal rock close south of it. Caution is advised (BC Sailing Directions).

We found Kenneth Passage an easy passage with lots of room to navigate. It is best used at or near slack.

Kenneth Point

Watson Island

Kenneth Passage

**Steamboat Bay** — N 50°56.593' W126°48.229'

Steamboat Bay

Not for Navigation

### Inset: Watson Island

Turnbull Cove, Nepah Lagoon, Yuki Bay, Roaringhole Rapids, Embley Lagoon, Watson Point, Claydon Bay, Watson Island, Claypole Point, Hoy Bay, Grappler Sound, Hopetown Passage, Burly Bay, Carriden Bay, Kinnaird Island

Not for Navigation

170

*Right: Kenneth Passage from the south, showing the route for navigating it.*

*Below left: The entrance to Nepah Lagoon with the tidal Roaringhole Rapids that keep boats at bay*

*Below right: Entering Kenneth Passage at the north end.*

*Bottom: Nimmo Bay in Mackenzie Sound. This is a fishing lodge where you may anchor off and visit for a possible dinner if space and timing allows.*

*Opposite page: Mount Stephens looms over Grappler Sound.*

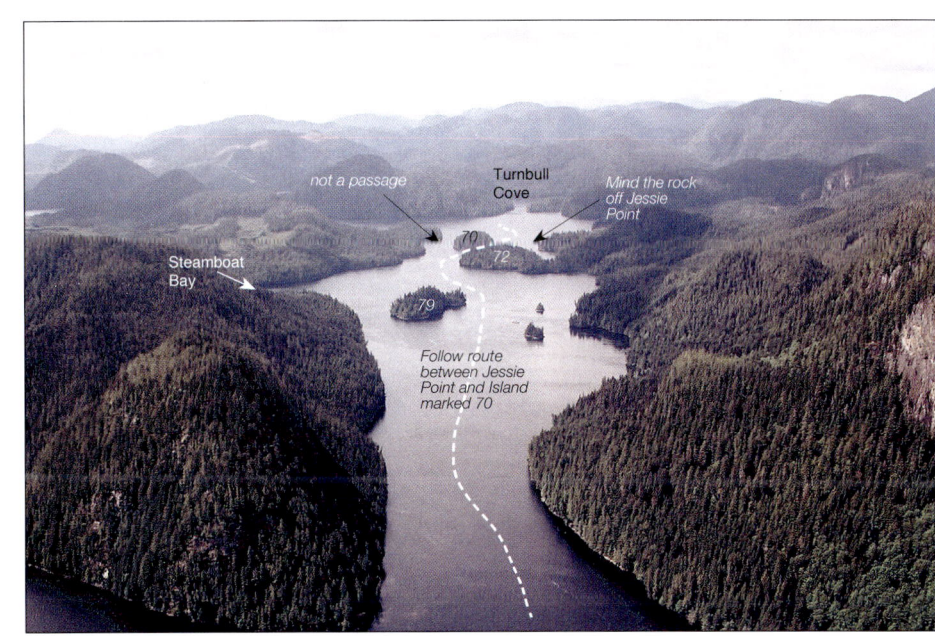

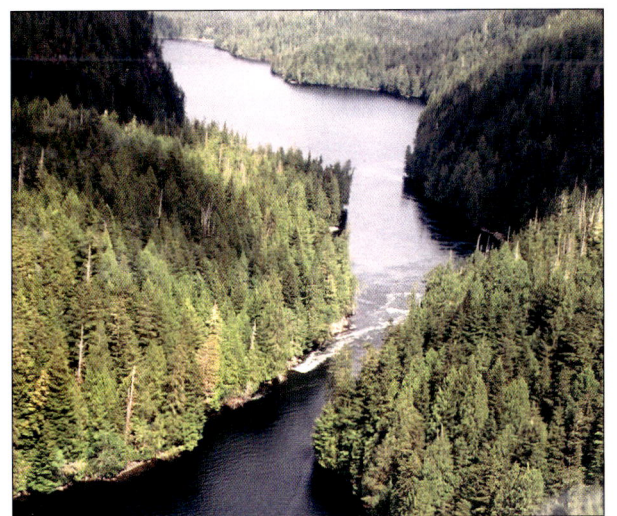

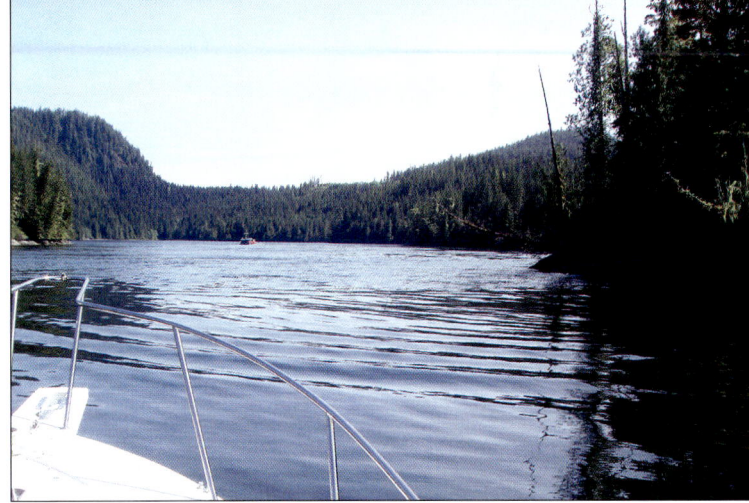

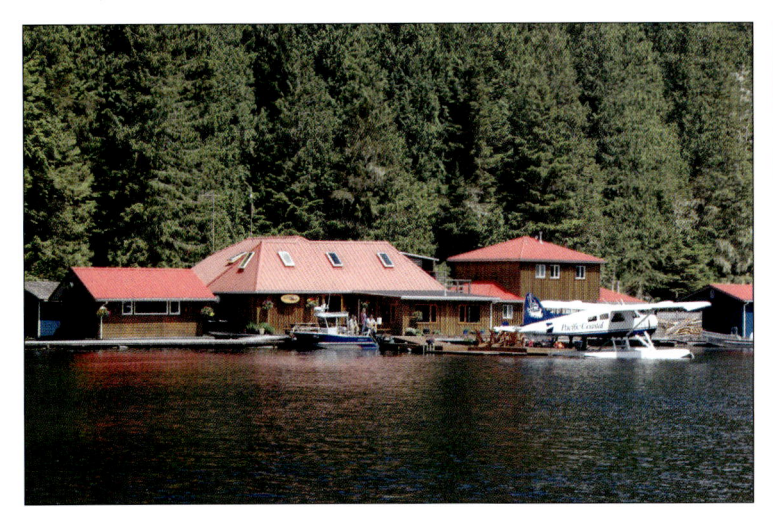

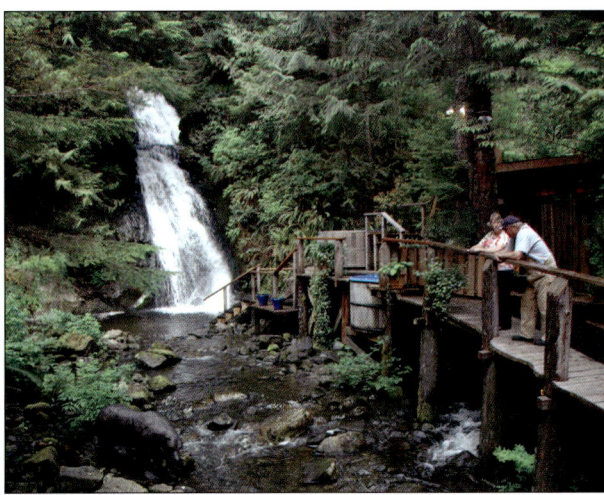

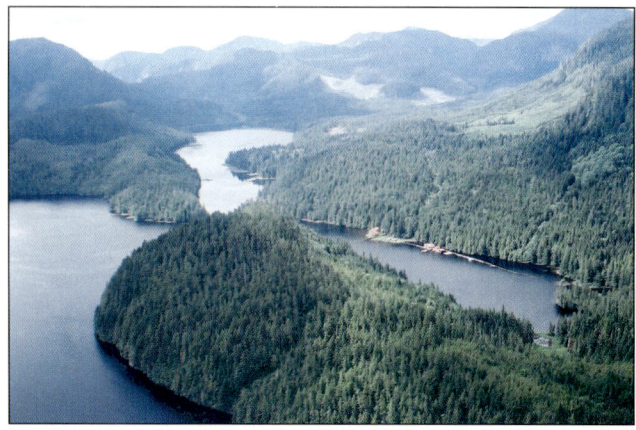

*Nimmo Bay, Little Nimmo Bay and the lodge. The larger bay or lagoon, is seen also in the inset photo below. The entrance is off Mackenzie Sound.*

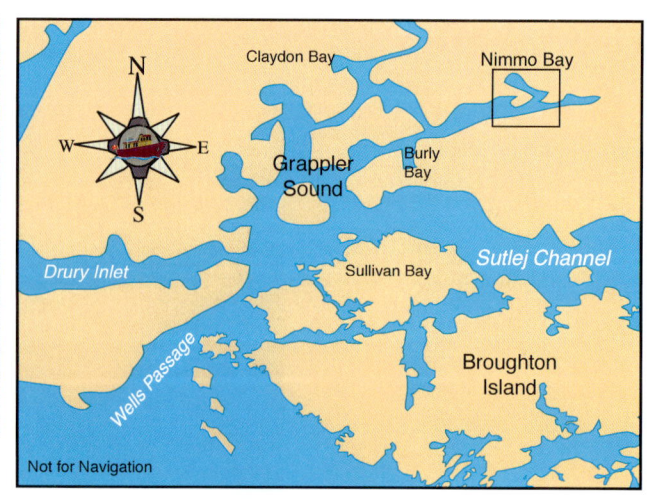

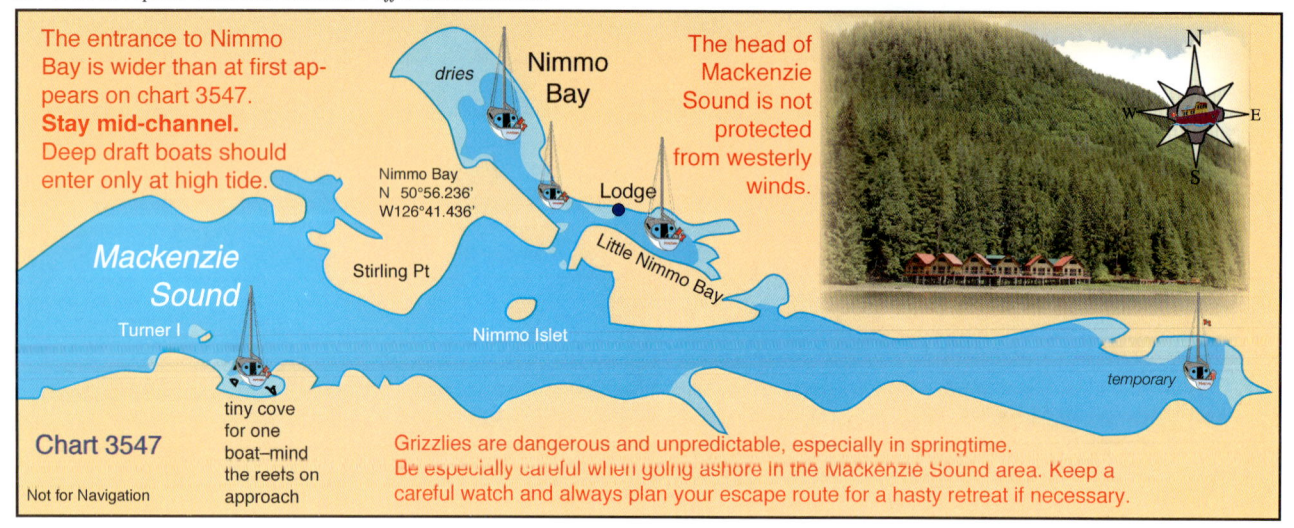

**The entrance to Nimmo Bay is wider than at first appears on chart 3547. Stay mid-channel. Deep draft boats should enter only at high tide.**

**The head of Mackenzie Sound is not protected from westerly winds.**

Nimmo Bay N 50°56.236' W126°41.436'

**Grizzlies are dangerous and unpredictable, especially in springtime. Be especially careful when going ashore in the Mackenzie Sound area. Keep a careful watch and always plan your escape route for a hasty retreat if necessary.**

## Steamboat Bay  chart 3547 (diagrams page 167, 170)

On the north side of Watson Island, Steamboat Bay offers anchorage and protection from easterlies. Getting to Steamboat Bay requires navigation through and into Kenneth Passage in currents of about 3 knots at most times. Faster boats will easily slip through with careful navigation, passing mid-channel off Jessie Point and taking care to avoid the submerged rock noted on the chart and the swirling currents it generates.

## Burly Bay  chart 3547 (diagram above and page 167)

Inside Mackenzie Sound at the east end of Hopetown Passage anchor in the large, somewhat exposed Burly Bay. It is a wide, windy bay but with protection from winds other than southeasterlies. We prefer the anchorage, small though it is, west of **Blair Islet**. A small area of land in the southeast corner of the bay is designated IR–owned by First Nations people. Adjacent to it is a tall ridge of granite that casts early morning shadow over the entrance to the anchorage and deflects some of the westerlies into the bay.

## Nimmo Bay  chart 3547

Once through the narrows of Kenneth Passage, the preferred destination is Nimmo Bay. Here you will find a flourishing fishing lodge used for fly-in guests but not designated a boating destination with overnight moorage unless space permits. The entrance to Nimmo Bay is not as challenging as it appears at first, with adequate water for a careful passage through. Avoid the rocks on the east shore by maintaining a mid-channel course. Once inside drop the hook in Little Nimmo Bay, but away from the activities of the fishing lodge. Be mindful of the winds that course in from the southeast and treat this as a temporary anchorage. Explore the entirety of Nimmo Bay in a small boat, being mindful of the mud flats and reefs as well as the pinnacle at the end of the narrows, where the larger Nimmo Bay opens to the northwest. There is a waterfall partly obscured by the forest reaching down to the water's edge near the head of Little Nimmo Bay. If you go ashore be prepared for possible encounters with bears.

For more secure anchorage return to Steamboat Bay or Turnbull Cove at the west end of Mackenzie Sound.

172

# Drury Inlet and Actaeon Sound

Chart 3547

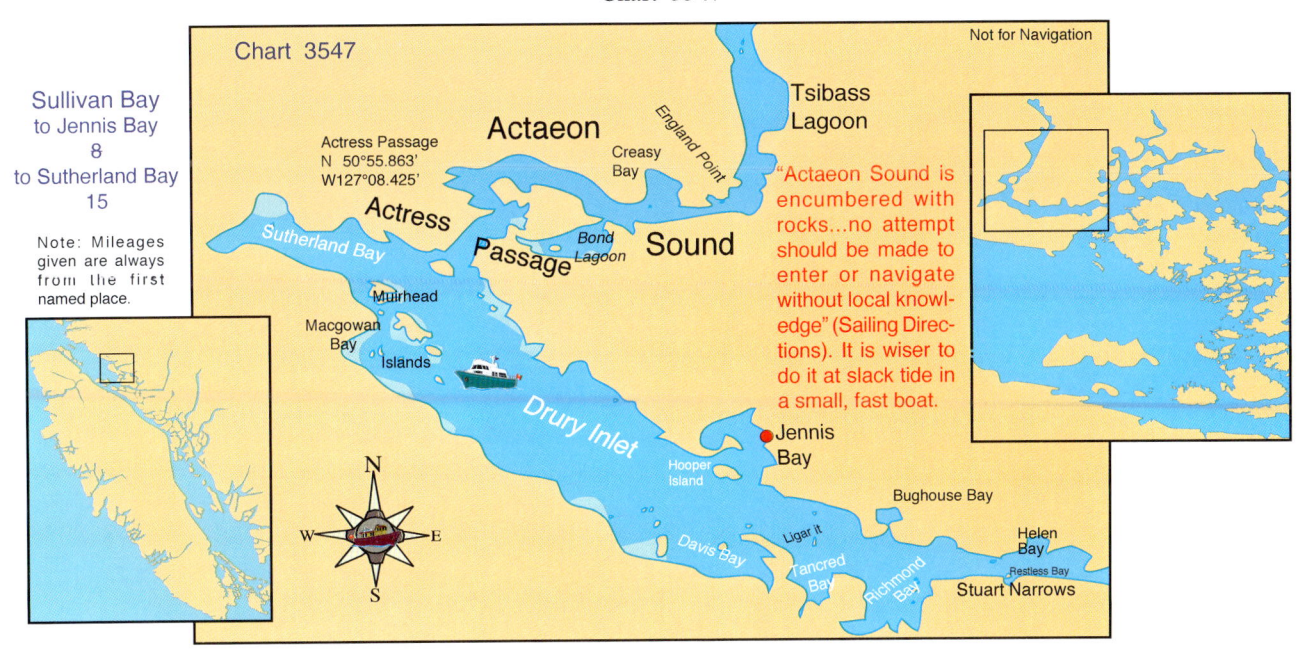

## Drury Inlet  chart 3547

Drury Inlet opens to the west off Grappler Sound where Wells Passage and Sutlej Channel meet near Sullivan Bay. Crossing from Sullivan Bay requires a short jaunt across Wells Passage, past Morris Islet and its adjacent rocks and into Stuart Narrows. Here you will often encounter currents of up to seven knots, flood or ebb. When accompanied by wind, conditions in this passage could be rough. On calm days and moderate tidal changes entry is normally quite easy. Pass Welde Rock to the south (north of the island that juts out from the south shore) and continue beyond. Take into consideration the current around Welde Rock at all times other than slack. Do not attempt to use **Restless Bay** as a passage. It is too obstructed (see diagram page 175).

Some mariners look for overnight places to call their own and drop the hook in **Helen Bay** (temporary) or **Richmond Bay**, while others go on to Jennis Bay and beyond. Going straight up Drury Inlet, pass to the north of Leche Islet. To enter Richmond Bay, travel southeast of the islet.

Richmond Bay affords protected moorage for a couple of boats in mild weather. Use the nook in the southwest corner when it is blowing from the southwest and the cove on the opposite side, southeast, for protection from easterlies. Avoid **Tancred Bay** where the wind simply will not allow you a good night's rest, if it is blowing from any direction.

Continue past the north side of Ligar Islet then turn into **Davis Bay**. That is if you are inclined to conduct an exercise in navigation. Travel carefully past Davis Islet, by way of a very narrow, shallow north passage or the easier south entrance. Mind the reef that protrudes from the shore opposite Davis Islet. Anchor in the shallows in the centre of the bay. Or simply cross Dury Inlet and visit Jennis Bay–the most recommended anchorage and a welcoming marina and lodge in this 12 nautical-mile-long inlet.

If you continue deeper into Drury Inlet skip the Muirhead Islands, leaving them to port (there is nowhere to anchor among them comfortably, although some mariners have reported finding temporary anchorage), and make your way into **Sutherland Bay**. Here you can anchor in shallow water over a muddy bottom in a depth of about 2 to 4 metres at low water (use chart 3547).

**Macgowan Bay** will not provide any protection as an anchorage either, but take your dinghy around the Muirhead

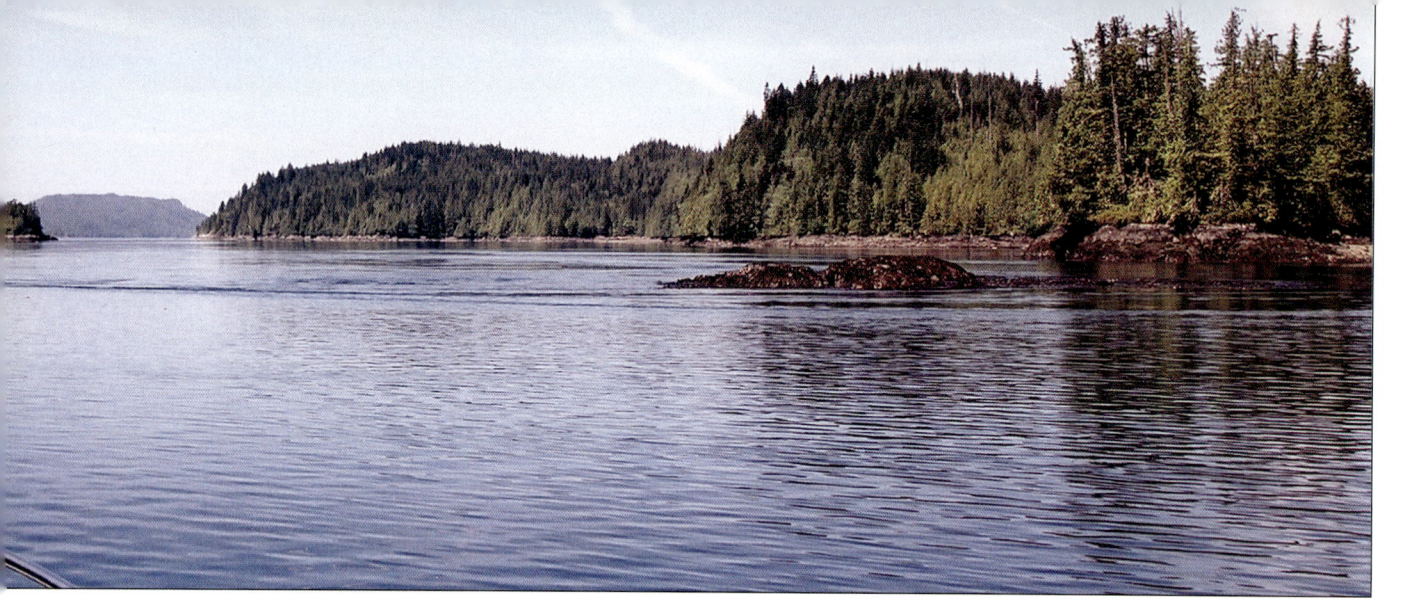

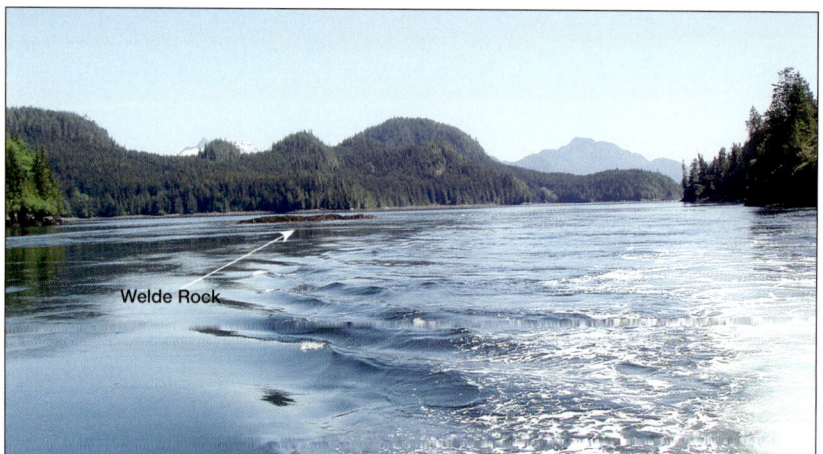

*Above: Stuart Narrows is guarded by Welde Rock–seen from the eastern approach. Keep to the south of it as you pass, even though from a distance, at first, it appears the passage is to the north. The current runs to 7 knots in Stuart Narrows, so time your entrance and departure for slack or near slack. Left: Pass Welde Rock cautiously. View from the west. Below: Stuart Narrows, entrance to Drury Inlet. This view shows the passage to Drury Inlet from the east with Morris Islet in the foreground at its entrance. Drury Inlet and Actaeon Sound are surrounded by mostly low lying terrain.*

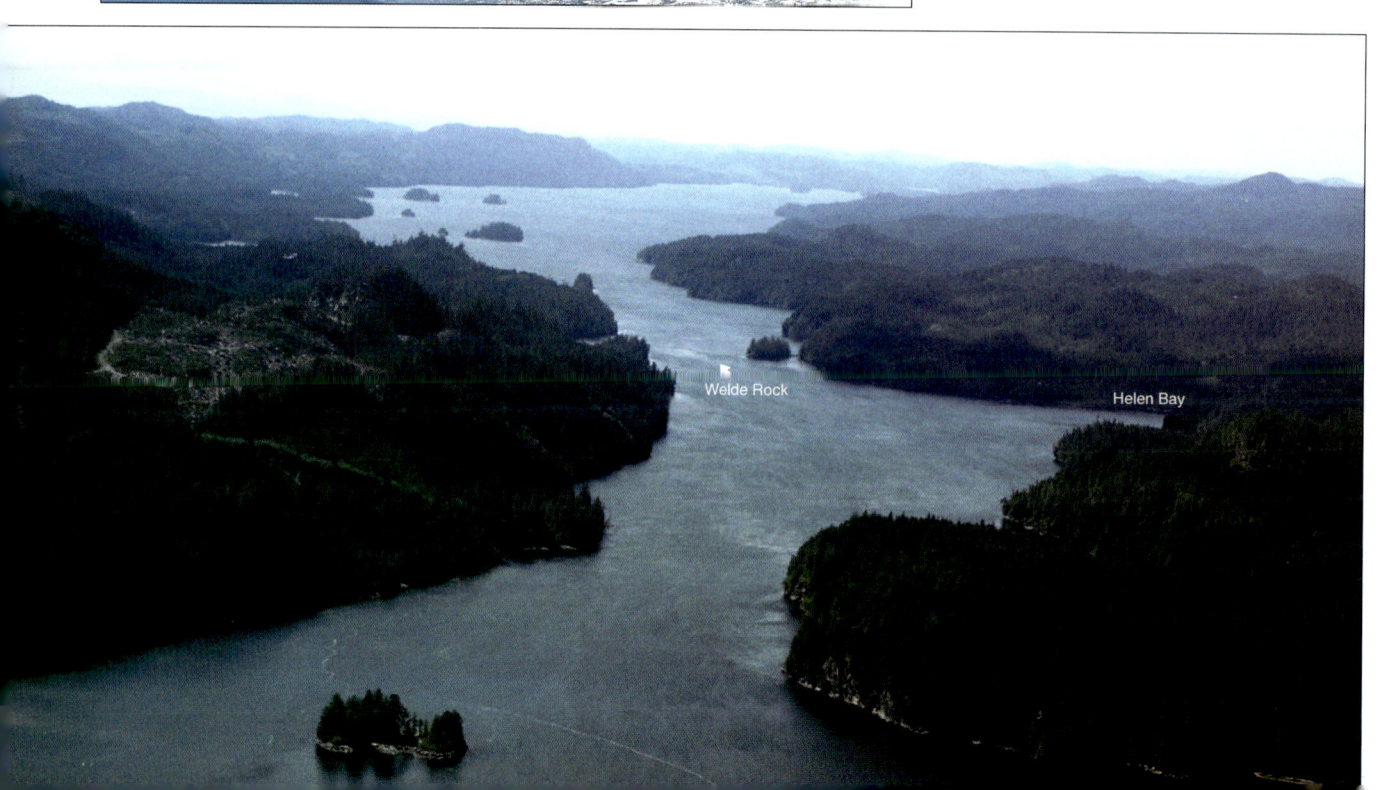

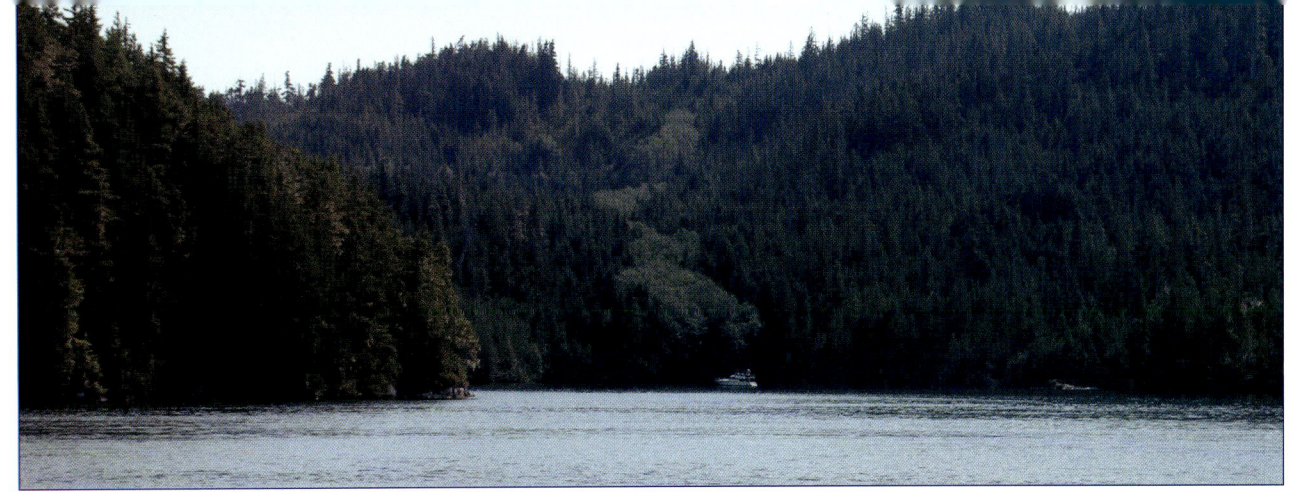

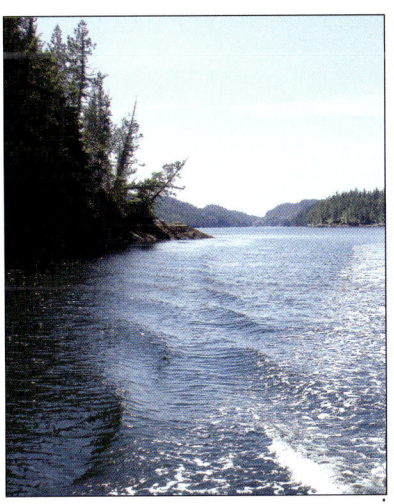

*Top: Anchored in Helen Bay that opens to the north off Stuart Narrows.*
*Above: Entering Actress Passage from Drury Inlet.*

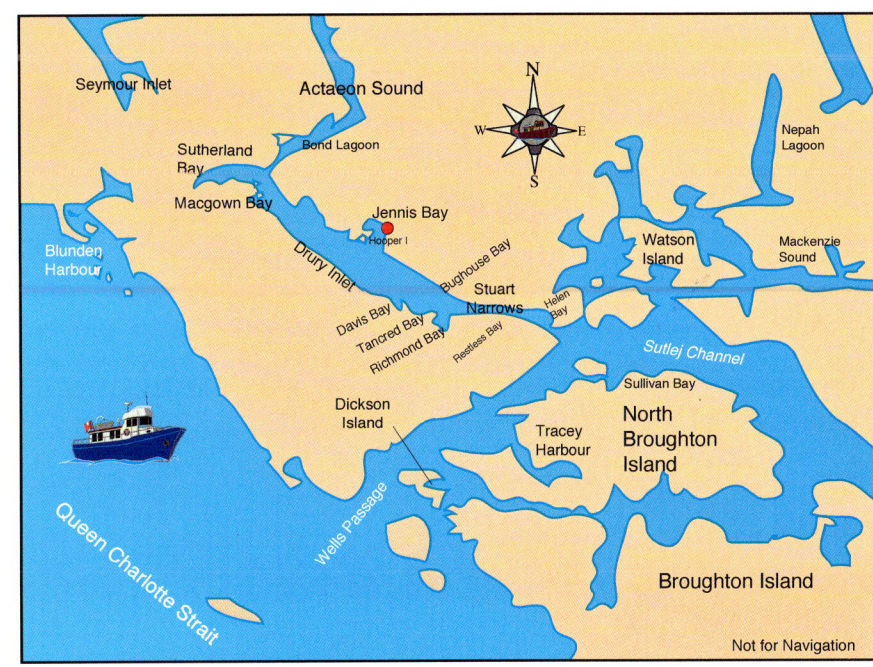

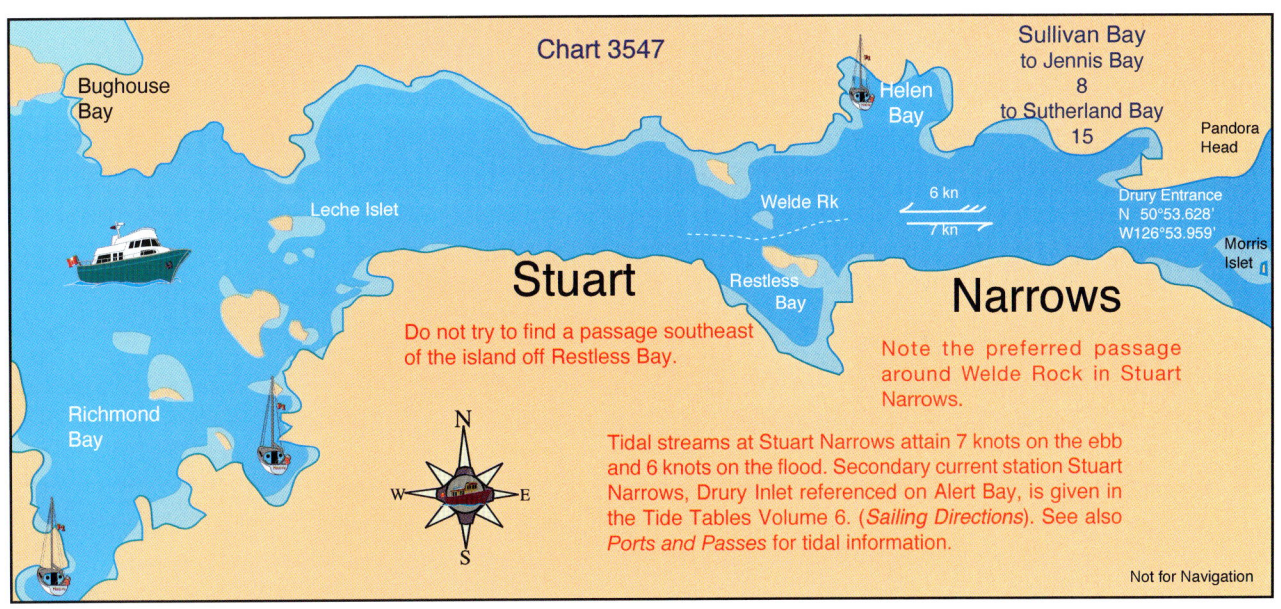

## Chart 3547

Sullivan Bay to Jennis Bay 8
to Sutherland Bay 15

Bughouse Bay, Leche Islet, Richmond Bay, Welde Rk, Restless Bay, Helen Bay, Pandora Head, Morris Islet

Drury Entrance N 50°53.628' W126°53.959'

6 kn / 7 kn

## Stuart Narrows

**Do not try to find a passage southeast of the island off Restless Bay.**

**Note the preferred passage around Welde Rock in Stuart Narrows.**

Tidal streams at Stuart Narrows attain 7 knots on the ebb and 6 knots on the flood. Secondary current station Stuart Narrows, Drury Inlet referenced on Alert Bay, is given in the Tide Tables Volume 6. (*Sailing Directions*). See also *Ports and Passes* for tidal information.

Not for Navigation

175

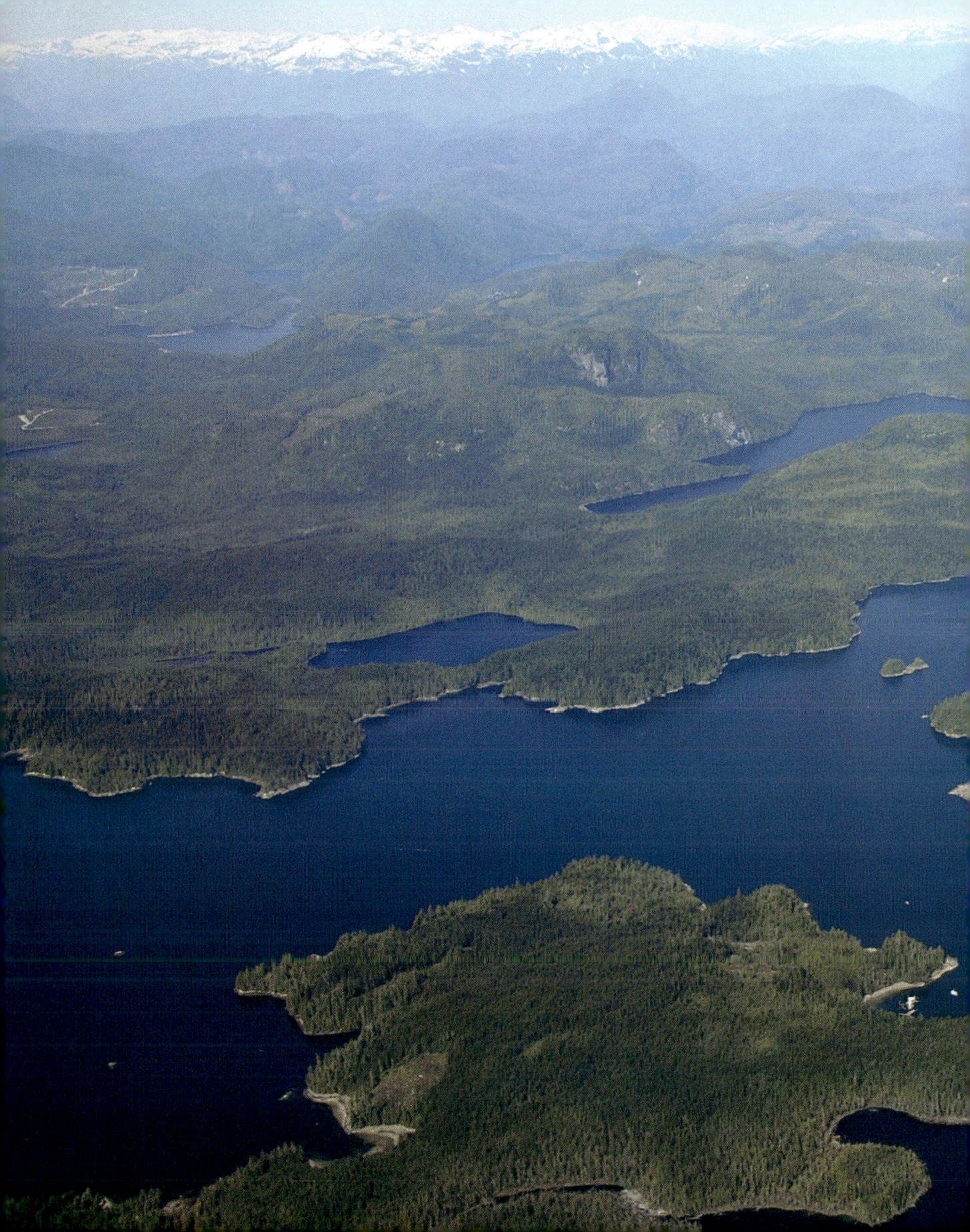

Welde Rk

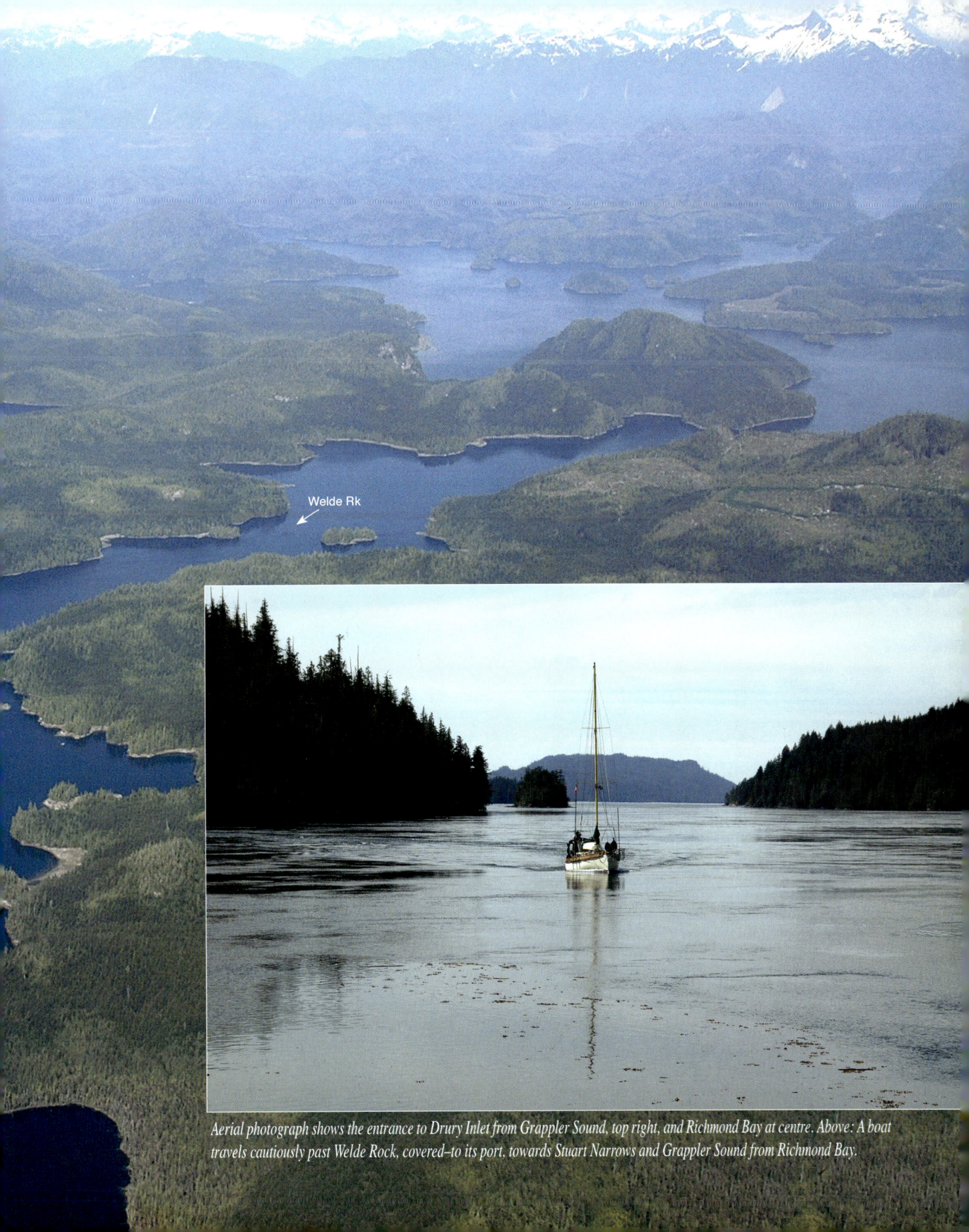

*Aerial photograph shows the entrance to Drury Inlet from Grappler Sound, top right, and Richmond Bay at centre. Above: A boat travels cautiously past Welde Rock, covered–to its port, towards Stuart Narrows and Grappler Sound from Richmond Bay.*

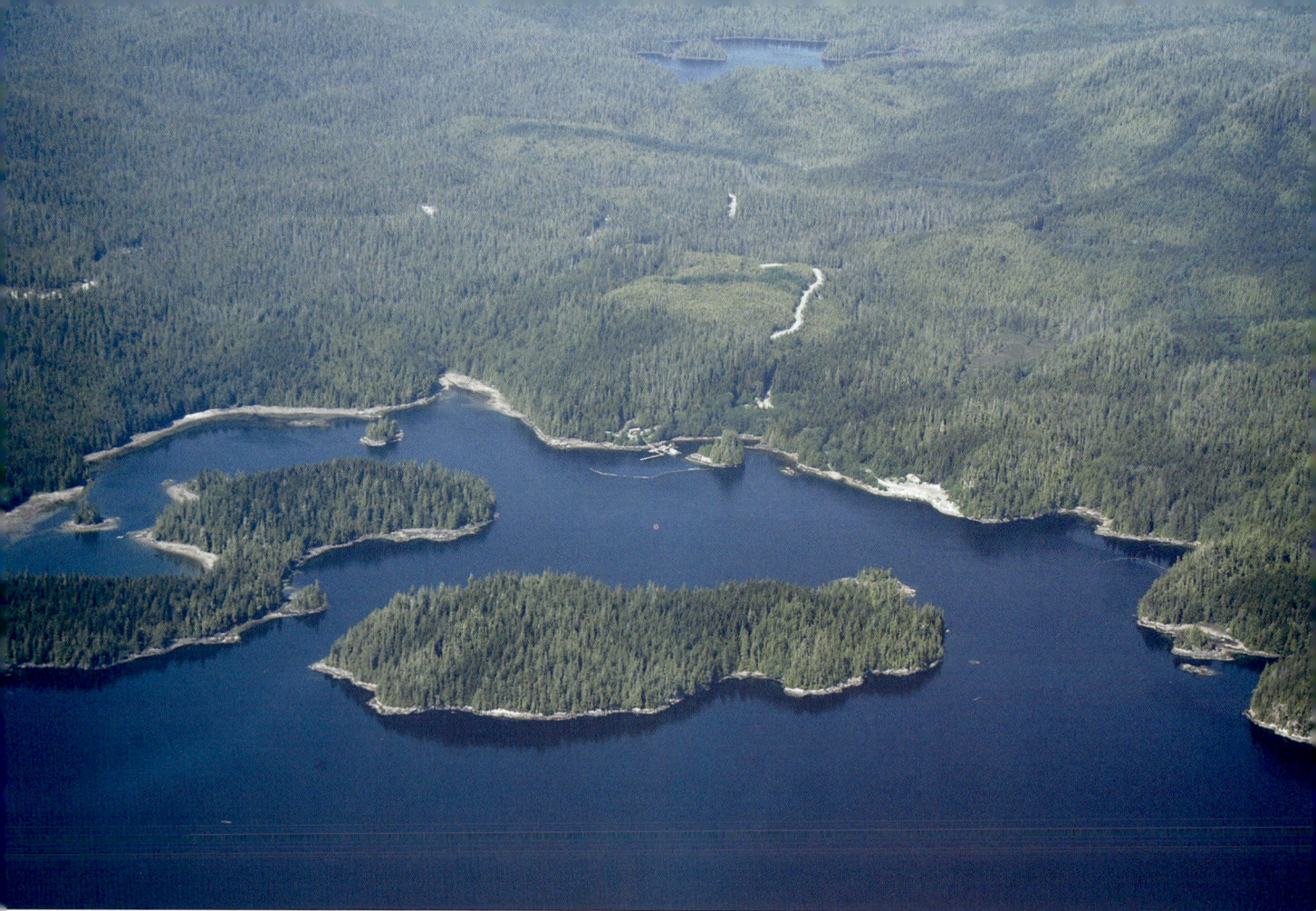

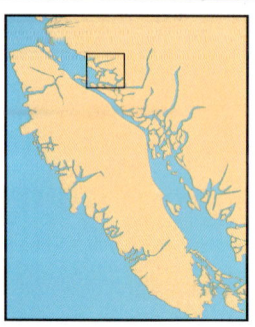

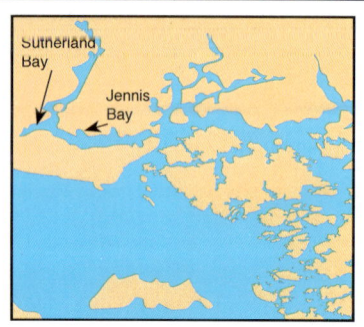

*Above: Jennis Bay with the lodge and marina floats at centre, and the favoured anchorage in the cove to its left.*
*Opposite, top: Anchored in the cove west of Jennis Bay Marina.*
*Opposite, bottom: The marina at Jennis Bay is sheltered from the weather and has cabins and a small community building. It was formerly a popular fishing lodge and private homestead. In recent years additions were made to improve its many features and functions as a marina.*

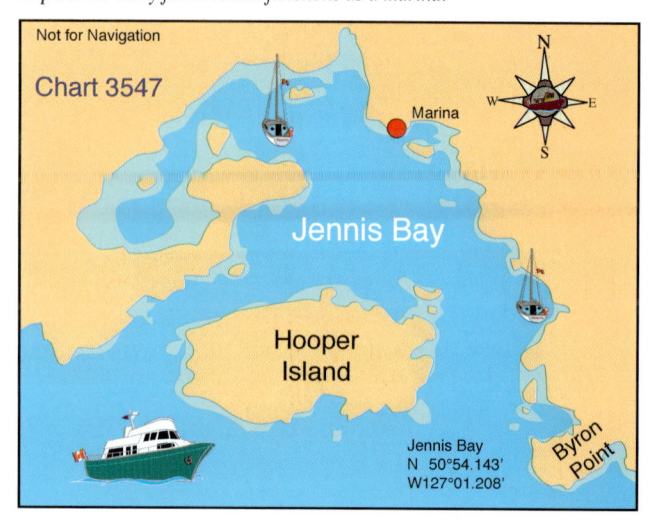

*From page 173*

Islands where, off the south passage, you will find a small beach and may catch sight of marine mammals and some interesting birds, including eagles and herons. Continue your poking about in and around the adjacent islands, being very cautious among the many rocks, pinnacles and reefs in the group. At the end of the inlet, at Sutherland Bay you are not that far from Blunden Harbour on the outside of the peninsula that separates Drury Inlet from Labouchere Passage in Queen Charlotte Strait. Many boaters looking for exercise love to walk trails such as the one that leads from Sutherland Bay to a small bay near the entrance to Blunden Harbour.

On the north side of Drury Inlet is sheltered Jennis Bay.

178

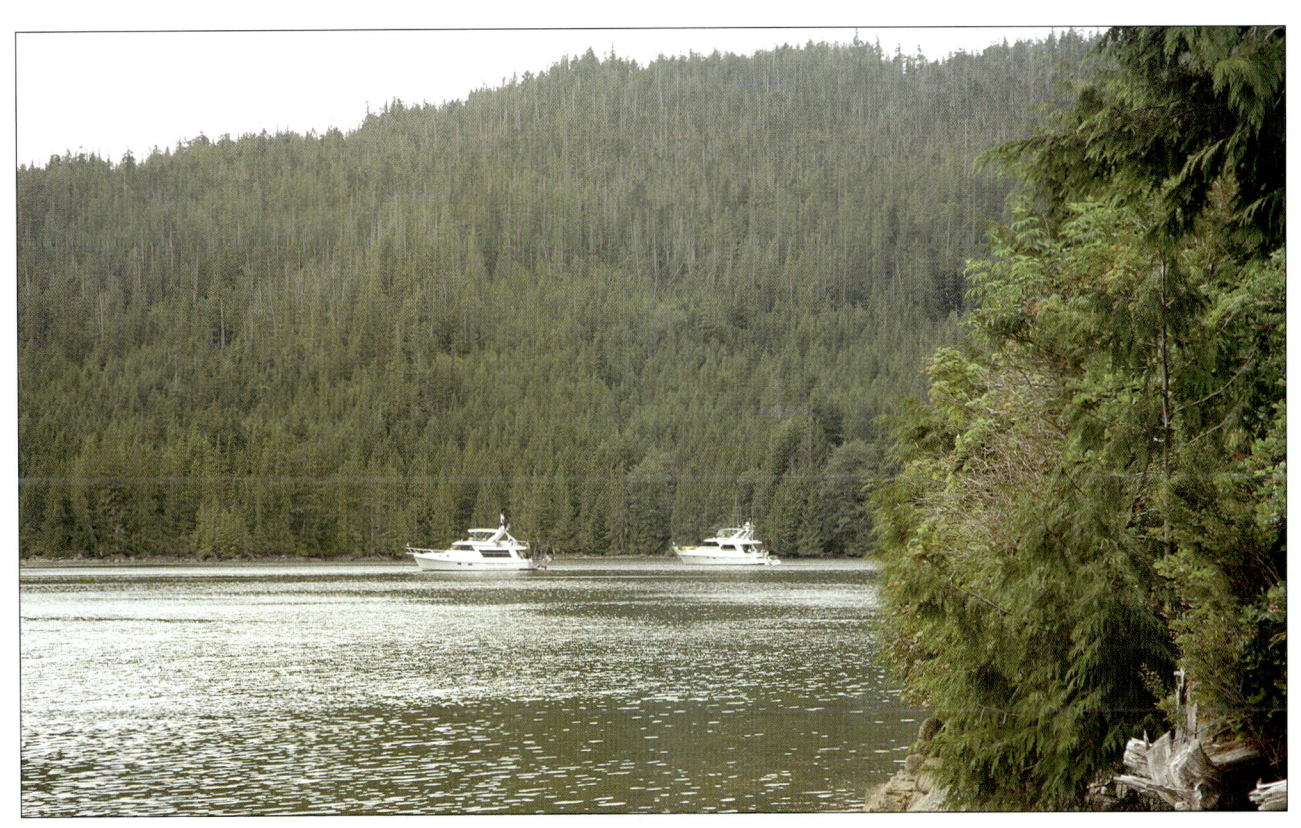

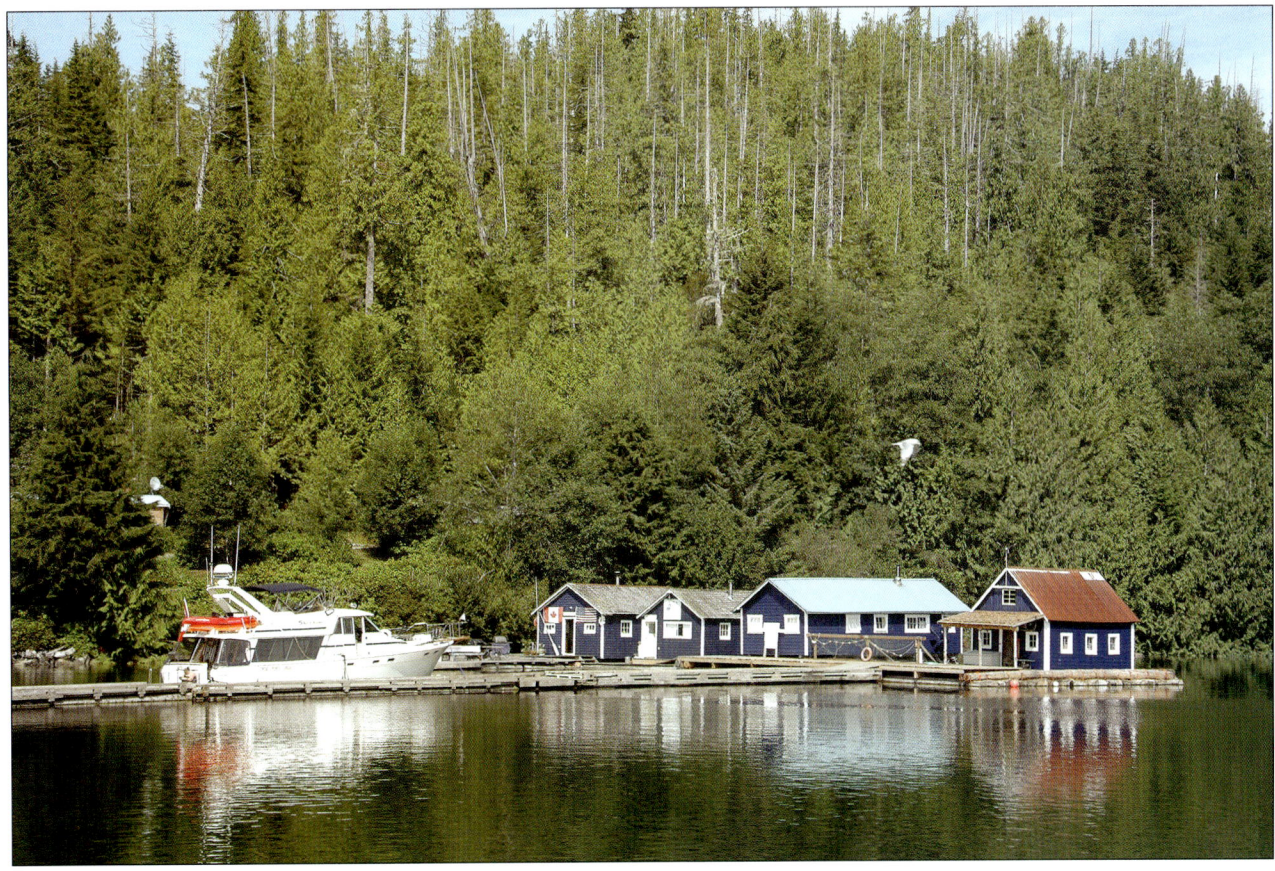

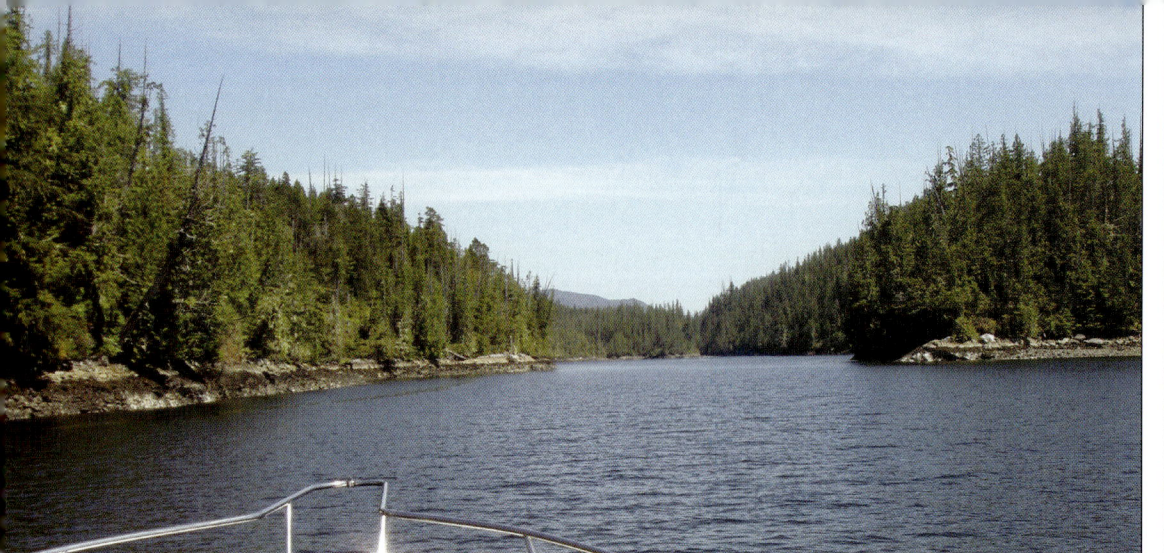

*Above: The north entrance to Actress Passage. It is wider than expected. Stay close to Dove Island and pass the small islet on its north side to avoid the rock protruding from the opposite shore. Then turn into the passage. The alternative route into Actress Passage is between two markers opposite the Muirhead Islands. Mind the reef near the rock in the middle of the channel southwest of Dove Island. Below: Jennis Bay Marina. Bottom, right: Inside Actress Passage, narrow sections and rocks. Use caution when the current is running. Right: The Muirhead Islands and the entrance to Actress Passage and Actaeon Sound.*

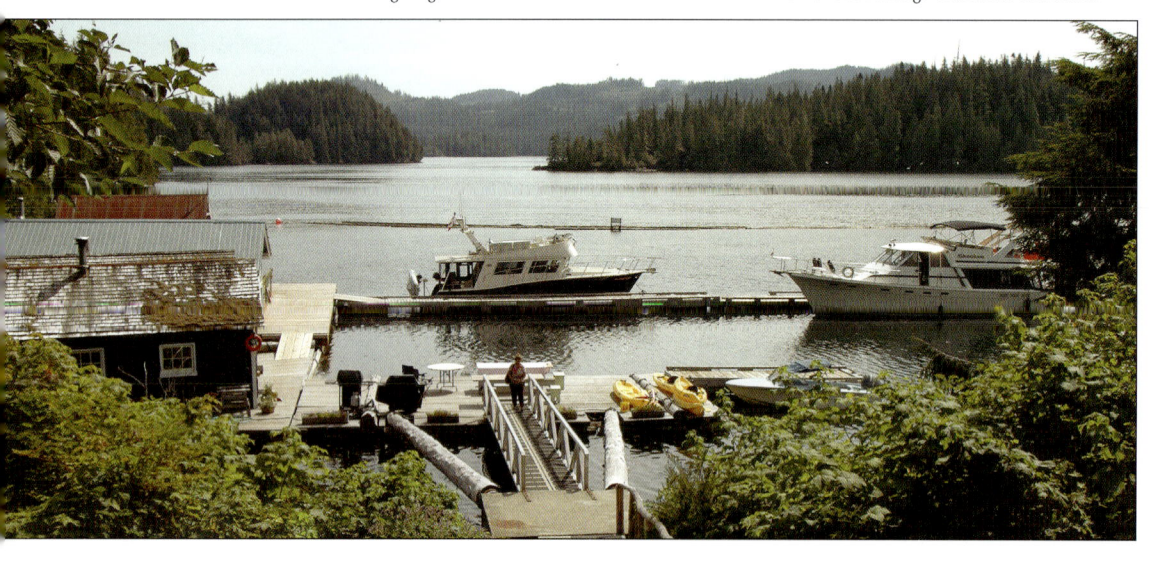

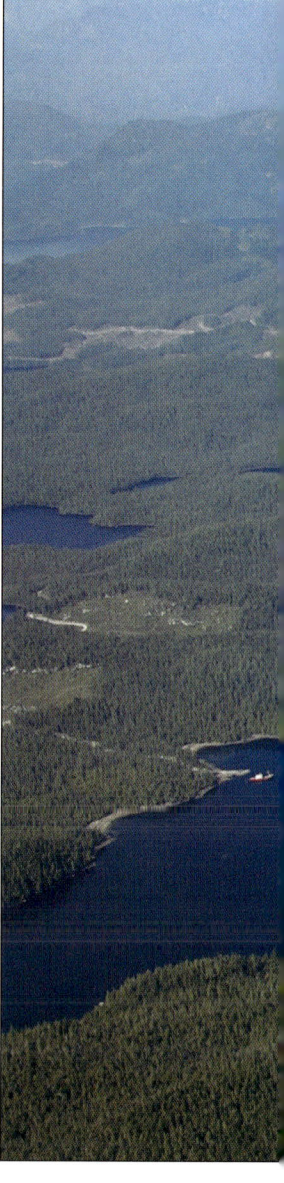

## Jennis Bay  chart 3547

The bay is the site of a popular marina and lodge. It was out of operation for a while after being a busy destination that catered to over-nighting mariners or visitors arriving at the lodge itself. It is now functioning as a favoured stop for visiting boaters.

The bay was once a thriving logging camp, long since abandoned, along with the adjacent shake mill. Logging still takes place in the bay but it is not obtrusive.

Some boat owners choose to anchor temporarily at the little cove directly opposite Hooper Island while others venture farther in and drop anchor in the lee of the peninsula and the rock north of it. Do not bother trying to enter the bay beyond this point as it is too shallow at the narrow entrance, all too often leaving boats dry until the next high tide.

## Jennis Bay Marina
PO Box 456 Port McNeill BC V0N 2R0
Phone 250-330-3076
*jennisbay@hughes.net*
*www.jennisbay.com*

The marina offers overnight guest moorage, rental cabins and a gift shop. The family that owns the facility has been upgrading its docks and structures to better accommodate visiting mariners. They offer eco-tourism, treasure hunting, trail hiking and bicycling.

Among the activities provided are kayak rentals and guided trail and lake excursions. At the marina there are special dining events and campfire get togethers. The marina welcomes children and pets.

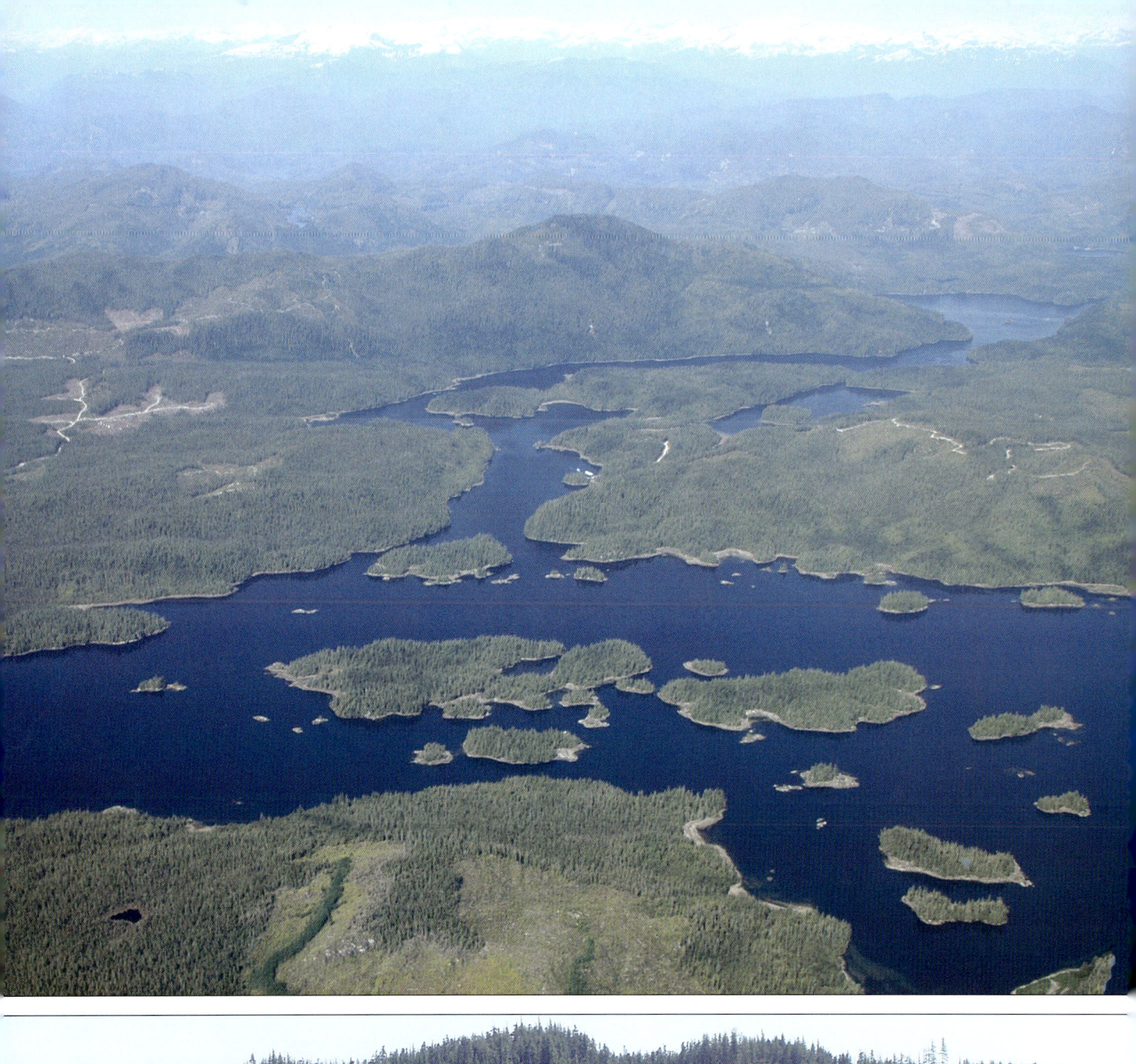

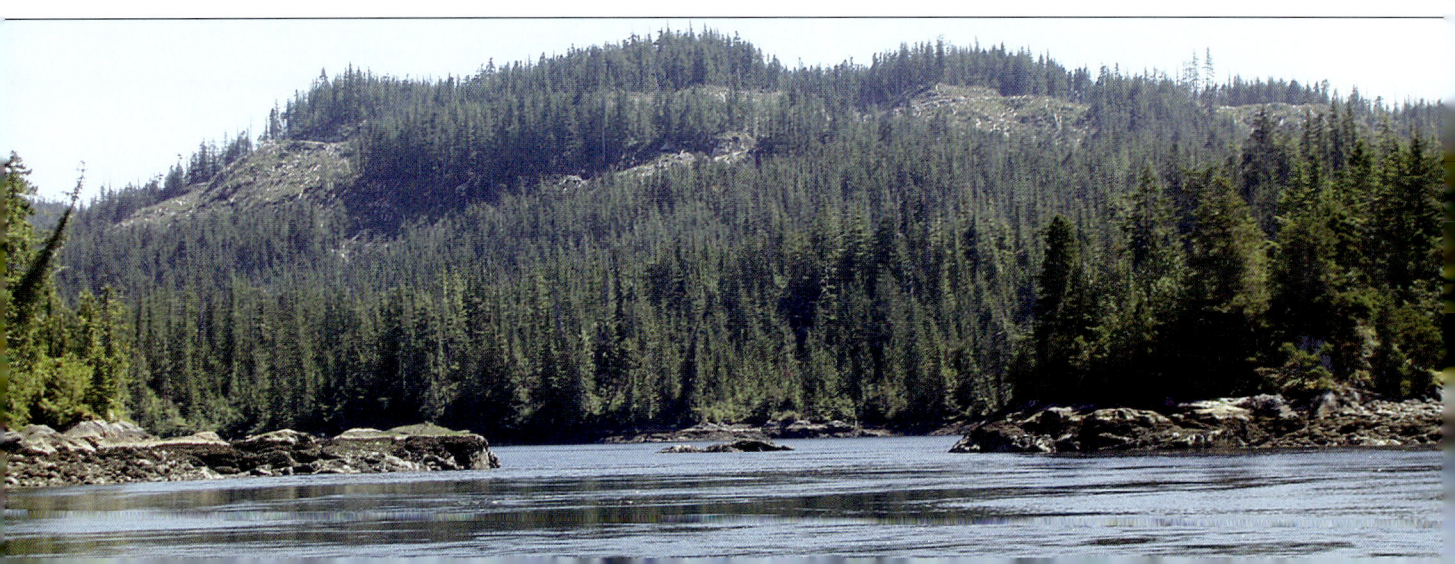

## Map annotations

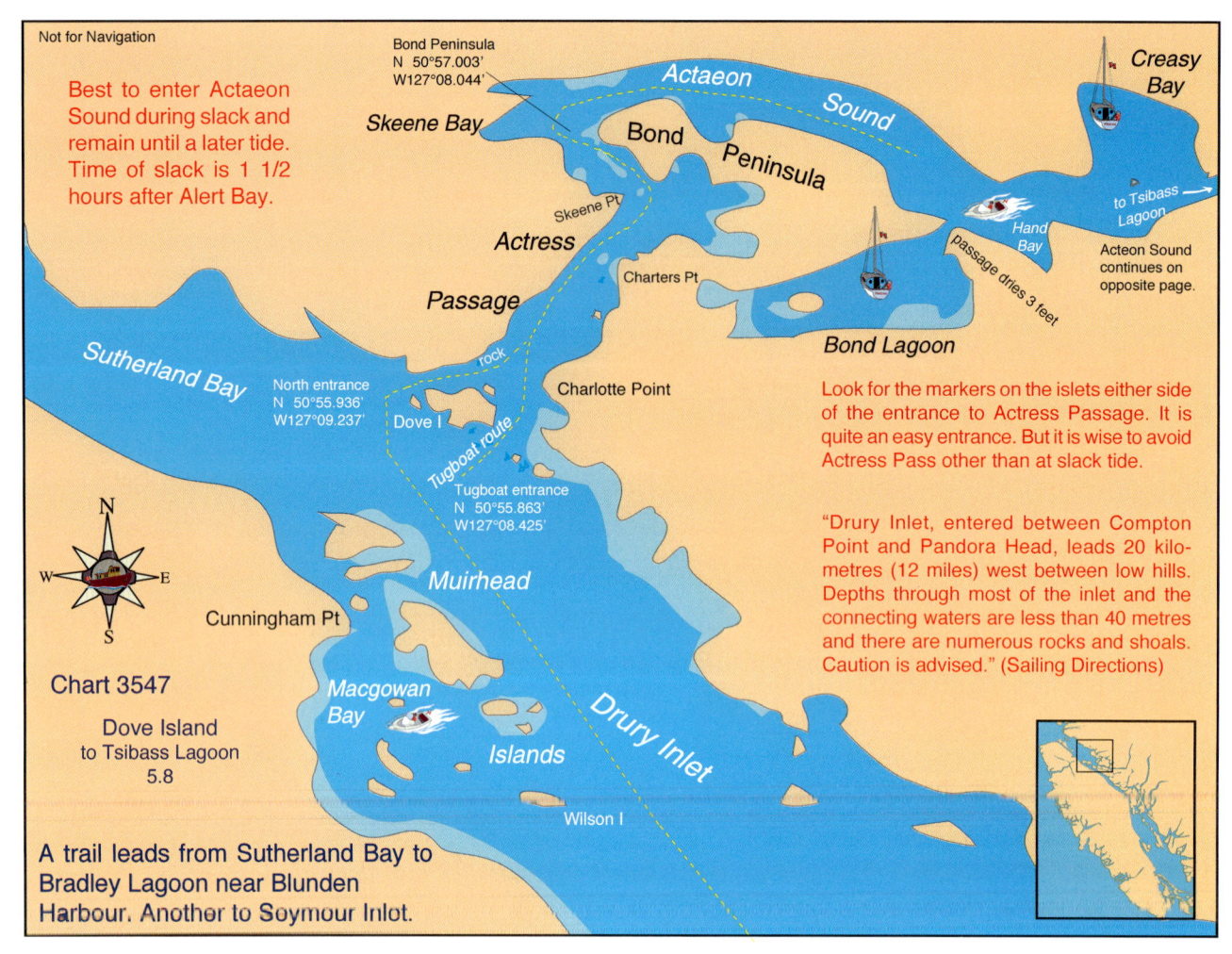

Not for Navigation

Best to enter Actaeon Sound during slack and remain until a later tide. Time of slack is 1 1/2 hours after Alert Bay.

Bond Peninsula N 50°57.003' W127°08.044'

Skeene Bay
Actaeon Sound
Creasy Bay
Bond Peninsula
Skeene Pt
Actress Passage
Charters Pt
to Tsibass Lagoon
Hand Bay
passage dries 3 feet
Acteon Sound continues on opposite page.
Bond Lagoon
Sutherland Bay
North entrance N 50°55.936' W127°09.237'
Dove I
rock
Charlotte Point
Tugboat route

Look for the markers on the islets either side of the entrance to Actress Passage. It is quite an easy entrance. But it is wise to avoid Actress Pass other than at slack tide.

Tugboat entrance N 50°55.863' W127°08.425'

Muirhead

Cunningham Pt

"Drury Inlet, entered between Compton Point and Pandora Head, leads 20 kilometres (12 miles) west between low hills. Depths through most of the inlet and the connecting waters are less than 40 metres and there are numerous rocks and shoals. Caution is advised." (Sailing Directions)

Chart 3547
Dove Island to Tsibass Lagoon 5.8

Macgowan Bay
Islands
Drury Inlet
Wilson I

A trail leads from Sutherland Bay to Bradley Lagoon near Blunden Harbour. Another to Seymour Inlet.

## Actaeon Sound  chart 3547

Actress Passage is for the careful, more adventurous exploring types who want to venture into Actaeon Sound. This involves some careful negotiation of tight waterways amid rocks and reefs at the north end of Actress Passage, off Bond Peninsula. Beyond that is almost 6 miles of inlet with open bays and an extremely narrow passage leading to **Tsibass Lagoon**. Take the dinghy with an outboard motor and explore. We went through Actress Passage at slack tide in our Monaro 27 powerboat. It was easier than expected but it was not long before the current picked up and we could see the potential for a troublesome ride, or a longer stay than planned.

The attraction is to conquer Actress Passage and find tranquility in Bond Lagoon. That is if you are up to its narrow, drying entrance. Read the *BC Sailing Directions* on the cautions associated with navigating into Actaeon Sound. They call for local knowledge when attempting the passage, and that speaks for itself.

Prior to my first visit, several mariners set me up for the inner workings of Actaeon Sound, stating that their best recalled experience was lying at anchor in Hand Bay for a short while, thereby avoiding the negotiation with mother nature to enter Bond Lagoon.

You can use the entrance to Actaeon Sound past the west side of Dove Island, being cautious of the rock shown on the chart just north of it. Veer to the east after passing Dove Island to avoid the rock.

Most skippers prefer to use the tugboat route on the east side of Dove Island off Charlotte Point, which is readily possible with some careful navigating. The entrance is east of Dove Island between two islets bearing markers.

Like any fast water it is best to travel through this waterway when the tides and currents are favourable. When passing between Charters Point and Skeene Point stay west of the rock in the centre of the passage. Then cross over towards the south point of the Bond Peninsula, navigating around to the north of the cluster of rocks and reefs that take up most of the channel. Follow the north shore after leaving Skeene Bay.

There are rocks in the narrower section of the passage. Markers along the way can be used for monitoring your passage. Use chart 3547 to navigate through the waterway.

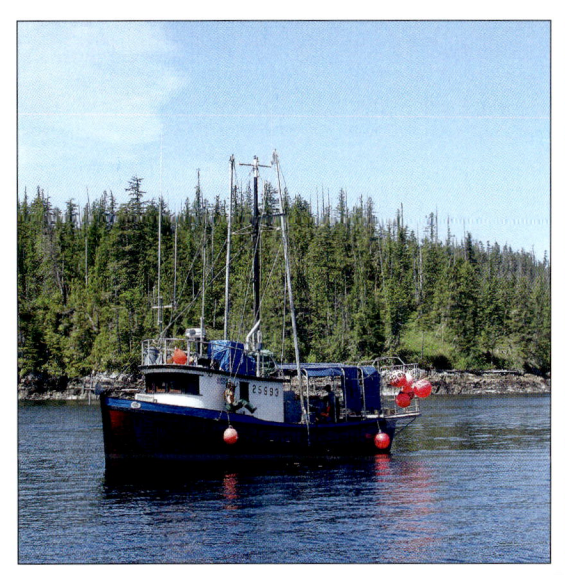

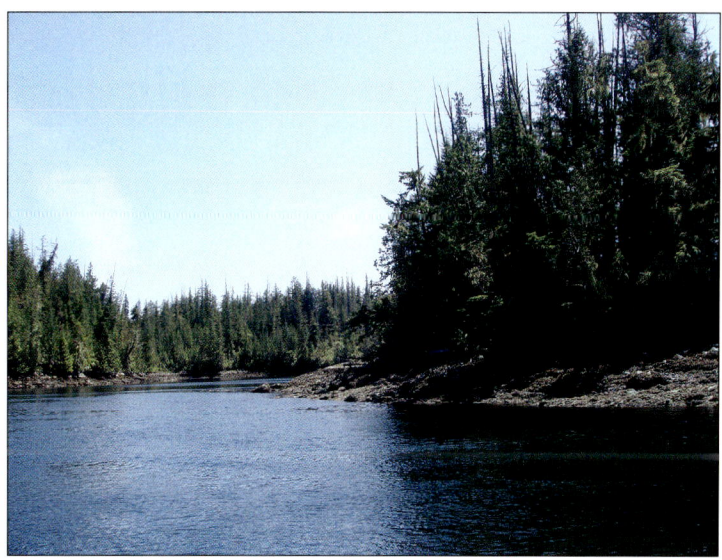

*Above left: A prawn boat checking traps at the entrance to Actress Passage in Drury Inlet. Above right: Behind Dove Island inside Actress Passage.*

**Bond Lagoon** is entered through a very narrow passage which dries one metre at low tide. You should have entered Actaeon Sound at high tide so entry to Bond Lagoon would be possible. Make your departure plans for high water if you plan to stay for any length of time. Anchorage is suitable anywhere in the deeper areas of the bay.

Mariners not wanting to be delayed in the lagoon can anchor at **Hand Bay.** There are other places to drop anchor in Actaeon Sound. Temporary anchorage may be taken in **Creasy Bay.** There is more secure overnight anchorage in 4 metres in the tiny unnamed cove protected by England Point. Creasy Bay was once a busy logging camp settlement and some remnants of pilings can still be found on the west shore against the beach.

## Tsibass Lagoon  chart 3547

Another protected anchorage is in the bay just before the narrow entrance to Tsibass Lagoon. This latter anchorage, just off a piece of First Nations land, is known to have good holding ground in easterly winds. The anchorages mentioned above are protected against winds from the west.

Tsibass Lagoon itself can be entered by smaller boats. There appears to be lots of good water inside the lagoon but the passage into it is too restricted to make it accessible for most boats. The entrance is about 30 metres long and a mere 7 metres wide at high water. At low tide it should not even be considered, unless you are exploring in a very small boat, preferably a runabout or dinghy.

After visiting Drury Inlet head south down Wells Passage for Queen Charlotte Strait and the run north along Labouchere Passage to Blunden Harbour, or spend some more time in the area, stopping at Tracey Harbour or Dickson Island.

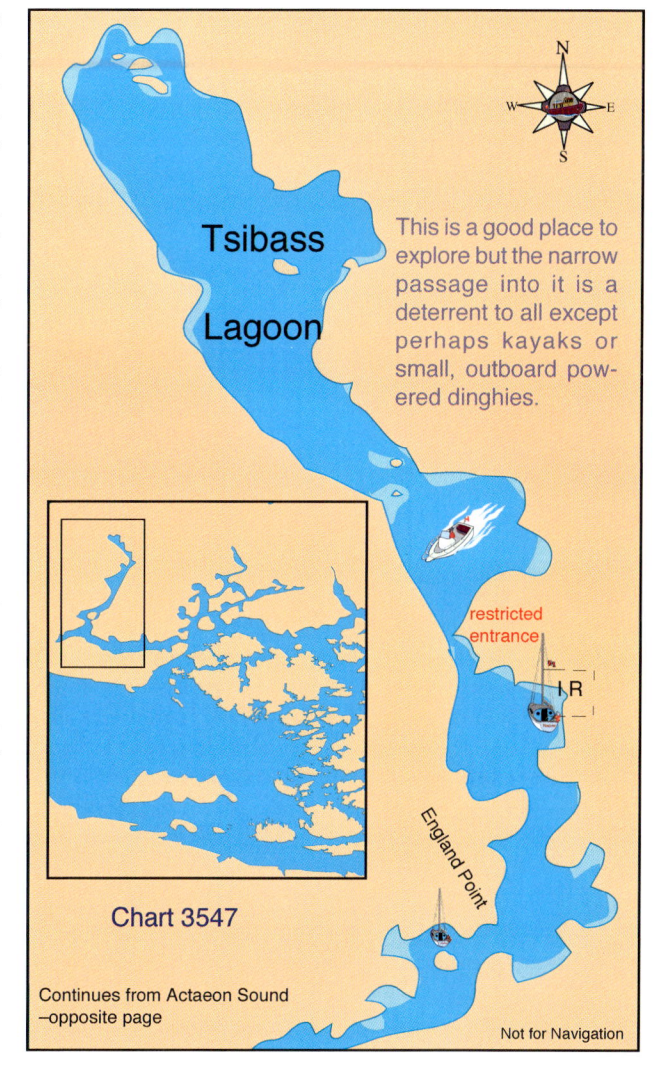

This is a good place to explore but the narrow passage into it is a deterrent to all except perhaps kayaks or small, outboard powered dinghies.

Chart 3547

Continues from Actaeon Sound —opposite page

Not for Navigation

183

# Wells Passage to Allison Harbour

## Leaving the Broughtons northbound

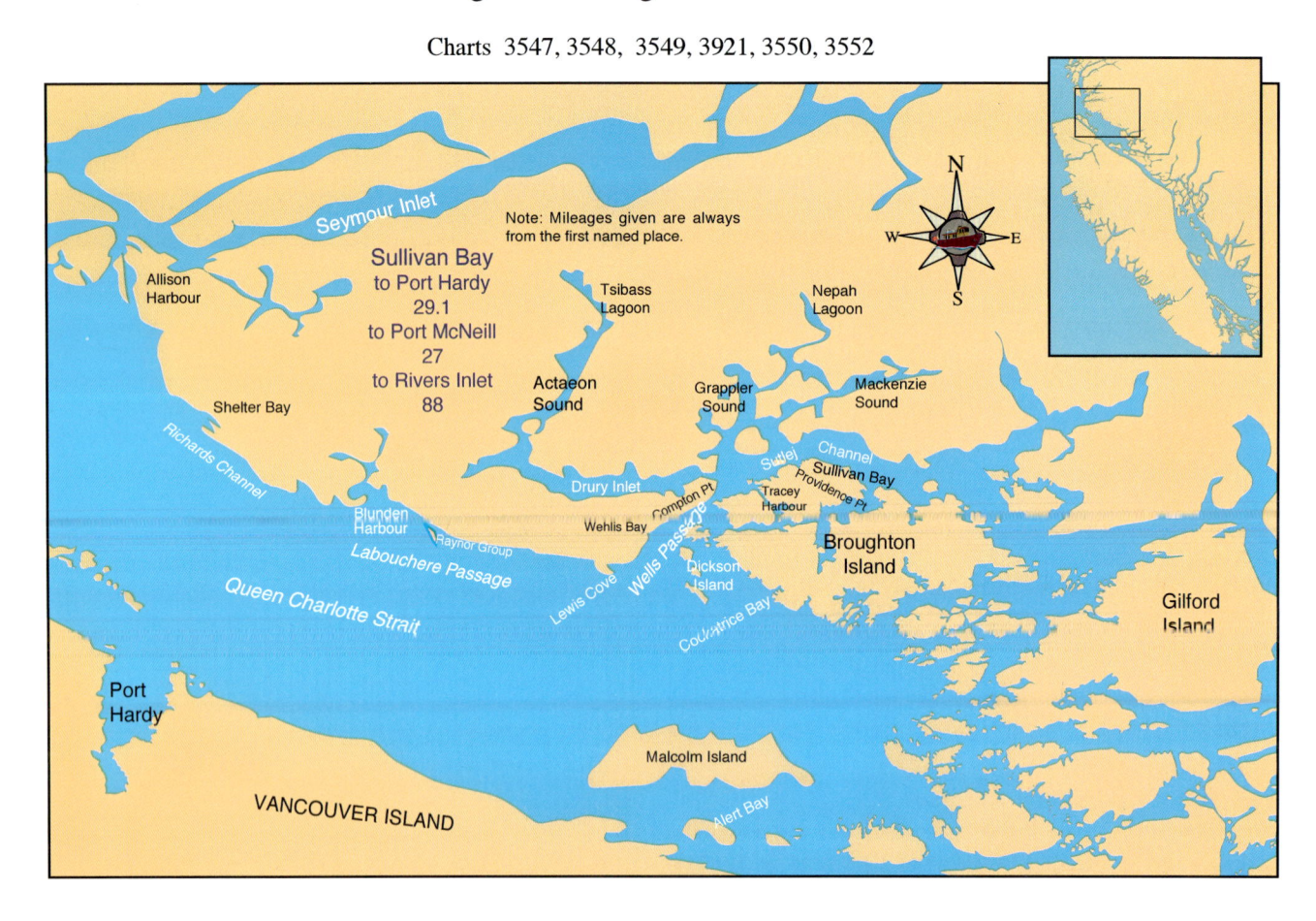

Charts 3547, 3548, 3549, 3921, 3550, 3552

Leaving the security of Dickson Island or Wells Passage en route to either Blunden Harbour or Allison Harbour and to Seymour Inlet and other ports off Queen Charlotte Strait, it is imperative that you check the wind conditions first. Strong westerly or northwesterly winds blowing in the strait can be most uncomfortable, even for salty sailors. Rolling swells often come down from Cape Caution and funnel through Richards Channel, and windy conditions pick up the seas again in the open waters of Labouchere Passage. We have passed across the lower portion of Queen Charlotte Strait in silky calm conditions at times, and stayed put in Wells Passage at others, due to stormy seas in the strait.

It is about 10 nautical miles from Wells Passage using La Bouchere Passage to Blunden Harbour, and about 18 beyond that to Allison Harbour. The route is along the east shore and past the Raynor Group of islands.

Fom Sullivan Bay, when you pass between Providence Point and Compton Point leaving Sutlej Channel or Grappler Sound you enter Wells Passage. The distance to Boyles Point where you enter Queen Charlotte Strait at Labouchere Passage is about 6 miles. In that stretch you have the option of continuing on the way to Blunden Harbour and Allison Harbour, perhaps, or taking shelter in one of several anchorages if the weather dictates you do so. The currents run to three knots in Wells Passage, with the effect of them strongest at the entrance to Gappler Sound.

184

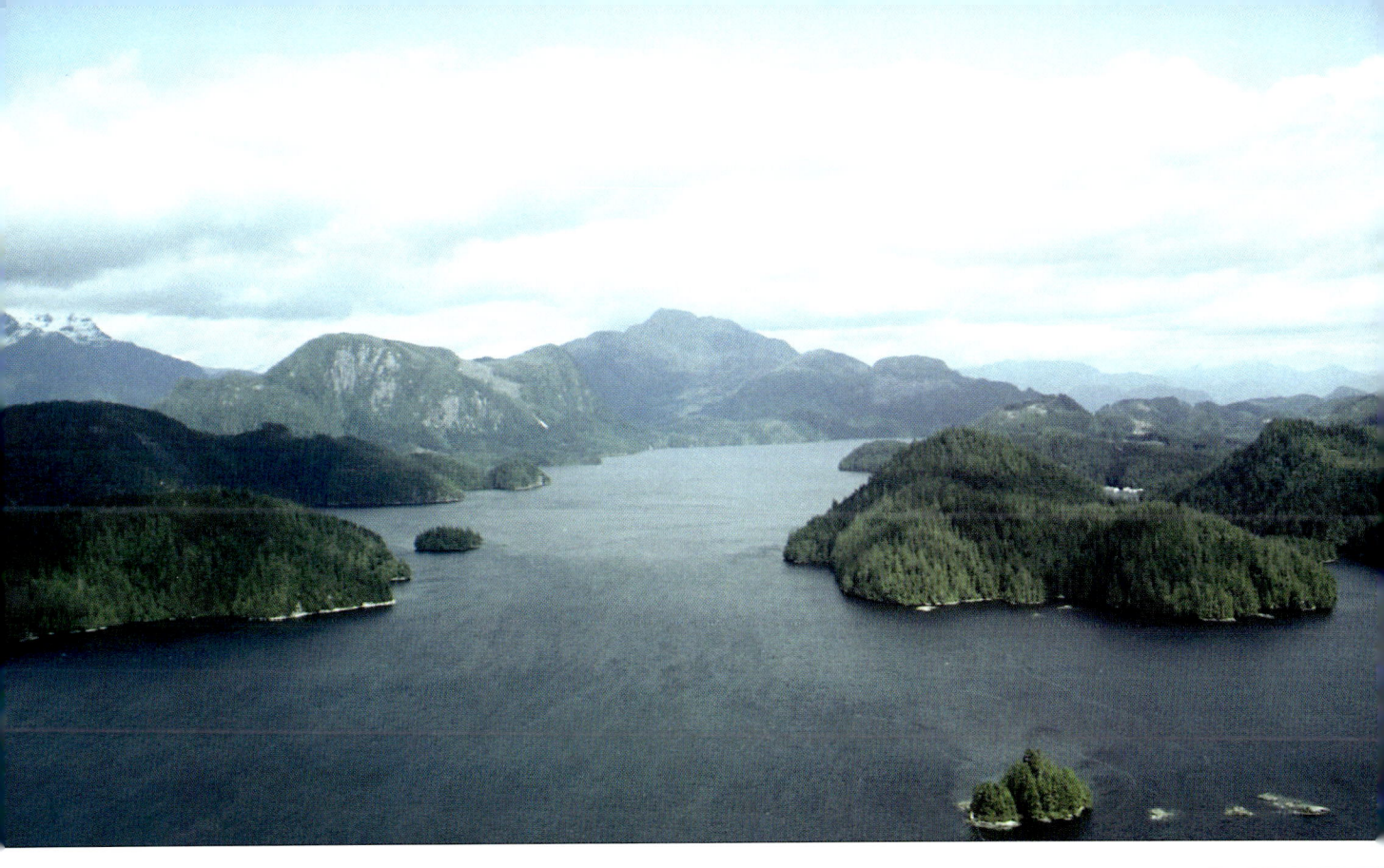

If you are venturing out into Queen Charlotte Strait you may feel the first signs of ocean swells that make their way up Wells Passage when winds are up. Pass by Wehlis Bay on the west side of Wells Passage, as it cannot provide shelter in any but the calmest conditions.

The first and largest harbour after Sullivan Bay is **Tracey Harbour** with its sheltered **Napier Bay** deep inside (see page 186). This inlet cuts into the southwest side of North Broughton Island with its entrance just south of Lambert Island and before Carter Passage. Star Rock on the north side of Tracey Harbour is to be considered if you follow its north shore. It is best to remain in the centre of the passage. Pass Wolf Cove and find temporary anchorage in **Freshwater Cove** or continue into the deeper reaches of Napier Bay.

Some mariners intent on continuing north choose to avoid the slightly out-of-the-way extra distance to an anchorage inside Napier Bay. They do this by taking shelter in Dickson Island's small bay at the entrance to Carter Passage, or even in the protection of that passage.

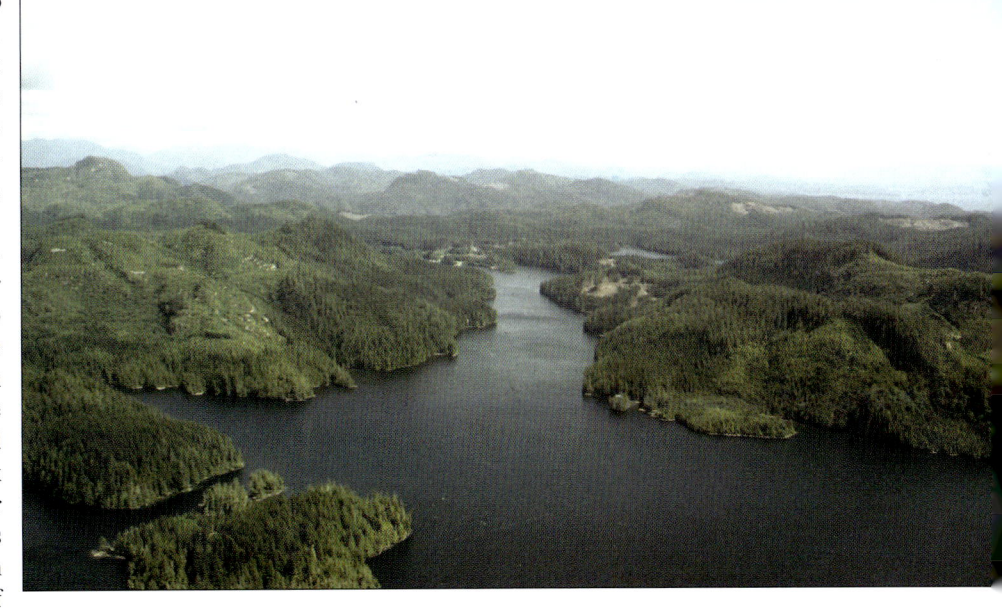

*Above: Tracey Harbour entrance with Lambert Island at left in the foregound. Napier Bay is at the east end of this narrow harbour.*

*Top: The north end of Wells Passage looking east, with Atkinson Island at the right serving as a breakwater to Sullivan Bay.*

185

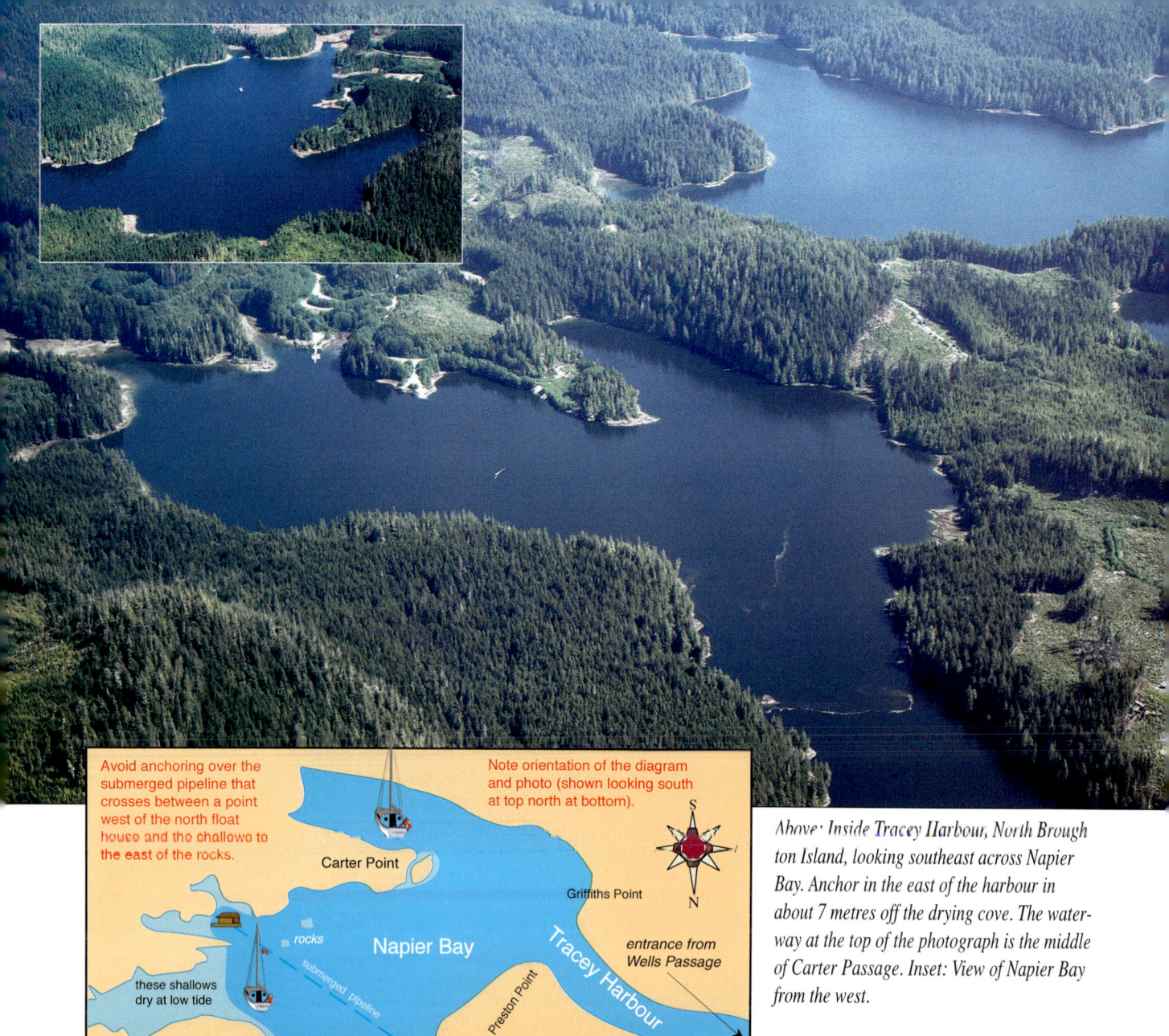

*Above: Inside Tracey Harbour, North Broughton Island, looking southeast across Napier Bay. Anchor in the east of the harbour in about 7 metres off the drying cove. The waterway at the top of the photograph is the middle of Carter Passage. Inset: View of Napier Bay from the west.*

- Avoid anchoring over the submerged pipeline that crosses between a point west of the north float house and the shallows to the east of the rocks.
- Note orientation of the diagram and photo (shown looking south at top north at bottom).
- Carter Point
- Griffiths Point
- rocks
- Napier Bay
- submerged pipeline
- these shallows dry at low tide
- Preston Point
- Tracey Harbour
- entrance from Wells Passage
- float houses
- North Broughton Island
- Freshwater Cove
- Chart 3547

## Tracey Harbour  chart 3547

Travel through Tracey Harbour into **Napier Bay**. There is good anchorage in the large basin at the east end just off a large drying flat.

A mud bottom and five fathoms of water make for good holding. There is also a small nook beyond Carter Point, which is preferred for a truly quiet anchorage. This is a good place to stop and spend time if you are waiting for good weather conditions before venturing into Queen Charlotte Strait.

Winds generally do not disturb the anchorage in Napier Bay, particularly in the shelter of Carter Point. However, this anchorage is not as sheltered as the one deeper inside the bay.

Watch for the rocks beyond the point, Several float homes are moored around the bay. These are private and should be respected as such.

A submerged pipeline runs across the bay near the head of the harbour, but it is possible to drop anchor well beyond it, off the drying ledge of the easternmost cove.

Some logging activity in the adjacent and nearby forest can be noisy at times. Anchoring in an area where logging is in progress can be disruptive. It can also be interesting, especially if you get to watch some heli-logging

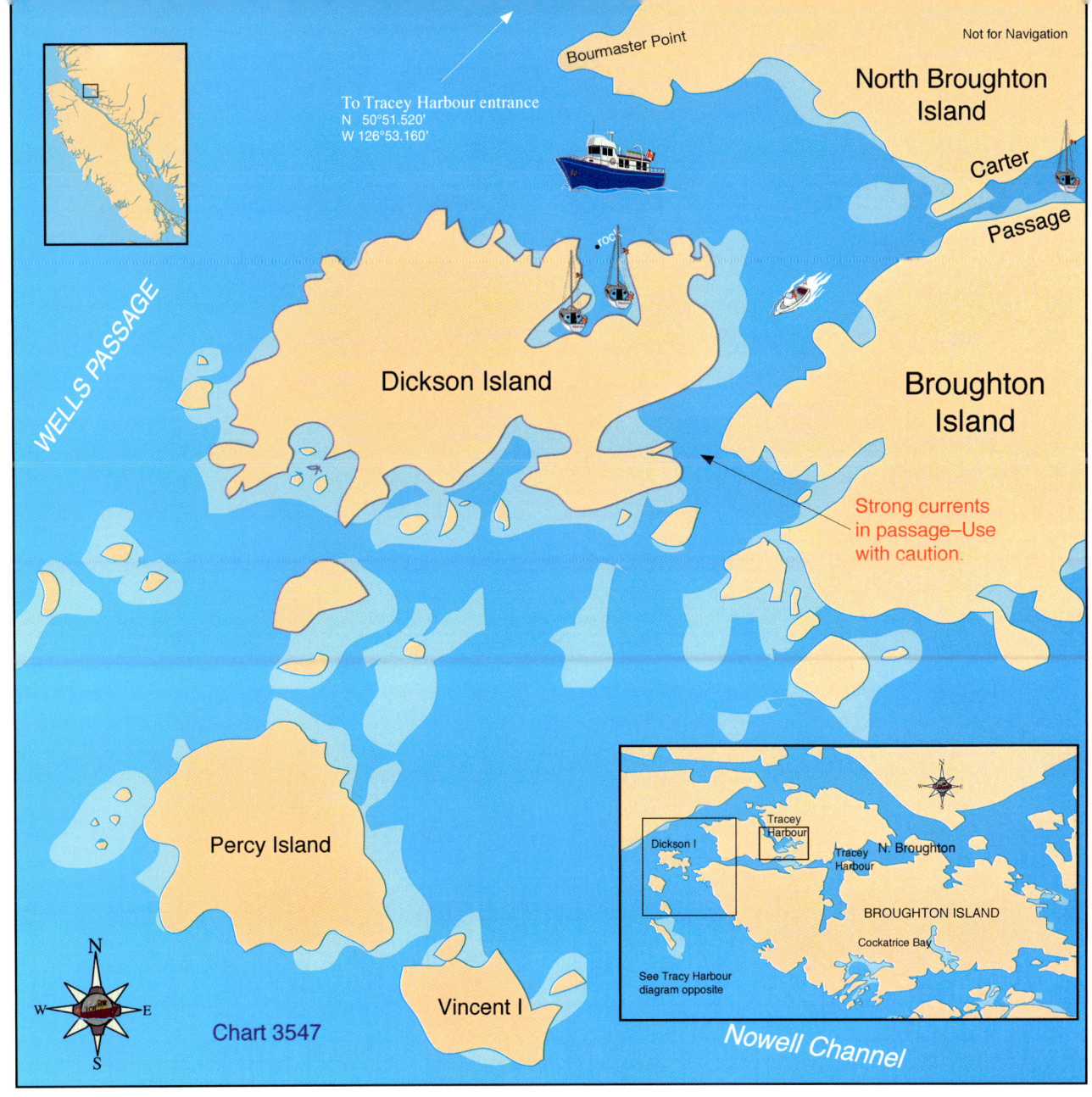

## Dickson Island chart 3547

Time your trip down Wells Passage from Sullivan Bay half an hour after Alert Bay tides as you do need to consider the three knot current caused by the tidal change. This current affects slow craft navigating around Dickson Island.

Dickson Island is a popular anchorage while awaiting suitable weather for departure to the open waters of Queen Charlotte Strait, crossing to Port Hardy and Port McNeill, or heading out to northerly destinations such as Blunden Harbour, Allison Harbour and Cape Caution to Rivers Inlet.

*Napier Bay in Tracey Harbour. The best anchorage is close to the drying ledge to the left of Carter Point. Stay clear of the submerged pipeline (see diagram opposite page).*

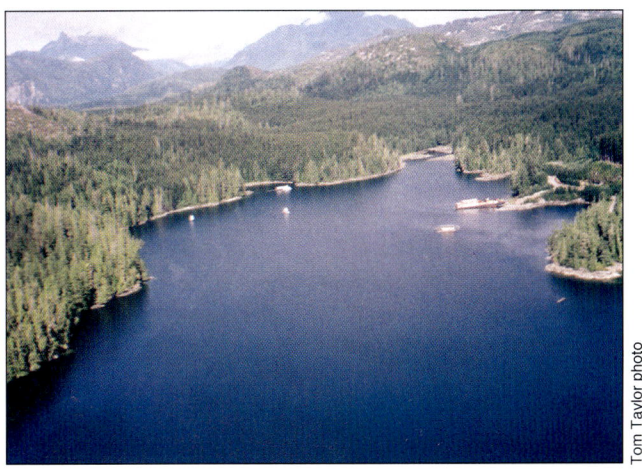

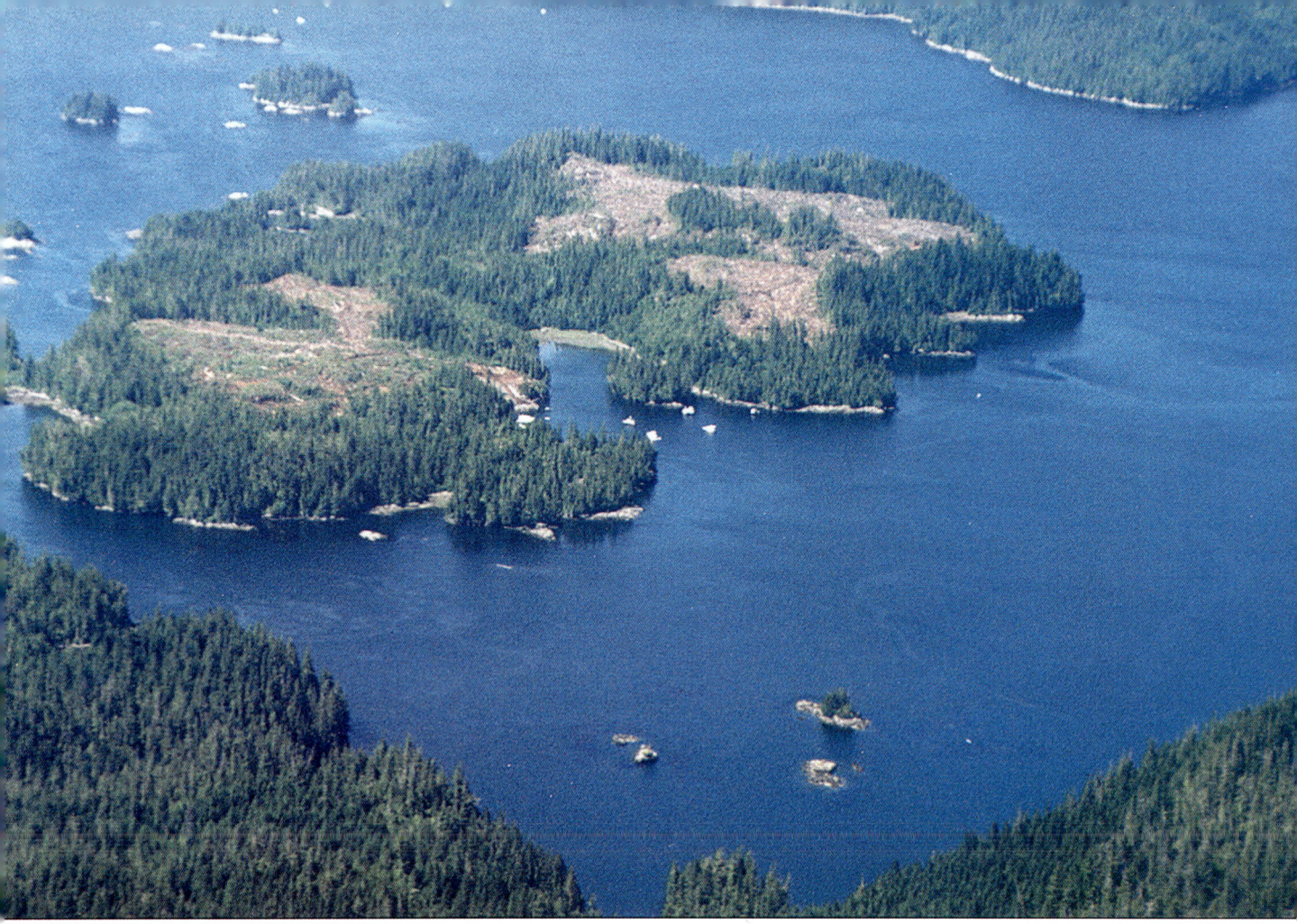

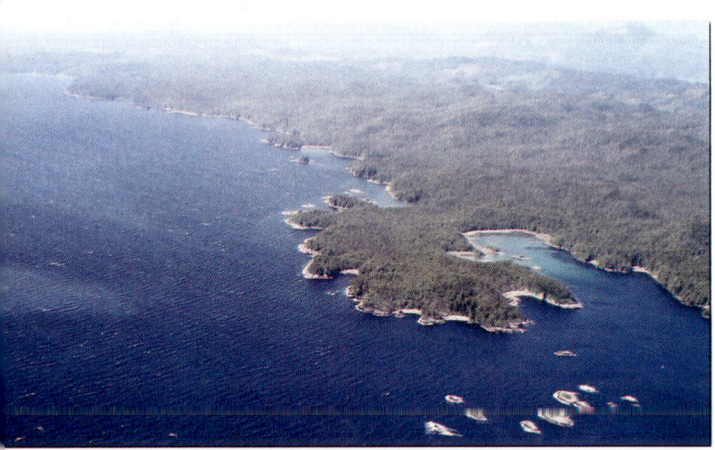

*Top: Dickson Island, like Sullivan Bay or Napier Bay, makes a good place to wait for suitable weather conditions in Queen Charlotte Strait. Above: Lewis Cove and Lewis Rocks (see also diagram opposite page) with the shore extending beyond towards Blunden Harbour. Duck into this cove if sea conditions prove unsuitable to continue after leaving the comfort of Wells Passage. Shelter here is only suitable as protection against westerly or northwesterly winds. Be very mindful of the rocks off the entrance.*

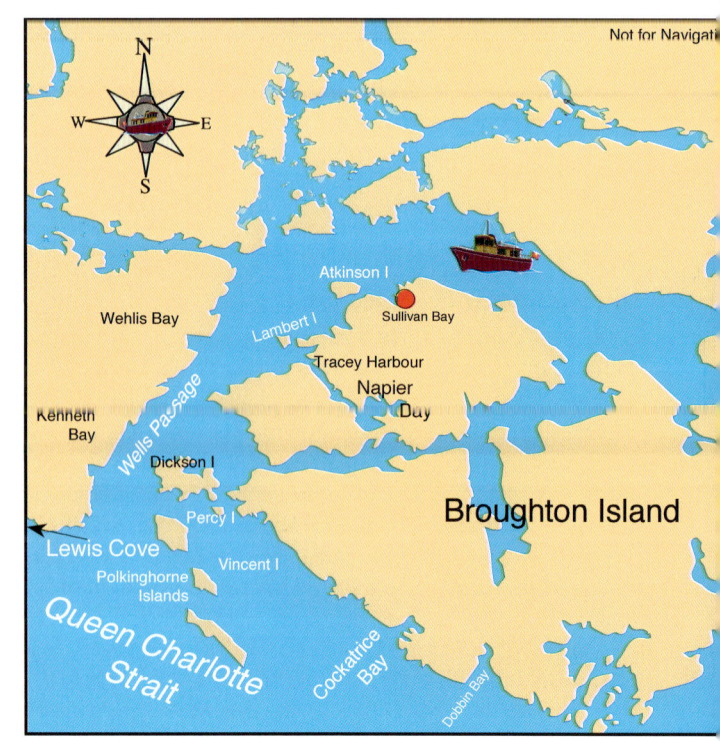

188

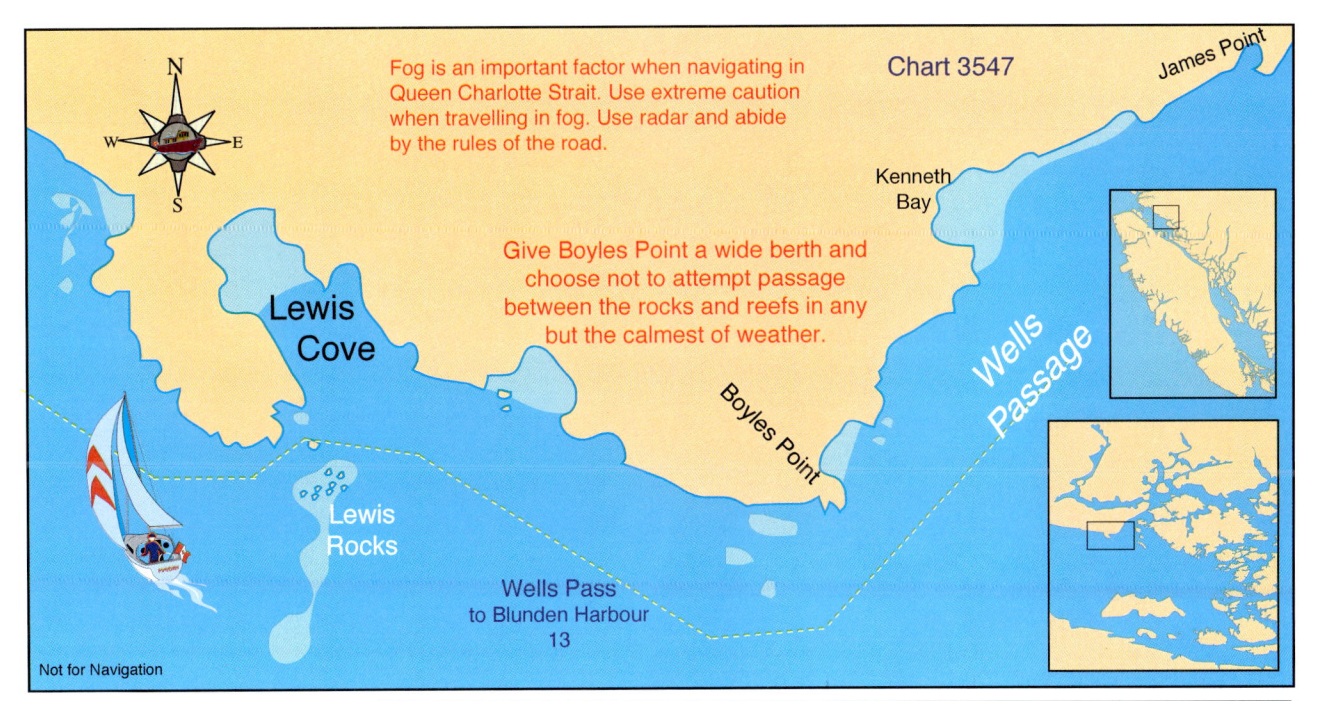

*Right: Calm conditions along the southwest side of Broughton Island on the outside of Wells Passage. In the distance are the Polkinghorne Islands beyond Cockatrice Bay. Dobbin Bay is just beyond the two islets. The photo was taken from above the entance to Fife Sound just west of Booker Lagoon. When it is like this in Queen Charlotte Strait, powering to Alert Bay, Port Hardy or Cape Caution is easy. But don't dally–weather can change quickly in these regions.*

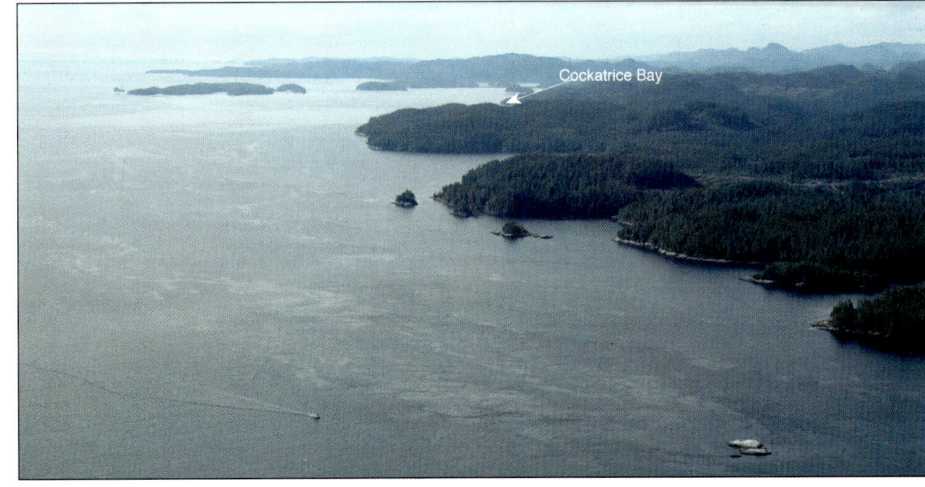

## Lewis Cove  chart 3547

Lewis Rocks afford protection from some westerly or northwesterly winds when navigating past Lewis Cove. If conditions are such that you need to take this sheltered route it is probably best to have stayed in Wells Pass in the first place. If you are caught in rising winds and rough seas in the strait, and are brave enough to venture to the inside of Lewis Rocks, you may find reduced wave action on the approaches to Wells Passage. You may choose to turn into Lewis Cove and wait for calmer conditions. However it is not recommended that you remain there overnight as it is useful only as a temporary stop. The best place to drop anchor is off the steep bluff at the west side of the cove. Mind the rock in the middle and the low rock off the point between the cove and Lewis Rocks. Passage is best to the west of that rock.

On the south shore of Broughton Island, just off Nowell Channel in Queen Charlotte Strait, **Cockatrice Bay** is exposed to the northwest winds, and the open waters of Queen Charlotte Strait. If you do stop here, once inside its inner basin you will find good shelter from most conditions. The anchorage is shallow and preferred by owners of small boats. Bypass this bay if you are looking for secure overnight anchorage. Entering it during rough conditions in the strait is a challenge and can be unnerving.

Cockatrice Bay is also the last resting place of the former luxury yacht *Maid of Orleans*. It once served the rum running trade before ending up on the Sunshine Coast as a barge, as did so many former beautiful sailing vessels, and then was moved to the Broughtons.

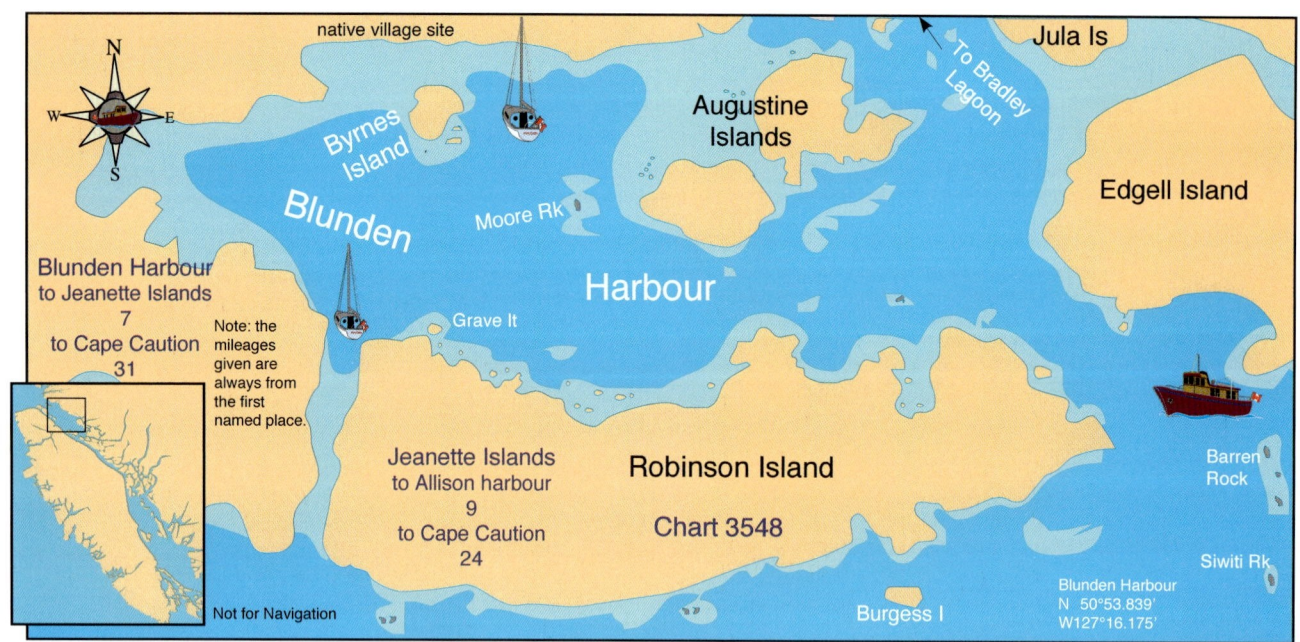

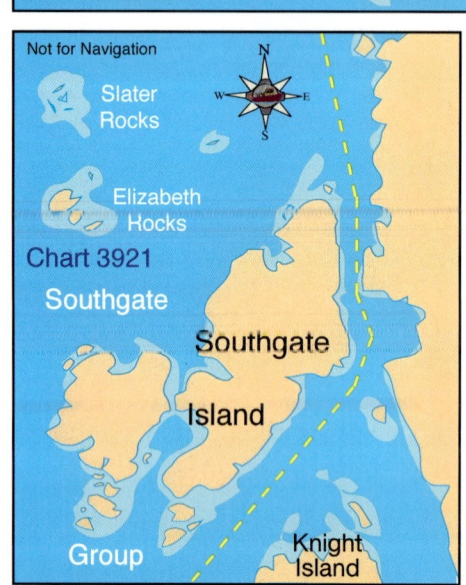

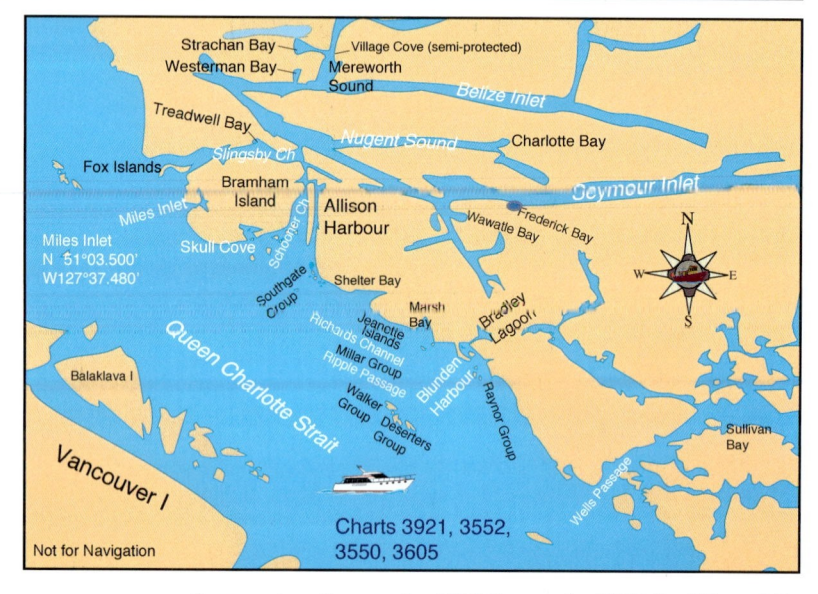

## Blunden Harbour chart 3458.

Entrance to Blunden Harbour is guarded by Siwiti Rock, and just beyond is Barren Rock and an adjoining reef. Pass Barren Rock to port (leaving the unnamed rocks and reef to starboard) and head for safe anchorage behind Moore Rock in the westernmost bay. A white sandy beach lies off the Augustine Islands and an old First Nations village north of the anchorage. Some years ago we went ashore very carefully on the opposite side of the basin at Grave Islet and found burial boxes in the trees. Bradley Lagoon opens from the northeast of the anchorage and can be explored in a small dinghy. A tidal falls that dries about 3 metres will keep you from entering at anything but a large high tide.

Blunden Harbour was named by Captain Pender in charge of surveying the area by HM Beaver in 1863 for Edward R. Blunden a master's assistant aboard HM Hecate.

When leaving Blunden Harbour northbound it is necessary to head out into the open waters of Queen Charlotte Strait. Follow a course around and staying well clear of the Browning Islands to avoid the rock off the south end. Then proceed up Richards Channel keeping offshore of the Jeanette Islands. It was at the Millar Group that Captain Vancouver ran aground in 1792. If you decide to venture through the passages between the islands and islets along this exposed coastline, be mindful of the tides and currents. The tidal current runs quite strongly through the Jeanette Islands. I have chosen to cruise by on the west side most times in the past, but the route through the islands is not difficult in calm conditions.

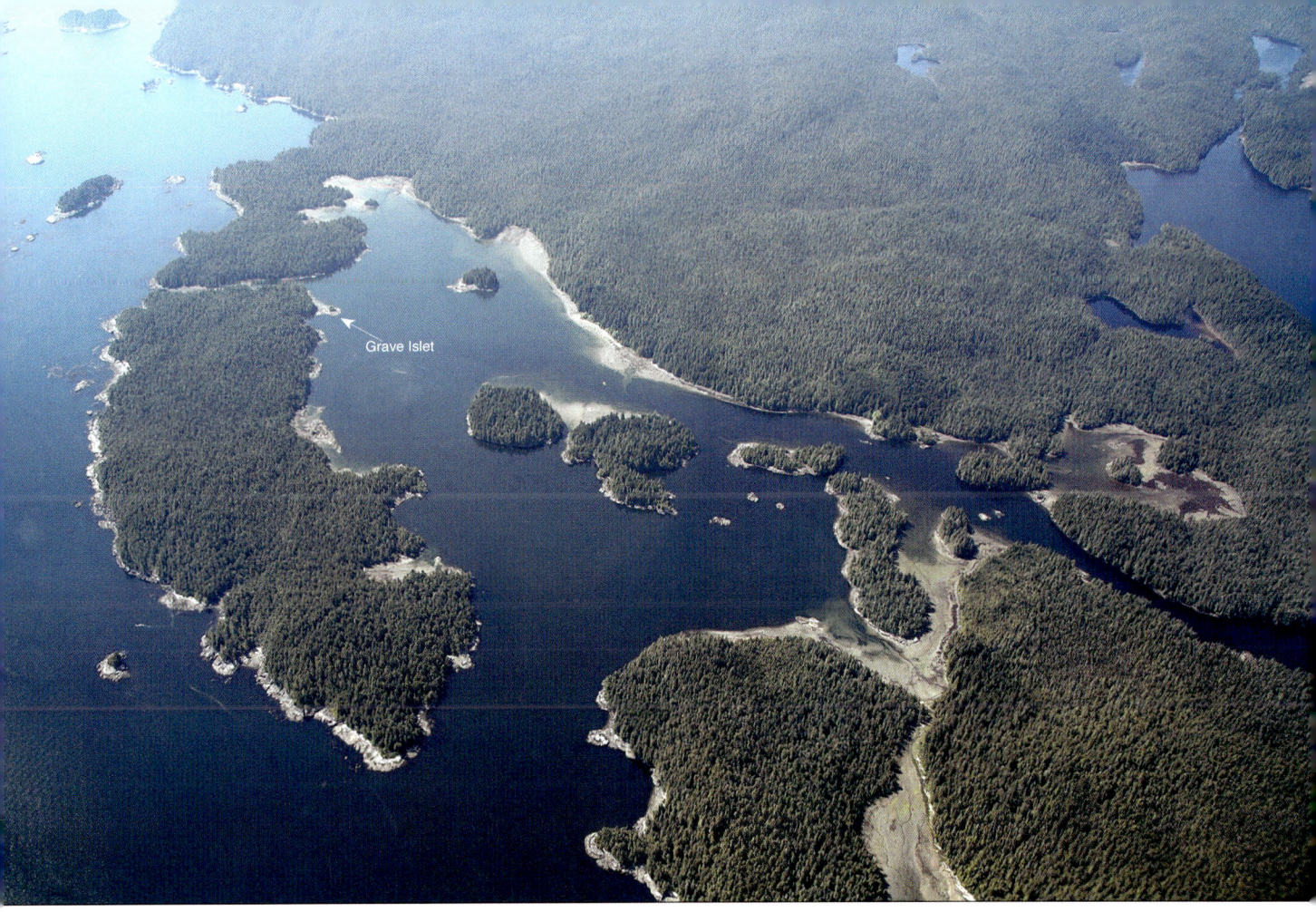

*Above: Blunden Harbour. The tiny Grave Islet close to the east side of Robinson Island was a native burial site. At one time it contained burial boxes in the trees. It is a sacred place that should be respected. Below: The Southgate Group near the entrance to Allison Harbour makes for scenic viewing. The passage between the group and the mainland may be used to access Allison Harbour from the south.*

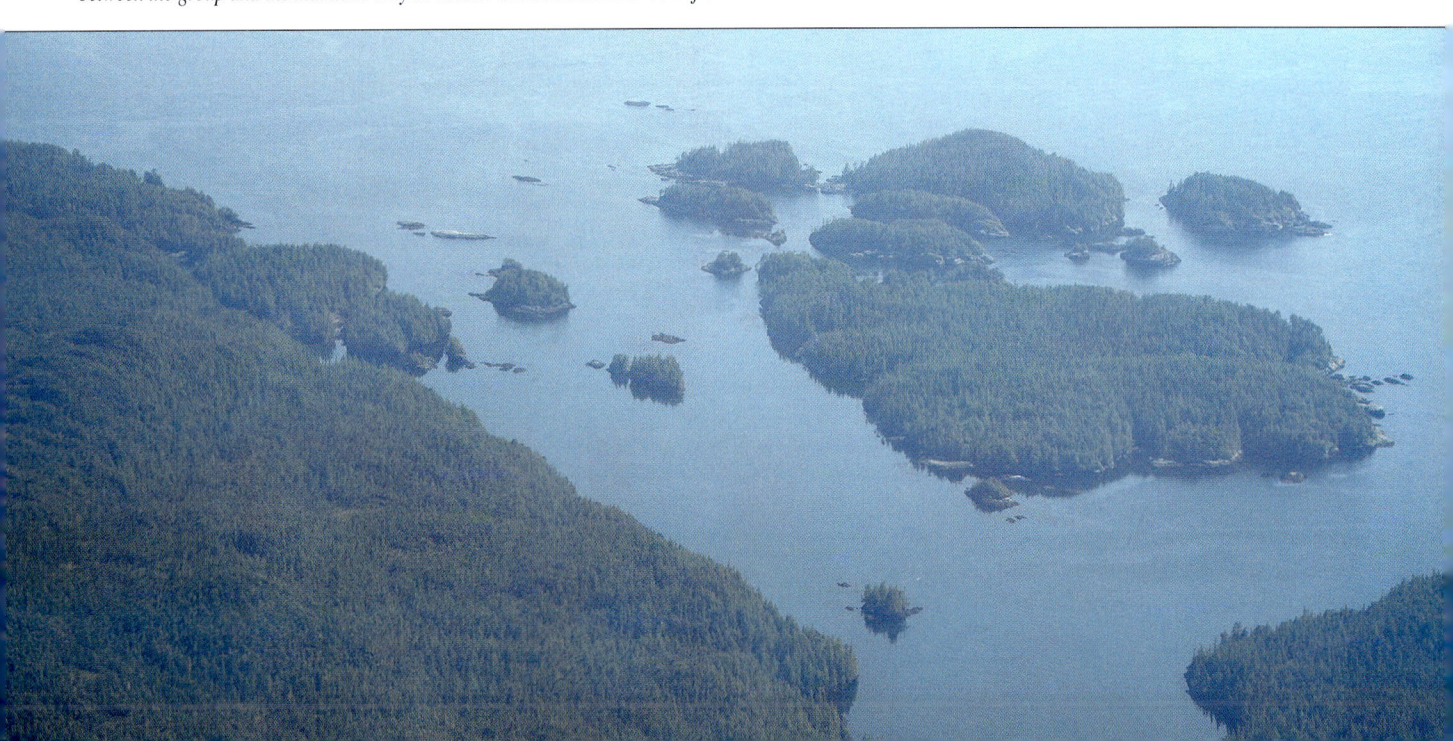

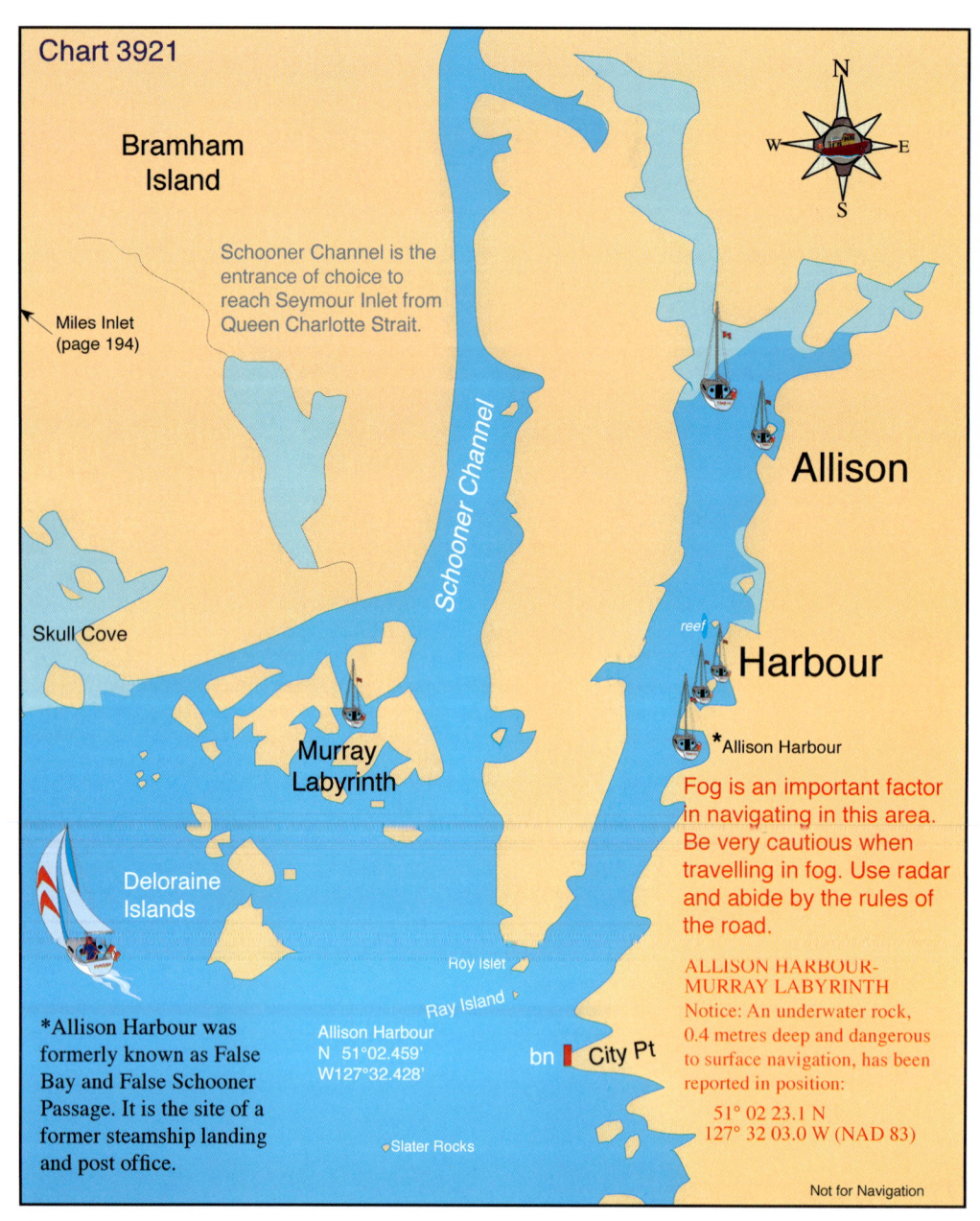

## Map Chart 3921

**Bramham Island**

Miles Inlet (page 194)

Schooner Channel is the entrance of choice to reach Seymour Inlet from Queen Charlotte Strait.

Schooner Channel

Skull Cove

Murray Labyrinth

Deloraine Islands

*Allison Harbour was formerly known as False Bay and False Schooner Passage. It is the site of a former steamship landing and post office.

Hoy Islet
Ray Island
Allison Harbour
N 51°02.459'
W127°32.428'

bn — City Pt

Slater Rocks

Allison Harbour

reef
*Allison Harbour

**Fog is an important factor in navigating in this area. Be very cautious when travelling in fog. Use radar and abide by the rules of the road.**

**ALLISON HARBOUR–MURRAY LABYRINTH** Notice: An underwater rock, 0.4 metres deep and dangerous to surface navigation, has been reported in position:
51° 02 23.1 N
127° 32 03.0 W (NAD 83)

Not for Navigation

---

Look for calm weather when travelling along the coast from Wells Passage to Allison Harbour and enjoy the gentle rise and fall of the swells.
Avoid trying to navigate rock-strewn waterways especially when the seas are rough. Give preference to Schooner Channel over Slingsby Channel to gain entry to Seymour Inlet.

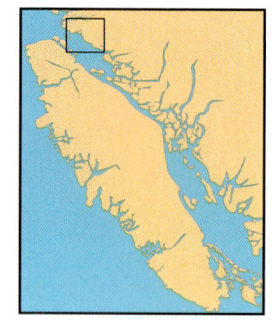

*Opposite top: The Jeanette Islands with Stuart Point and Marsh Bay showing at right. Opposite bottom: Allison Harbour and Schooner Channel with the Murray Labyrinth lower left. Use Schooner Channel with caution when entering Seymour Inlet. Refer to large scale chart 3921. Inset: Allison Harbour with the Murray Labyrinth and Deloraine Islands in the foreground.*

---

## Allison Harbour  charts 3921, 3550, 3552.

If you want to stop between Blunden Harbour and Allison Harbour try **Marsh Bay** or **Shelter Bay**, which afford temporary anchorage in fair weather. I prefer to run all the way to Allison Harbour, making passage around the Southgate Group or through the narrow gap dividing them from the mainland shore. This passage is accessed around the west and north of Knight Island. The alternative is to use Harris Island as a reference point and travel around the Southgate Islands to the north using charts 3550 and 3921.

Beyond Allison Harbour there is **Skull Cove** on the south side of Bramham Island. It can be reached by passing through a channel between the **Murray Labyrinth** and the **Deloraine Islands**. It is not recommended as an anchorage unless the weather is very settled. There is a sheltered anchorage in the midst of the islands of Murray Labyrinth and a temporary one just north of the east side of the Deloraine Islands.

Continuing north around the outside of Bramham Island takes you to a favourite anchorage at **Miles Inlet**. This fairly large but narrow inlet opens off the exposed waters of Queen Charlotte Strait two miles to the west of Skull Cove. Anchor at the junction of the T-shaped bay in about 6 metres.

If you travel up the east side of Bramham Island you will use Schooner Channel to reach the Nakwakto Rapids and the entrance to Seymour Inlet. This is the recommended route into Seymour Inlet, particularly when travelling from the south.

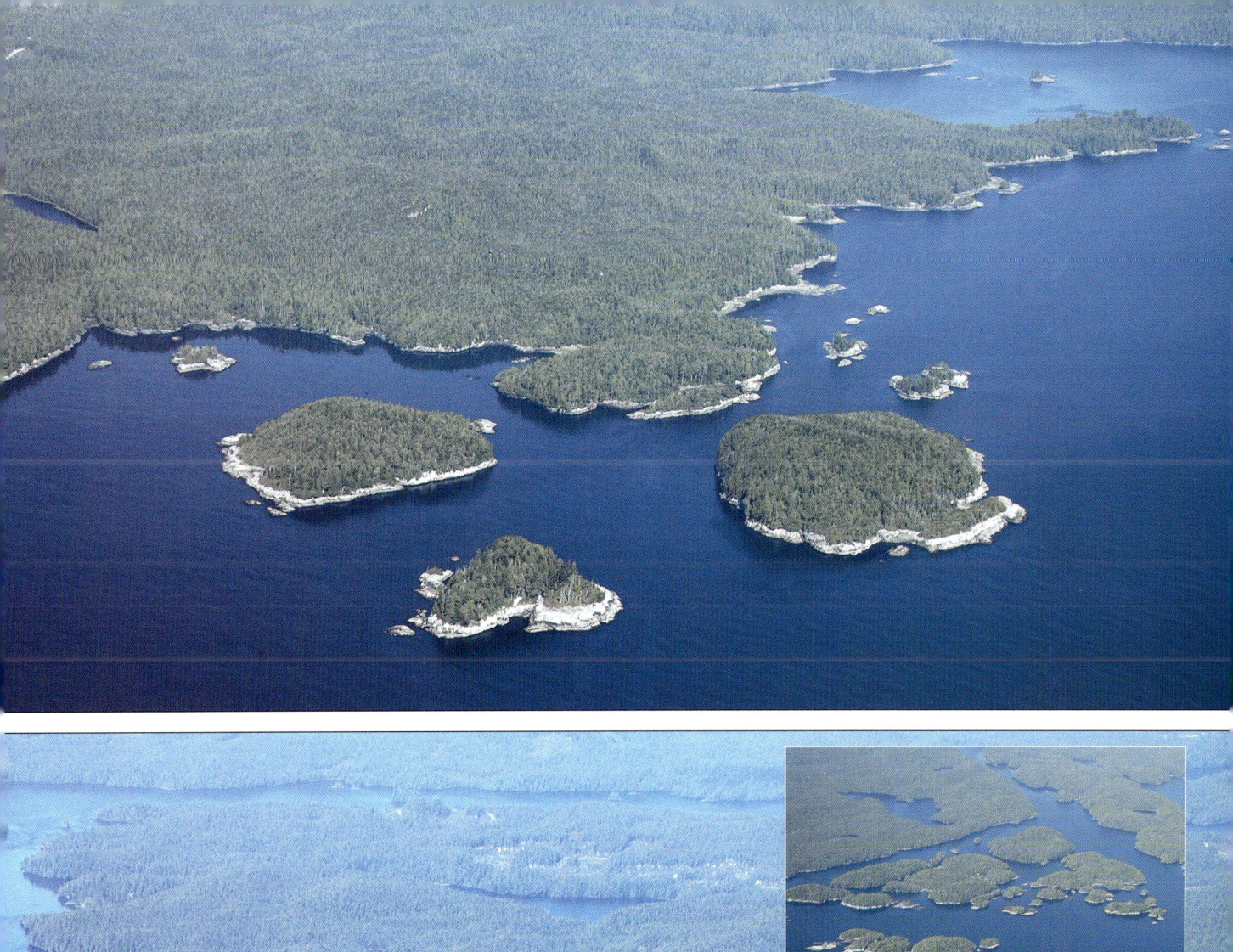

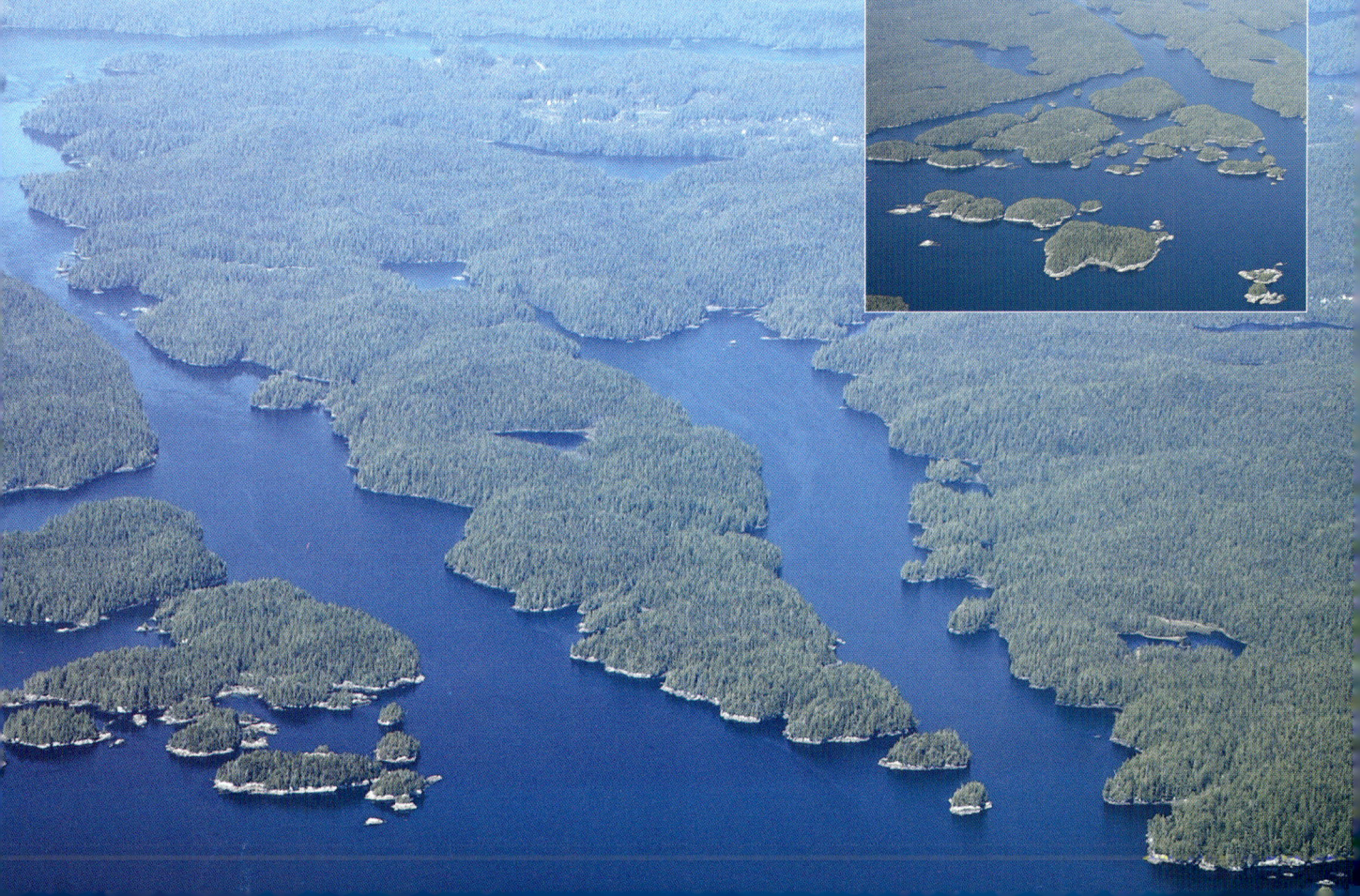

# Seymour Inlet

## Through the Nakwakto Rapids
## with David Hoar and Noreen Rudd

Charts 3552, 3550, 3921, 3605

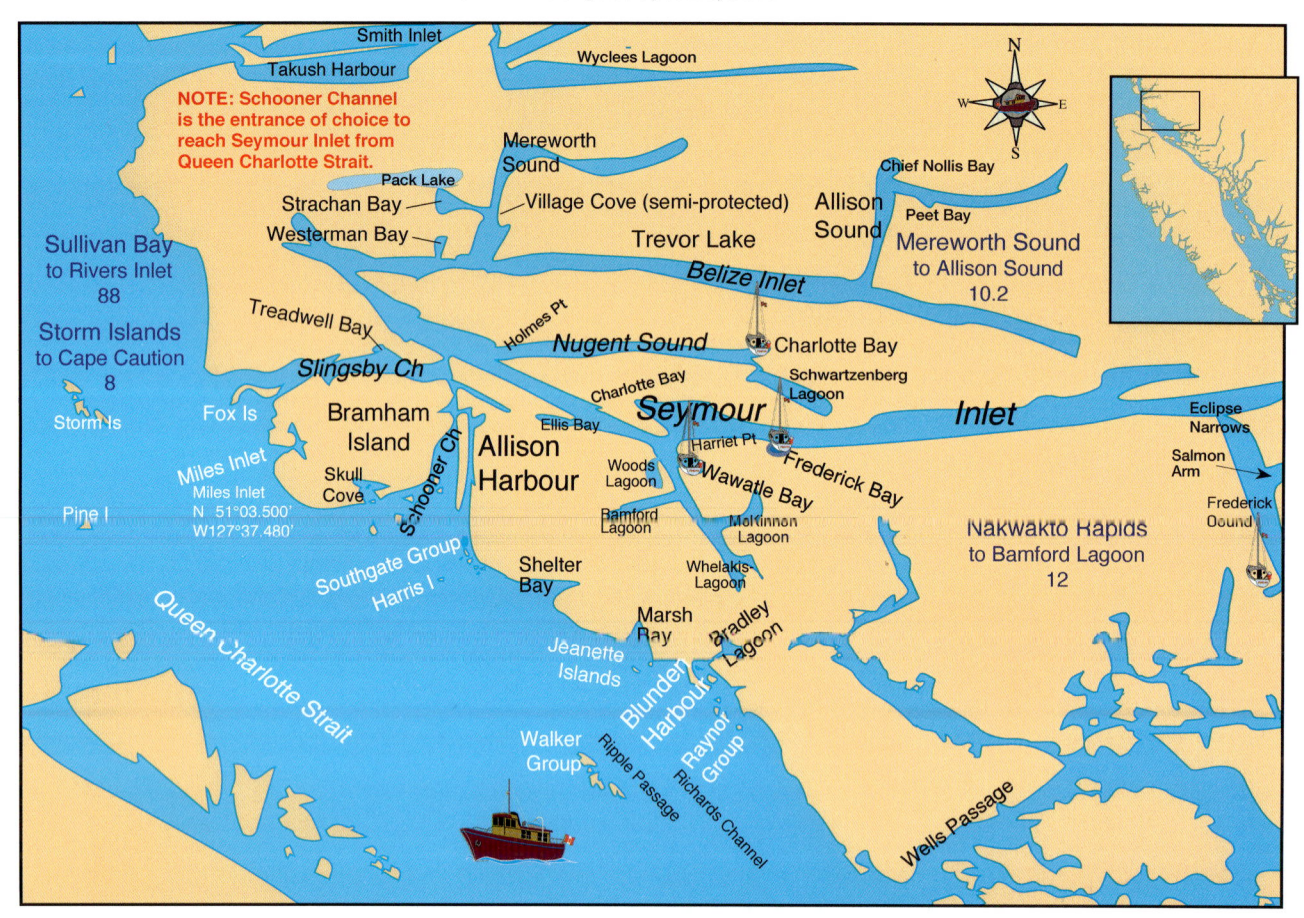

### Seymour Inlet chart 3550, 3552

Entering Seymour Inlet by way of Slingsby Channel requires passing the Fox Islands and dealing with turbulence during the ebb against the westerly swell. Currents run at 10 knots and mariners are advised to avoid Slingsby Channel in adverse weather. The Fox Islands do not offer any sheltered anchorage. Continuing beyond Treadwell Bay you are faced with the renowned Nakwakto Rapids currents which can run in excess of 16 knots. Use Nakwakto only at completely slack tide. Anchorage can be taken at the north end of Schooner Channel or at Treadwell Bay while awaiting transit.

**Treadwell Bay** is the anchorage of choice when waiting for the right conditions at Nakwakto Rapids or for good weather in Queen Charlotte Strait. The bay lies in the lee of Anchor Islands and provides secure anchorage.

Seymour Inlet opens beyond Nakwakto Rapids into 90 nautical miles of waterways that reach almost to Wakeman Sound and fall only a little short of connecting with Drury Inlet, Actaeon Sound (Tsibass Lagoon) and Nepah Lagoon.

It is vital that mariners follow the cautions of the Hydrographic Service charts when entering Seymour Inlet. The currents through Nakwakto Rapids are every bit as dangerous as they are said to be. Eddies and whirlpools, overfalls and foaming seas will overwhelm the sturdiest of small to medium boats and certainly present severe problems for larger

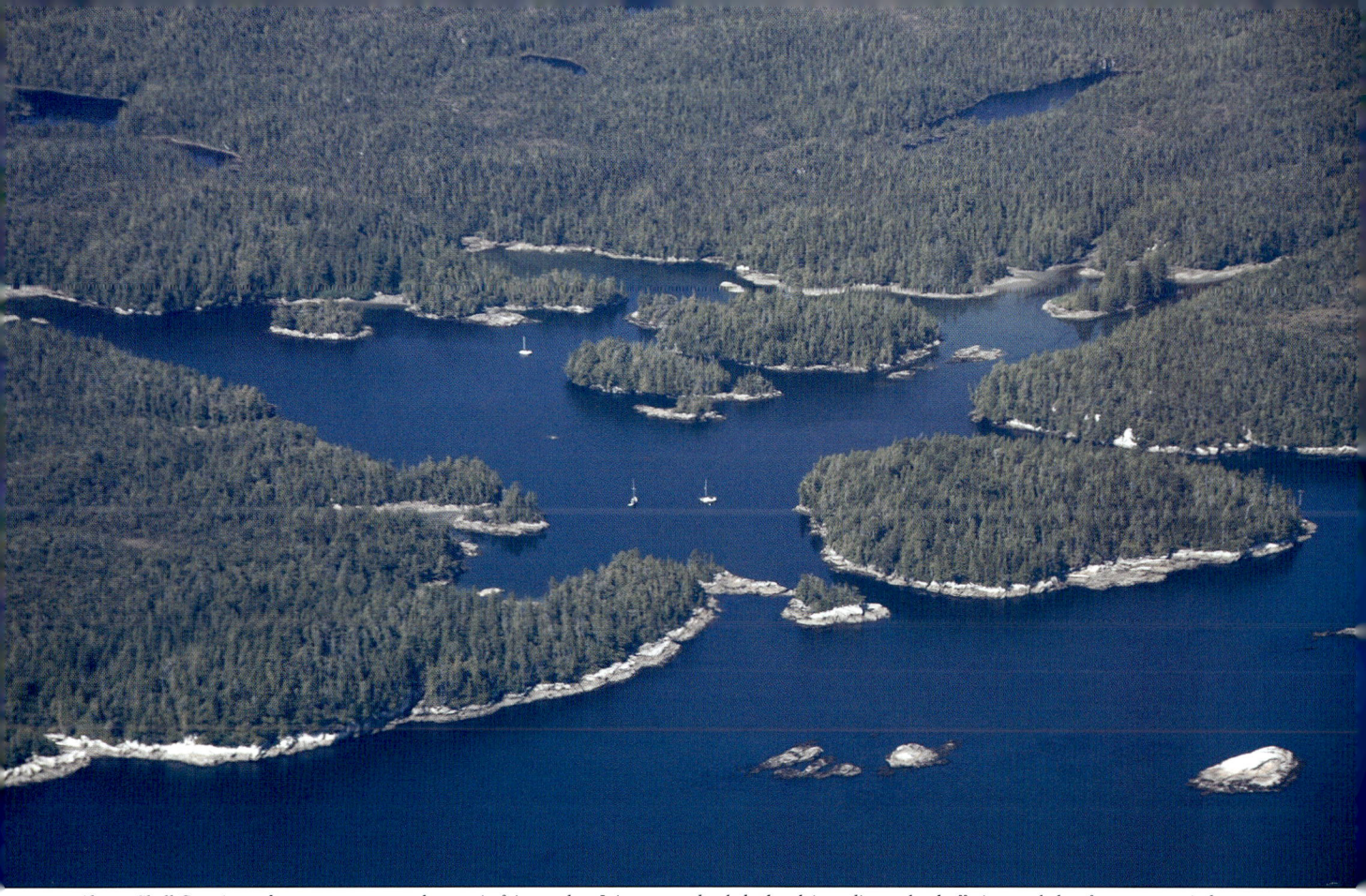

*Above: Skull Cove is used as a temporary anchorage in fair weather. It is protected only by low lying adjacent land offering no shelter from strong winds.*

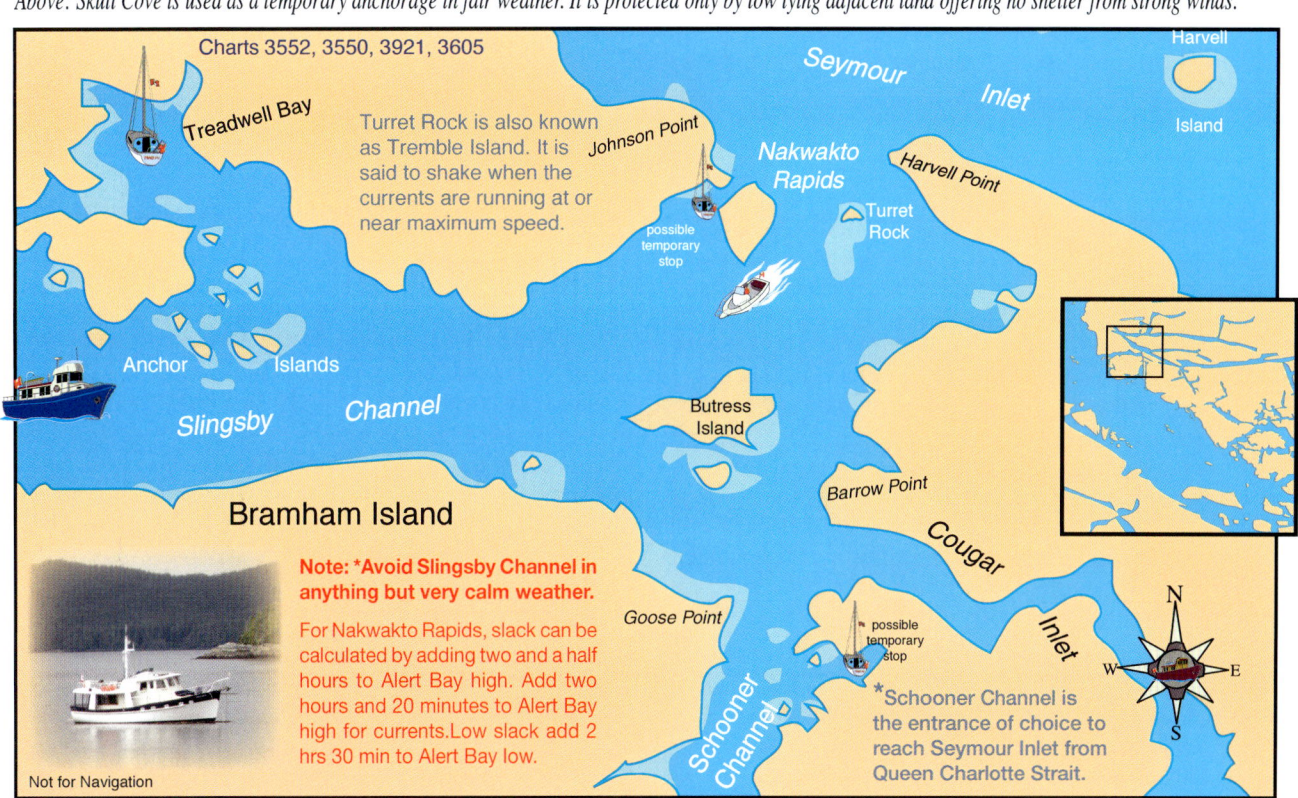

Charts 3552, 3550, 3921, 3605

Treadwell Bay

Turret Rock is also known as Tremble Island. It is said to shake when the currents are running at or near maximum speed.

Johnson Point

Seymour Inlet

Nakwakto Rapids

Harvell Point

Harvell Island

Turret Rock

possible temporary stop

Anchor Islands

Slingsby Channel

Butress Island

Bramham Island

Barrow Point

Cougar Inlet

**Note: *Avoid Slingsby Channel in anything but very calm weather.**

For Nakwakto Rapids, slack can be calculated by adding two and a half hours to Alert Bay high. Add two hours and 20 minutes to Alert Bay high for currents. Low slack add 2 hrs 30 min to Alert Bay low.

Goose Point

possible temporary stop

Schooner Channel

*Schooner Channel is the entrance of choice to reach Seymour Inlet from Queen Charlotte Strait.

Not for Navigation

195

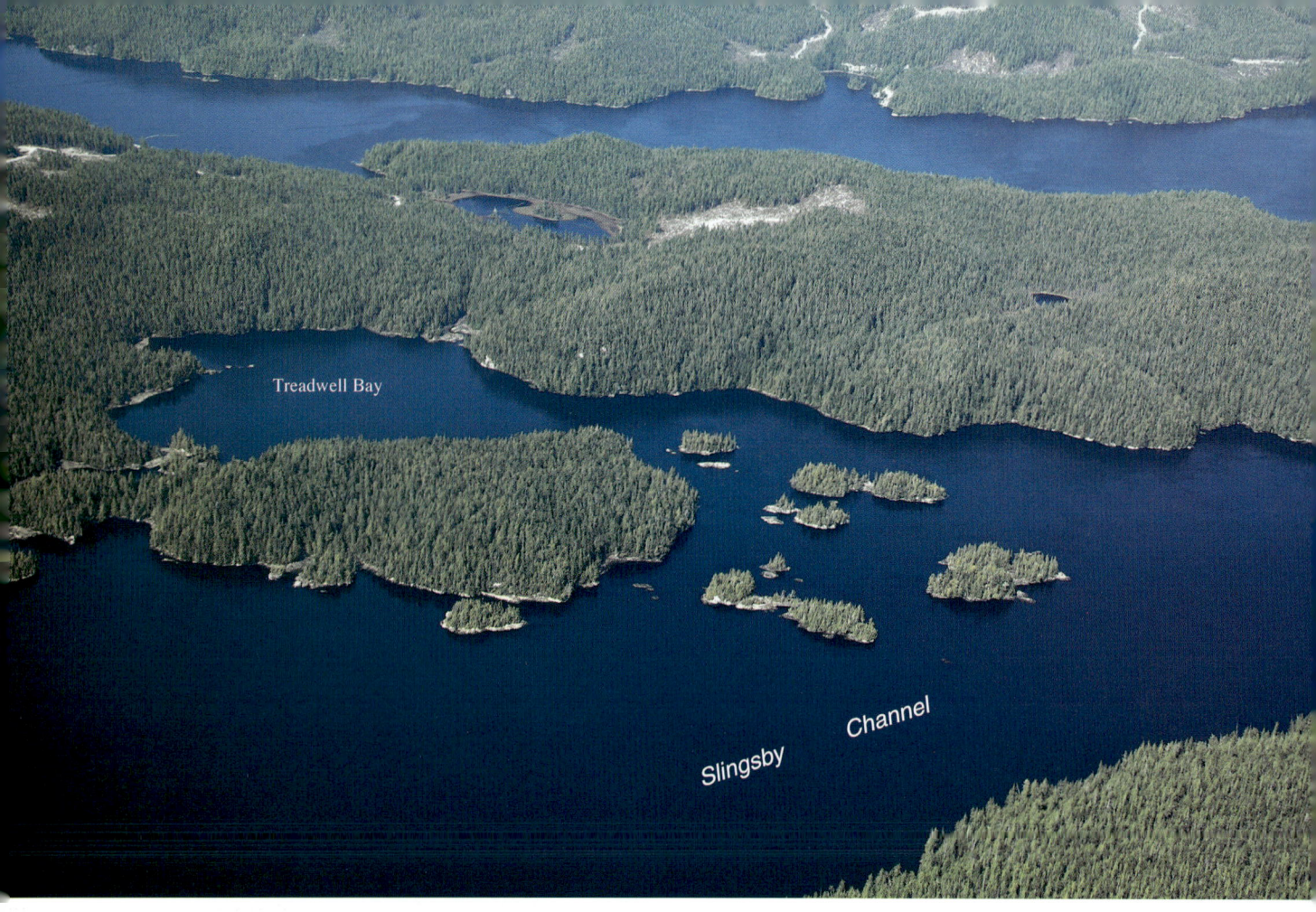

Treadwell Bay

Slingsby Channel

*Left: Turret Rock at Nakwakto Rapids in Slingsby Channel—near slack tide. Opposite centre, bottom and far right: The water picks up speed following the very brief slack tide interval at Nakwakto Rapids.*

Scuba divers love to explore the waters around Slingsby Channel. However, they have the shortest time in which to do so at the height of slack.

Once inside Seymour Inlet you have the option of exploring Belize Inlet, Nugent Sound, Mereworth Sound and Seymour Inlet itself.

Since the relatively recent charting of the area and the publication of chart 3552 by the Canadian Hydrographic Service many mariners have ventured beyond the intimidating entrance to Seymour Inlet. At the advice of several people familiar with Seymour Inlet there are some half a dozen bays inside which afford possible anchorage and exploration.

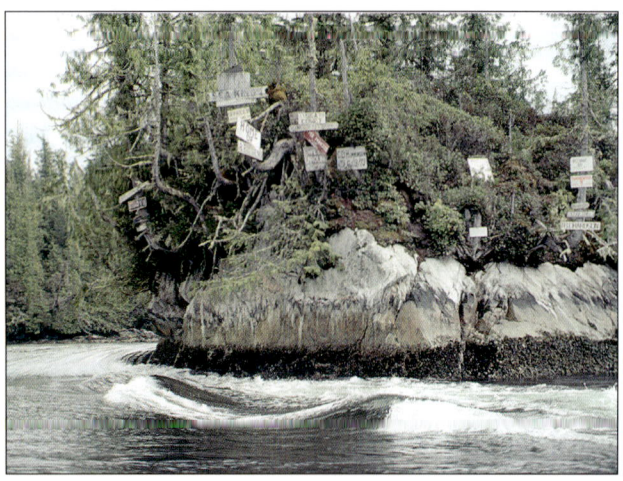

vessels. At or near the peak of the tidal rush no boats should attempt the passage.

If you approach the rapids from Schooner Channel you may wait in a small anchorage opposite Goose Point. If you find yourself in the rapids and the currents are too much for you even at a calculated safe time, try taking shelter in the lee of Johnson Point behind the small island opposite Turret Rock, but only during the ebb tide.

The most recommended anchorages are at **King Bay** in Seymour Inlet and **Westerman Bay** in Belize Inlet with a caution against westerly or southwesterly winds. **Village Cove** in Mereworth Sound affords shelter only from the east. Good anchorage in easterlies is found at **Charlotte Bay**. Other anchorages are found at **Wawatle Bay** adjacent to Harriet Point and **Frederick Bay** farther along Seymour Inlet.

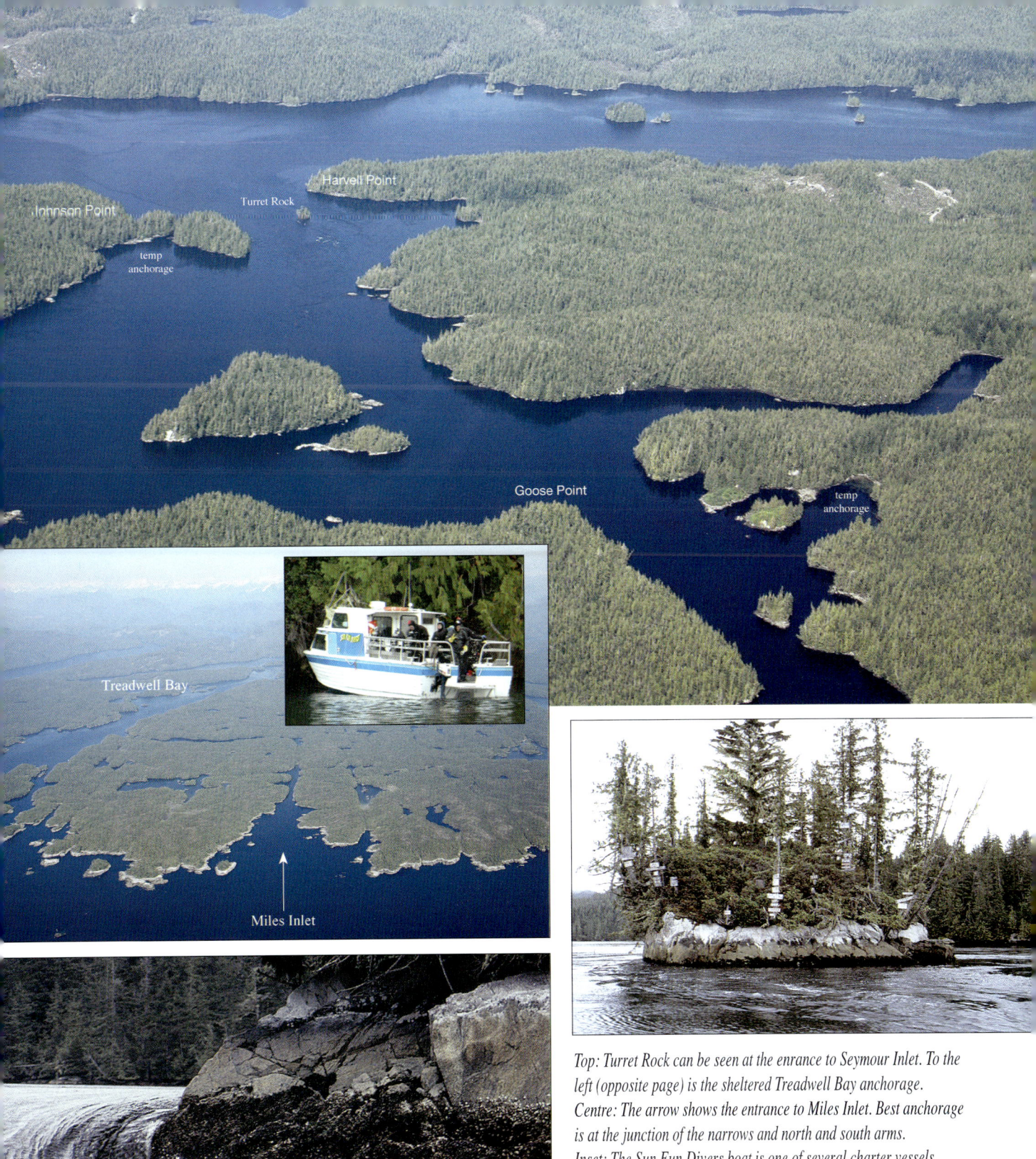

Top: Turret Rock can be seen at the enrance to Seymour Inlet. To the left (opposite page) is the sheltered Treadwell Bay anchorage.
Centre: The arrow shows the entrance to Miles Inlet. Best anchorage is at the junction of the narrows and north and south arms.
Inset: The Sun Fun Divers boat is one of several charter vessels that take divers to the Nakwakto Rapids for some fast-water diving experiences. Turret Rock photographs above, left and opposite lower courtesy of Jett Britnell.

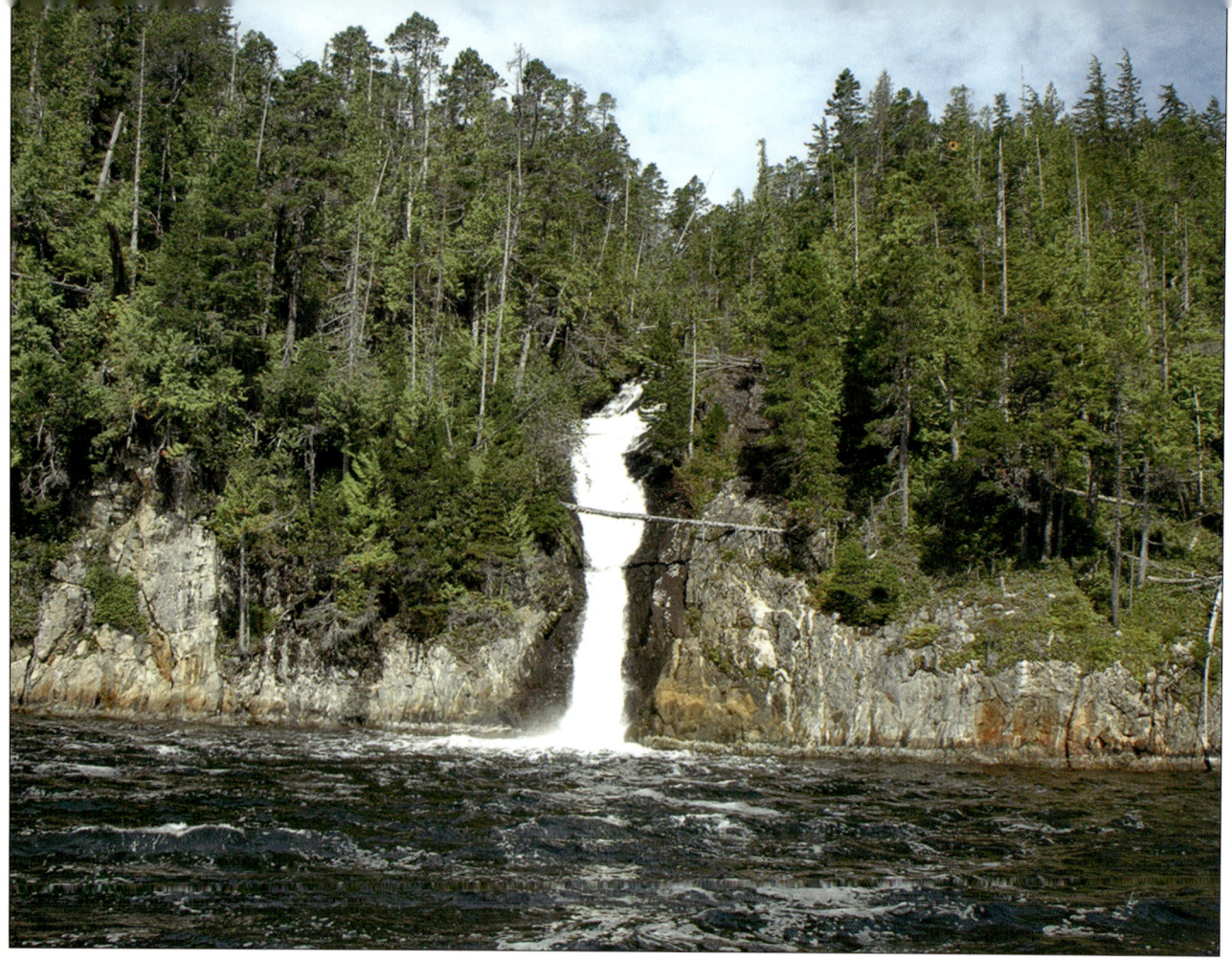

## Behind Nakwakto Rapids  chart 3552

The vision of a rapids that, during spring tides can attain ebb flow rates in excess of 14 knots, generates a mental, if not a physical barrier, for many. Yet, behind these tidal rapids there lies a recent history of mining, logging and simple living that dates back before the turn of the last century and even older evidence of indigenous peoples pre-dating this. There are also some well preserved and spectacular rock paintings that seem to document early contact. A tribal group from inside the rapids relocated to establish the native village in Blunden Harbour, ostensibly to facilitate trade with the large ships travelling the coast. Once you have read the Tide and Current Tables for Nakwakto Rapids you will realize these are just like all the other coastal rapids and they have periods of slack water each day when a dugout canoe or row boat could easily transit the narrows.

What are you waiting for? Slack water of course!

Once you decide to head for the narrows do not be surprised to encounter other vessels in the vicinity, as the tides dictate travel and activities within Seymour Inlet. In addition to those in transit, you may see dive charter boats waiting for slack water in back eddies as this is a dive destination with some unique fauna.

Approaching from the south, it is just over four miles from a good anchorage in Skull Cove to the narrowest point in the rapids at Tremble Island. If you enter from Slingsby Channel in the north, good anchorage can be found in the small cove to the west of **Treadwell Bay** behind the west end of **Anchor Islands**, that are less than 2.5 miles from Tremble Island. Once you pass Tremble Island, festooned with boards bearing boat names, turn north towards Belize Inlet and Mereworth and Allison Sounds or south towards Nugent Sound and Seymour Inlet. If you were to travel to the ends of each arm of the inlet, and back, you would cover over 100 miles in either direction; clearly you will need time and sufficient fuel to explore all the possibilities.

South of Harriet Point at Seymour's entrance, there is a network of lagoons, best left for dinghy exploration. There is almost 15 miles of additional exploration once you pass Harriet Point; however, you do not want to be like the vessel we heard calling a mayday from atop a rock in Woods Lagoon entrance on a falling tide. You are likely miles from the closest assistance, which could be the other side of a tidal rapids in full flow. When examining a chart of this area you will note that most of these inlets run east-west. As a consequence there can be inflow-outflow wind effects, influenced by conditions in the interior of the province.

Afternoon and late night outflow winds can be strong and the long narrow inlets with steep walls will cause funnelling winds at narrow points. Under these circumstances it is advisable to make transits early in the day and seek anchorages accordingly. Most of the complex of inlets and sounds are deep and good anchorages are not plentiful; however, the detail on chart 3552 is good and can be used to design a route that will have secure stops at each destination.

There are numerous waterfalls, and during times of heavy rain the waters are a bronzy colour and it is difficult to see submerged dangers, so use caution. Although the currents in the Nakwakto Rapids are extreme, the actual tidal range is relatively small, seldom exceeding six feet, so keep this in mind while anchoring and exploring some of the shallower lagoons.

If you head north, it is about seven miles to **Westerman Bay** and a further six miles to a beautiful pocket anchorage in the southwest corner of **Strachan Bay**. There is much evidence of past logging and some recent activities with heli-logging going on in places. These activities may once again be reactivated when the lumber industry revives. From here you can explore by dinghy and perhaps catch a trout in the Pack Creek mouth.

Just outside the mouth of Pack Creek there is a float community consisting of one individual (Buck) who has been there for over 12 years, the more recent years alone after Charlie Chilson passed on in 2004. During the summers Buck nurtures strawberries and tomatoes and feeds a menagerie of wild freeloaders. He always welcomes visitors.

During the late August salmon migration, at Pack Creek and at other creek mouths, you will often see active jumpers and might be lucky enough to tempt one to a spinning lure. Mereworth Sound is a good day trip from Strachan Bay as it is deep and lacks sheltered anchorages. You can find anchorage near the midden on the northwest corner of **Village Cove**, or possibly at a suitable place where you can shore tie farther up the sound while you explore.

Continuing farther into Belize Inlet and Allison Sound you can obtain satisfactory overnight anchorages in **NE Chief Nollis Bay** or **Peet Bay**. The latter will provide better shelter from gusty outflow winds that sometimes come down off the steep bare rock faces. Just before the entrance to Allison Sound there is a notch on the north shore of Belize that is very steep to and on the underside of the overhanging

*Right, top: Buck in Strachan Bay. Right: Pictographs in Belize Inlet. Just before the entrance to Allison Sound there is a notch on the north shore of Belize Inlet that is very steep to and on the underside of the overhanging rock face can be found the beautiful ochre coloured pictographs (located at 51° 07.499' N x 127° 08.980' W).*
*Opposite top: Trevor Lake Falls in Belize Inlet.*

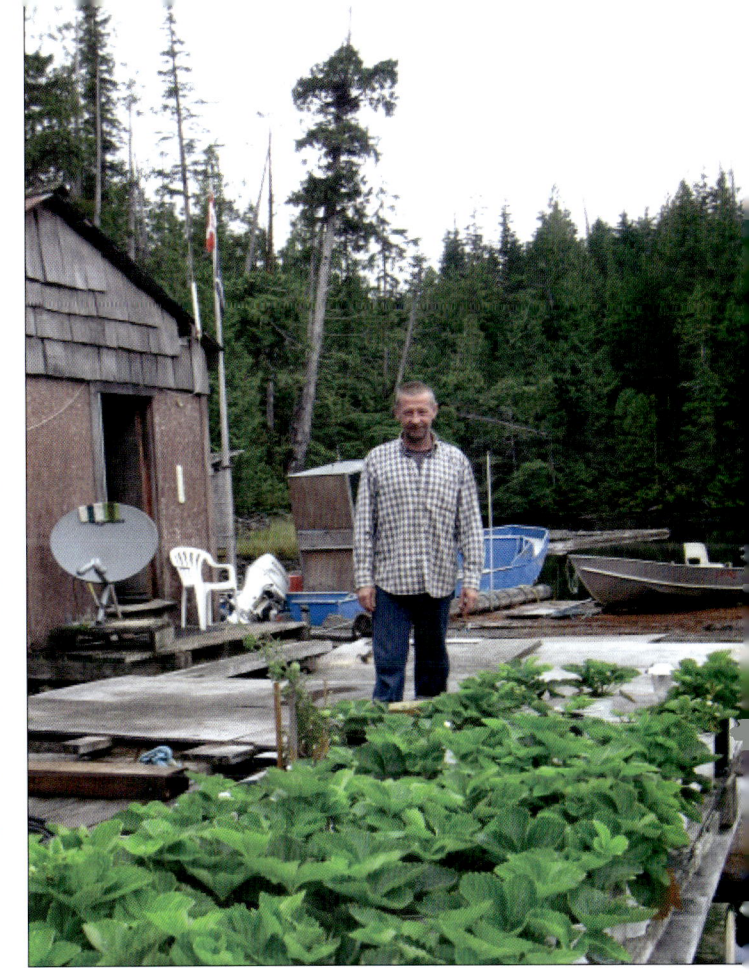

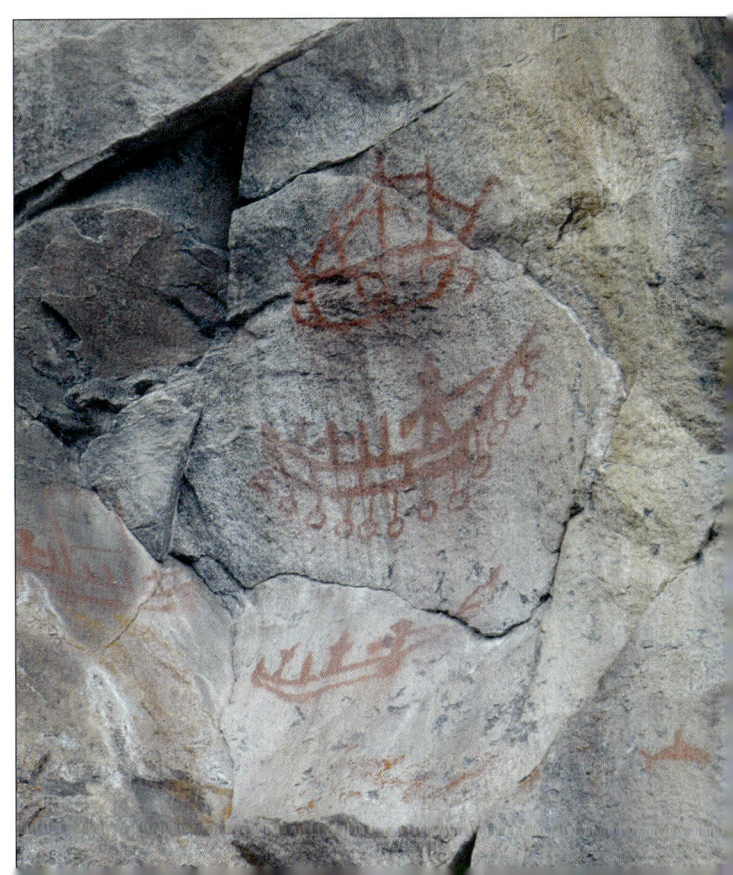

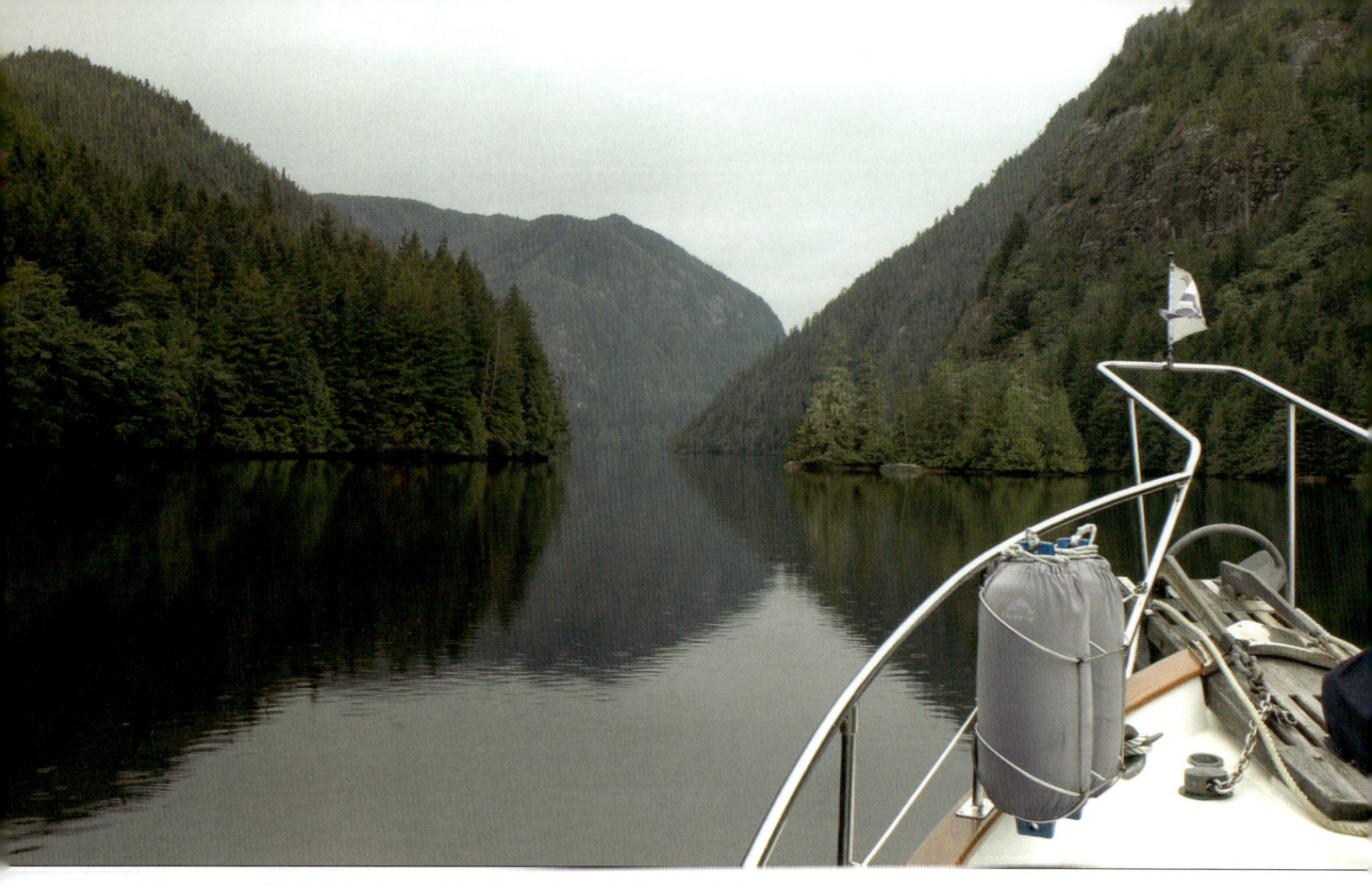

rock face you will find the beautiful ochre coloured pictographs (51° 07.499' N x 127" 08.980' W). As you proceed up the narrow channel into Allison Sound, the chart indicates adequate depth either side of the small mid channel island; however, we have only transited the east side and can only vouch for ample depth there.

Turning south from the Nakwakto Rapids entrance it is about one mile to Holmes Point (one of the old native sites) and three miles farther up Nugent Sound to a narrows where there is an anchorage to the northwest. Although afternoon outflow winds may build in this area, the holding is good and it provides a secure spot to explore deeper into Nugent Sound. Directly south of the narrows at Nugent Creek, 'ruins' are noted and you can explore this site and farther back to Schwartzenberg Lagoon entrance. If you are feeling 'peckish', keep in mind that these deep fjord-like waters provide ideal habitat for shrimp and prawns.

About four miles south of Holmes Point is **Charlotte Bay**, the 'Meeting Place' for early residents behind Nakwakto. It provides good anchorage across from the intricate waters of Ellis Bay and three miles short of Harriet Point, the entrance to Seymour Inlet. You can also find anchorage in the southeast corner of **Wawatle Bay** and use it as a base if you venture by dinghy into the lagoons to the south.

Exploring deeper into Seymour Inlet it is about 22 miles to Eclipse Narrows, the entrance to Frederick Sound and Salmon Arm. It is over 30 miles to the head of Frederick Sound where there is good anchorage. About 16 miles into Seymour Inlet along the north shore that is essentially devoid of anchorages you will stumble upon the delightful 'Jesus Pocket', a local name for the tight shallow cove between Safety Cove and Dine Point.

Although it is only just large enough for a couple of boats, few boats venture to it and you will probably find yourself alone. The head of Seymour Inlet is about 15 miles away. This makes a nice day trip from the cove as anchorages are limited. If you plan to depart from this location to make slack water at Nakwakto, you will have to take into account a run of about 25 miles.

The history and miles of waterways behind the rapids are monumental. Perhaps it is best to make Belize and Seymour Inlets a destination in themselves with an open agenda. It is worthwhile examining the salmon fishing regulations and making this trip in concert with the returning salmon.

**This section, on Seymour Inlet, has been provided by David Hoar and Noreen Rudd, well known coastal cruisers and authors of Cooks Afloat.**

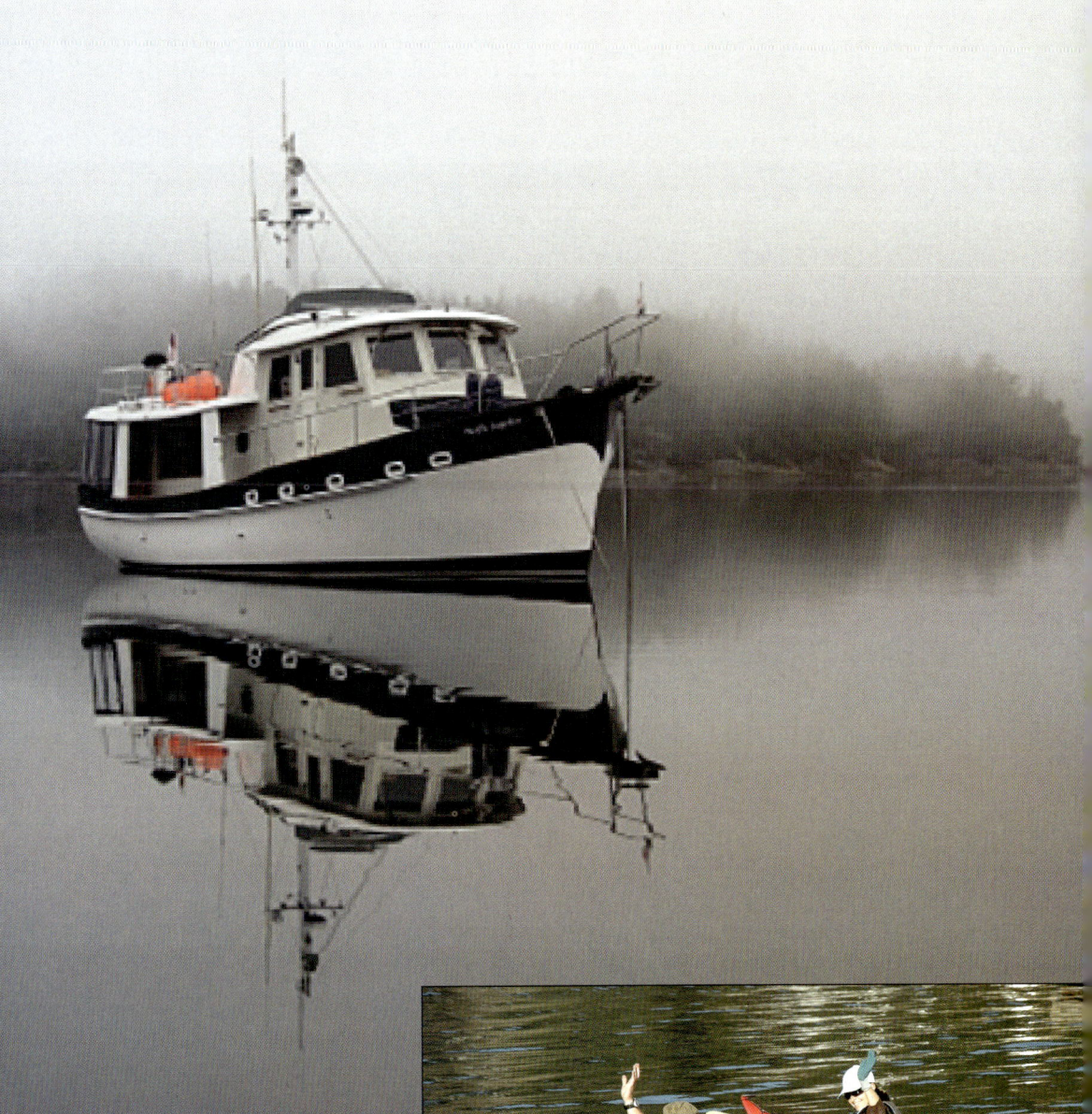

*These kayakers were met by the authors at Nakwakto and again in Port Hardy, Campbell River, Ganges and Victoria. They are from Basque country in Spain where he is a fire fighter and she is a lawyer. They were on a two month trip from Alaska to Victoria via kayak, car, and bicycle and were delighted at the pristine beauty of trhe BC coast, and especially the solitude of Seymour Inlet and its approaches.
Above: The authors' boat in Blunden Harbour.
Opposite: Cruising into Allison Sound.*

# Broughton Strait to Port Hardy

## Queen Charlotte Strait
## Havannah Channel to Alert Bay via Johnstone Strait

Charts 3546, 3548

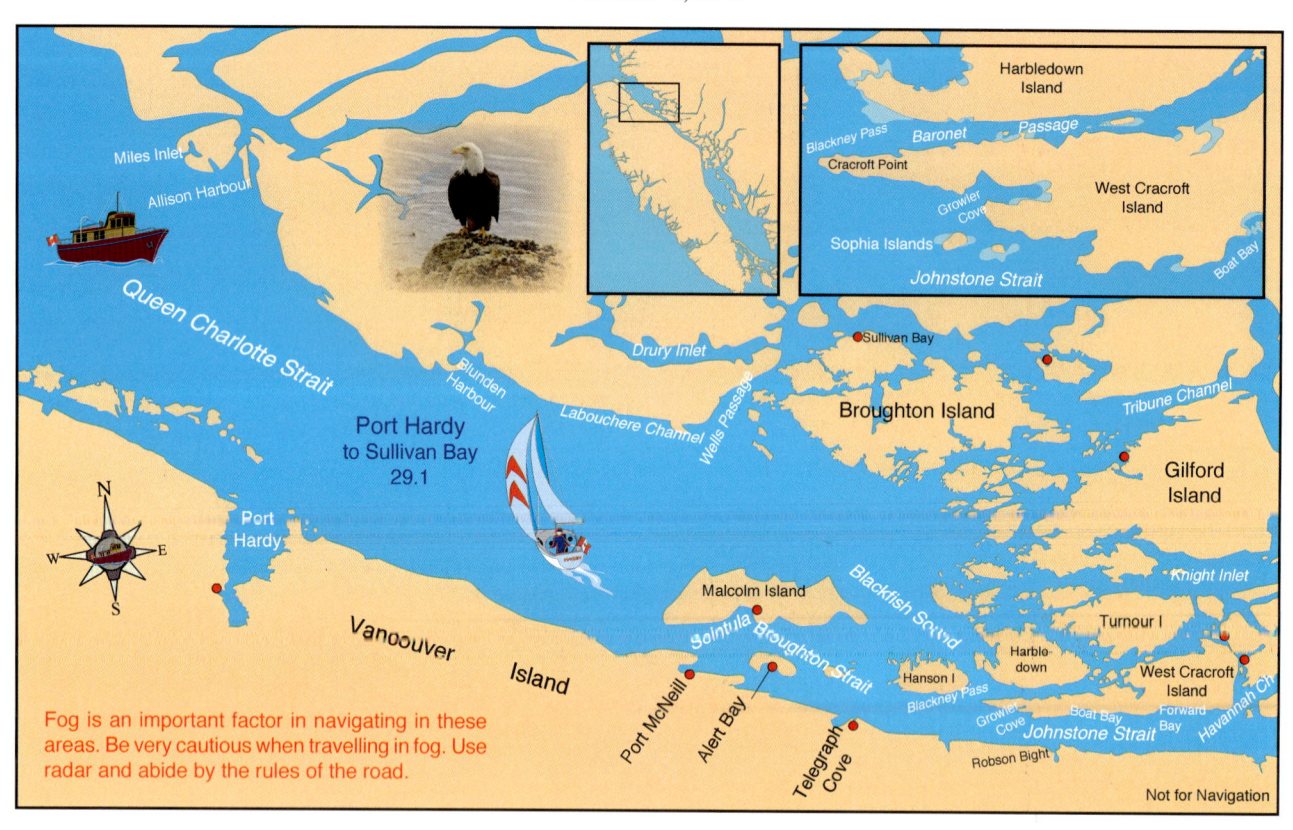

Fog is an important factor in navigating in these areas. Be very cautious when travelling in fog. Use radar and abide by the rules of the road.

From Havannah Channel, where you had the opportunity to turn off to Port Harvey and Minstrel Island, Johnstone Strait continues west between Vancouver Island and West Cracroft Island. Most vessels continue along the north shore of the strait passing Escape Reef on the inside or the outside, past **Forward Bay** and then beyond to **Boat Bay**. This latter bay (see page 88) was once a busy community. Today it sees the occasional activity, mostly the coming and going of whale watchers, both those involved in the scientific and behavioural study of the animals and those out simply to see them.

On the opposite side of Johnstone Strait is Robson Bight, a principal habitat for killer whales. This is an ecological reserve for the whales and has been declared such for the purpose of education and research. It is strictly forbidden for boaters to go into the preserve area. The preserve includes the shoreline, adjacent waters and the abutting forests. The whales move across Johnstone Strait and in and out of the bight area constantly. Whale watching may be conducted without entering the ecological area.

Do not chase after whales in order to get close to them. If you happen to be in their path simply stop and turn off your engines if it is safe to do so. Keep a minimum distance of 100 metres from whales at all times.

If the westerlies are making it too uncomfortable to continue to Blackney Passage take temporary shelter in behind the Bush Islets. Larger craft may be comfortable in the partially exposed north part of Forward Bay if smaller craft are anchored in the sheltered area adjacent to Bush Islets.

As you continue along Johnstone Strait you will pass the Sophia Islands and the entrance to **Growler Cove** (see page 88). You can do so on the inside or the outside, but if you do go inside of them you will have to emerge back onto your former

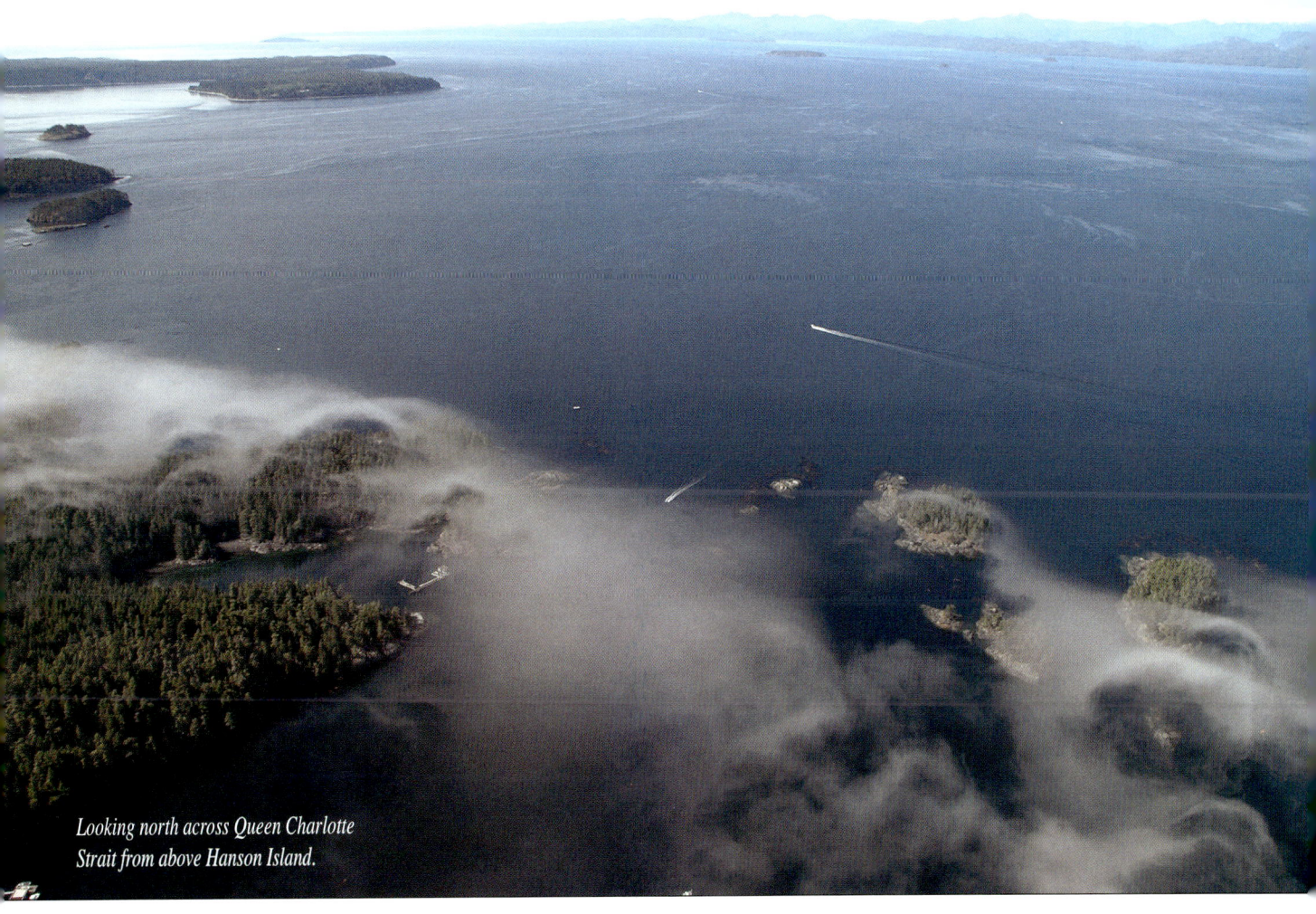

*Looking north across Queen Charlotte Strait from above Hanson Island.*

path in any event because of Baron Reef near Cracroft Point, at the end of West Cracroft Island. Be mindful of a 4 knot flood tidal stream out of Blackney Passage as you approach the pass. The currents make this a popular spot for fishing and observing eagles and whales. It is also a good spot for scuba diving at slack tide, with careful planning. Expect a 5 knot flood or ebb at maximum in the passage itself and about the same if you continue on into Blackfish Sound.

## Blackfish Sound  chart 3546

If you turn off Johnstone Strait into Blackney Passage your journey takes you either up Baronet Passage to Minstrel Island or west towards Malcolm Island and Alert Bay through Blackfish Sound along the north side of Hanson Island.

## Broughton Strait  chart 3546

From Blackney Passage to the beginning of Broughton Strait is a matter of simply cruising along the south side of Hanson Island. Where Johnstone Strait ends in the west, Broughton Strait continues. It runs from Weynton Passage (opposite Telegraph Cove) at its eastern end to Queen Charlotte Strait in the west. The channels and islands abutting the Strait are worth a slow sight-seeing passage or anchoring among them and gunkholing about in a small boat. Stop at centres such as Alert Bay and explore the fascinating Ecological Reserve (formerly known as Gator Gardens) on the hill above the town. See also **Plumper Islands** page 108.

## Beaver Cove  chart 3546

This large, exposed cove is seldom used by mariners. The bay does not offer protected moorage. The first settlement at Beaver Cove was established in 1917, complete with wharf, pulp mill and sawmill. It was built by the Beaver Cove Lumber and Pulp Mill Company. Some 30 families made Beaver Cove their home in the 1930s.

It is also the terminus of the Englewood Railway line which continues to function today. On its west shore the remnants of the former town of Englewood are testament to the heyday of logging activity. The floathouses and cabins at East Bay on the east side of the cove still remain occupied but in a state of relative disrepair. Beaver Cove was named after the Hudson's Bay Company paddle wheeler *Beaver*.

Beyond Beaver Cove, across Broughton Strait, you will find moorage and facilities at Alert Bay. Prior to reaching Beaver Cove from Johnstone Strait, the settlement at Telegraph Cove is picturesque and full of local history.

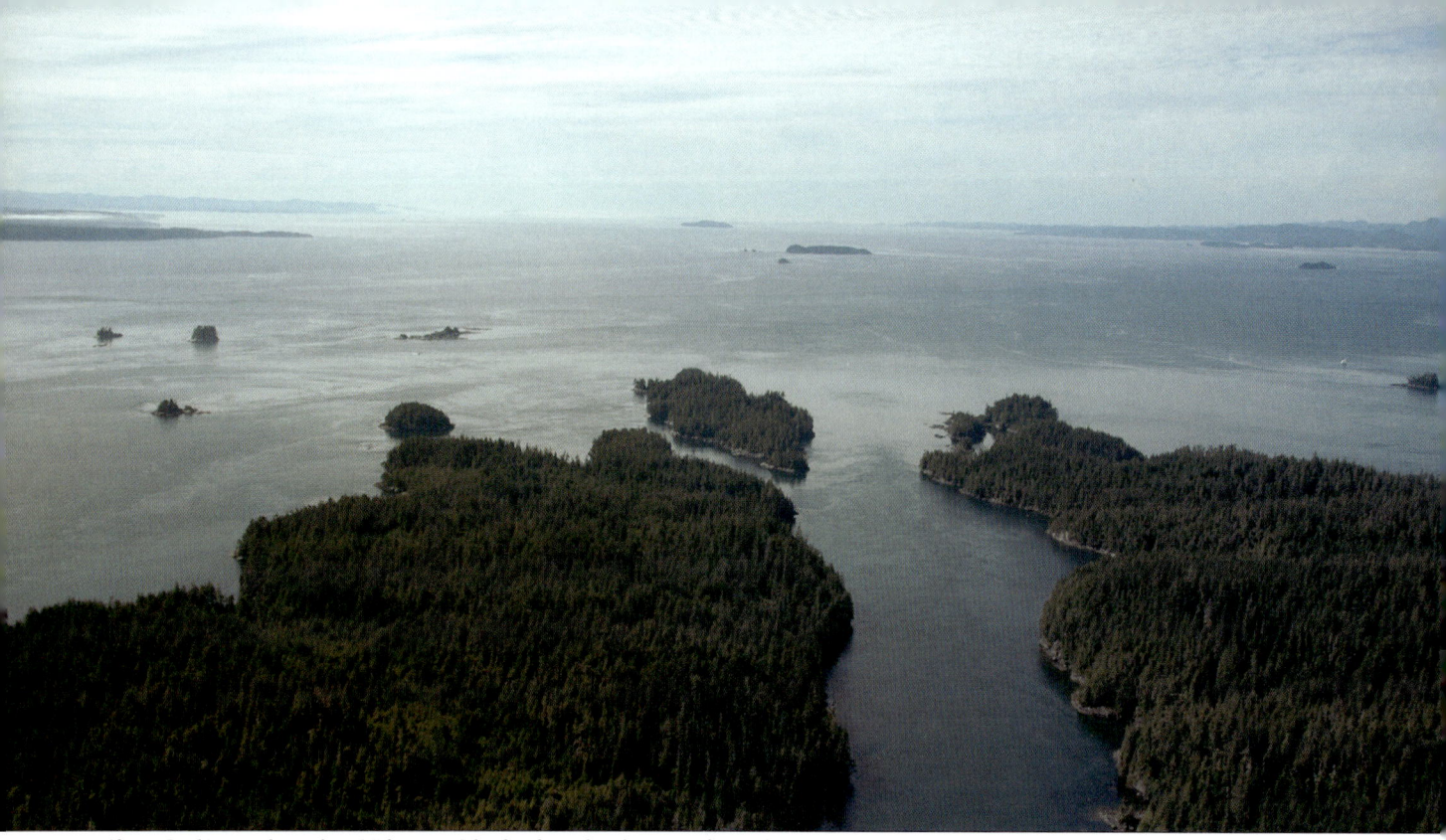

*Above: Looking northwest from Midsummer Island and Knight Inlet across the southeast reaches of Queen Charlotte Strait.*

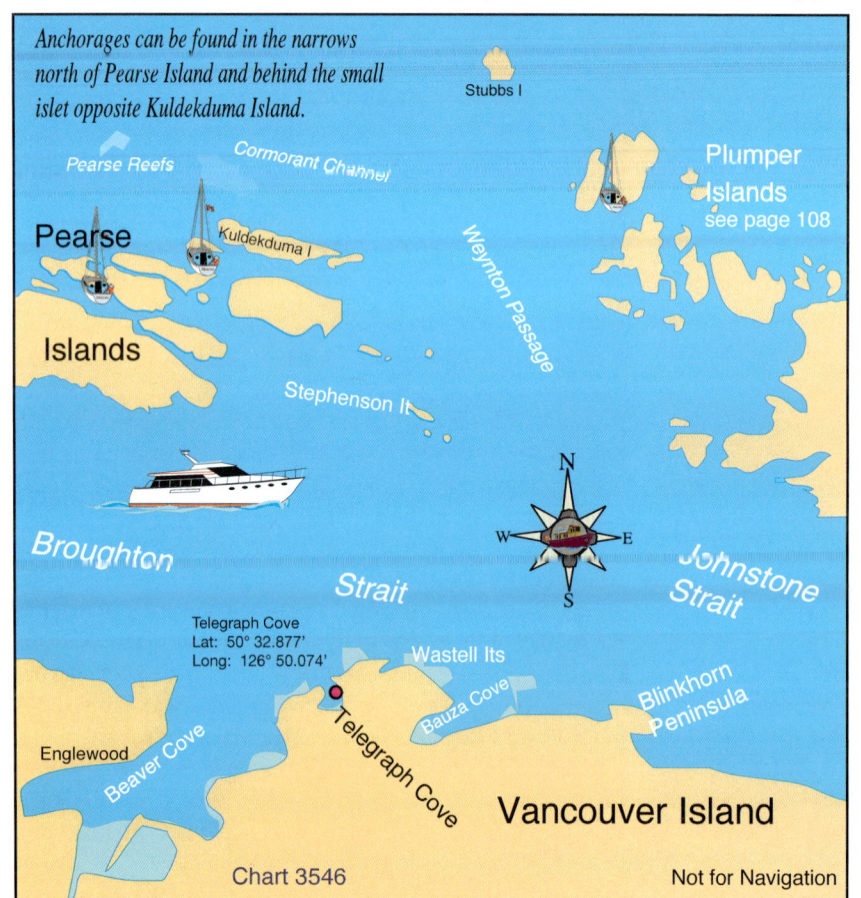

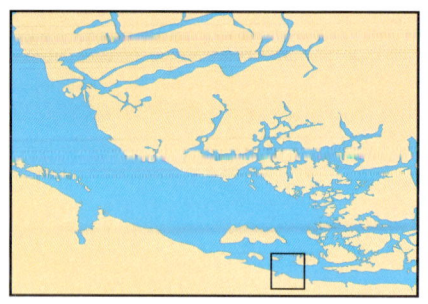

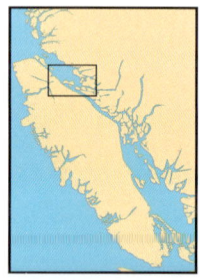

Anchorages can be found in the narrows north of Pearse Island and behind the small islet opposite Kuldekduma Island.

Stubbs I
Pearse Reefs
Cormorant Channel
Pearse
Kuldekduma I
Plumper Islands
see page 108
Islands
Weynton Passage
Stephenson It
N W E S
Broughton Strait
Johnstone Strait
Telegraph Cove
Lat: 50° 32.877'
Long: 126° 50.074'
Wastell Its
Bauza Cove
Blinkhorn Peninsula
Englewood
Beaver Cove
Telegraph Cove
Vancouver Island
Chart 3546
Not for Navigation

*Below: Thanks to Canadian Flight Centre, Boundary Bay, for the use of the Citabria aircraft shown below for the acquisition of many new aerial photographs used in this edition.*

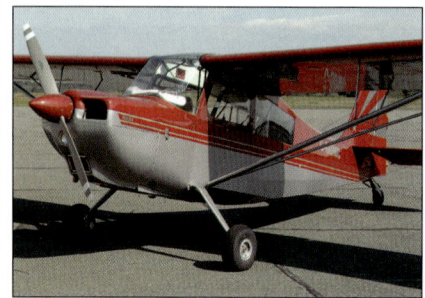

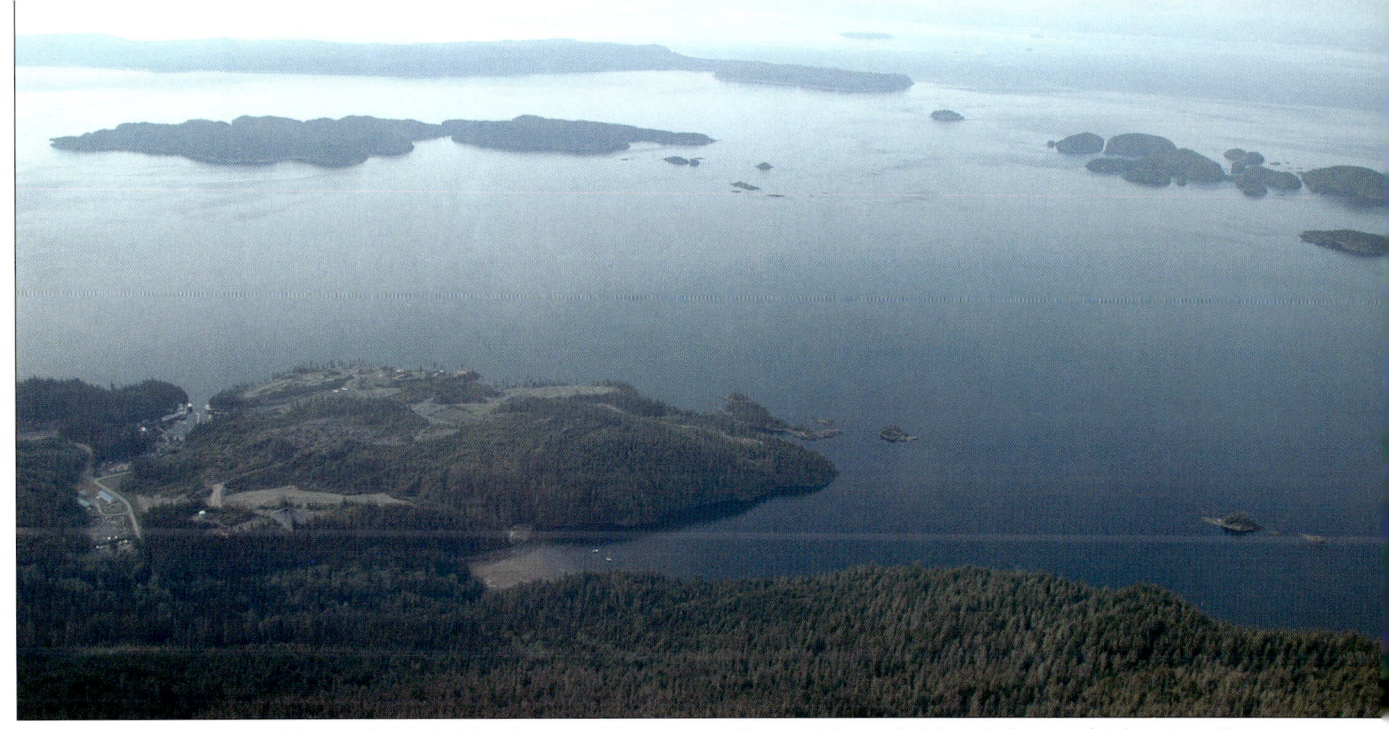

*Above: The Plumper and Pearse Islands with Malcolm Island beyond and Bauza Cove and Telegraph Cove to the left, in the foreground. Below: Krista Houston (centre) and Catherine Wykes (bottom) were helpful in the acquisition of photographs. Thanks to Grizzly Helicopters, and West Coast Helicopters, we were able to fly out of Port McNeill to photograph some of the nearby passages and islands. It's a trip worth doing as an orientation excercise, if you plan to cruise in the Broughton Islands.*

## Telegraph Cove  chart 3546

A fairly narrow entrance, about 60 metres wide, gives access to the cove. This is one of the coast's jewels for visitors. The main attraction here is the boardwalk and buildings adjacent to the fuel dock. A store at the head of the dock sells art, gifts and souvenirs, catering particularly to the whale watching trade. It is part of Stubbs Island Charters which runs whale watching vessels out of the cove. A trip with this organization is well worthwhile as it practically always produces whale sightings and there is a wealth of information about whales provided by the crew.

As you enter the cove there is a small dock to your starboard that serves as a gas dock and landing for drop off and pick up. A ramp leads up to the boardwalk set onto tall pilings with the main feature being the old Broughton Lumber and Trading Company building, known also as the freight building. This building was altered from the original with an 18 metres extension to accommodate a special exhibit as part of a museum and whale interpretive centre. It houses a collection of whale and other mammal skeletons which were partly the doing of Jim Borrowman, long time resident of Telegraph Cove and the man behind one of the earliest whale watching businesses in British Columbia. The extension was added after the centre came into possession of a 17.5 metre fin whale, which had been hit by a cruise ship in 2002. The whale was undetected and still attached to the bow when the ship docked in Vancouver.

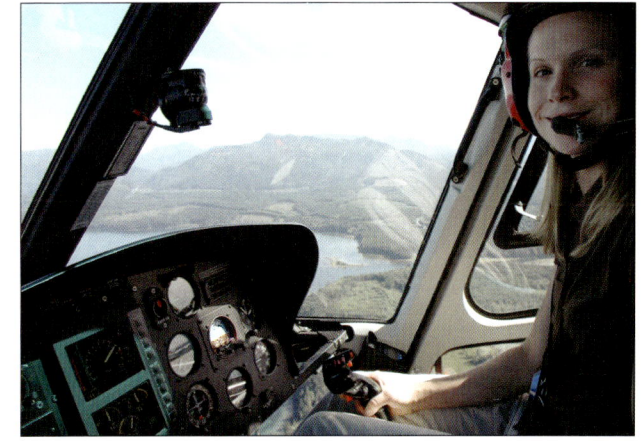

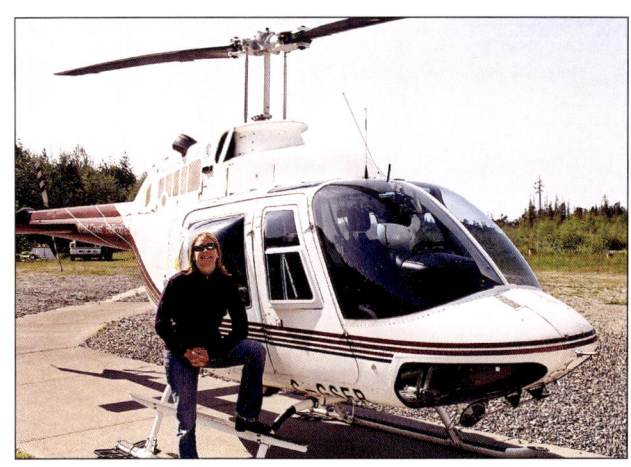

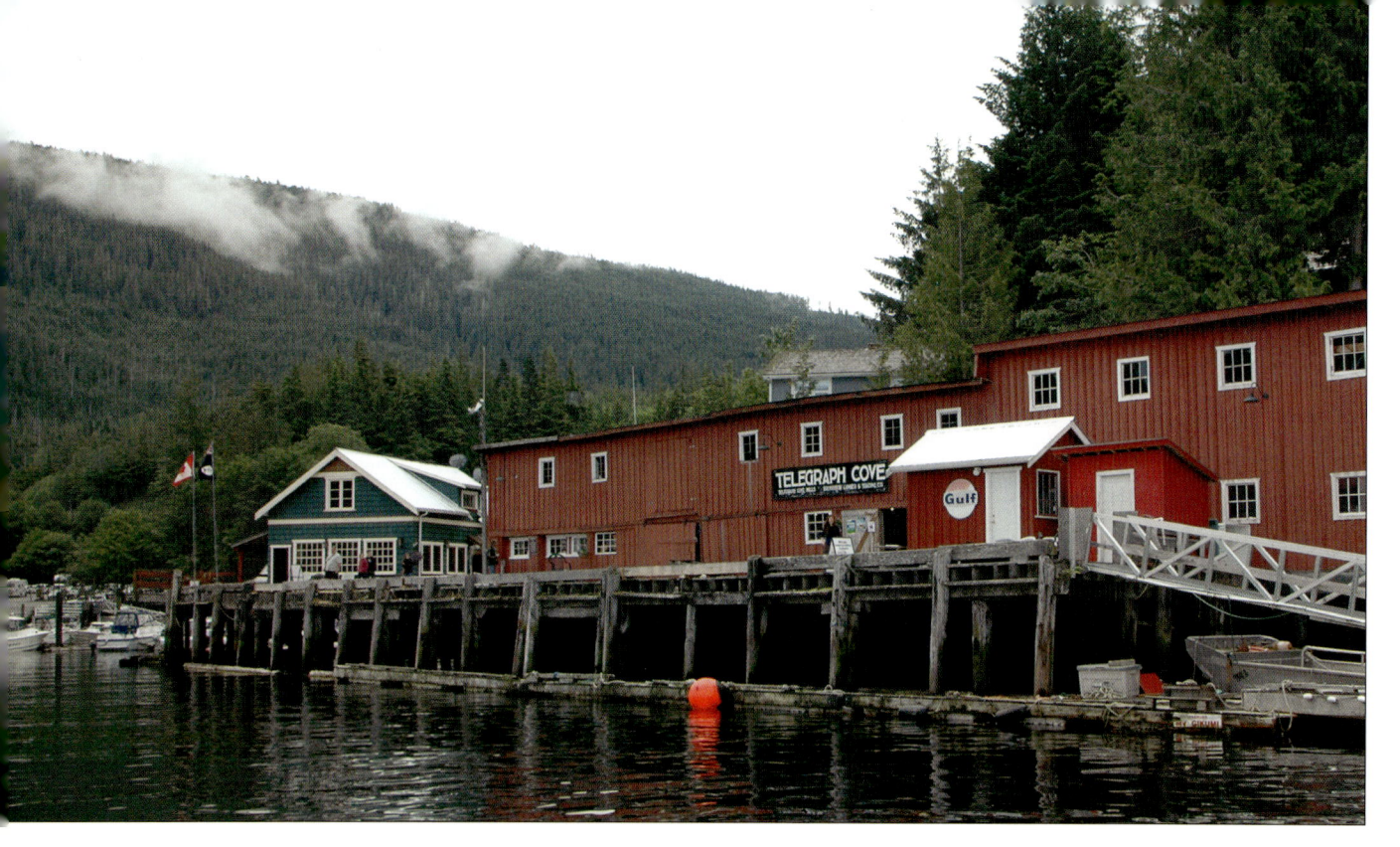

Telegraph Cove's historic boardwalk curves around the cove, passing another building that was once an old saltery, but now accommodates a store, a pub and a large restaurant. Historic cabins and houses flank the rest of the walk leading to a landing with general store, offices and lodgings. To port there is a resort complex with marina and RV campground and a small launch ramp. This facility is not so much for transient mariners as it caters specifically to its resort guests and trailer boats, mostly those brought in by guests. On the opposite shore from the landing is Telegraph Cove Marina, with facilities for transient boats and a new, large launch ramp. The marina includes side tying for larger craft and ample slips for boats to about 10 metres.

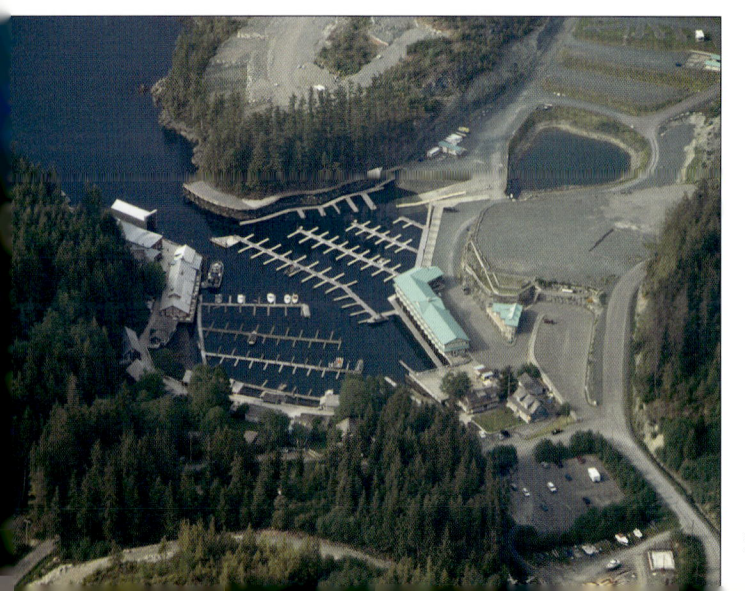

## Telegraph Cove Marina  VHF 66A  chart 3546
P.O Box 2-8 Telegraph Cove, BC V0N 3J0
Ph 250 928-3163   Fax 250-928-3162
email: reservations@telegraphcove.ca  www.telegraphcove.ca
This marina offers 50, 30 and 20 amp power and water at the dock. It has pumpout, laundry, showers, washrooms, RV park and accommodation and a 16 metre wide launching ramp. There is a landing with gift, snack and food stores.

## Telegraph Cove Resorts
Telegraph Cove BC V0N 3J0
Phone 250-928-3131
The resort runs the gas dock and has a small launch ramp. There is a restaurant and pub at the cove, also art and souvenirs for sale. The Whale Interpretive Centre has displays of mammal skeletons—two types of whales, a sea otter, sealion and dolphins. Other amenities at Telegraph Cove include a convenience store, books, charts and produce. Fuel is available at the entrance to the cove–gasoline only. Other services include grizzly bear watching, fishing charters and tours. Nearest diesel and all services are available at Port McNeill.

*Top: Telegraph Cove with its historic buildings along the water's edge. The red building is the museum and whale interpretive centre.*
*Left: Aerial shows the dock layout and entrance to Telegraph Cove.*
*Opposite: Historic buildings on stilts are a feature of the cove.*

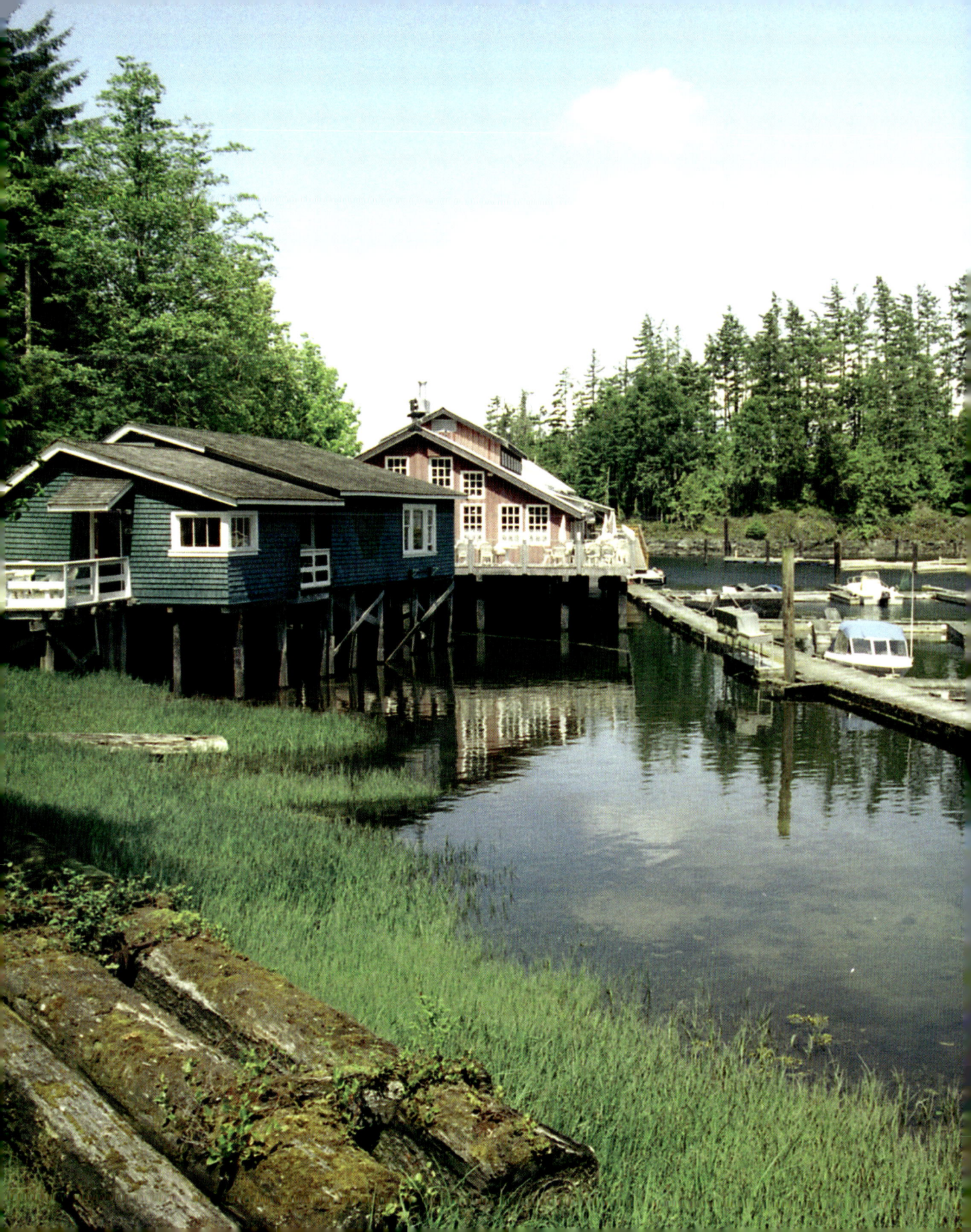

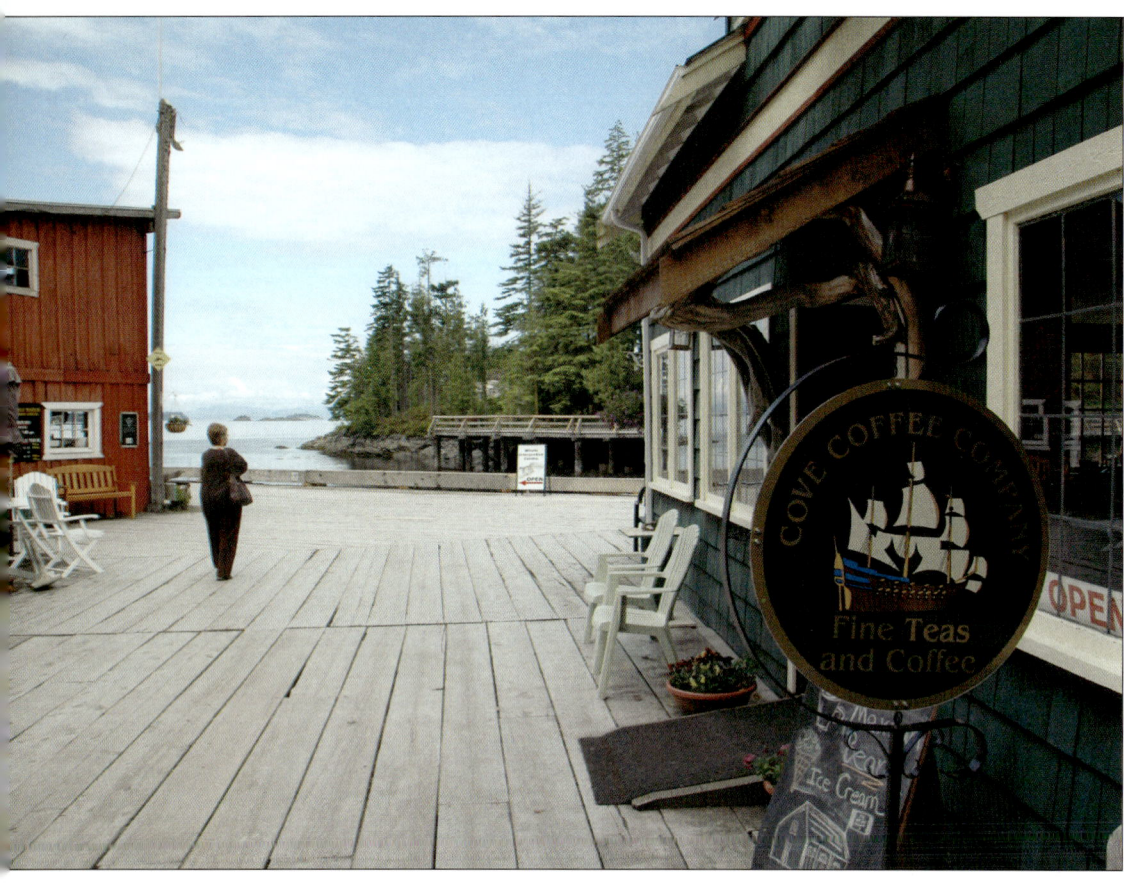

*Left: When it shines it really shines at Telegraph Cove. The cove faces across Broughton Strait to the Pearse and Plumper Islands and Weynton Passage.*

*Bottom left: Jim and Mary Borrowman and the whale bone collection in the Interpretive Centre at Telegraph Cove. Jim Borrowman is a pioneer of the whale watching business on the coast. Bottom right: The boardwalk at the Cove.*

*Opposite page: Views of the Cove showing the Whale Interpretive Centre and the marina docks adjacent to the boardwalk buildings.*

Historically Telegraph Cove is of special interest. In 1894 a sawmill was established at the Cove, well before it was given its present name. The mill was built by the cove's original settler, Alfred Marmaduke Wastell and we found his son Fred still living there the first number of times we visited Telegraph Cove. A telephone station was built in 1911 to connect the northern parts of Vancouver Island to Campbell River.

We have enjoyed visits to Telegraph Cove since the 1970s when the store was still the rustic old place it must have been in the early days. In it were typical hardware items and some marine supplies. The same structure houses a more refined store now, with art and gifts among the wares on display, but there is still a trace of the original store's ambience. The houses along the walk have signs describing their history. One of the buildings at the cove is said to have been the hospital in Simoom Sound at one time. There are other historic buildings, appropriately posted with signage telling of their history.

The floats at Telegraph Cove are mostly for small sport fishing craft. They accommodate the vessels brought in by trailer and launched at the head of the bay or at the larger ramp to the east of the bay. There is some space for larger vessels at the main dock deep inside the cove.

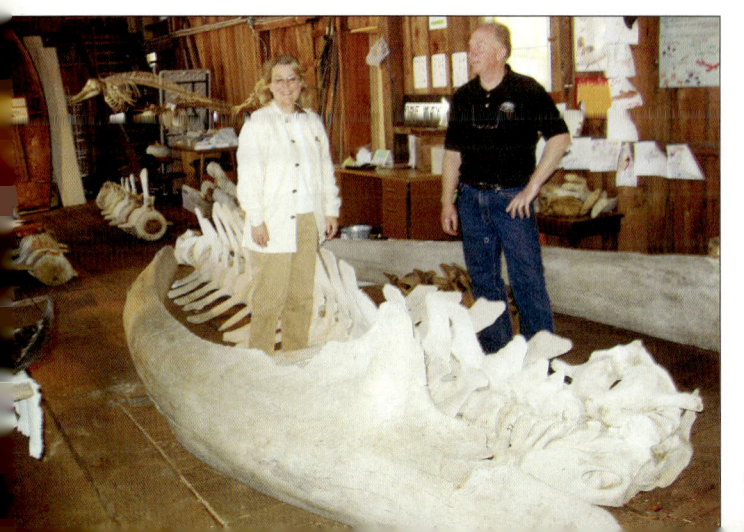

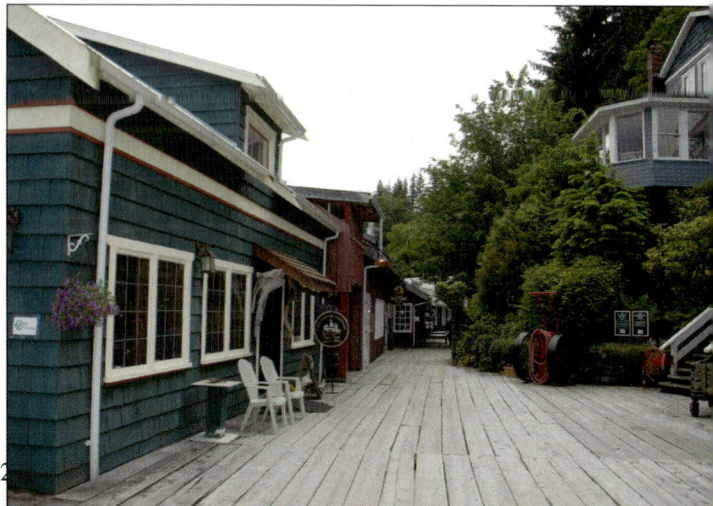

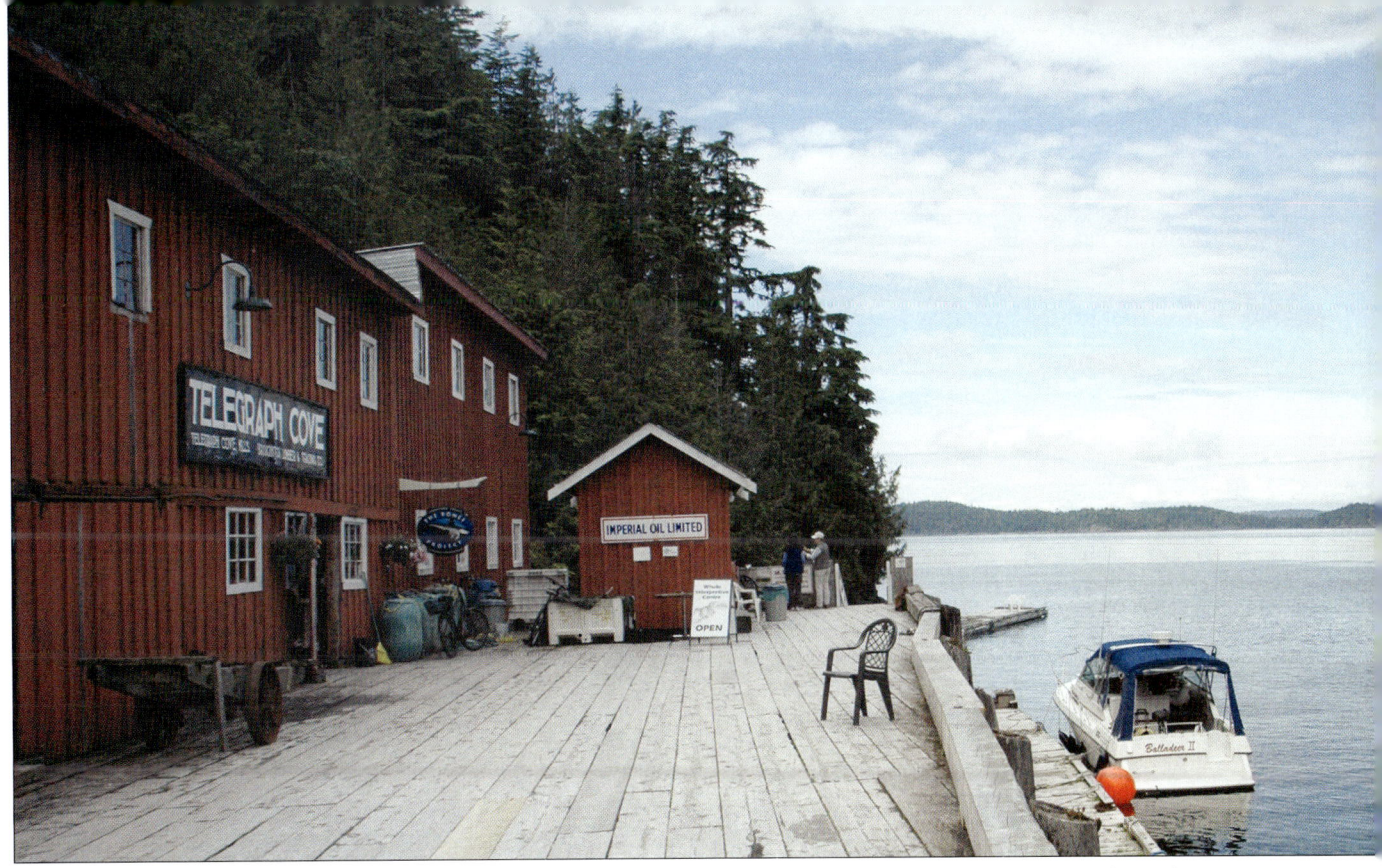

*The Whale Interpretive Centre was established to increase public awareness about marine mammals in the area and the threats facing them. Its 'Bones Project' exhibit includes complete skeletons of various species, including two types of whale, a sea lion, seal, dolphin and otter. You can also see the jaw bones of a blue whale, the largest animal ever to inhabit the earth.*

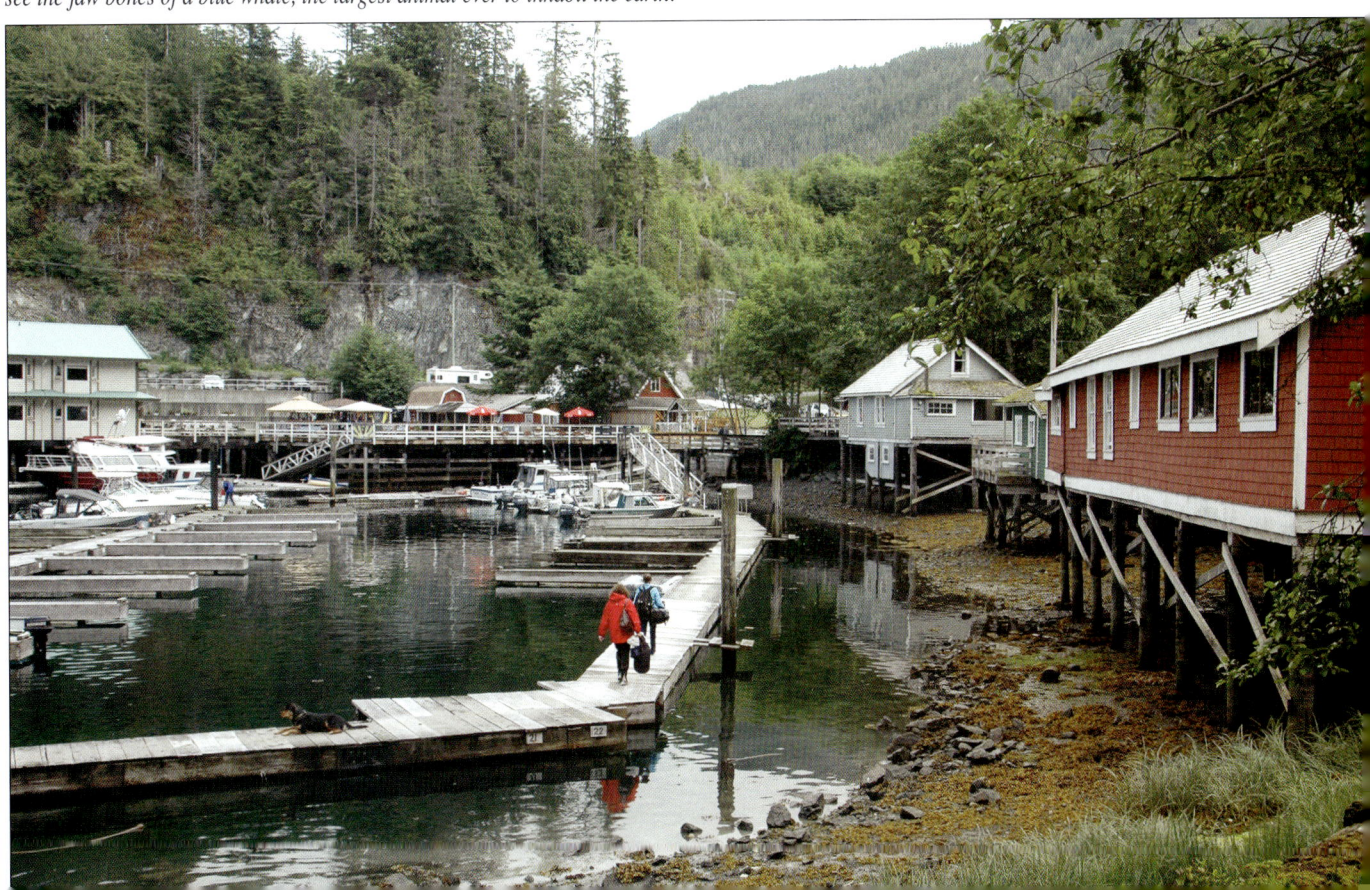

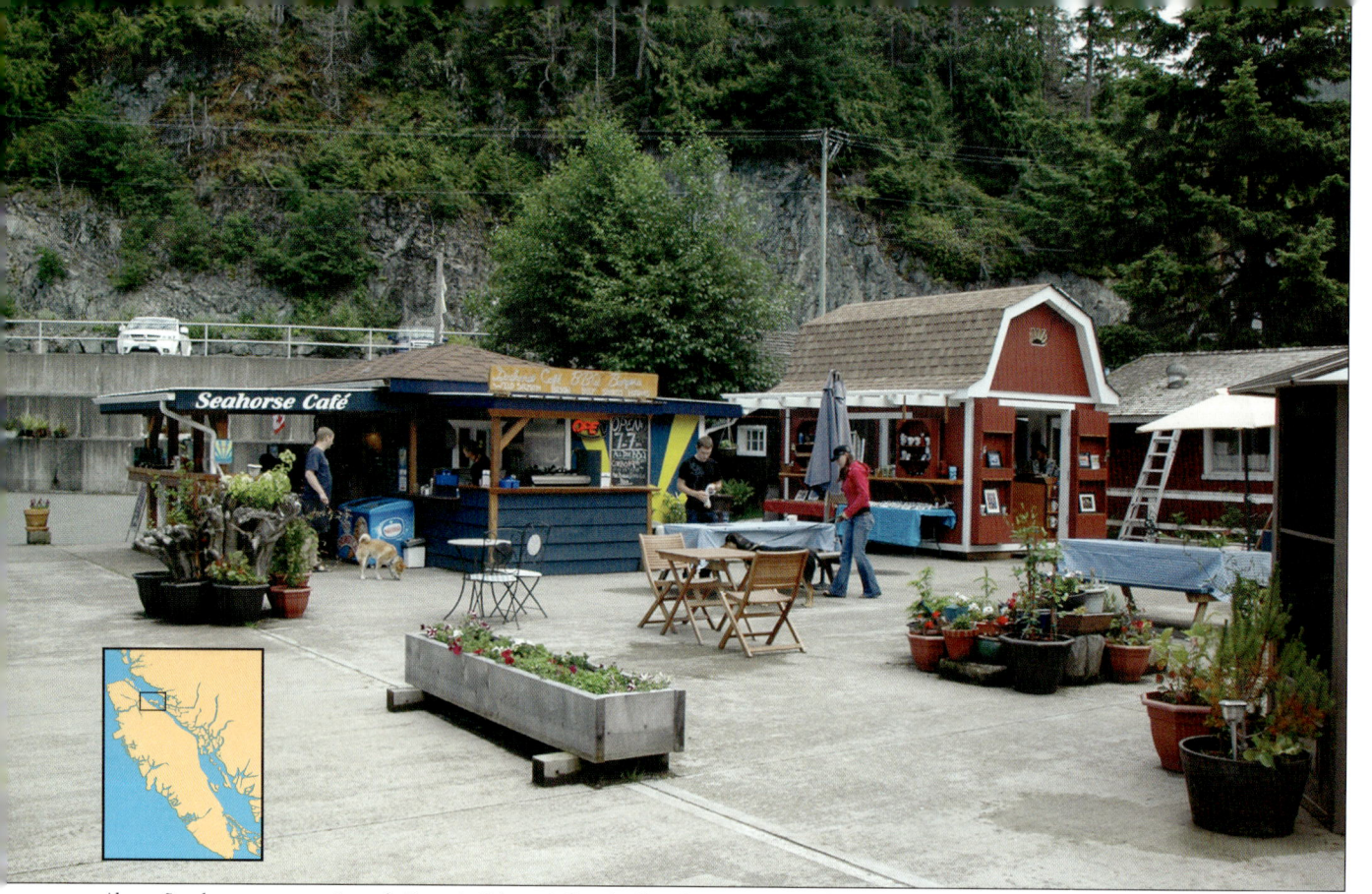

*Above: Snacks, treats, souvenirs and gifts at the Telegraph Cove landing. Opposite page top left: View of some of the historic structures and the small craft floats at Telegraph Cove. Far right, top: The shoreside end of the walkway and the general store at Telegraph Cove.*

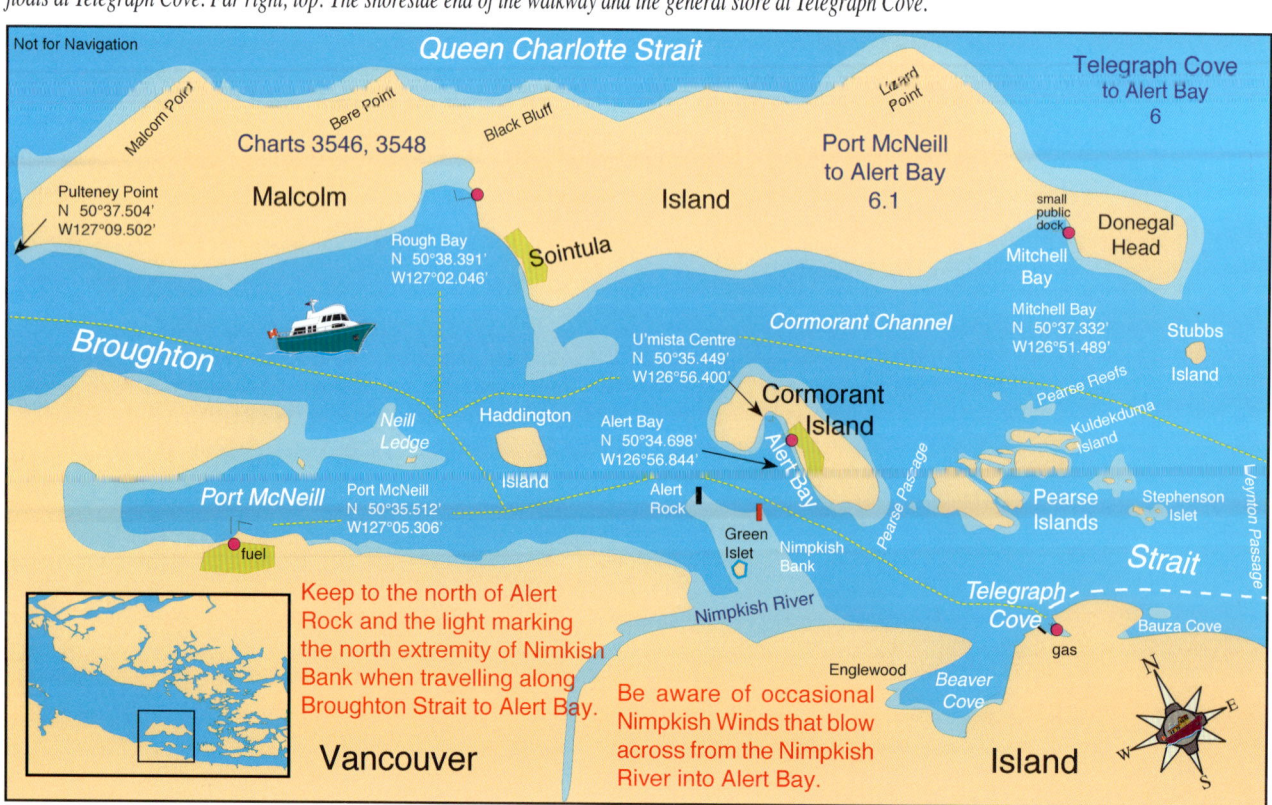

---

**Queen Charlotte Strait**

Not for Navigation

Telegraph Cove to Alert Bay 6

Malcom Point • Bere Point • Black Bluff • Lizard Point

**Charts 3546, 3548**

Port McNeill to Alert Bay 6.1

small public dock

Pulteney Point
N 50°37.504'
W127°09.502'

**Malcolm** **Island**

Donegal Head

Rough Bay
N 50°38.391'
W127°02.046'

Sointula

Mitchell Bay

**Broughton**

Mitchell Bay
N 50°37.332'
W126°51.489'

Cormorant Channel

Stubbs Island

U'mista Centre
N 50°35.449'
W126°56.400'

Pearse Reefs

**Cormorant Island**

Kuldekduma Island

Neill Ledge

Haddington

Alert Bay
N 50°34.698'
W126°56.844'

Alert Bay

Pearse Passage

**Port McNeill**

Island

Alert Rock

Pearse Islands

Stephenson Islet

Port McNeill
N 50°35.512'
W127°05.306'

Green Islet

Nimpkish Bank

**Strait**

Weynton Passage

fuel

**Telegraph Cove**

Bauza Cove

Keep to the north of Alert Rock and the light marking the north extremity of Nimkish Bank when travelling along Broughton Strait to Alert Bay.

Nimpkish River

Englewood

Beaver Cove

gas

Be aware of occasional Nimpkish Winds that blow across from the Nimpkish River into Alert Bay.

**Vancouver** **Island**

210

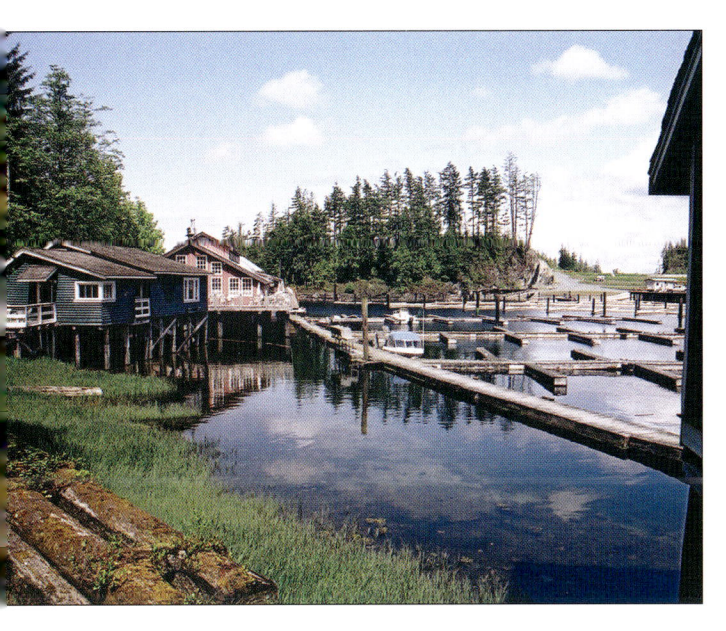

West of Telegraph Cove is **Beaver Cove**. This is an open bay with a fairly deep anchorage close to shore. It is a bay we usually pass by as a place to stop because of the log booming, which means the likelihood of sunken logs and debris that could snarl anchors and rode. Beaver Cove reflects a long history on the coast. It was settled in the early 1900s by the Beaver Cove Lumber and Pulp Company that established a small town, complete with hotel and a large wharf for deep draft ships.

A sulphate mill and a shingle mill were built later towards the head of the bay, and lodging facilities were provided for Japanese and Chinese workers. The charted settlement of Englewood was named after two men who built a sawmill there in the mid-1920s. If you travel by road into Telegraph Cove you will pass the old mill and its trestle along the flats of the Kokish River that flows into the cove. In recent years the company has been owned and operated by the Canadian Forest Products company. We have used a crude ramp on the shores of Beaver Cove to launch a small boat for the purpose of scuba diving in the nearby islands.

### The Pearse Islands  chart 3546

These beautiful islands are part of a provincial marine park. The eastern portion of the islands, including Stubbs Island, comprise Cormorant Channel Park. We have dropped anchor among the Pearse Islands with caution, being mindful of the currents, but have remained only long enough to enjoy the beauty of a fading sunset over dinner before moving on to a more protected overnight moorage. Scuba divers find lots to see underwater among these islands, choosing slack tides and relatively calm nooks out of the main stream of tidal flows. One spectacular dive site is at nearby Stubbs Island where the duration of slack for a quick dive is a mere five to ten minutes.

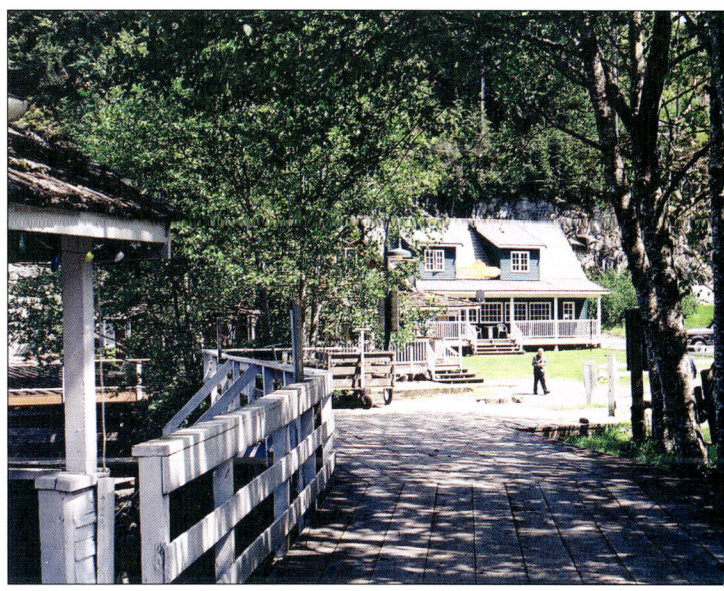

In calm conditions navigating around the Pearse Islands provides a grand view of sea and sky, mountains and the islands themselves. In rough conditions it is wise to remain in the main channels and seek shelter without undue delay. Weynton Passage is wide and easily navigated, but it is full of rocks and reefs just off Stephenson Islet and among the Pearse Reefs north of Kuldekduma Island.

During tidal rips it can be difficult to distinguish tide rip waves from reefs, so use your charts diligently and stay well clear, especially west-northwest of Pearse Reef, where an isolated drying rock lies unmarked well out into Cormorant Channel.

We have cruised around the north end of the Pearse Islands and have always made sure to do so only in fair to good conditions. Our destination, from Stubbs Island, on more than one occasion, using that route, was Alert Bay.

Use a bearing from the north side of Stubbs Island to the north end of Cormorant Island. Follow it until well into the centre of the northern extremity of Pearse Passage before turning down the passage for a run past Gordon Bluff and into Alert Bay. Alternatively take a bearing on the east end of Kuldekduma Island and cruise close up to it before turning along its shore, then skirt the Pearse Islands into and through Pearse Passage.

Keep clear of the shallows around the southeastern end of Cormorant Island as you approach Alert Bay.

### Bauza Cove  chart 3546 (see photo page 205)

This cove lies in the lee of Bauza Islet just east of Ella Point and Telegraph Cove. It affords some sheltered anchorage in about 20 metres for small craft. Enter with care either side of the foul ground around Bauza Islet.

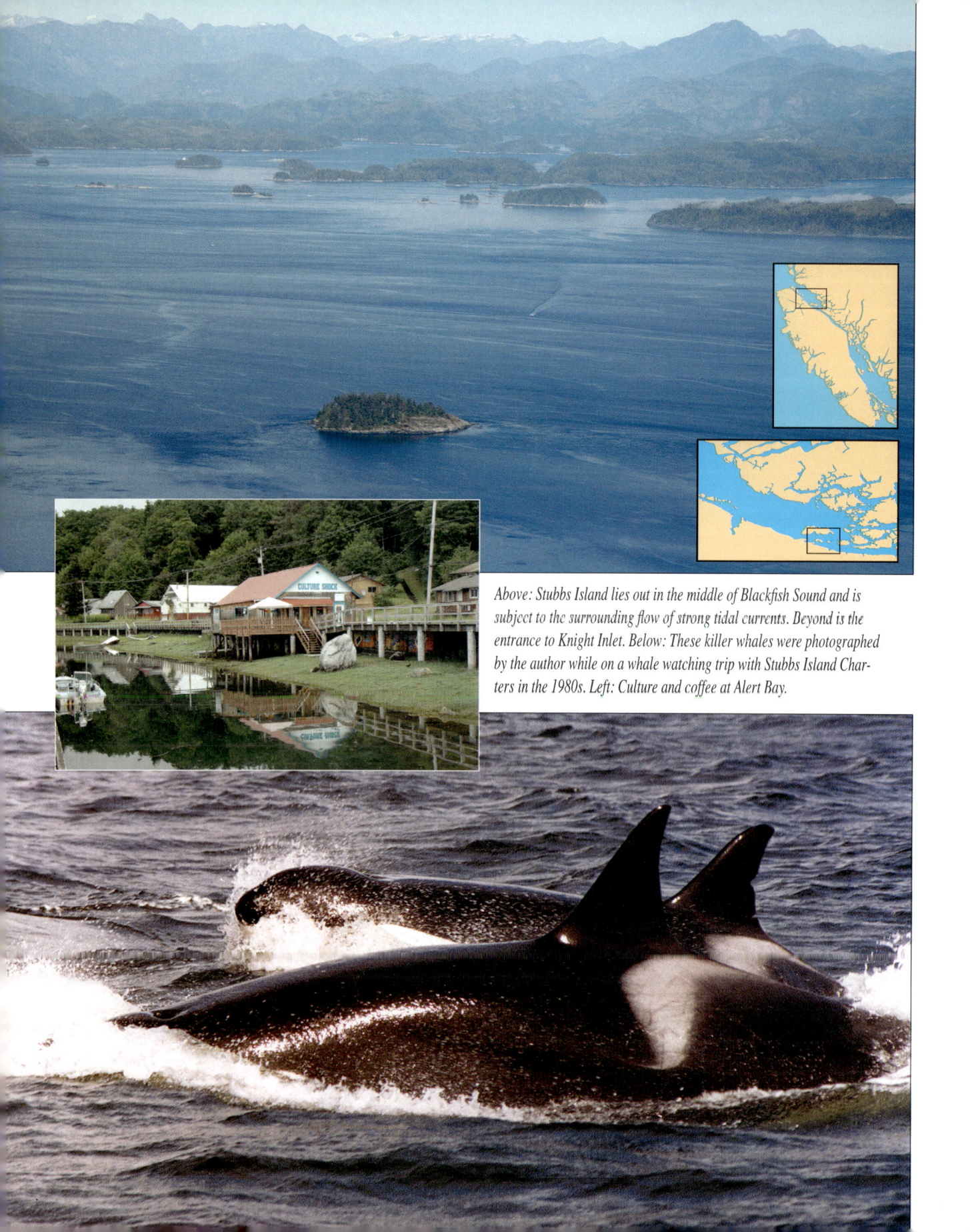

*Above: Stubbs Island lies out in the middle of Blackfish Sound and is subject to the surrounding flow of strong tidal currents. Beyond is the entrance to Knight Inlet. Below: These killer whales were photographed by the author while on a whale watching trip with Stubbs Island Charters in the 1980s. Left: Culture and coffee at Alert Bay.*

*Alert Bay was named for the Royal Naval vessel HMS Alert which conducted surveys in the area about 1860.*

N 50° 34.698'
W 126° 54.844'

*Looking north over Cormorant Island.*

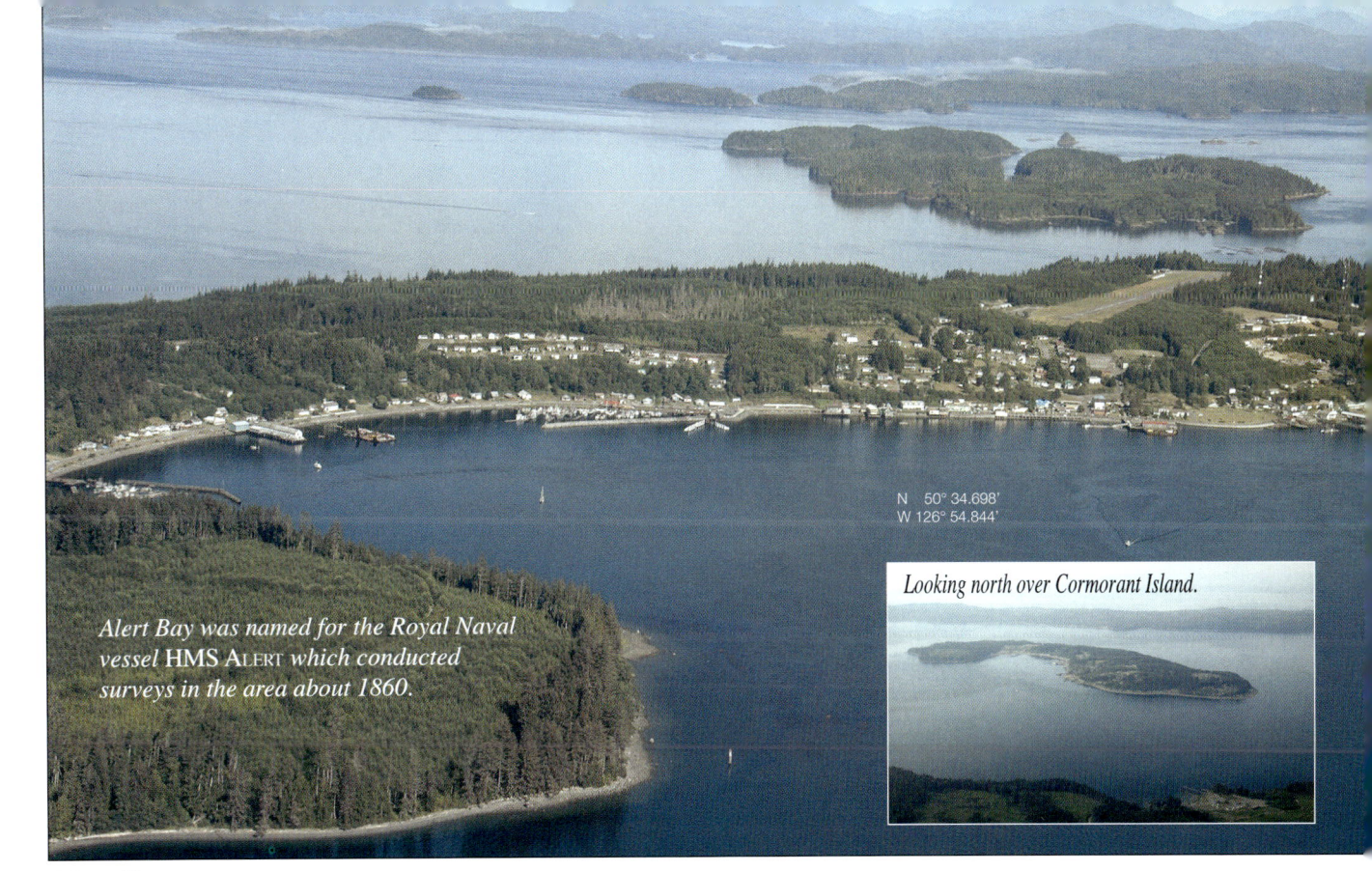

## Alert Bay  chart 3546

Alert Bay attracts mariners as a stop for replenishment and an opportunity to go ashore for some exercise as they travel on the way to points north, or south home again. For many, Alert Bay is a final destination on their northward travels.

It is a short distance, about 6 nautical miles, from Telegraph Cove to Alert Bay. You can travel in an almost straight line aimed at the southwestern tip of Cormorant Island from the entrance of Telegraph Cove, and you will arrive directly in Alert Bay. Be mindful of the shallow waters off the southeastern shore of Cormorant Island and of marine traffic in the area, especially if it's foggy and you are running only by GPS and compass. It would be beneficial to have radar if you are going to travel in fog.

The first dock you come to is a small public dock at the foot of a wharf at the south end of Alert Bay. Beyond that is the boat harbour adjacent to the ferry dock, and at the north end of the bay the docks of the U'mista Cultural Centre.

The *Sailing Directions* recommends using the traffic separation scheme in Broughton Strait. We have found this a good idea, particularly off Alert Bay and around Haddington Island where there are shoals lying adjacent to the passage and flood and ebb currents run at up to 4 knots in various directions. Ferries and slow moving tugs with long tows travelling eastbound face possible difficult navigation around the south side of Haddington Island because of the dogleg in the passage caused by Neill Ledge (see charts 3546, 3548). Vessels

*Top: Alert Bay showing the main harbour at centre of the photo. Note the large air strip. Bottom: U'mista Cultural Centre docks.*

entering this waterway sometimes will choose to take the opposing side of the channel for ease of manoeuvering.

Pleasure boat operators should be diligent, and considerate of commercial traffic. Keep to the north of Alert Rock and the light marking the northern extremity of Nimpkish Bank when travelling along Broughton Strait off Alert Bay.

There is a ferry service operating among the islands of Broughton Strait. The crossings are between Port McNeill on Vancouver Island, Alert Bay on Cormorant Island and Sointula on Malcolm Island. Although the routes are shown on the chart, due to the currents and the geography of the area the ferries may ply varying courses. Use the tide table predictions for Alert Bay.

If you enter Port McNeill you will not feel the effects of the tidal streams in Broughton Strait. The set is oblique

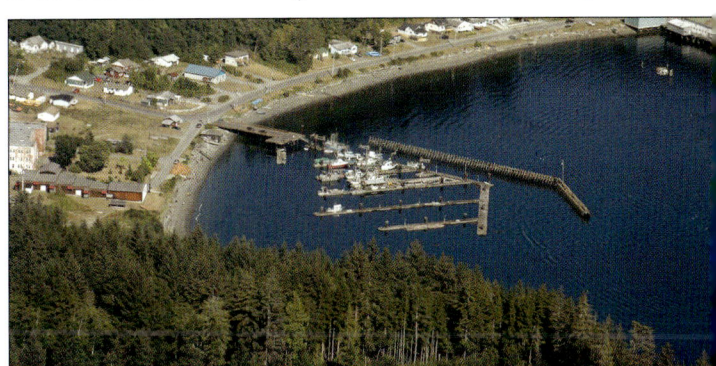

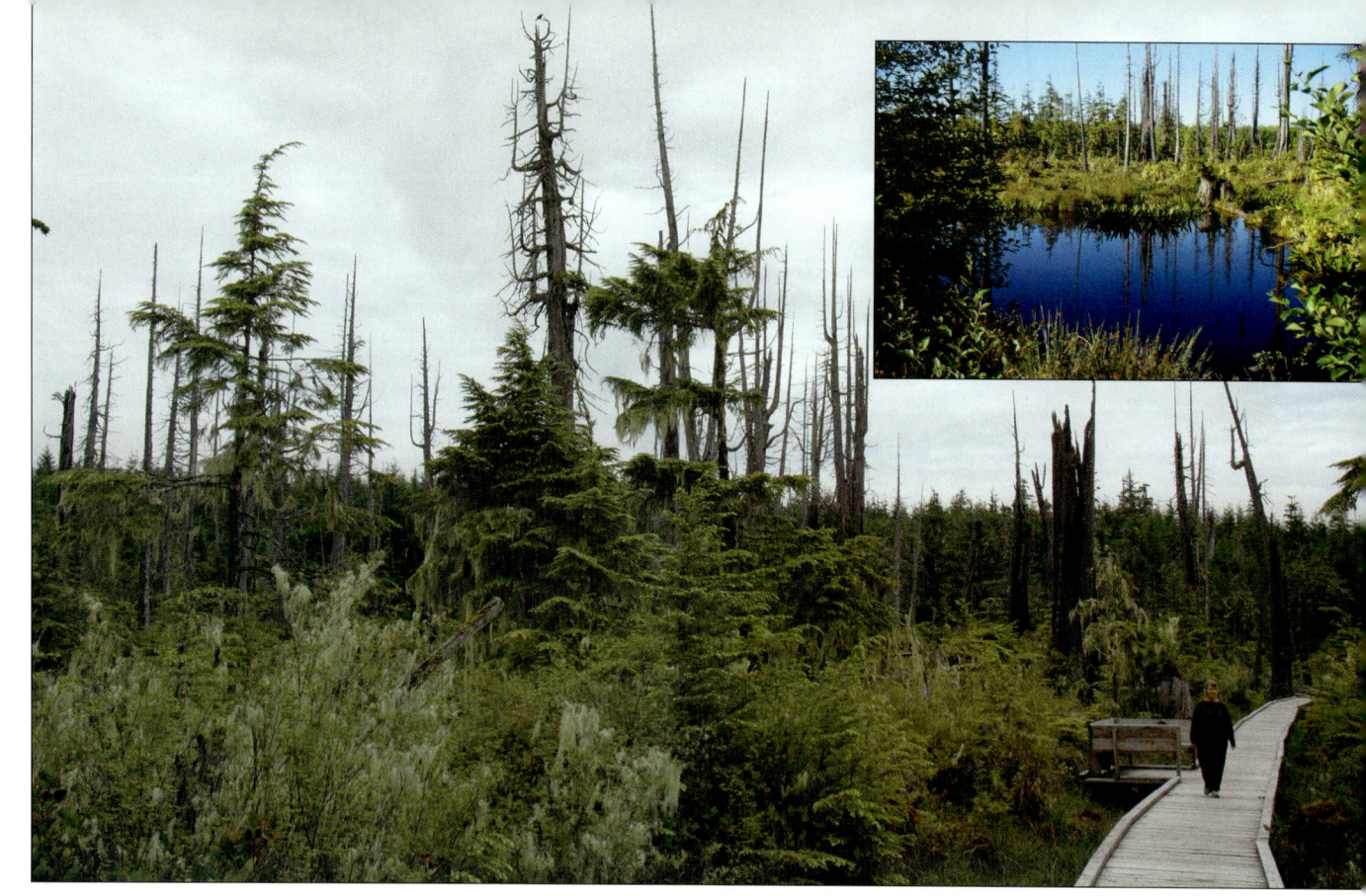

*Above. The Ecological Park at Alert Bay with its boardwalk, craggy trees and 'witches' hair' covered shrubbery.*

across Neill Ledge, says the *Sailing Directions*, and on a strong flood tide there is often a strong counter-current to the east of Alert Bay setting west along the south shores of the Pearse Islands.

Winds can be strong in the area but shelter is always available in Port McNeill, Alert Bay or Sointula. Dock facilities for pleasure craft are very good at Port McNeill, with a pick of docks at Alert Bay and more, spacious docks at Sointula.

In **Alert Bay** there are several choices for possible tie up. The small dock at the south end of the bay is suitable for one large or two or three smaller boats. It is rather exposed and not ideal for docking during strong 'Nimpkish' winds, which sweep across the bay from the Nimpkish Valley on Vancouver Island. But for a quick stop and a walk up to the nearest stores or across to view the totems at the 'Namgis' burial ground it will do. Visitors are asked to not trespass into the burial grounds.

We have used the south dock in the past when heading up the hill to the Ecological Park. This preserve, formerly known as Gator Gardens, has been embellished over the years since our earlier visits and now has a network of wooden pathways through the everglade-like shrubbery.

Cruising into the bay, beyond this dock, you will find the large Alert Bay harbour behind a breakwater. In the northern corner of the bay is another dock, sheltered by a breakwater in front of the U'mista Cultural Centre.

The Alert Bay Boat Harbour is the public dock where you are most likely to find moorage. The marina provides limited services but has shore power. Power plugs are 20 amp with an available 15 amp supply. This is primarily a fishing harbour so expect it to be busy with commercial vessels. Two fingers are allocated for pleasure craft use and chances are you will have to raft up. We have tied alongside fishing boats after verifying that they are not going to move before our planned departure. Fishermen generally do not object to having recreational boats raft up to them. Anchorage off Cormorant Island is in the north corner of Alert Bay.

From the harbour it is a short walk to the nearest shops and uptown facilities. Several restaurants in Alert Bay offer a variety of menus. There is a restaurant located almost opposite the south dock while a couple of others are closer to the centre of the village. A picturesque gift store and coffee shop, the Culture Shock, is on the new boardwalk, overlooking the public harbour, near the centre of town. It offers cultural experiences and instruction on cedar weaving, fish barbequeing and story telling.

The U'mista Cultural Centre is well worth a visit. Among the interesting items it has on display are repatriated artifacts, native coppers, ceremonial regalia and masks, and permanent exhibits of traditional ethnobiology of the Kwakwaka'wakw First Nations people.

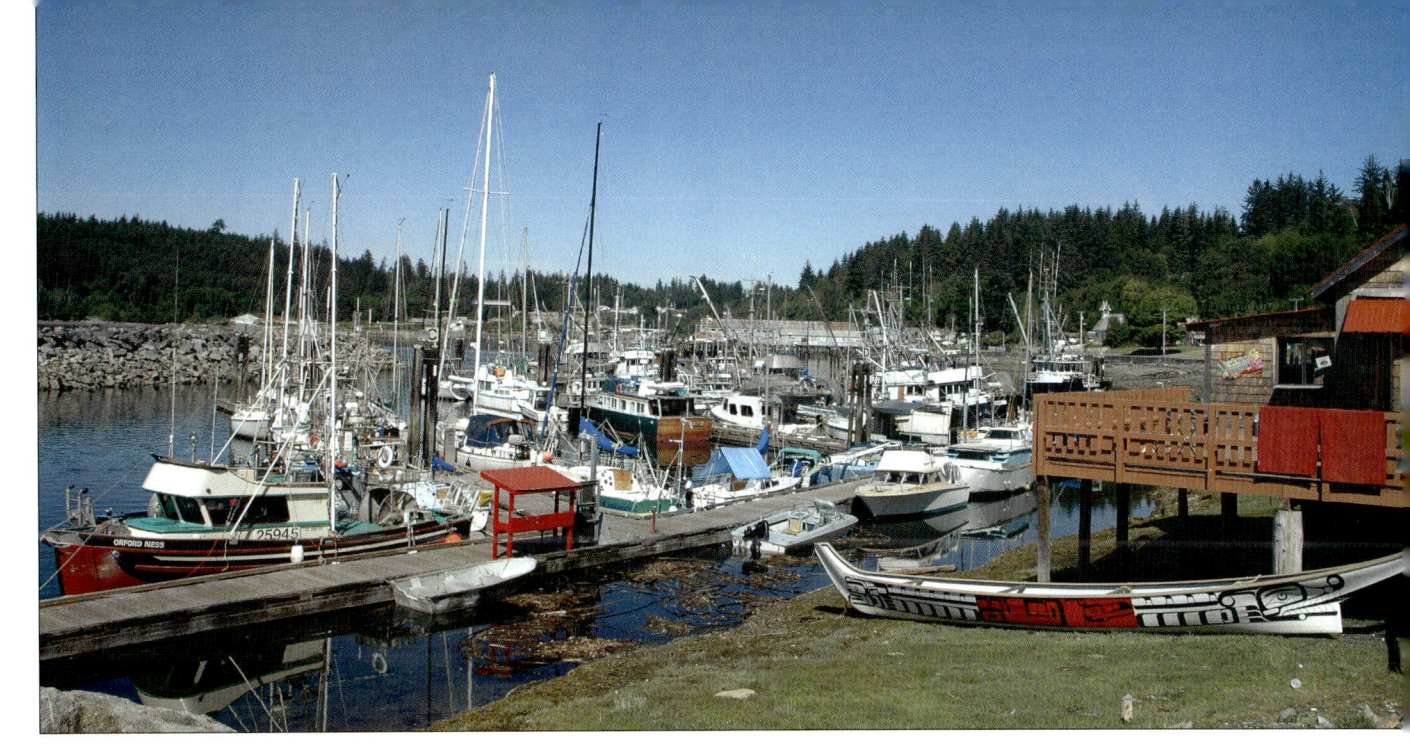

*Above:* Use the main harbour for protected overnight moorage. Many commercial vessels will be found tied up at this marina but rafting is allowed and there are often open spaces available. Check with the harbourmaster for directions to available moorage.
*Right:* A BC Ferry leaves a foggy Alert Bay for Port McNeill. *Below:* A wharf at the south end of the Alert Bay waterfront. This dock is exposed to Nimpkish winds coming in from Vancouver Island.

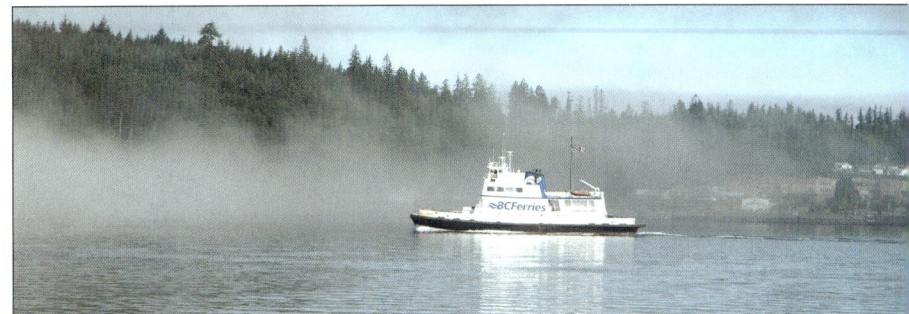

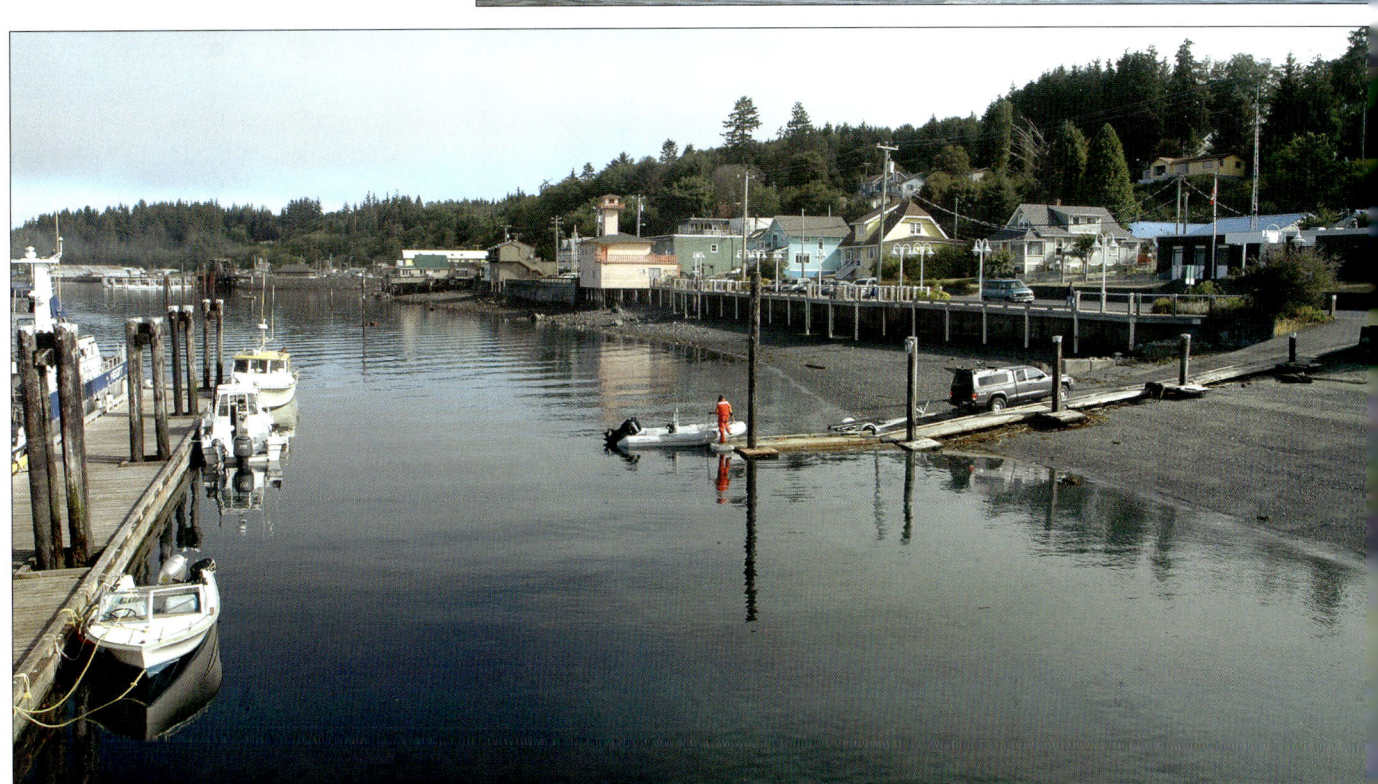

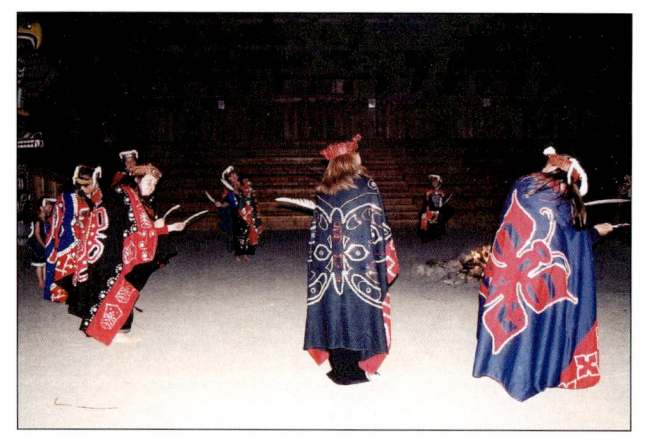

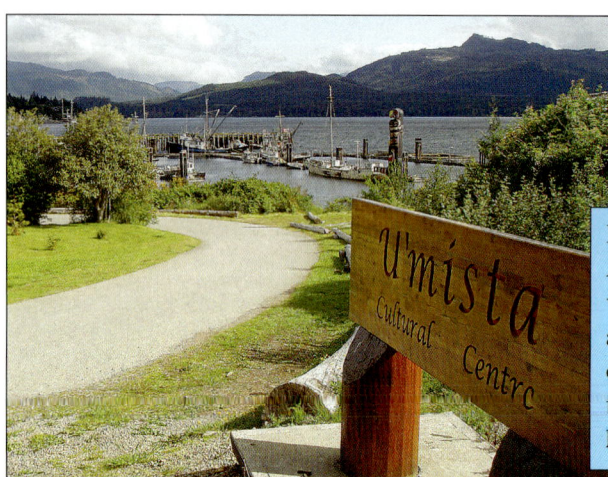

Bird watchers love Alert Bay for its many varieties of birds, and fishermen thrive on the good salmon fishing, particularly in late August.

*Top, left: The T'sasata Cultural Group performs Thursdays through Saturdays in summer, dancing in the Big House. Arrangements to view the dancing and the interior of the Big House should be made through the U'mista Cultural Centre. Above left: View of the marina at the Cultural Centre. Above right: The tallest totem pole in the world stands outside the Big House. Opposite page: The Alert Bay burial grounds near the east end of the village. Totems weather and fall and new ones are erected, a First Nations tradition allowing poles to return to nature. The old school building at Alert Bay is at bottom left.*

The Cultural Centre also houses segments of the exhibits that were shown at Expo '86 in Vancouver, and other interesting artifacts in the Potlatch Collection. There is a gift shop which exports and distributes First Nations art, carvings, silver and gold jewelry and other local products.

Alert Bay boasts the tallest totem pole in the world. It is 52 metres tall. You will find it next to the Big House a short walk up the hill behind the U'mista Cultural Centre.

Until fairly recently, we found that few people were aware of the existence of the ecological park at Alert Bay. However, with the amount of attention the area has been receiving lately it has become a favoured attraction for boaters and tourists.

The very name that it enjoyed in the earlier years, Gator Gardens, seems to indicate that this attraction is somewhat misplaced here in British Columbia. In name and character it is more like something you would expect to stumble across on a tour of Florida. It is a marshy, swampy glade complete with large still pools of water afloat with the massive leaves of various forms of vegetation, and sprouting large sprays of skunk cabbage. Wooden walkways have been erected across the park to allow access for easy walking and viewing.

The most prominent feature of the park is its incredible trees, which appear to have been struck by lightning at one time. These massive trees are broad and tall and mostly scarred and craggy with eerie looking branches, and cracks and splits appearing as though they were the inspiration for the tale of Sleepy Hollow. Three nature trails through the park provide viewing of bald eagles and crows. It is a paradise for bird-watchers and botanists. Cedar snags, hemlocks and pine trees draped with 'Witches Hair' moss give the park its eerie charm and beauty.

The park is located on top of the hill at the south side of Alert Bay. An easy walk to the Alert Bay campground from the public marinas takes you to the ecological park. The route begins in the village and ends up alongside or near the M.O.T transmitter station and the entrance to the park.

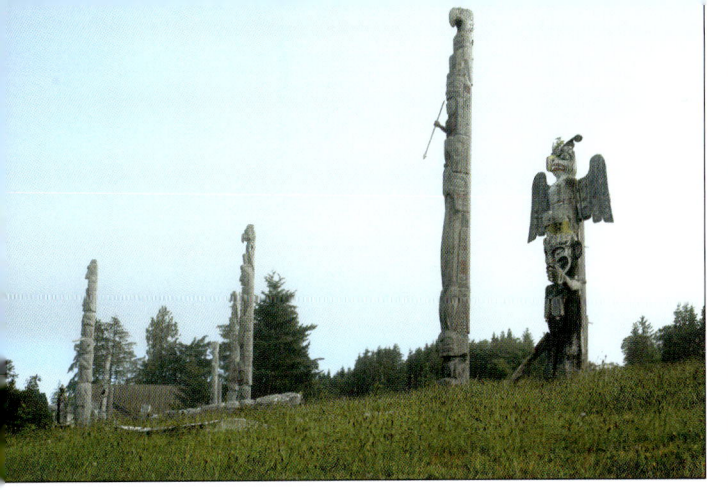

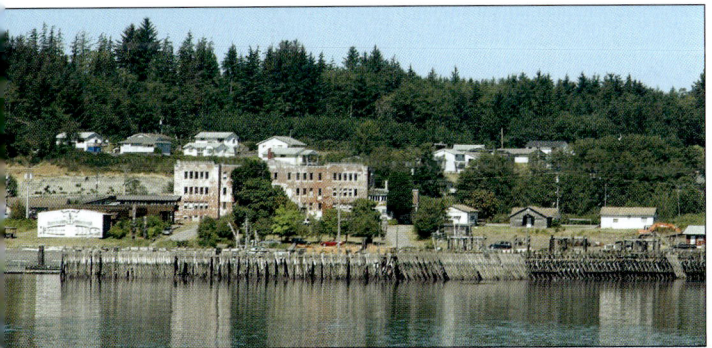

### Alert Bay public docks

Wharfinger 250-974-5727. Fax 250-974-5470.
*email: boatharbour@alertbay.ca. www.alertbay.ca*
At the main public dock there is 20 amp power. Water is available at the docks. There is no marine fuel at Alert Bay so supplies should be taken on at Port McNeill, Echo Bay, Lagoon Cove, Port Hardy or Sullivan Bay. Most services are available at the village of Alert Bay including rustic hotels, restaurants, grocery and hardware stores, books, charts, produce and credit union bank machine and ferry service between Alert Bay, Port McNeill and Sointula.
The Alert Bay Visitor Centre can be reached at 250-974-5024. email: info@alertbay.ca

> ## U'mista Cultural Centre:
> PO Box 253 Alert Bay, BC. V0N 1A0.
> Phone 250-974-5403.
> *email: info@umista.ca   www.umista.org*
> It is open to the public throughout summer all week from 9 am to 5 pm and in winter, weekdays only, 9-5.
> Regular scheduled flights to or from Port Hardy, Campbell River, Vancouver and Seattle are available at Port McNeill. BC Ferries runs Port McNeill–Alert Bay.
> Alert Bay is serviced by a paved 870 metre foot airstrip.

You may be lucky when visiting Alert Bay and experience some calm, sunny weather. If not, watch the currents and sea conditions that sweep around the northern channel on the way to Port Hardy or the open northern reaches of Johnstone Strait. In windy conditions it is usually possible to sneak around the south end of Cormorant Island and through the rock-lined channels and islets in the area of Weynton Passage.

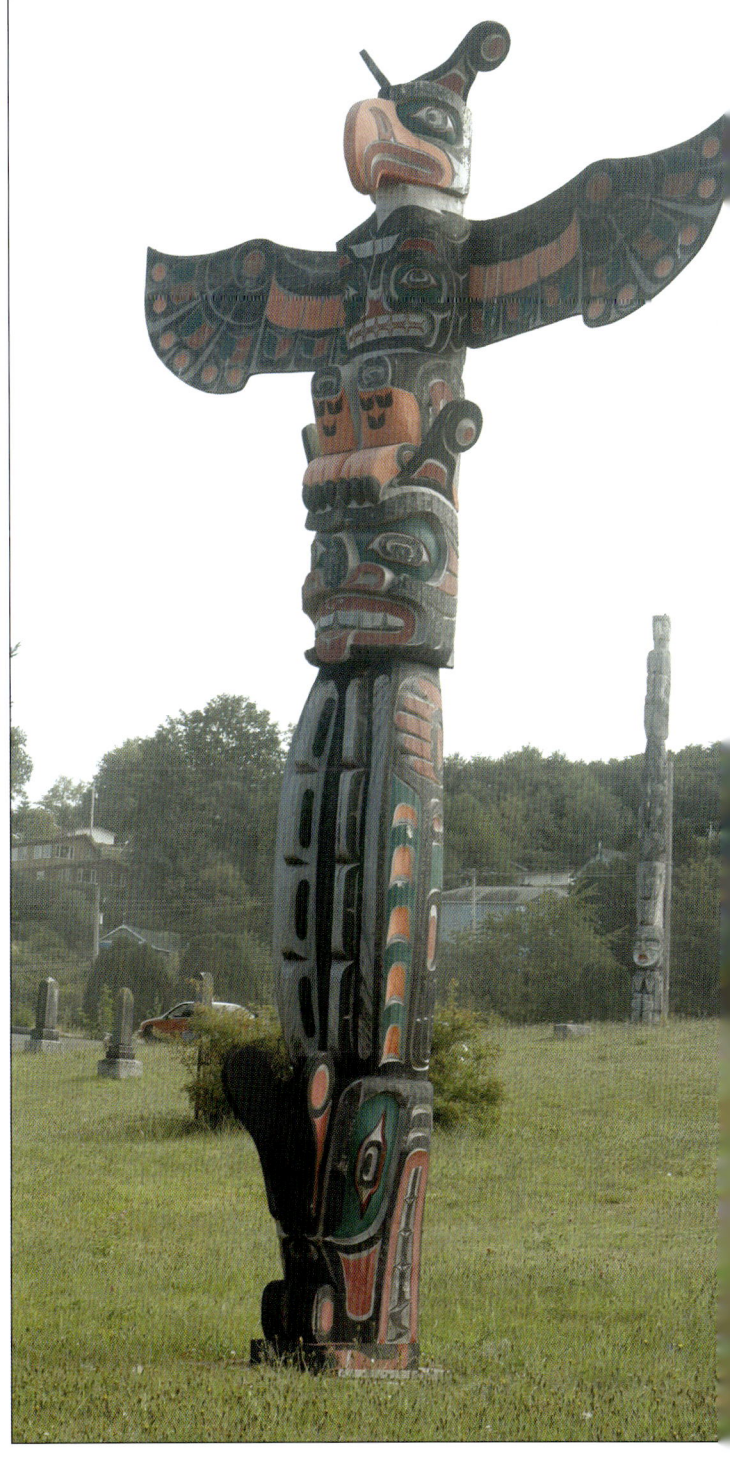

We once took shelter for two days in the Plumper Islands while the wind raged. However, the gap between the two islands where we stopped, is not always a suitable anchorage for more than a temporary stay because the current rips through quite fast, especially at high tides (see page 108).

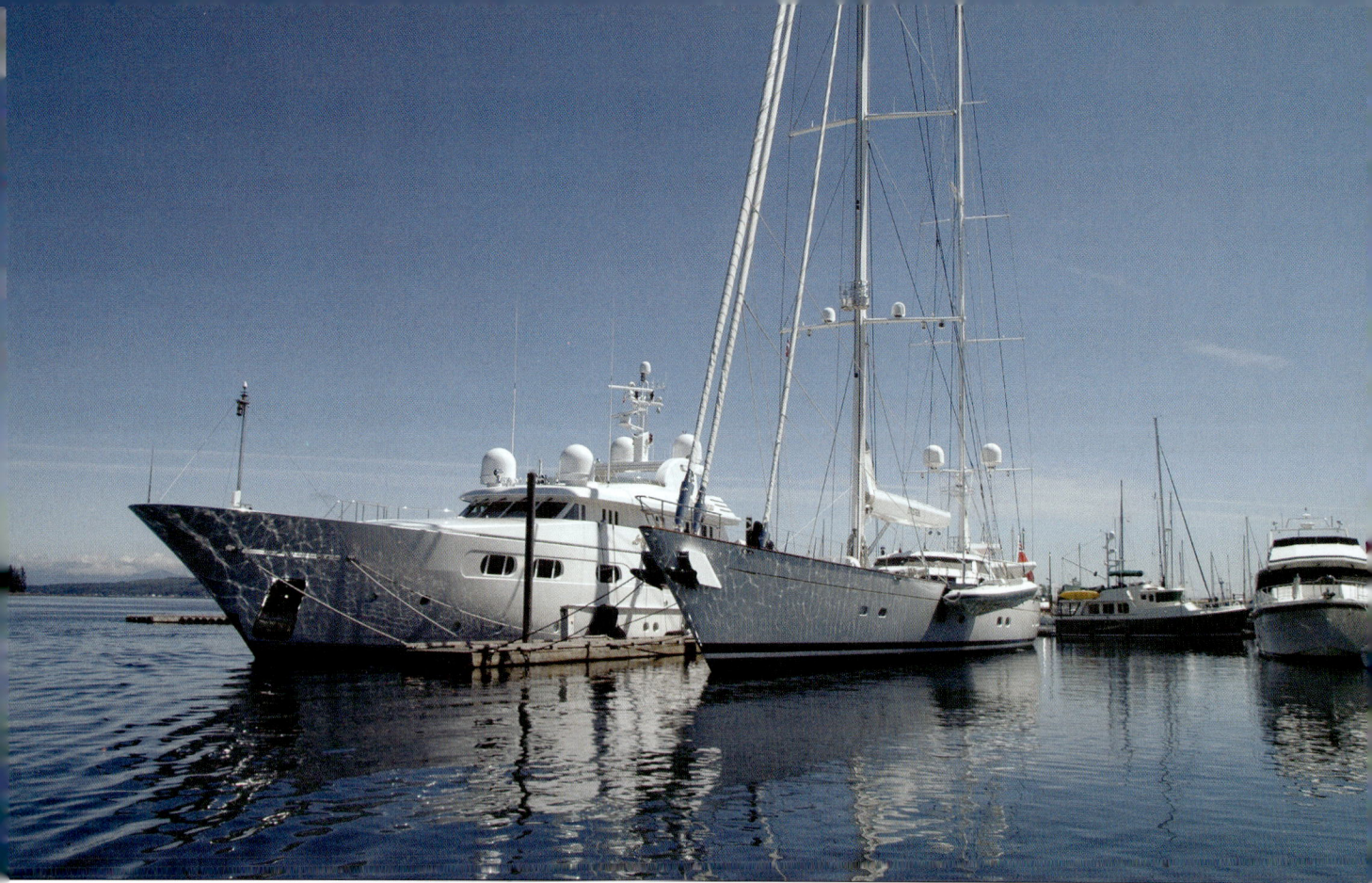

*Above: Large vessels are catered to at the Port McNeill Fuel Dock and Marina. Overleaf: The waterfront at Port McNeill—photo courtesy of Steve Jackman.*

## The Port McNeill Fuel Dock and Marina

PO Box 488, 1488 Beach, Port McNeil BC V0N 2R0
Phone 250-902-8128 or 250-956-4044
*email: sjackman@portmcneill.com*
*www.portmcneill.com*

This facility has been, for many years, the well-known fuel dock at Port McNeill, serving the marine and aviation industry. It has expanded in recent years to offer increasing amounts of dock space for transient vessels. It is a popular stop for gas, diesel, avgas and propane. Power at the dock is available in 100, 50 (120/208v), 30 and 20 amps. Water is available at the docks. Free computer use is available at the laundry.

The Mackay Whale Watching charter boat loads at this dock for whale and bear watching. Also for scuba diving and other watersports activities.

Grizzly Helicopters and Pacific Coastal Airlines are stationed here and offer services to the logging industry, Broughton Islands residents and the tourism sector. The local launch ramp is located at the head of the dock. There is a well-stocked hardware store at the marina and a marine store nearby. Uptown Port McNeill has restaurants, grocery stores, gift shops, hotels and a variety of service stores.

Information Centre 250-956-3111

## Port McNeill Boat Harbour

PO Box 1389, Port McNeil BC V0N 2R0
Ph 250-956-3881  Fax 250-956-2897
*email: pmharbour@telus.net   www.portmcneillharbour.ca*

Power at the dock is 100, 50, 30 and 20 amps. Water is available at the public docks plus sewage pumpout. showers, laundry and washrooms. The marina accepts garbage and oil for disposal. The marina has a calm-water loading dock. Bear and whale watching excursions are available with Mackay Whale Watching. Adjacent is the ferry terminal for Alert Bay and Sointula. Regular scheduled Pacific Coastal Airlines flights to Port Hardy, Campbell River, Vancouver, Seattle.

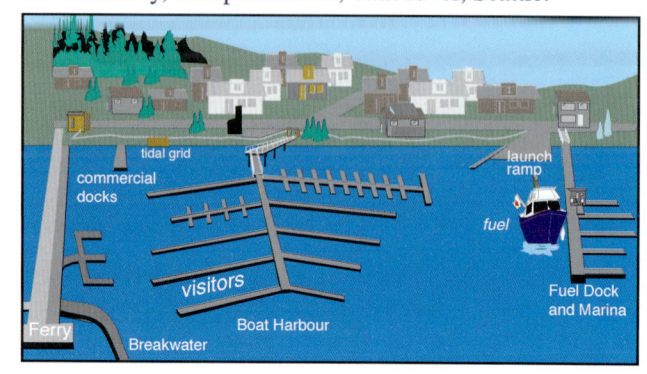

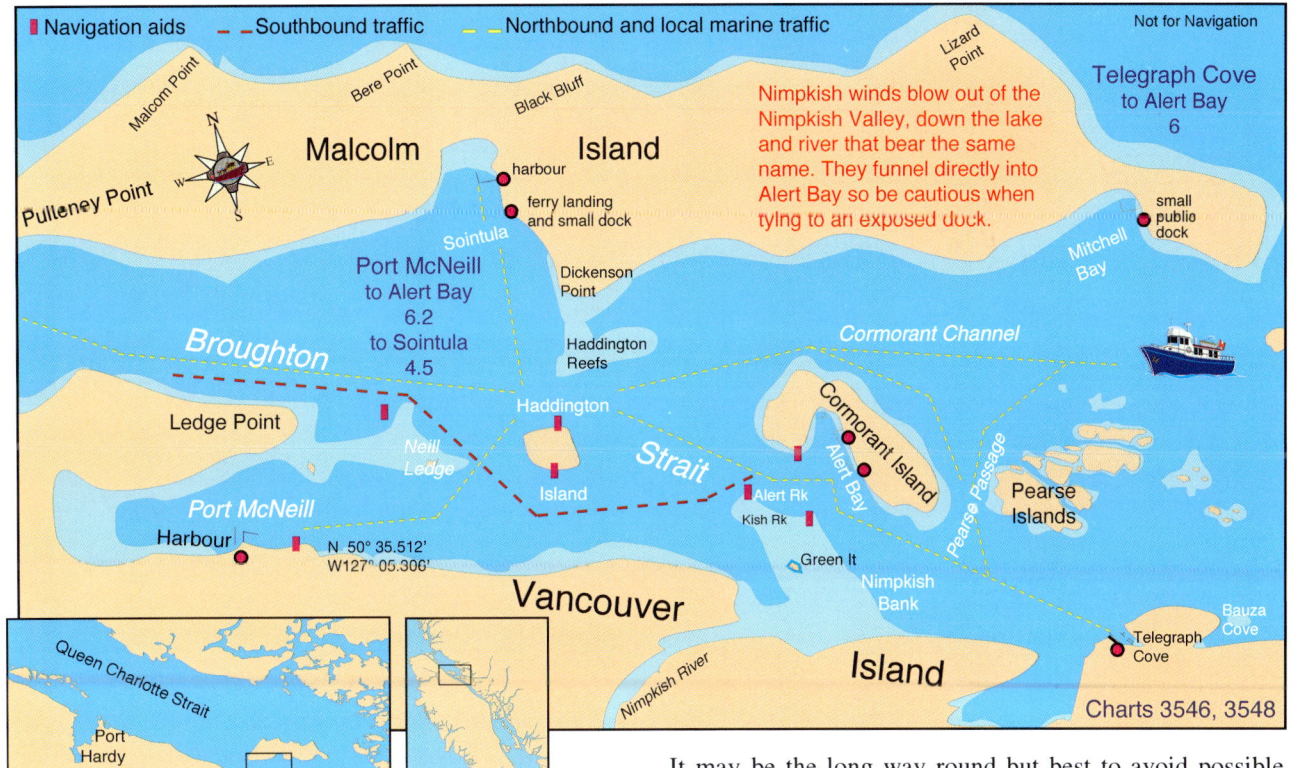

## Port McNeill chart 3546

It is an easy run from Alert Bay to Port McNeill. The waters are generally protected although windy conditions can lump up the seas in Broughton Strait. Out of Alert Bay the ebbing tide drains from the north part of the bay or floods in around Yellow Bluff and off down Broughton Strait. These currents are normally no stronger than 3 knots, so make your way westward towards the wide mouth of Port McNeill.

As stated earlier, there is a traffic separation system in place around Haddington Island. You are supposed to use the system even in a pleasure craft, although when there are no large vessels or tugs encumbered by a tow you may see some boats run opposite the traffic direction. If there are any vessels approaching Haddington Island you are obliged to pass north of it in Haddington Passage, being mindful of Haddington Reefs, and cross the traffic separation lane at right angles. All the reefs and shoals are well marked with buoys. Travel towards the Vancouver Island shore keeping clear of the buoyed rock off the west shore of Haddington Island and of Neill Ledge off Ledge Point. Travelling eastbound simply use the south route off Haddington Island.

Coming into Port McNeill from the north do not be tempted to cross Neill Ledge unless you know the waters very well. We always travel up to Haddington Island and cut past the reef marker on the west side then turn into the port only when well abeam of the centre of it. It may be the long way round but best to avoid possible danger of running aground. However, there is adequate water for those who know the way through. By keeping clear of Neill Ledge and other shallow spots you can avoid serious turbulence on the surface, particularly when it is windy over water against the tidal flow. Enter Port McNeill and proceed at leisure to one of the marinas berthing mostly pleasure craft, behind the breakwater.

The port has seen a big increase in recreational marine traffic in recent years since its docks and waterfront were enhanced. Vessels cruising to and from Alaska frequently use it as a provisioning and fueling stop. The fuel dock marina at Port McNeill has been built to accommodate larger yachts. If the marinas are busy and there is inadequate room to accommodate your vessel anchor across the bay in the lee of Ledge Point and commute to the docks by dinghy.

Grizzly Helicopters, West Coast Helicopters, and Pacific Coastal Airlines offer scenic flights to the local villages and settlements in the islands. This is also an alternative and appealing means of seeing those places as a side trip from the air while cruising in the area. Port McNeill has a number of restaurants and the most convenient of them are located on the waterfront. These include the Sportsman Steak and Pizza and Gus's Pub offering mediterranean dishes. The McNeill Inn features more standard fare. One particularly fine restaurant is at the Haida Way Motor Inn at the top end of town. Here the Northern Lights restaurant serves up some scrumptious seafood dishes and has a wide variety of other foods ranging from hamburgers to dietary delights.

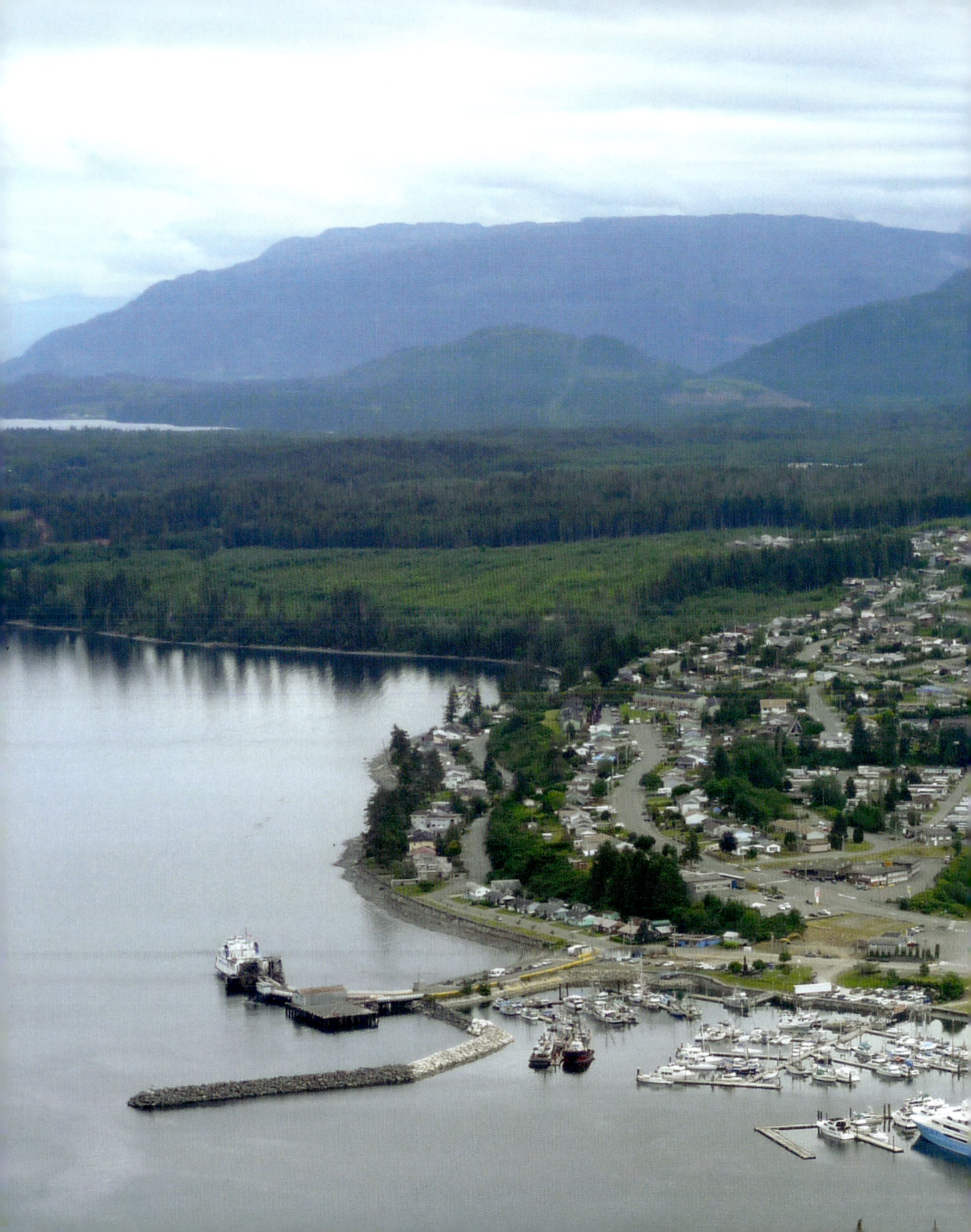

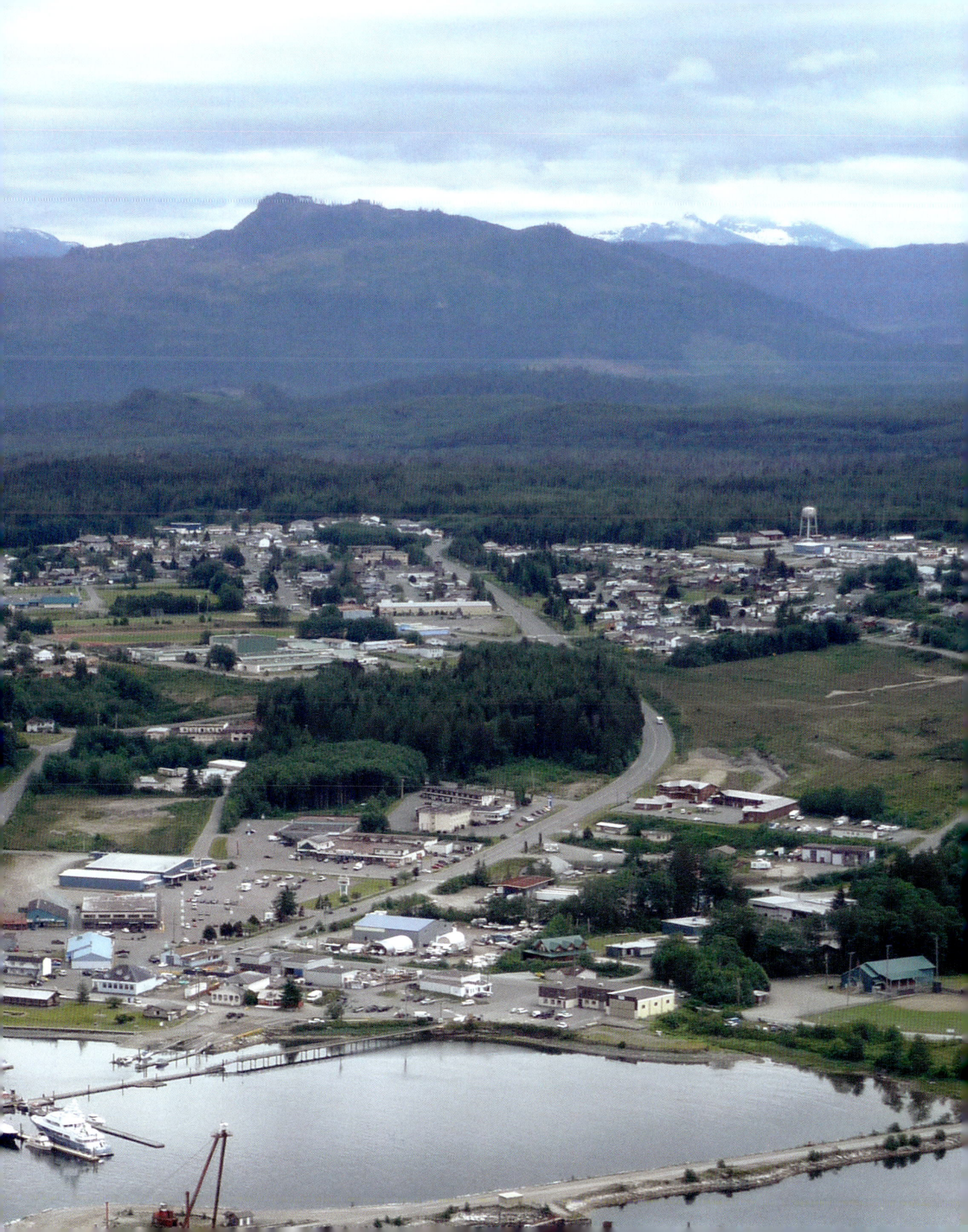

**Charts 3546, 3548**

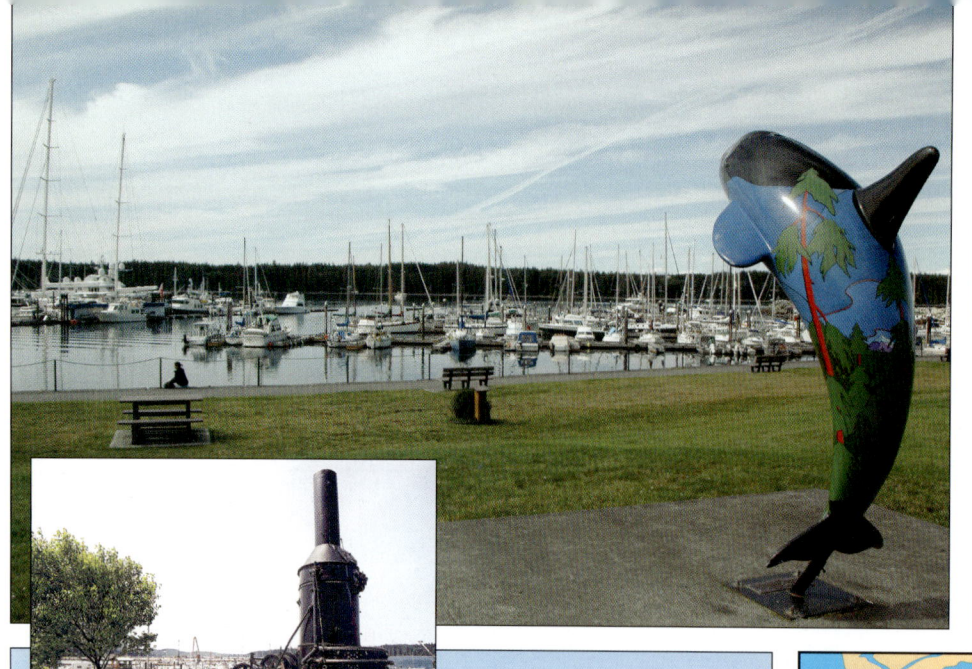

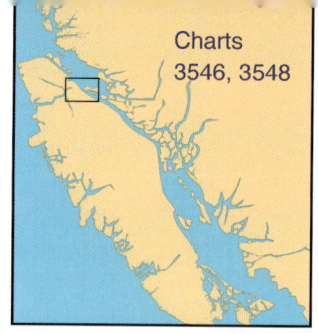

Port McNeill was founded as a logging camp, originally referred to as Dickie's Camp before it grew into a town. Then it was named for Captain Willaim McNeill of the Hudson's Bay Company.

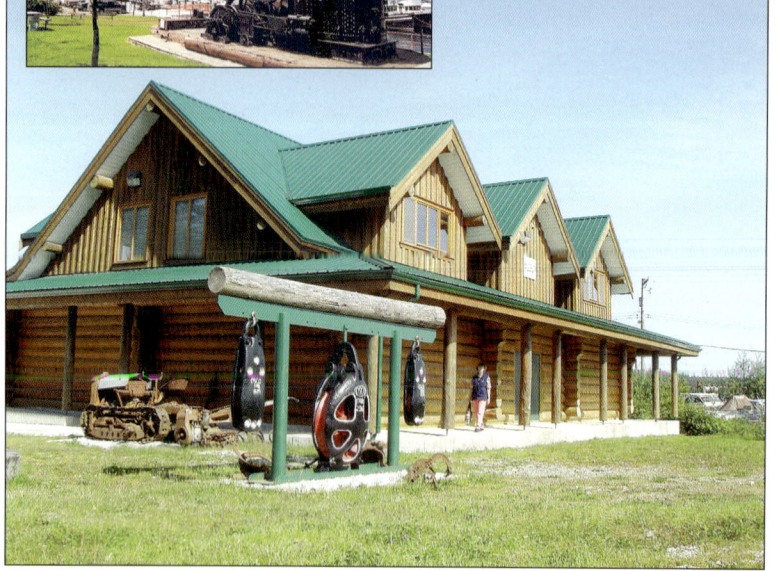

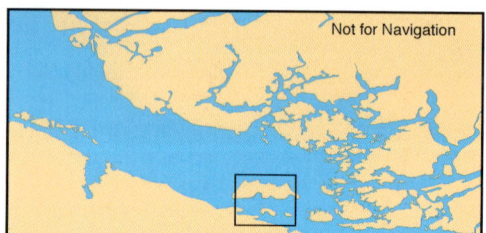

Not for Navigation

*Top: Overlooking the marina at Port McNeill. The inset steam donkey was used at Huaskin Lake until replaced by diesel. Left: The museum and tourism offices in Port McNeill. Bottom: A John Horton painting of Bruce and Nancy Jackman's boat at anchor in the Broughton Islands. The Jackmans are the owners of the fuel dock and marina and adjacent hardware store at Port McNeill.*
*Below: Port McNeill taxi, the way to reach the airport. For an interesting road trip, rent a car and drive to Fort Rupert and Port Hardy if you are not planning to stop there by boat. Along the way take in the world's largest burl, a 350-year-old giant of 22 tons. The First Nations village of Fort Rupert is a thriving art centre (page 227).*

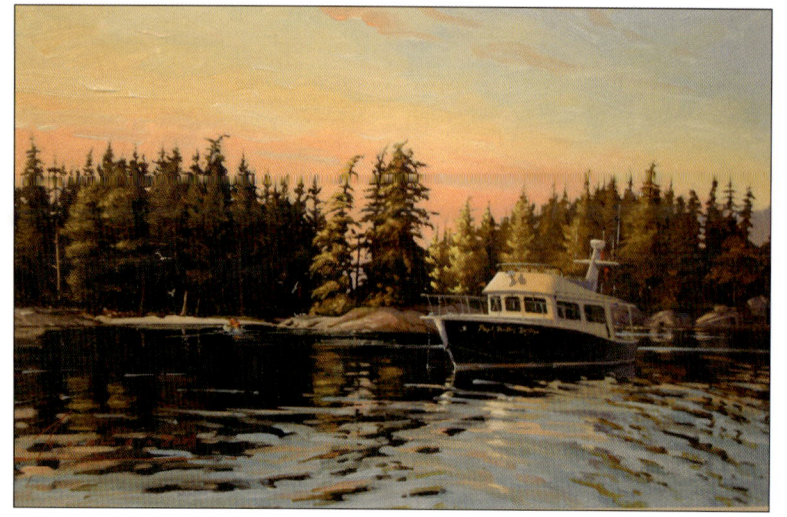

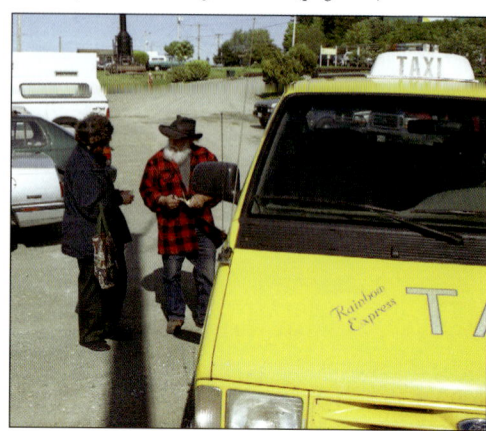

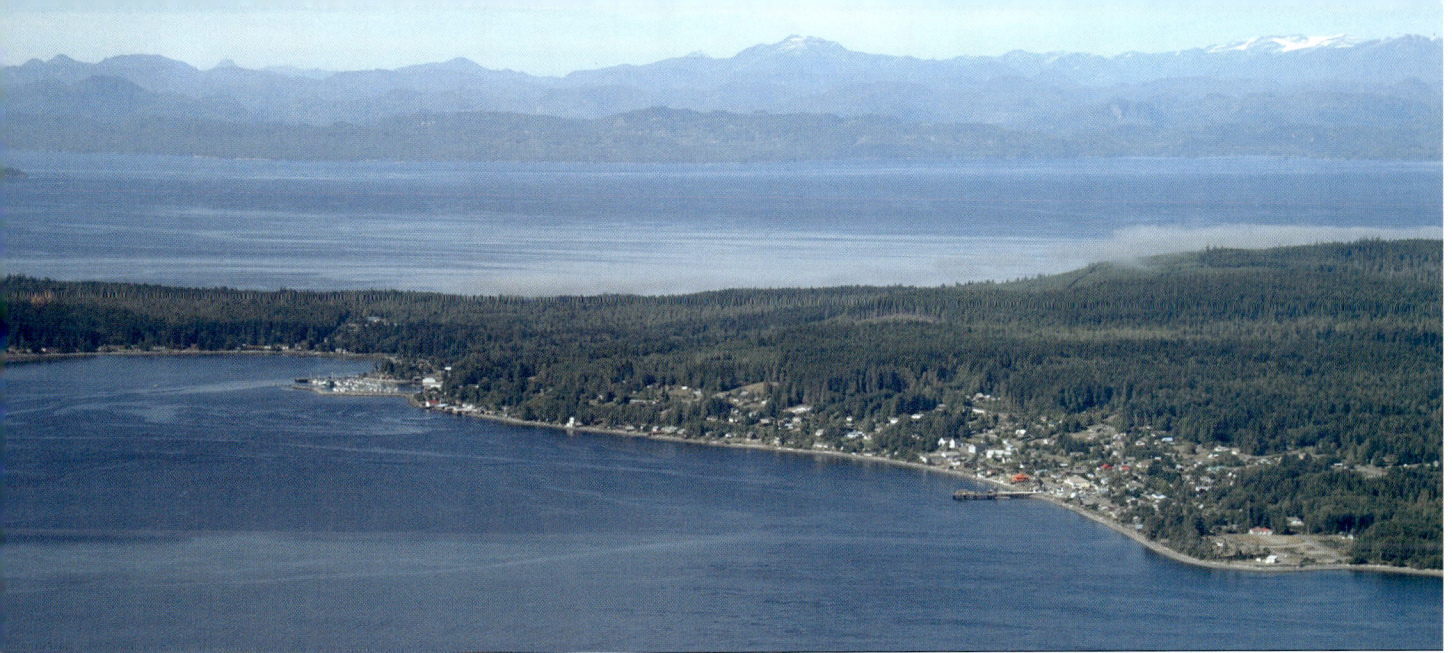

*Sointula Harbour on Malcolm Island.*

## Malcolm Island  chart 3546

Malcolm Island sits like a massive breakwater to the north of Cormorant Island. In 1900 Finnish settlers arrived at Malcolm Island as part of a colonization effort. They were there to fish, log and farm, but in about five years the settlement was disbanded as a company, which by then had been taken over by the Sointula Co-op that still exists today with only a few of the descendants occupying the island, along with the inevitable newcomers. The name Sointula means 'Harmony' in Finnish.

Malcolm Island does not offer much in the way of protective shelter for mariners other than the large harbour at Rough Bay. We always enjoyed the time spent at Rough Bay, which lies about a mile northwest of the settlement of Sointula. The *Sailing Directions* suggests small craft anchorage can be obtained a short distance southwest of the breakwater light in about 13 to 18 metres. That is relatively open water and should be used as an anchorage only if weather permits. The bay dries extensively at low tide, so check depths carefully.

Pleasure boat owners looking for recreational craft facilities and amenities will find these at Rough Bay public harbour. Enter at the north end of the bay. The marina is protected by a substantial breakwater. If the fishing fleet is out you will find many empty slips. The harbour manager, Lorraine Williams, runs the facility efficiently. A hamburger stand is located alongside her office. If you want the use of laundry, showers and washrooms tie up at the dock to the north after entering past the breakwater. Visitors are invited to tie up at either north or south docks.

The harbour has been dredged to a depth of 3 metres. Its floats range from 60 to 116 metres in length. There are two sections to the marina, one to the north and the other to south as you enter beyond the breakwater. The two sets of docks do not

## Sointula Harbour
## Malcolm Island Lions Harbour Authority

Harbour Office PO Box 202,
Sointula BC. V0N 3E0   Ph/Fax 250-973-6544
email: milha@cablerocket.com   www.sointulainfo.ca
Tourism Association phone 250-973-2001.

This harbour has all typical public dock amenities: power is 30 and 20 amp; water is available at the docks as well as laundry, showers and washrooms. There is a farmers market in summer. Try one of the burgers or the fish and chips at the Burger Barn. A nearby shipyard offers haul outs and boat repairs. Nearby there are B&Bs and a stroll into Sointula will take you to the museum, bakery, Sointula Gallery and Bistro—dock alongside ferry landing in calm conditions (or call 250-974-7172 for service to boat or a ride from marina). Free use of wifi and computer in store. Bicycles are available at the marina for free use riding to the stores and eateries. Nearby co-op hardware and general store and bank machine. Other services are available at Port McNeill or Alert Bay.

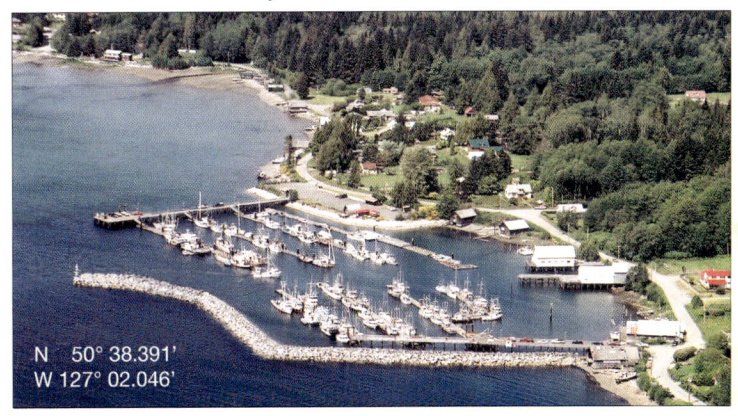

N  50° 38.391'
W 127° 02.046'

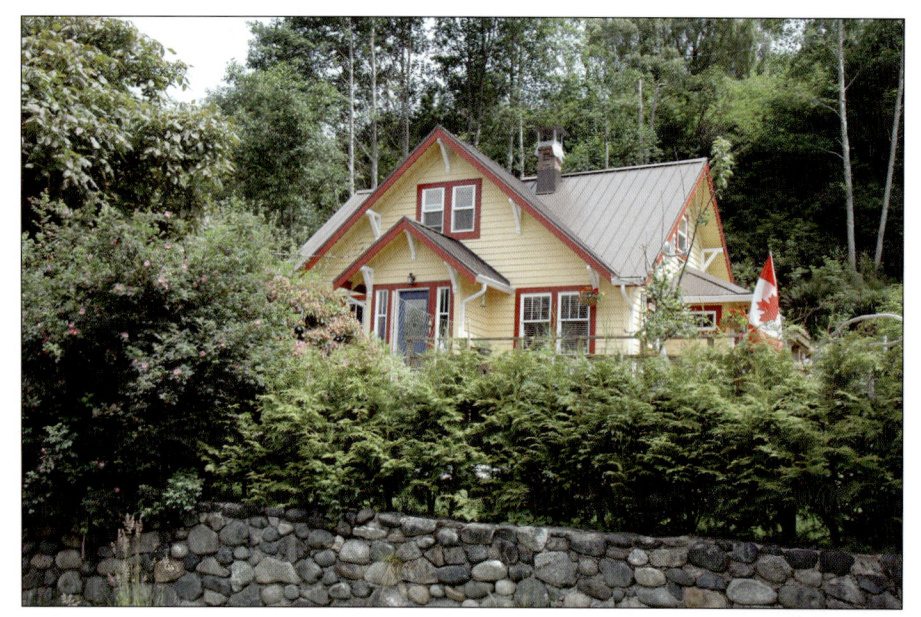

*Left: A walk or bicycle ride into Sointula from the harbour will provide an opportunity to view some of the charming houses and possibly meet up with local artists and other residents. This is one of the picturesque houses seen in the village.*
*Below, left: The Burger Shack at the harbour is known for its burgers and fish and chips. It has a take out window and a separate building overlooking the harbour for patrons to sit out of the rain or sun.*
*Below: A visit to the local museum near the ferry landing is worthwhile.*

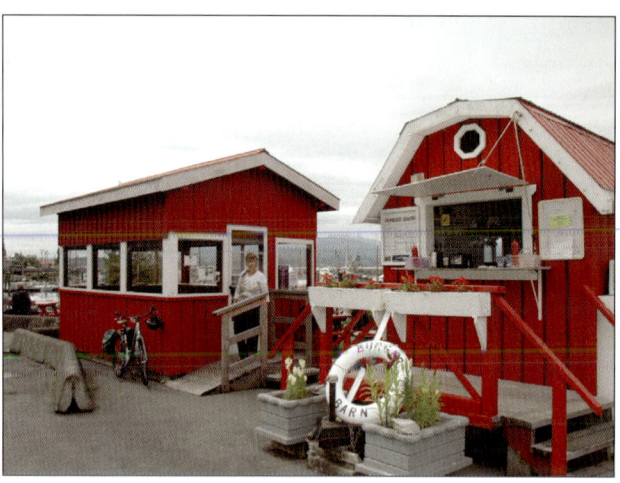

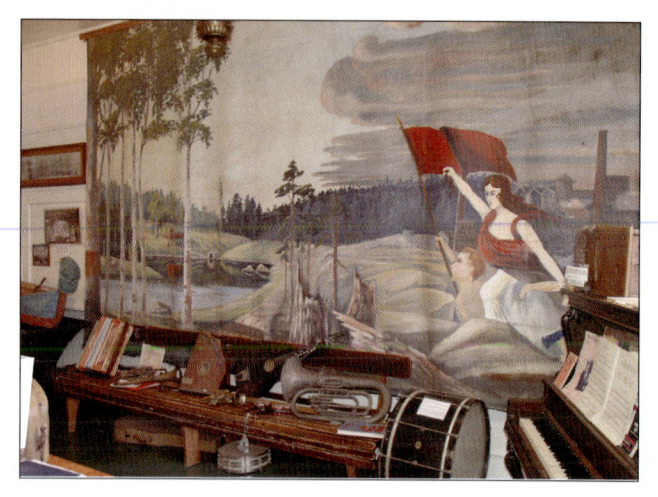

connect other than by land. The docks to the south have fewer amenities but are a shade closer to Sointula. Facilities for boat maintenance include oil and garbage disposal and recycling.

We docked and walked ashore to visit the hardware store at the head of the wharf. As you walk to the town note the quaint houses and properties, the art and craft galleries and other character homes all lending to the charm of the place.

The shipyard frequently has boats on the ways, with their bows almost hanging right over the main road. About a mile down the road there is a co-op food store at the village of Sointula. Opposite the co-op there is a public wharf and ferry landing where brief stops are possible in small to medium size boats. At the head of the ferry dock there is bistro and gallery and a bakery as well as the island's tourism office.

A prominent building in Sointula is the museum, where you can learn about the people and history of the island. It is located at the north end of the village, and worth the stop.

On the far side of the island, poking into Queen Charlotte Strait is Bere Point which is the location of the island's campgrounds. There is a walking trail to Bere Point and another to the water tower from the museum. Walking along the shore it is possible to see whales rubbing on the beaches during their regular migrations through the area.

Charter floatplanes fly in and out of Sointula frequently and therefore the adjacent waters are designated a water aerodrome. Watch for the coming and going of float planes and also of the ferry from Alert Bay and Port McNeill.

The Haddington Reefs run out into Haddington Passage from Dickenson Point (page 219) at the central south tip of Malcolm Island. These present a considerable hazard to navigation and mariners are advised to give them a wide berth.

**Mitchell Bay** lies at the east end of Malcolm Island. It has a public dock with a 113 foot float that is used mostly by local boat owners, usually with commercial craft.

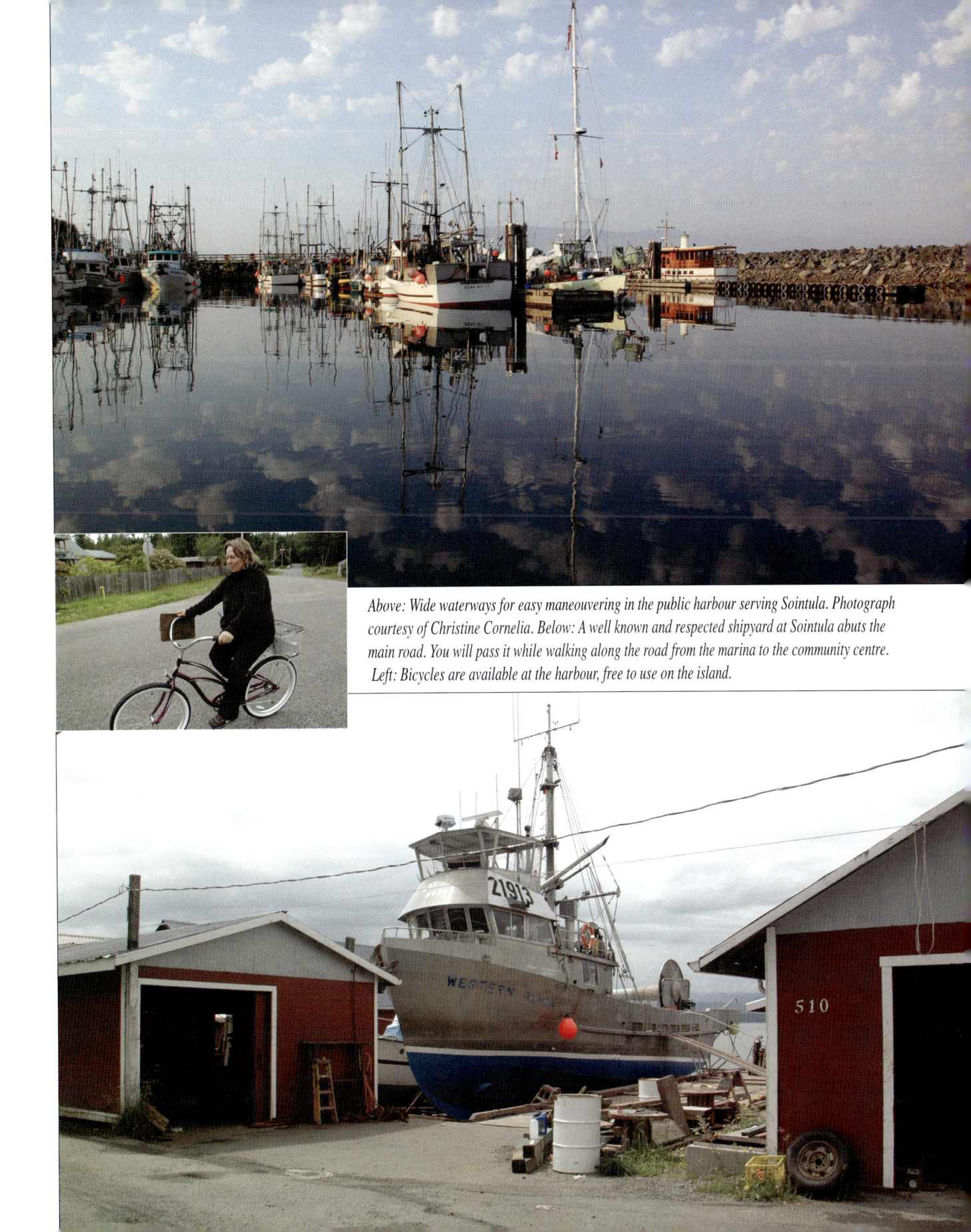

*Above: Wide waterways for easy maneouvering in the public harbour serving Sointula. Photograph courtesy of Christine Cornelia. Below: A well known and respected shipyard at Sointula abuts the main road. You will pass it while walking along the road from the marina to the community centre. Left: Bicycles are available at the harbour, free to use on the island.*

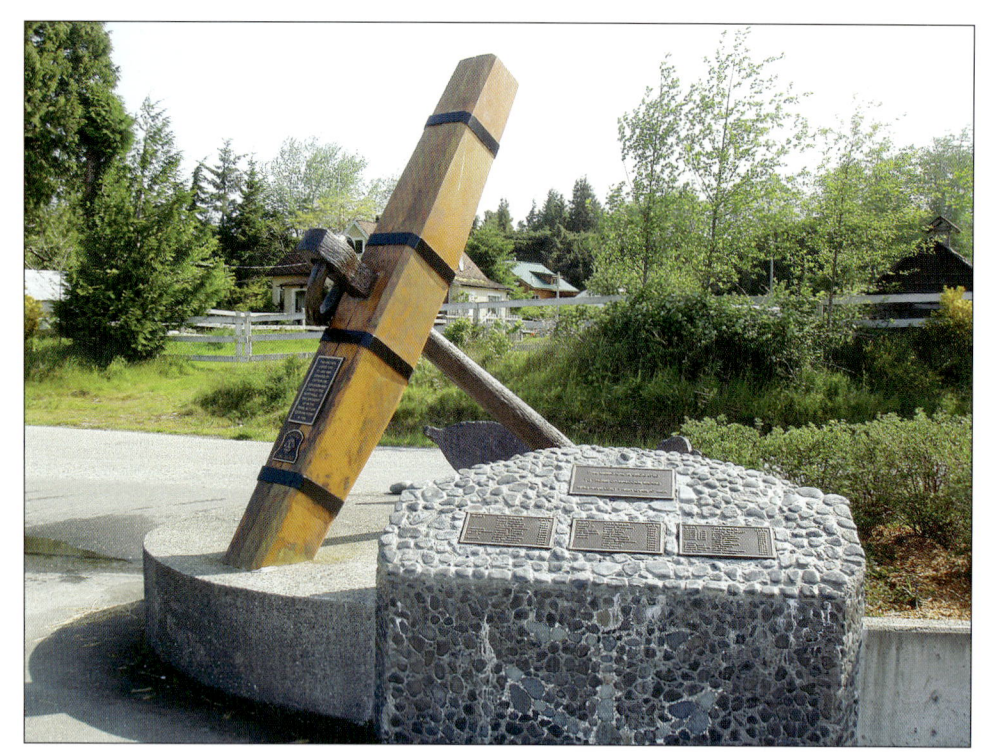

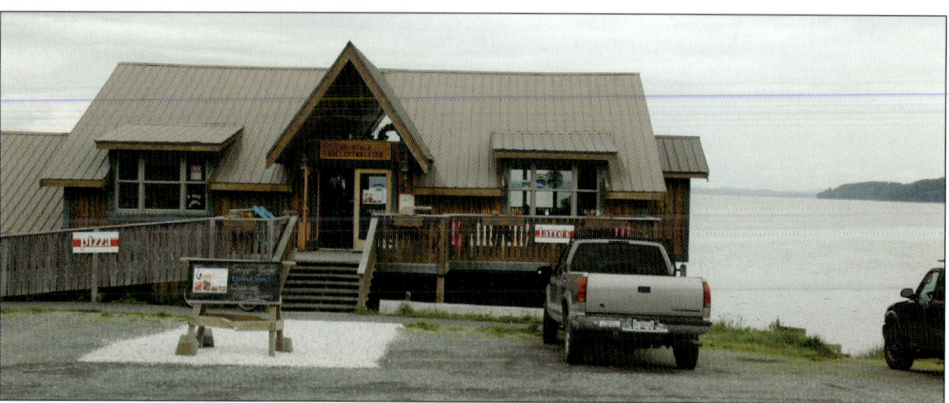

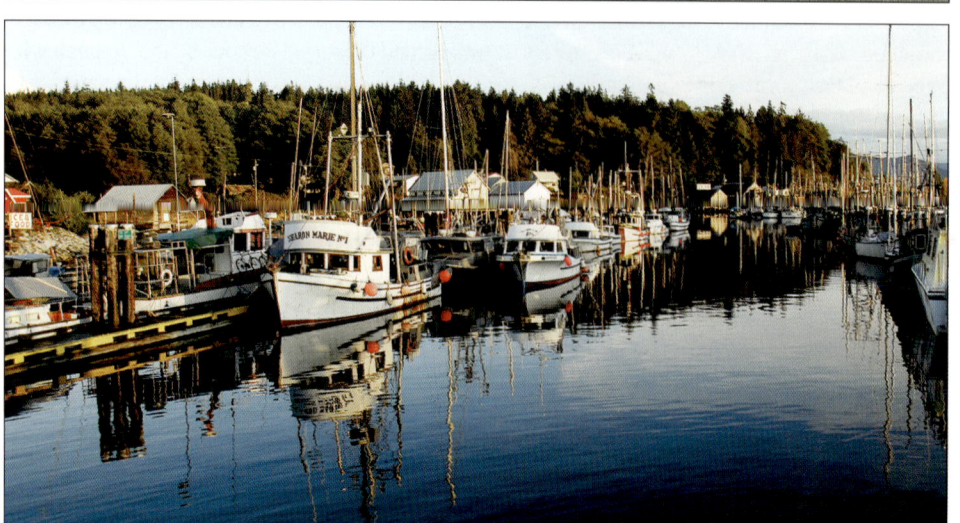

*Left: This anchor is set into concrete as part of the Fishermen's Memorial at Sointula. It was pulled up by a Sointula fisherman in fishing nets off Estevan Point on the west coast of Vancouver Island and is believed to be from one of Captain Cook's ships.*

*Below: Carla with Deb Wiggins of the local tourism office and artist at Sointula Bistro and Gallery.*

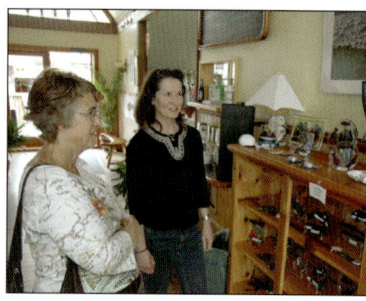

*Centre, left: The restaurant at the ferry terminal in Sointula serves meals and has a gallery as well as available internet.*

*Bottom: View of the harbour at Sointula. The north docks are closer to the marina facilities than the south docks. However, the south docks are slightly closer to the town of Sointula making the walk to the stores a little shorter. Courtesy Christine Cornelia.*

If you are heading for the museum, bakery or one of the stores at Sointula, you will find that the local community is very hospitable and will readily stop to offer you a ride if they are driving between the harbour and the town. There are also freely available bicycles at the harbourmaster's office.

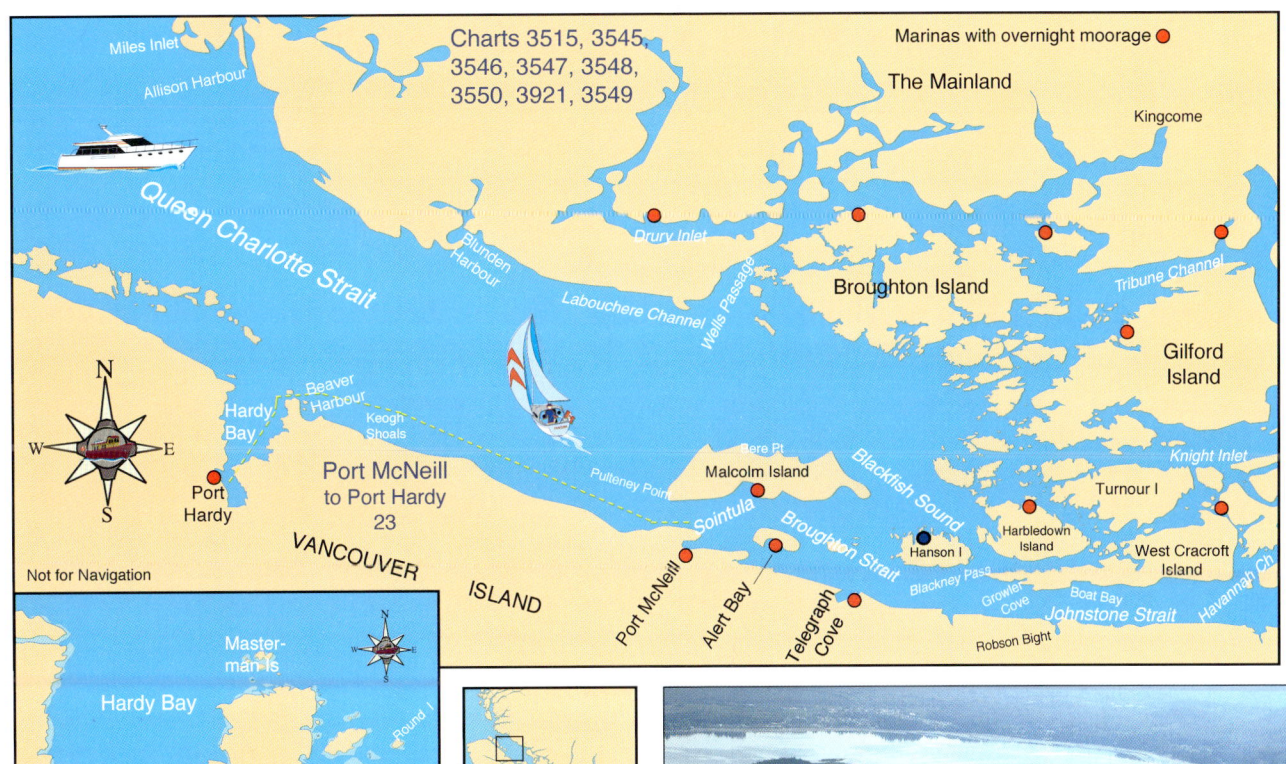

## Broughton Strait to Port Hardy  chart 3548

When you leave Alert Bay, Sointula or Port McNeill for the passage to Port Hardy use chart 3546. Clear Neill Ledge off Port McNeill by passing across Neill Ledge, but only if you are certain of your chart reading. At low tide kelp clearly shows the reefs. The safest bet is to travel around the marker west of Haddington Island and proceed past Pulteney Point. There is also a large kelp bed just beyond this point. It is usually rougher in shallow water so keep well clear of it. Time your passage when seas are calm and likely to remain so until you reach the shelter of Port Hardy. In strong northwesterlies the seas coming down this section of the coast can provide a taste of what to expect in open waters. For Port Hardy, follow a direct course past Keogh Shoals and Round Island, or to enter Beaver Harbour follow the shoreline staying close to Deer and Eagle Islands past Thomas Point (see page 232).

## Beaver Harbour  chart 3548

There is plenty of good water in the channels around the Cattle Islands in Beaver Harbour. The popular anchorage lies in the shallows just off the west side of the islands in 4 to 6 metres over a muddy bottom, to the northeast of Cormorant Rock. Beaver Harbour is the place of an historic stop by early explorers. It was named Guemes Harbour by the Spanish who anchored there in 1792 and made contact with the natives. In later years a fort was built by the Hudson's Bay Company. The First Nations village of Sa-hees (Tsa<u>x</u>is), which is still referred to as **Fort Rupert**, was the first permanent white settlement in Kwakwaka'wakw Territory.

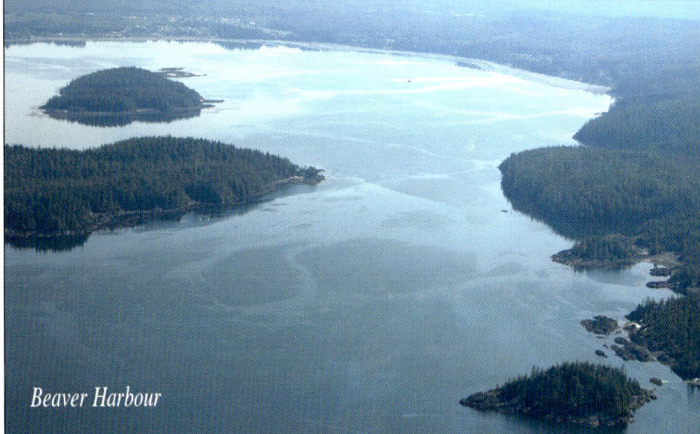

If you bypass Beaver Harbour and are in Port Hardy for a while find the time to make your way to Fort Rupert to view the art of its First Nations people. Some of the coast's finest works come from this renowned artist community.

The distance from Pulteney Point to Masterman Islands, just beyond Beaver Harbour is about 12 nautical miles, from Sointula's harbour in Rough Bay, about 15 nautical miles. To Port Hardy pass either side of Masterman Islands, taking care to avoid the indicated rock by passing around the north side of the 10 metre islet on the east side of the passage.

228

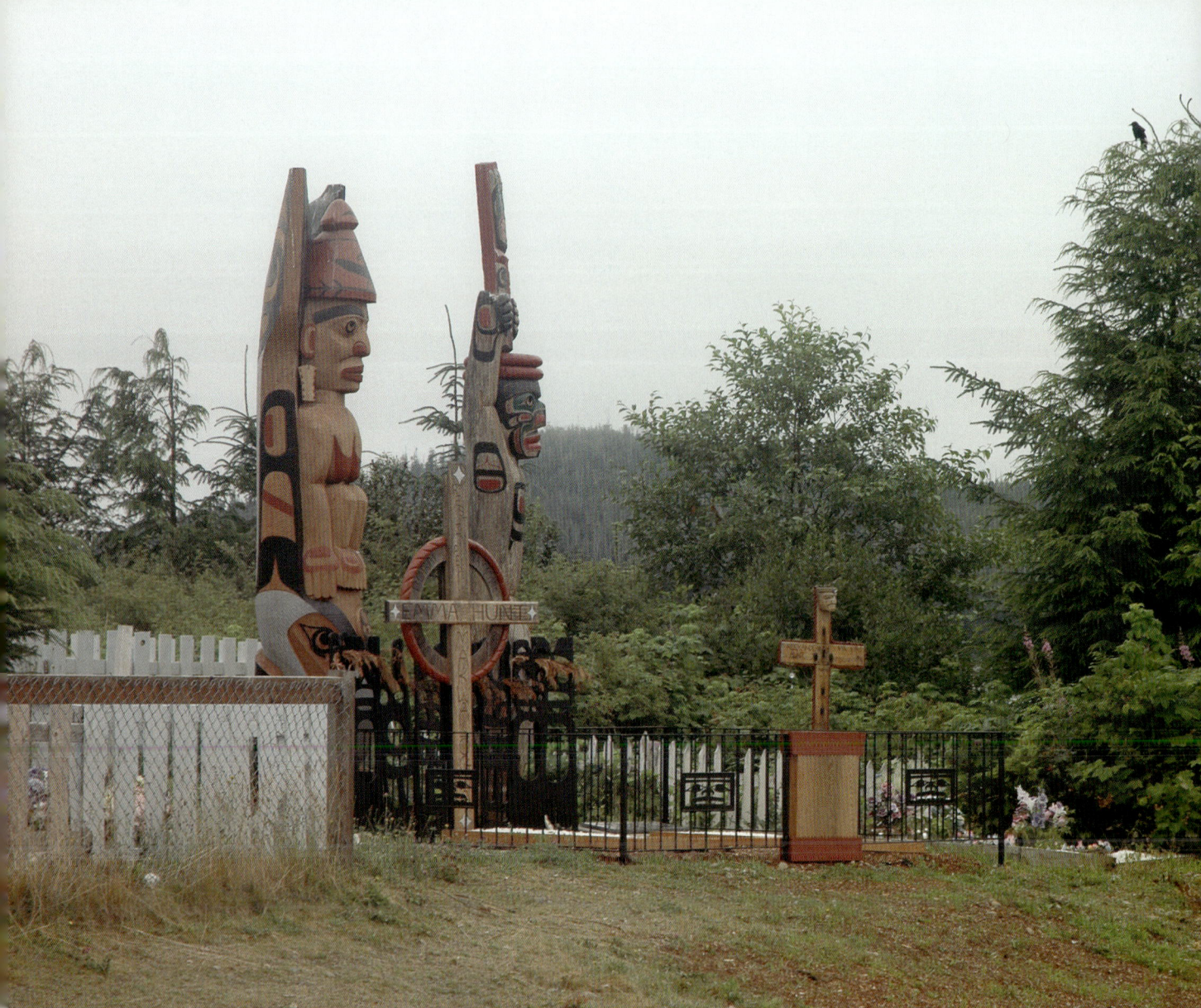

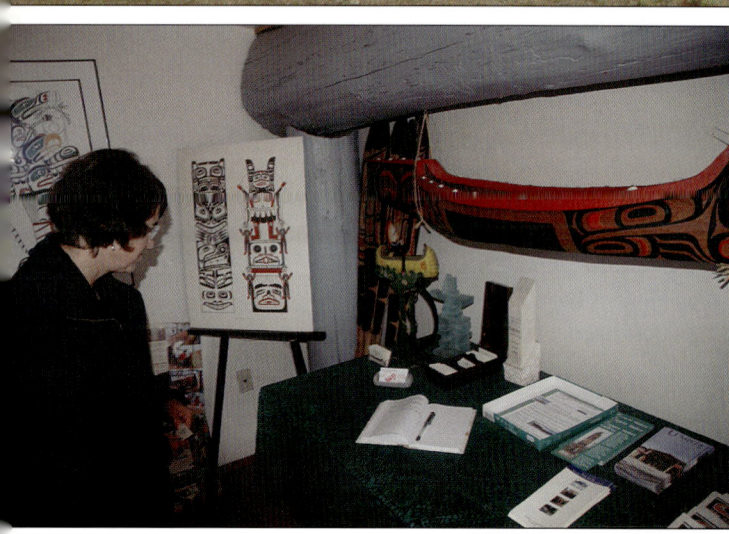

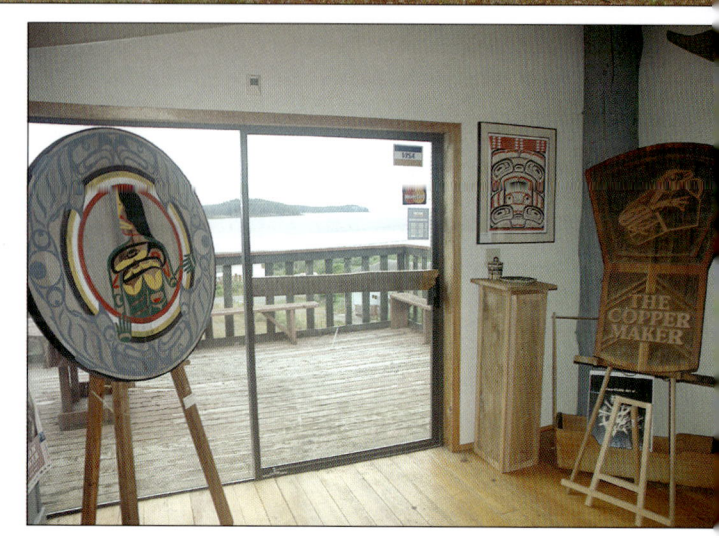

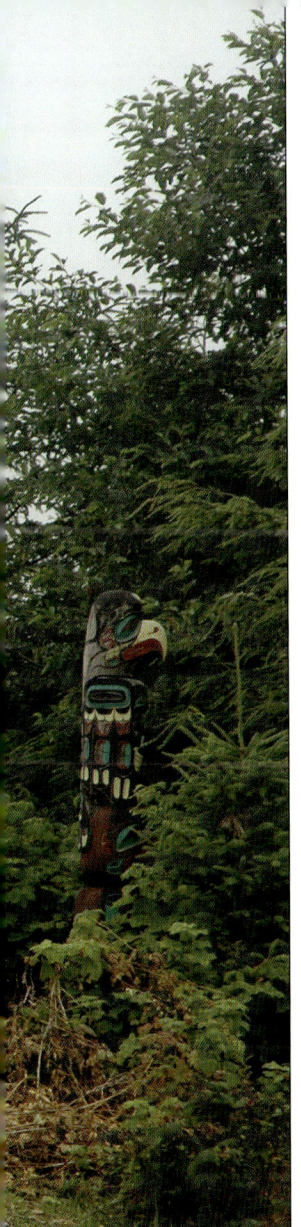

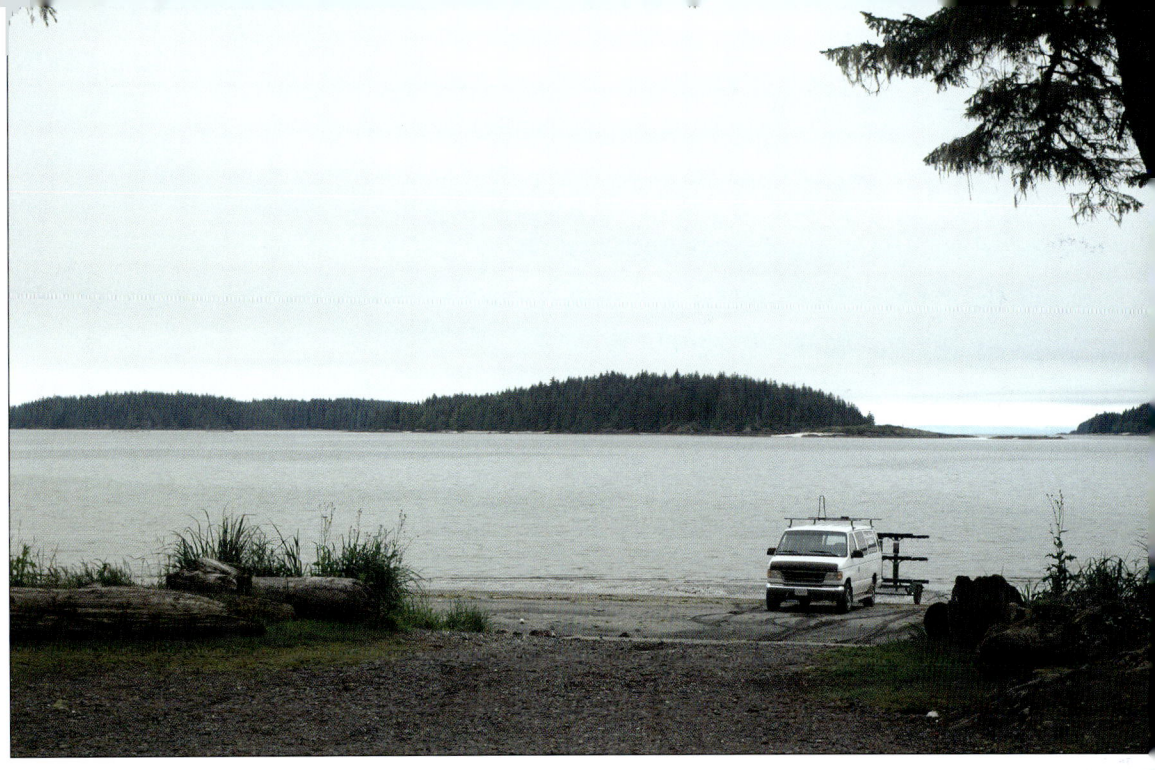

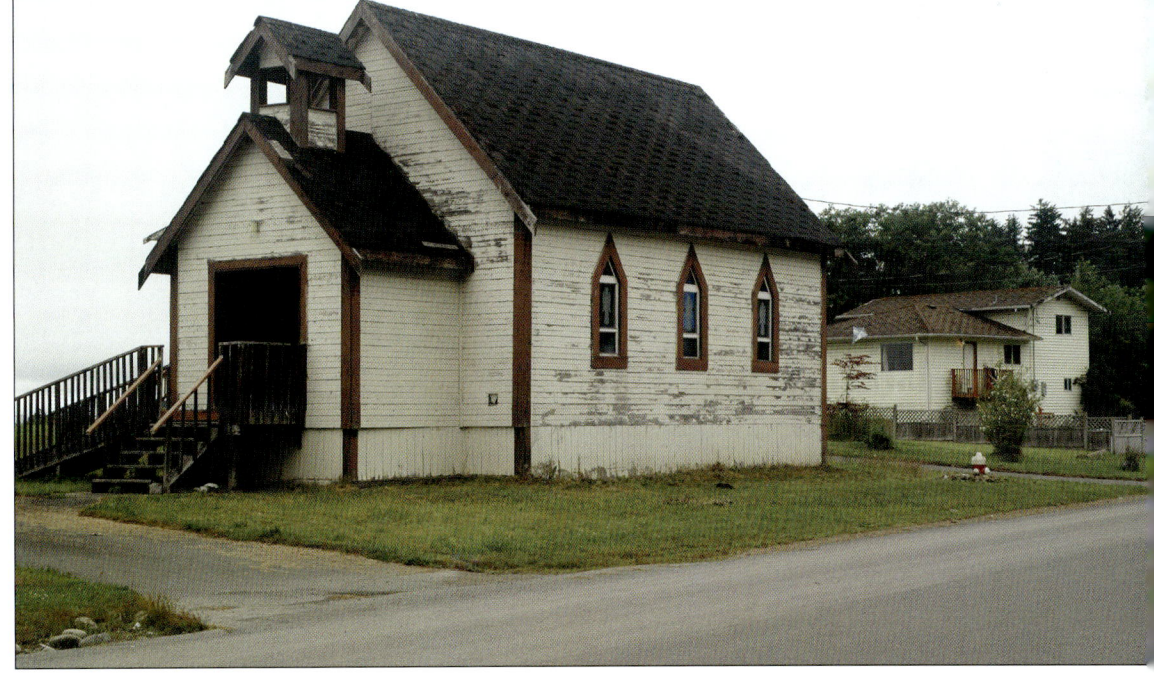

*At historic Beaver Harbour the village of Fort Rupert (Sa-hees or Tsaxis) is the home of the Kwakiutl, a member of the Kwakwaka'wakw people of the Northwest Coast of British Columbia. It was one of the places visited by the Spanish in 1792. Anchor out and go ashore to visit the Coppermaker Gallery of Calvin Hunt.*

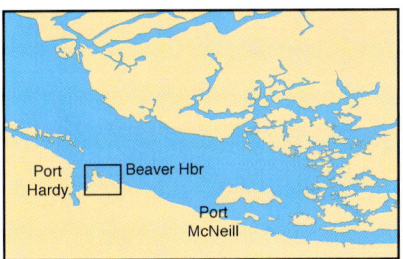

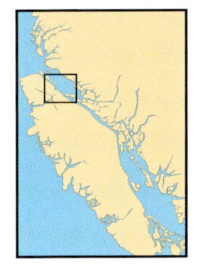

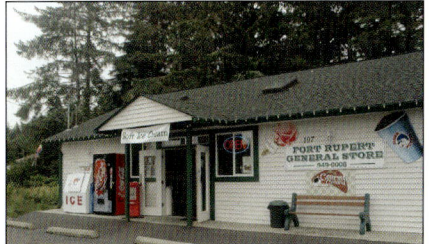

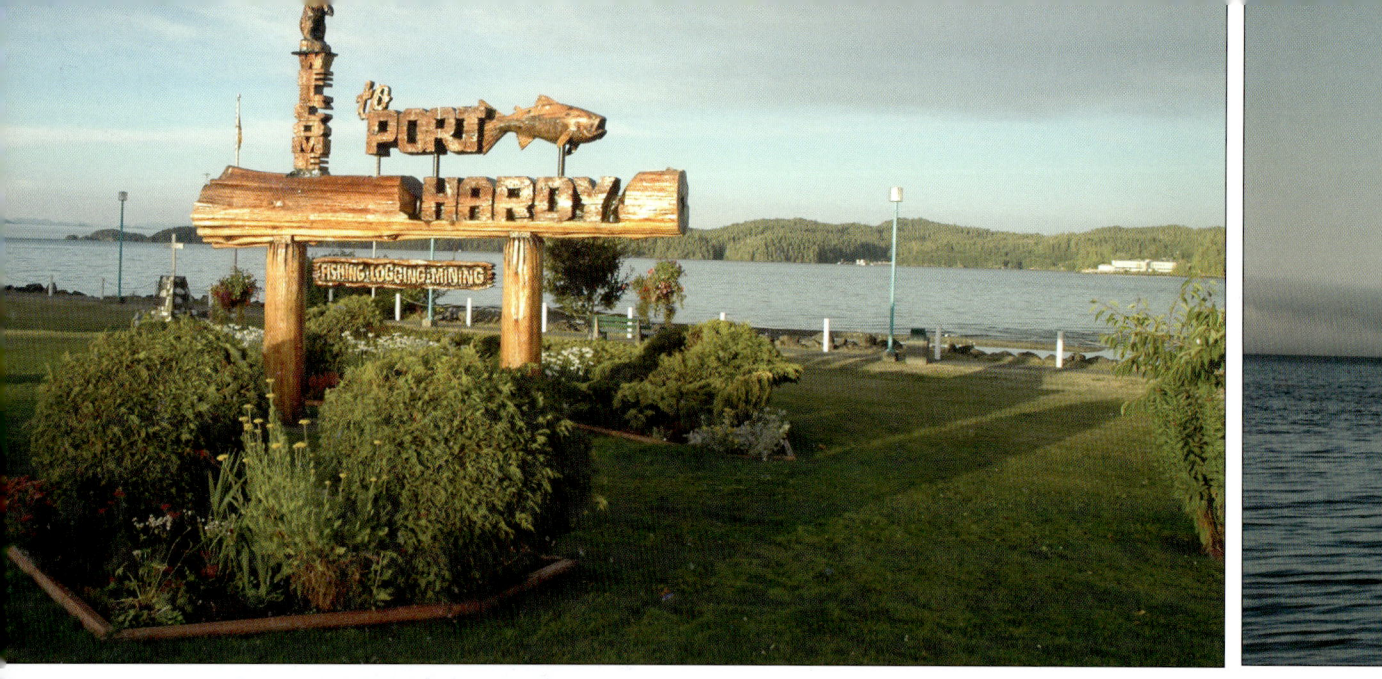

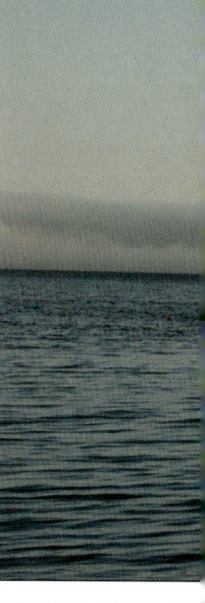

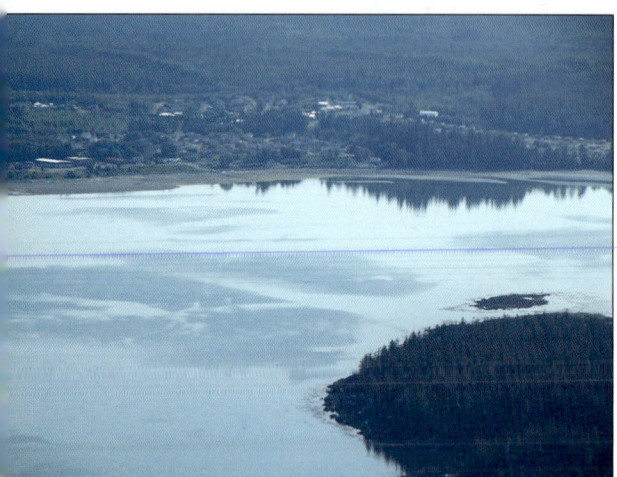

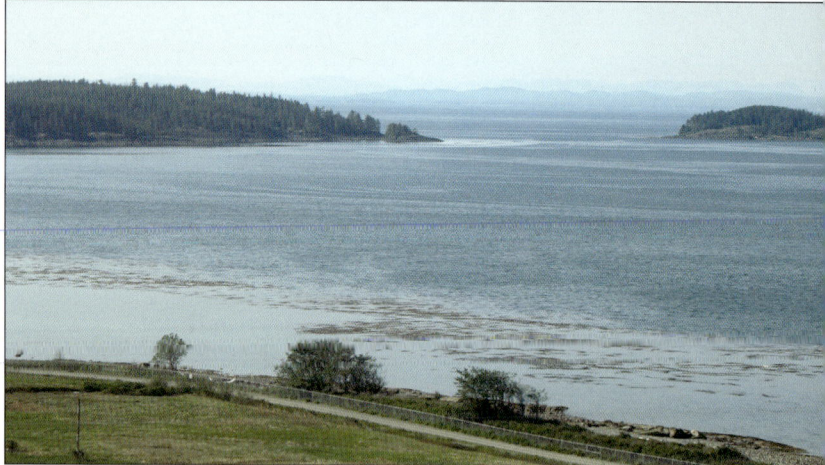

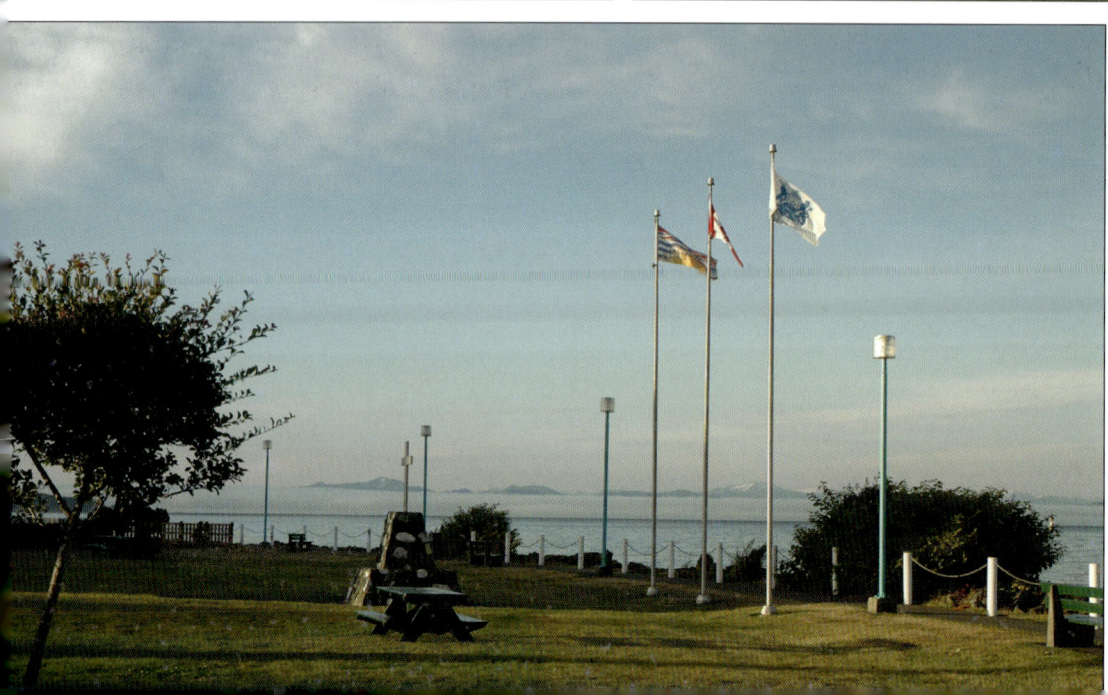

*Views of Port Hardy and Beaver Harbour. Top left: a park on the waterfront at the entrance to Port Hardy with a view of the terminal for the BC Ferries north coast run in the background.
Centre: Beaver Harbour with a view over Cattle Islands towards Fort Rupert (above left), and a glimpse of the outer reaches of Beaver Harbour with Round Island to the right. Flags fly at Port Hardy, bottom left.
Top right: Vessels tied up at the outer dock in Port Hardy.*

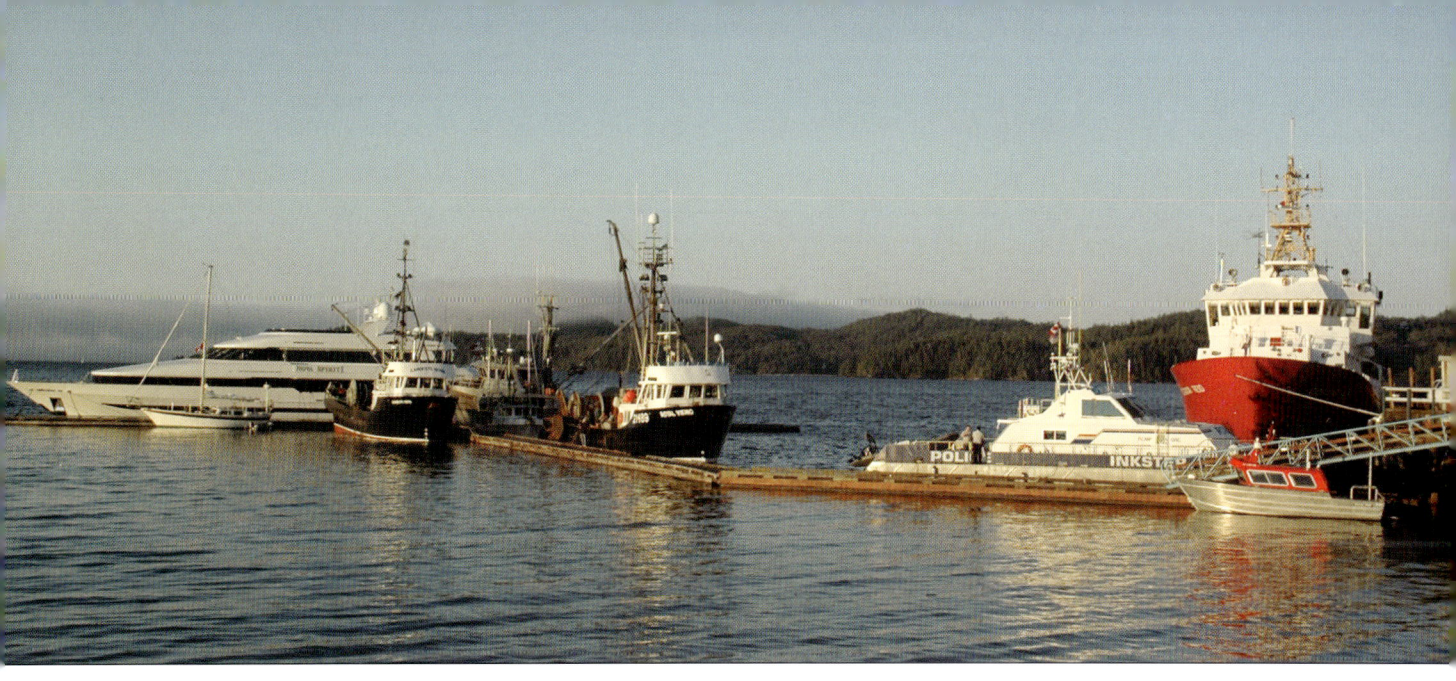

### Port Hardy  charts 3548, 3744

Port Hardy is the point of departure for destinations beyond the north end of Vancouver Island: Cape Caution, Rivers Inlet, Hakai Pass and on to Prince Rupert and Alaska. It is also the jumping off point to the west coast of Vancouver Island via Cape Scott. This very status makes it a town that cannot be overlooked. Along with Port McNeill, it is where cautious mariners stop to replenish fuel, inspect their boats prior to the run 'over the top' (of Vancouver Island) and to effect whatever repairs are necessary to ensure a safe journey. Vessels also stop here to reprovision their food supply, fill prescriptions, replace outdated charts and discuss the timing of crossing the Nawhitti Bar, the shallows beyond Bull Harbour at the north end of Goletas Channel.

Port Hardy centre is a relatively short walk away from the Quarterdeck Marina and adjacent public dock, but cab service is available. The town is a major commercial and residential centre with engineering services, boat works, repair facilities and grocery stores. The town has banks, grocery stores, pharmacy, general stores, hardware stores, speciality, clothing and art and crafts stores. It also has a hospital, post office, hotels and motels and other service businesses catering to the local community and visitors. Apart from a pub at the marina there is an eclectic array of dining establishments in Port Hardy. Malone's Oceanside Bistro actually is not on the waterfront but rather located on the hillside overlooking the town. A fresh fish store next door, Hardy Boys Smoked Fish, supplies fresh fish as well as live crab and lobster. You can make reservations at Malone's, call or visit the Hardy Boys, order a selection of fresh seafood and it is delivered to Malone's for preparation for dinner. Also visit the Sportsman Steak House in the town centre.

Port Hardy has two marinas which can be most accommodating. The public dock has lots of moorage when the fishing fleet is out, but when it is in, the docks are often crammed with fishboats. Another public dock is located on the approaches to the inner harbour. It is exposed to open Hardy Bay, but during summer it can be a pleasant stop for overnight moorage because of its downtown waterfront location.

> One year, due to fog, we sat in Port Hardy for three days. Then under protest from fellow travellers against further delay, we set out despite the fog. We were to travel to Bull Harbour, cross the Nawhitti Bar and head for Cape Scott and the west coast of the island to Winter Harbour. The fog was dense. Under radar we pulled out of Port Hardy and cautiously crept along the coast in calm seas. It turned out well, fortunately, and we reached the safe shelter of Bull Harbour easily. Several fishing boats passed close by in Goletas Channel. We failed to see them, other than on radar, when they passed within less than 100 metres of us. We timed the crossing of Nawhitti Bar so that we were not even aware of any current, which can be felt quite strongly during tidal exchanges.

*"The bulk of the Seagate wharf (out front Port Hardy) is usually not put in place until at least June some time. No reservations can be made here but the wharfinger comes to collect each evening. The dock has no power or water but there is a loading dock nearby where water can be obtained. It can get rough on the outer dock in SE or N and NE winds, particularly on the outer part of the dock.*

*You will probably find dock space (rafting) at the city docks across from the Quarterdeck. In the busy times and most of the summer, it is advisable to reserve ahead for Quarterdeck."* –David Whitworth

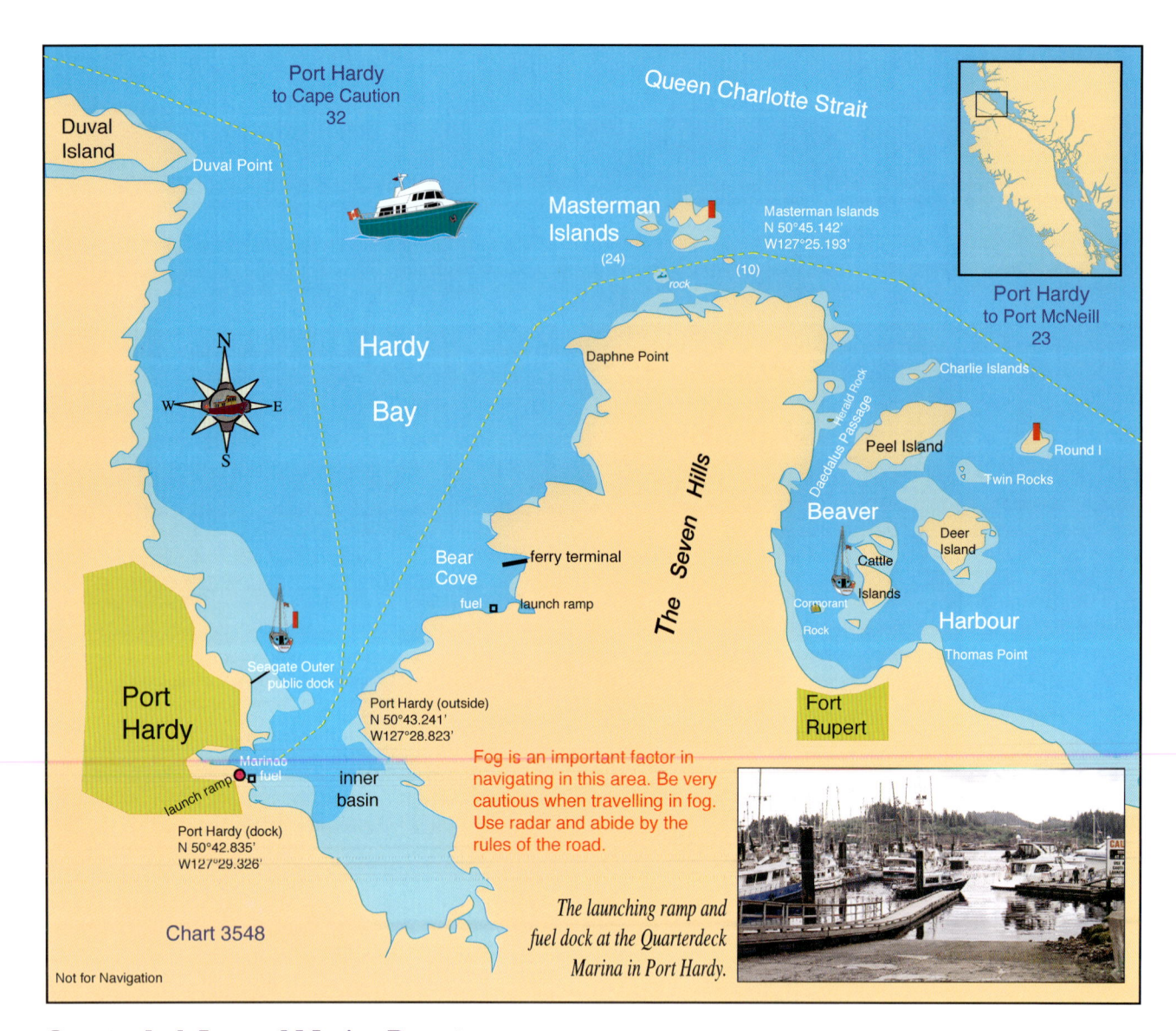

## Quarterdeck Inn and Marina Resort
PO Box 910, 6555, Hardy Bay Road
Port Hardy BC V0N 2P0
Ph 250 949-6551  Fax 250 949-7777
info@quarterdeck.net  www.quarterdeckresort.net
Boats to 150 feet can be accomodated at the Quarterdeck. Power supply at the dock is 50, 30 and 15 amp. Water, gas and diesel are available at the adjacent fuel dock. The marine store is located at the marina. Boat repairs are available.

## Port Hardy Harbour Authority
6600 Hardy Bay Road PO Box 68
Port Hardy BC V0N 2P0
Ph 250-949-0336  Fax 250-949-6037
phfloats@cablerocket.com  www.haa.bc.ca
Check for slips at the public dock, which are available especially when the fishing fleet is out. The launch ramp is between the two marinas.

## Port Hardy & District Chamber of Commerce
email: phcc@island.net  www.ph-chamber.bc.ca
All services are available at Port Hardy. Uptown facilities include hospital, pharmacy, hotels, restaurants, grocery stores, hardware stores, service stations and all amenities. Ask about grocery delivery to your boat.
At the marinas ask about available mechanics, ships ways, fishing, whale and bear watching charters.
There is a launching ramp at the inner harbour.
The ferry terminus for Prince Rupert and the Discovery Coast is located at Bear Cove in Hardy Bay.
There is a fuel dock at Bear Cove near the ferry terminal.
Regular scheduled Pacific Coastal Airlines flights are available to Campbell River, Vancouver and Seattle.

The Quarterdeck Inn and Marina Resort, alongside the inner public docks, will happily provide transient moorage, and gas and diesel fuel. There is a well-stocked marine store at the Quarterdeck and a large hotel on the property, a suitable place to meet up with guests who are looking for accommodations as part of a plan to fly in and meet up with you. I.V's (say Iveys) pub and restaurant at the resort is a busy place and meals are available at most hours. Here you can relax in the comfort of the pub with its nautical decor and atmosphere, just steps away from your yacht.

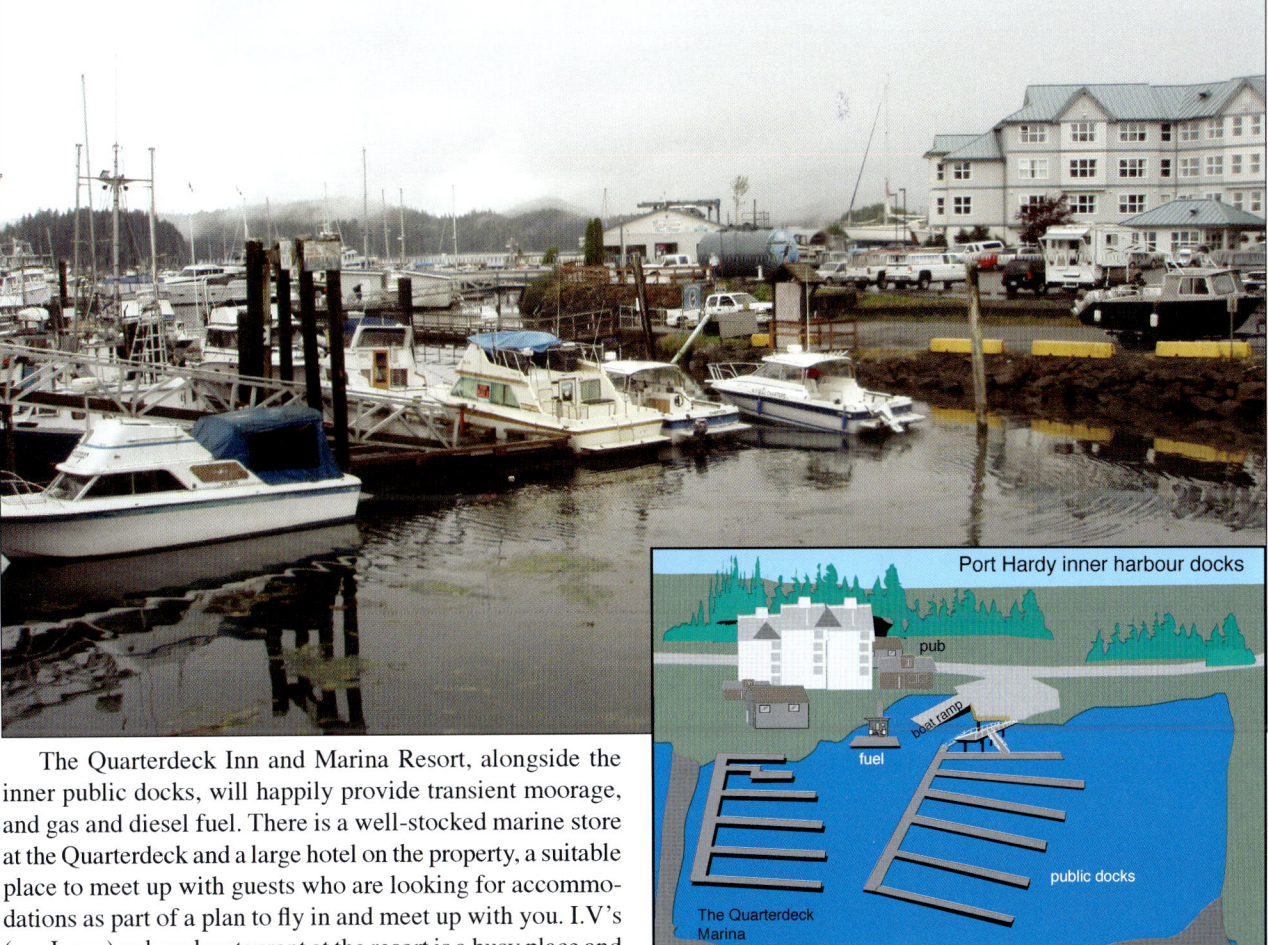

As you leave Port Hardy you may be inclined to hug the western shore if you are planning to travel north. Travel slightly eastward for awhile to avoid the reef that reaches far into the bay. Use the large scale inset on chart 3548. This is also the chart for approaching Port Hardy from the south.

Port Hardy serves as the southern terminal for the North Coast ferry. This service runs beyond Vancouver Island to Prince Rupert, just south of the Alaska panhandle. The regular arrival of passengers and vehicular traffic at Port Hardy produces a flow of visitors to all points of interest in the foregoing areas every summer. Cruise ships passing through the area provide a spectacular sight as well as a possible navigational hazard of which to remain clear, especially in fog.

The Port Hardy area enjoys tourism created by the ferry service, whale and bear watching opportunities, trailerable boat launching, fishing and transient moorage. Plans to visit Port Hardy and Port McNeill sometimes requires reservations at the marinas. The author's marine guides *Anchorages and Marine Parks* and *Docks and Destinations* provide more anchorage and moorage information with phone numbers and details of available facilities.

### God's Pocket

There is a popular scuba diving lodge on Hurst Island. It is 10 miles from Port Hardy in Christie Passage off Goletas Channel (chart 3549). The dock is small but a brief stop if space permits could be rewarded with a pleasant visit with convivial owners and their underwater adventuring guests.

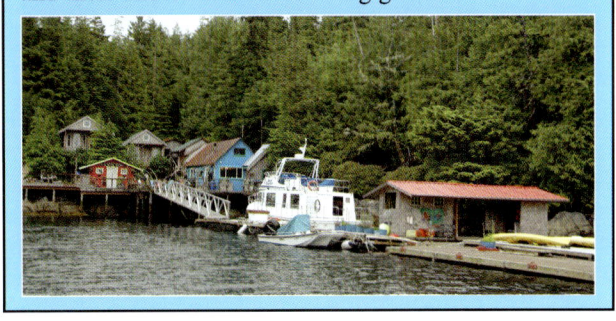

*Top: The waterfront at Port Hardy's inner harbour is busy with the public docks lying alongside a large private marina, the Quarterdeck. Both welcome overnight visitors. Fuel is available alongside the launch ramp as well as on the approaches to the inner harbour. Above: God's Pocket.*

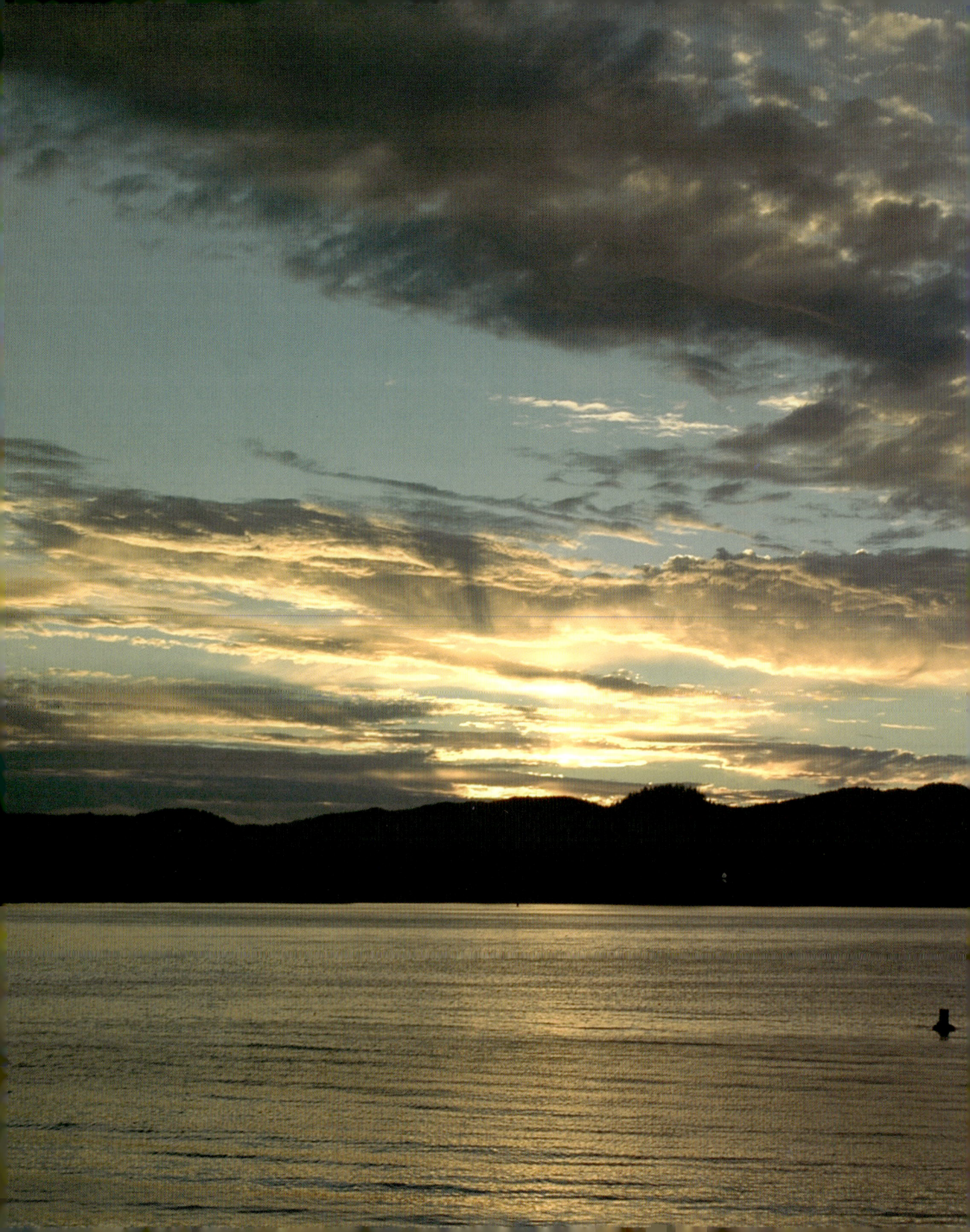

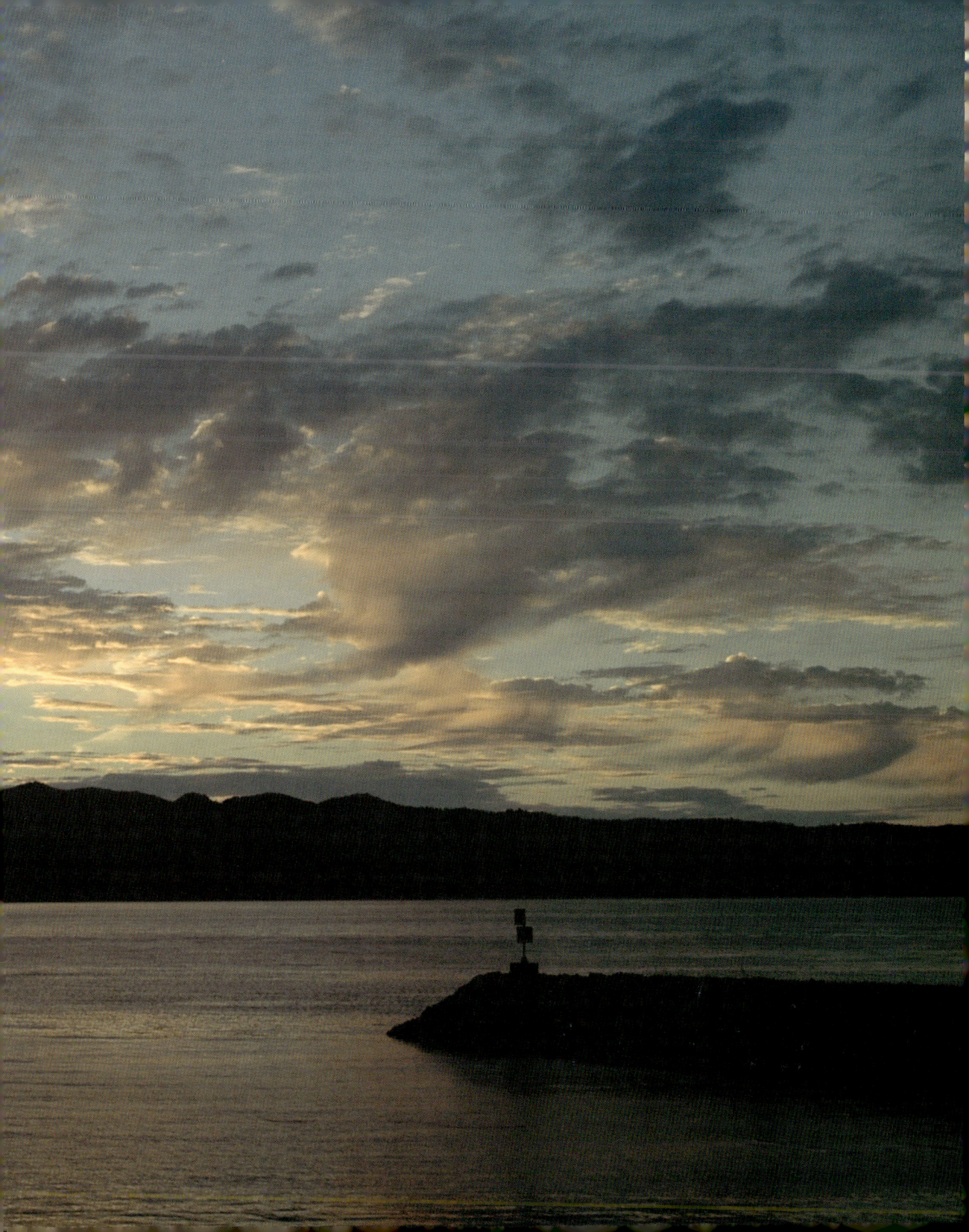

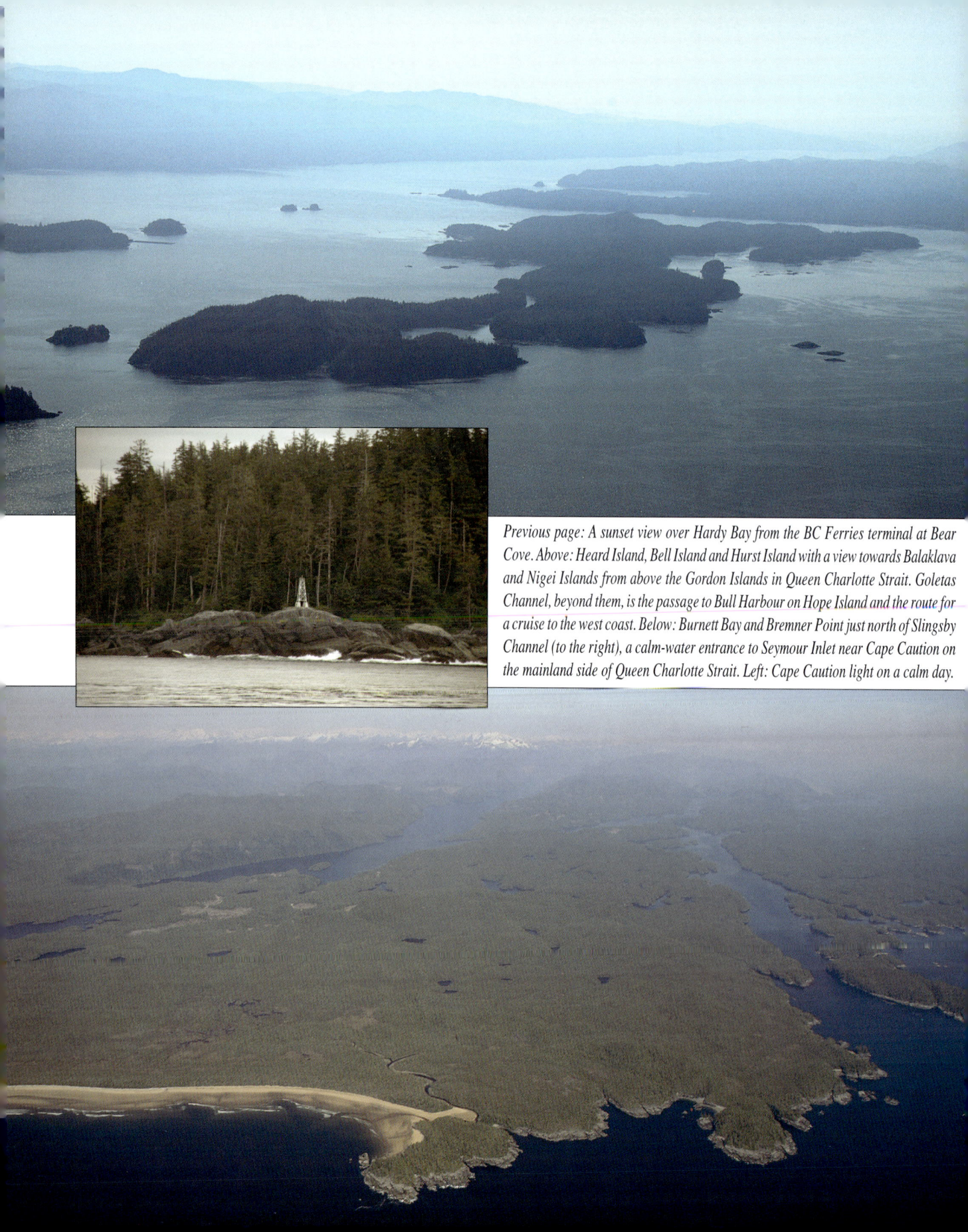

*Previous page: A sunset view over Hardy Bay from the BC Ferries terminal at Bear Cove. Above: Heard Island, Bell Island and Hurst Island with a view towards Balaklava and Nigei Islands from above the Gordon Islands in Queen Charlotte Strait. Goletas Channel, beyond them, is the passage to Bull Harbour on Hope Island and the route for a cruise to the west coast. Below: Burnett Bay and Bremner Point just north of Slingsby Channel (to the right), a calm-water entrance to Seymour Inlet near Cape Caution on the mainland side of Queen Charlotte Strait. Left: Cape Caution light on a calm day.*

# Cape Caution to Hakai Pass

## Rivers Inlet from Wells Passage on the Mainland or from Port Hardy on Vancouver Island

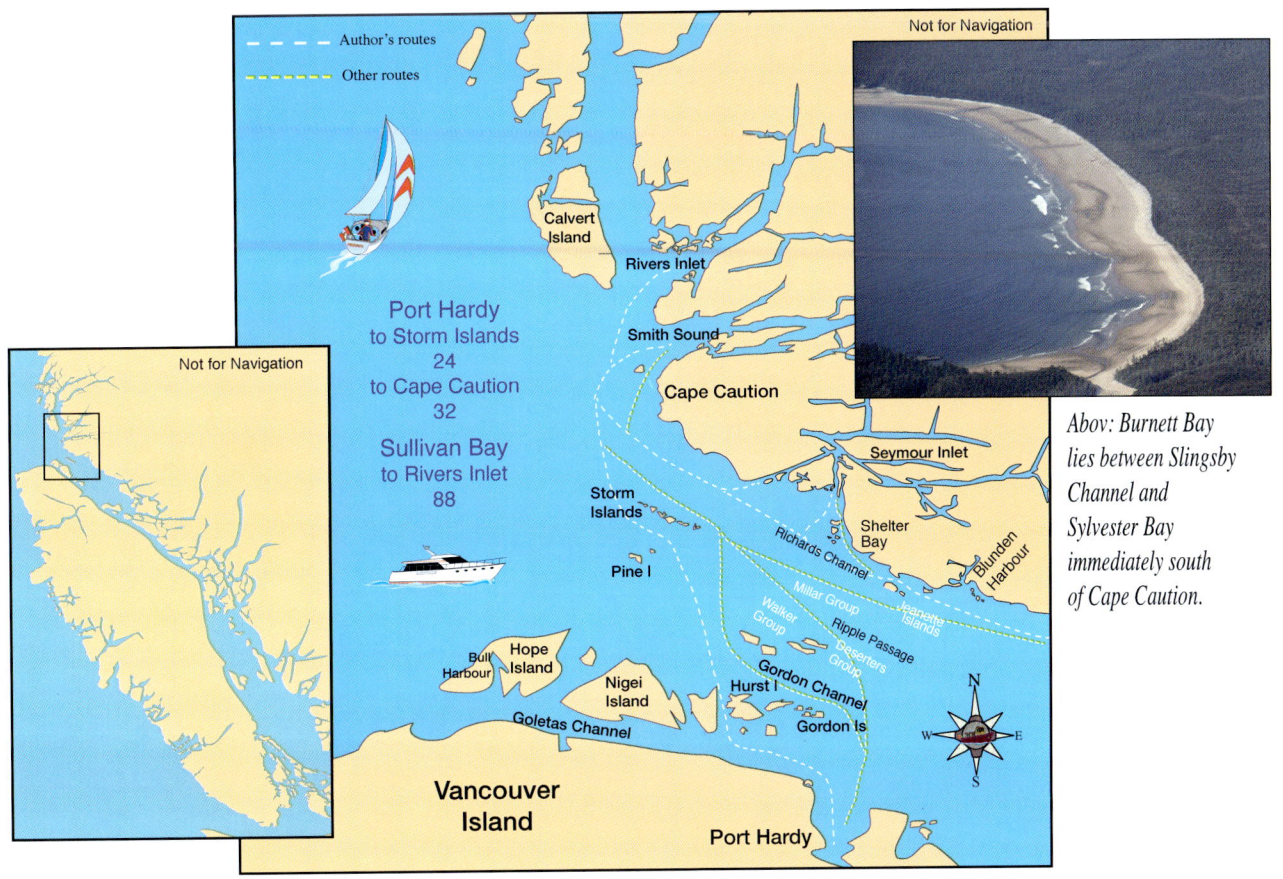

Charts 3550, 3934, 3931, 3598, 3806

*Abov: Burnett Bay lies between Slingsby Channel and Sylvester Bay immediately south of Cape Caution.*

The passage around Cape Caution should be taken with great care. Weather should be monitored in advance of the trip. Not only should the mariner assess the conditions at the point of departure but also at the destination as well as points en route. Listen to the VHF weather channel for current conditions at Cape Caution as well as at Egg Island. Take note of the forecast as well and wait for diminishing seas before your departure. If the barometer is falling rapidly that is not the time to leave. Rather stay where you are in a safe harbour and plan your departure for when conditions are improving. Watch for fog. If you are running on radar and GPS you can comfortably do the trip in calm weather, but you will enjoy it much more if you can see the islands and land features as you travel. It is safer that way as well.

Leaving Wells Passage, after a visit to the Broughton Islands, pass south and west of Lewis Rocks or enter Lewis Cove to the east of them if you need to wait for suitable weather. Following the mainland coastline, proceed along

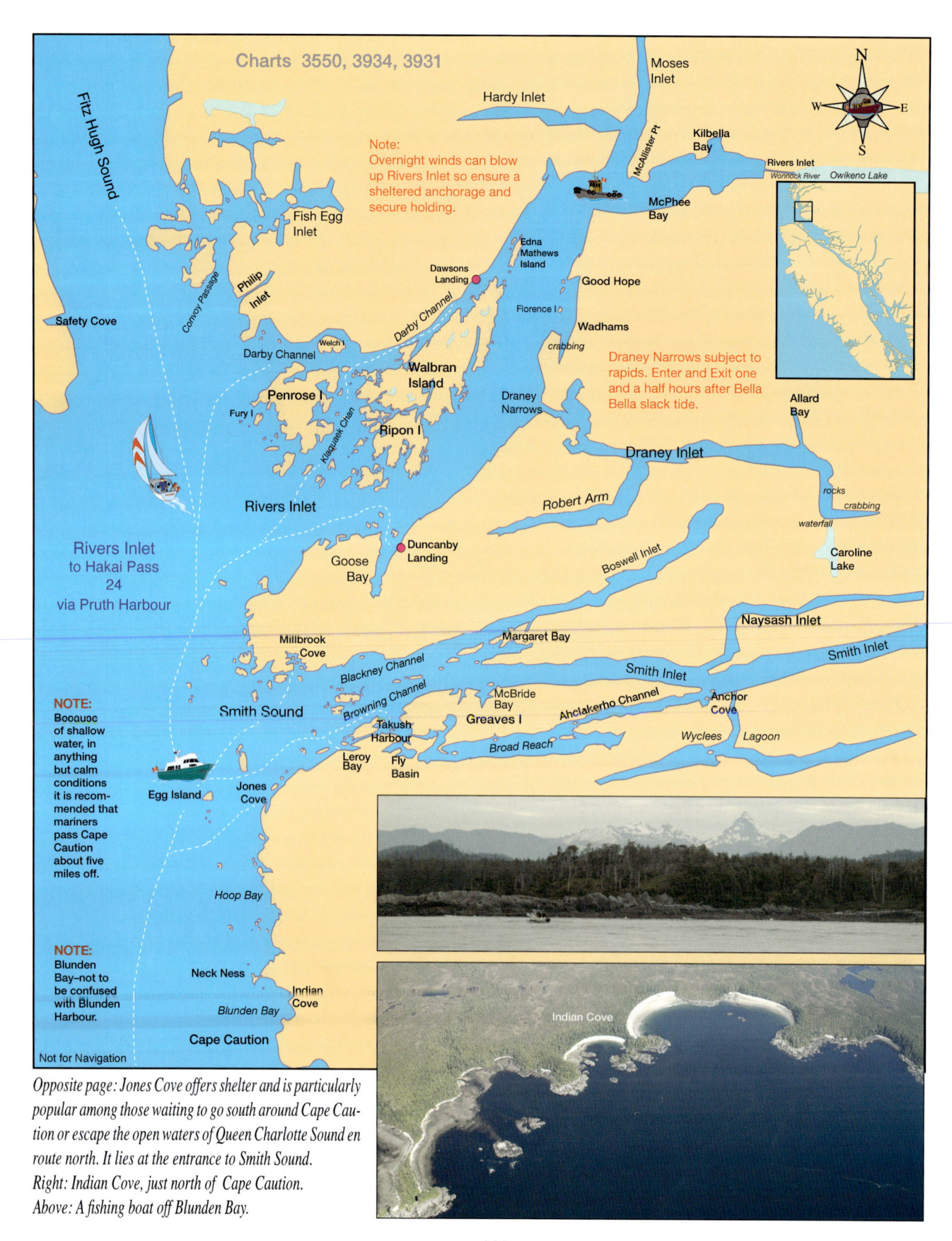

**Charts 3550, 3934, 3931**

**Note:** Overnight winds can blow up Rivers Inlet so ensure a sheltered anchorage and secure holding.

**Draney Narrows** subject to rapids. Enter and Exit one and a half hours after Bella Bella slack tide.

Fitz Hugh Sound
Hardy Inlet
Moses Inlet
McAllister Pt
Kilbella Bay
Rivers Inlet
Wannock River — Owikeno Lake
McPhee Bay
Fish Egg Inlet
Edna Mathews Island
Dawsons Landing
Good Hope
Convoy Passage
Philip Inlet
Florence I
Safety Cove
Darby Channel
Wadhams
crabbing
Welch I
Walbran Island
Penrose I
Draney Narrows
Allard Bay
Fury I
Ripon I
Klaquaek Chan
Draney Inlet
rocks
crabbing
Rivers Inlet
Robert Arm
waterfall
Caroline Lake
Rivers Inlet to Hakai Pass 24 via Pruth Harbour
Goose Bay
Duncanby Landing
Boswell Inlet
Naysash Inlet
Millbrook Cove
Margaret Bay
Smith Inlet
Smith Inlet
Blackney Channel
McBride Bay
Anchor Cove
**NOTE:** Because of shallow water, in anything but calm conditions it is recommended that mariners pass Cape Caution about five miles off.
Smith Sound
Browning Channel
Greaves I
Ahclakerho Channel
Takush Harbour
Broad Reach
Wyclees Lagoon
Egg Island
Leroy Bay
Fly Basin
Jones Cove
Hoop Bay
**NOTE:** Blunden Bay—not to be confused with Blunden Harbour.
Neck Ness
Indian Cove
Blunden Bay
Cape Caution

Not for Navigation

*Indian Cove*

*Opposite page: Jones Cove offers shelter and is particularly popular among those waiting to go south around Cape Caution or escape the open waters of Queen Charlotte Sound en route north. It lies at the entrance to Smith Sound.*
*Right: Indian Cove, just north of Cape Caution.*
*Above: A fishing boat off Blunden Bay.*

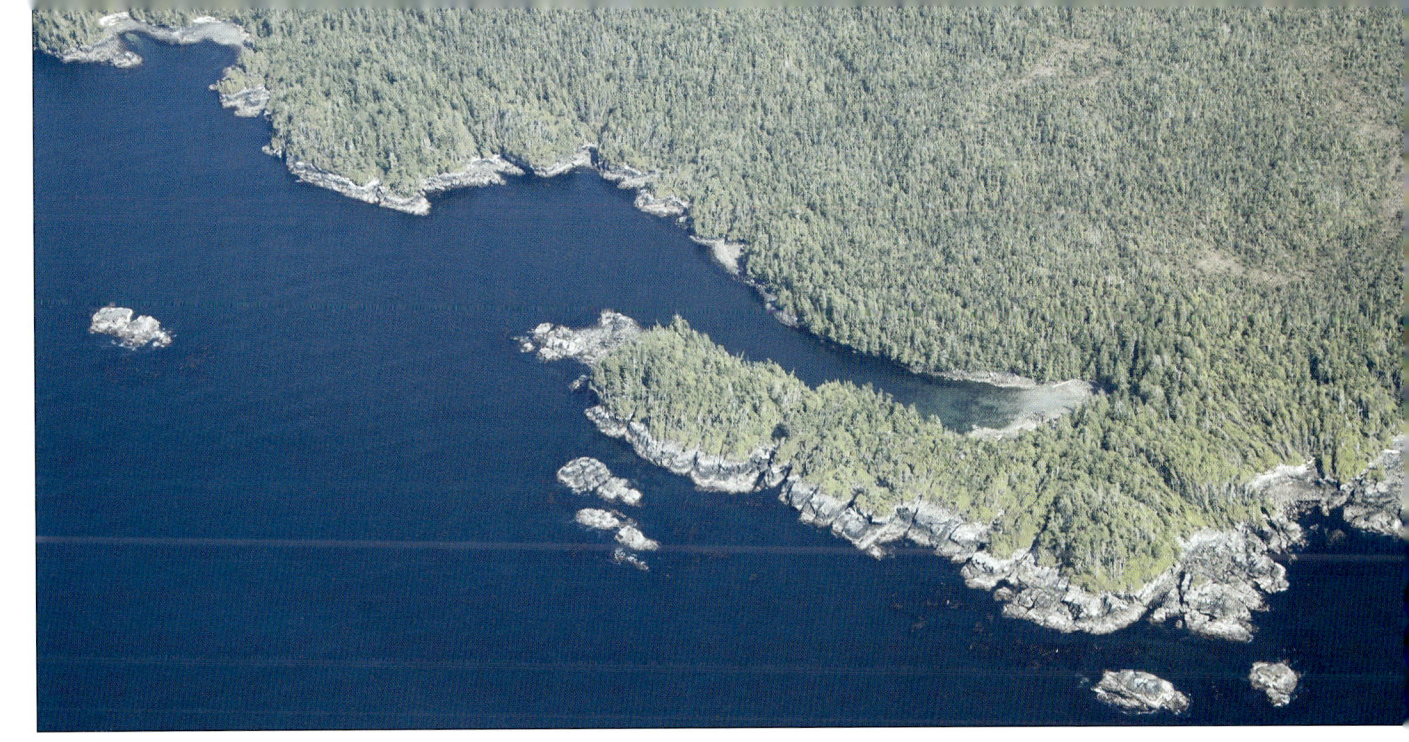

Richards Channel to Blunden Harbour and on to Allison Harbour via the Southgate Group as described in a previous chapter. If you are planning to visit Seymour Inlet go to page 194, or continue north towards Cape Caution taking a course east of McEwan Rock. In any but very calm seas, navigate in deeper water, giving Burnett Bay a fairly wide berth and heading for deeper water on the approaches to Cape Caution. Stay beyond the 20 fathom mark. If seas allow and you want to stop awhile to relax and enjoy being at Cape Caution, Indian Cove is reported to be a suitable anchorage.

Keeping several miles off Cape Caution head for Egg Island en route to Rivers Inlet. If you are going into Smith Sound pass to the southeast of Egg Island and continue through Alexandra Passage to a sheltered anchorage such as Jones Cove, Takush Harbour or Millbrook Cove.

North of Cape Caution there are numerous anchorages and nooks in which to take shelter. However, many of these are deep and care should be taken to avoid relying on your ground tackle in strong winds. Make sure you have enough scope, and use stern tying to shore as a means to avoid dragging anchor. Designated marine parks often include shallower and safer anchorages. Use your discrimination when choosing an anchorage, taking into account its exposure to wind and currents.

When travelling from Port Hardy to Cape Caution, use Goletas Channel and Christie Passage or Browning Pass. We favour the route past God's Pocket in Christie Passage. A small anchorage offers shelter from rough conditions and provides a place to wait for improved weather. The small lodge at Gods Pocket caters to scuba diving groups and may have some meals for transient visitors. Passing Scarlett Point, we head for Pine Island and the north end of the Storm Islands, passing to the west of them or between Pine and Tree Islets. We have travelled right through the Storm Islands in calm conditions, finding passage where the depths were suitable and the watwerway clear of obstacles.

## Jones Cove, Smith Sound  charts 3550, 3934, 3931

Jones Cove may be considered as a place to stop for

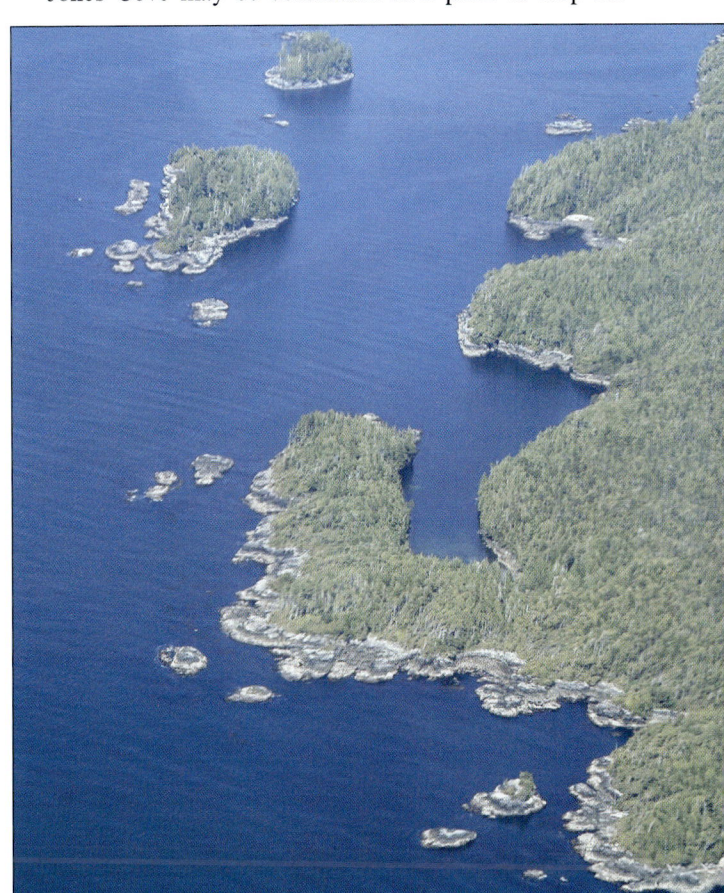

## Map Labels

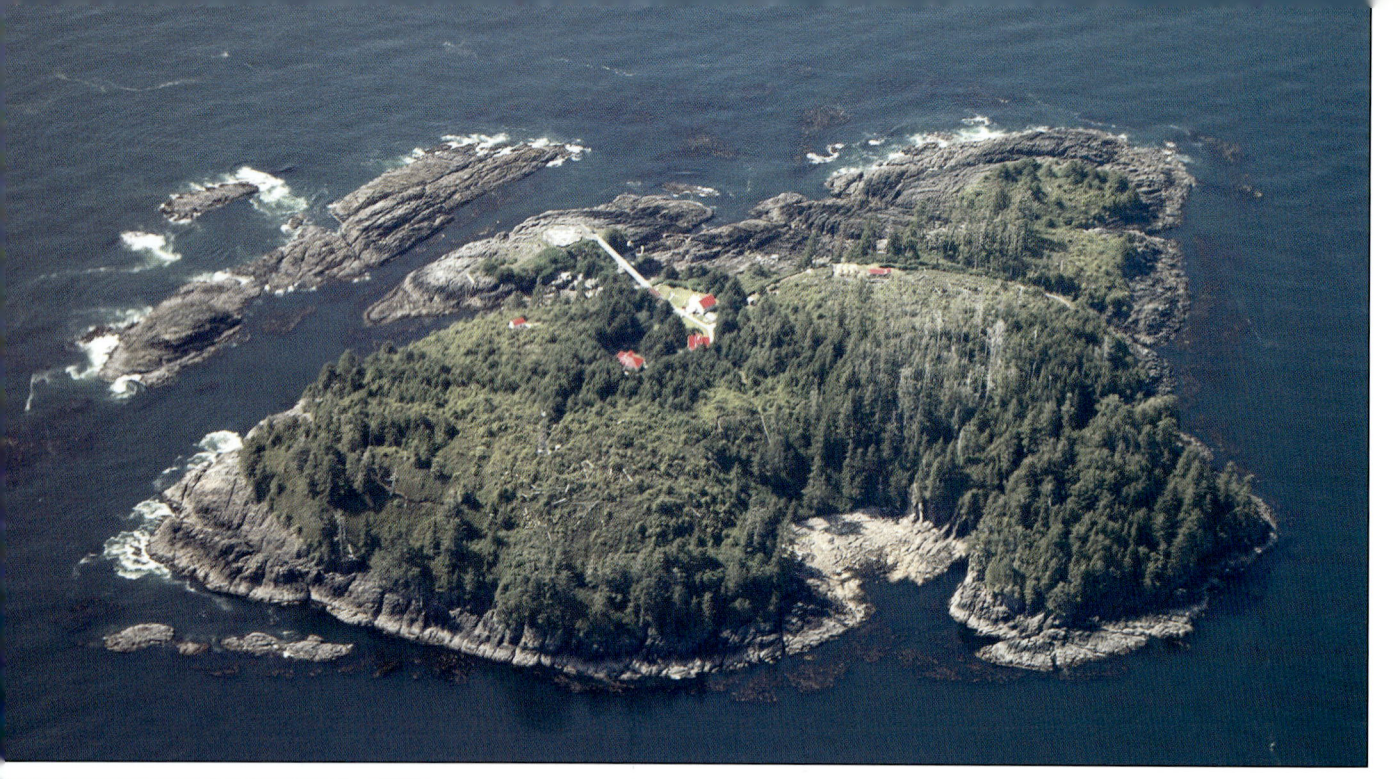

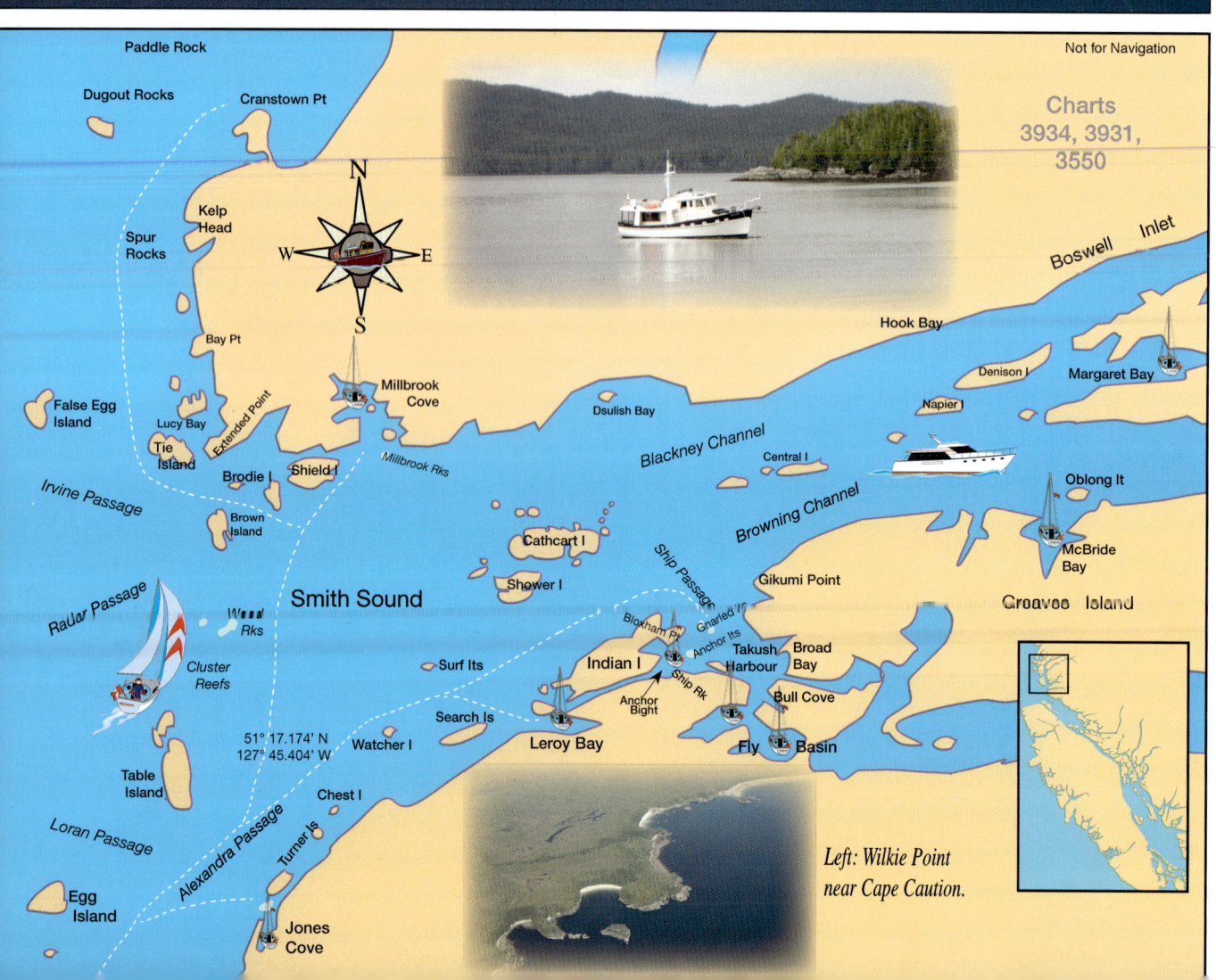

**Charts 3934, 3931, 3550**

Not for Navigation

Paddle Rock
Dugout Rocks
Cranstown Pt
Kelp Head
Spur Rocks
Bay Pt
False Egg Island
Lucy Bay
Tie Island
Extended Point
Brodie I
Shield I
Millbrook Cove
Millbrook Rks
Brown Island
Irvine Passage
Dsulish Bay
Boswell Inlet
Hook Bay
Denison I
Margaret Bay
Napier I
Blackney Channel
Central I
Browning Channel
Oblong It
McBride Bay
Cathcart I
Shower I
Ship Passage
Gikumi Point
Greaves Island
Radar Passage
Wood Rks
Smith Sound
Bloxham Pt
Gnarled I
Anchor Its
Ship Rk
Takush Harbour
Broad Bay
Cluster Reefs
Surf Its
Indian I
Anchor Bight
Bull Cove
Search Is
51° 17.174' N
127° 45.404' W
Watcher I
Leroy Bay
Fly Basin
Table Island
Chest I
Loran Passage
Egg Island
Alexandra Passage
Turner Is
Jones Cove

*Left: Wilkie Point near Cape Caution.*

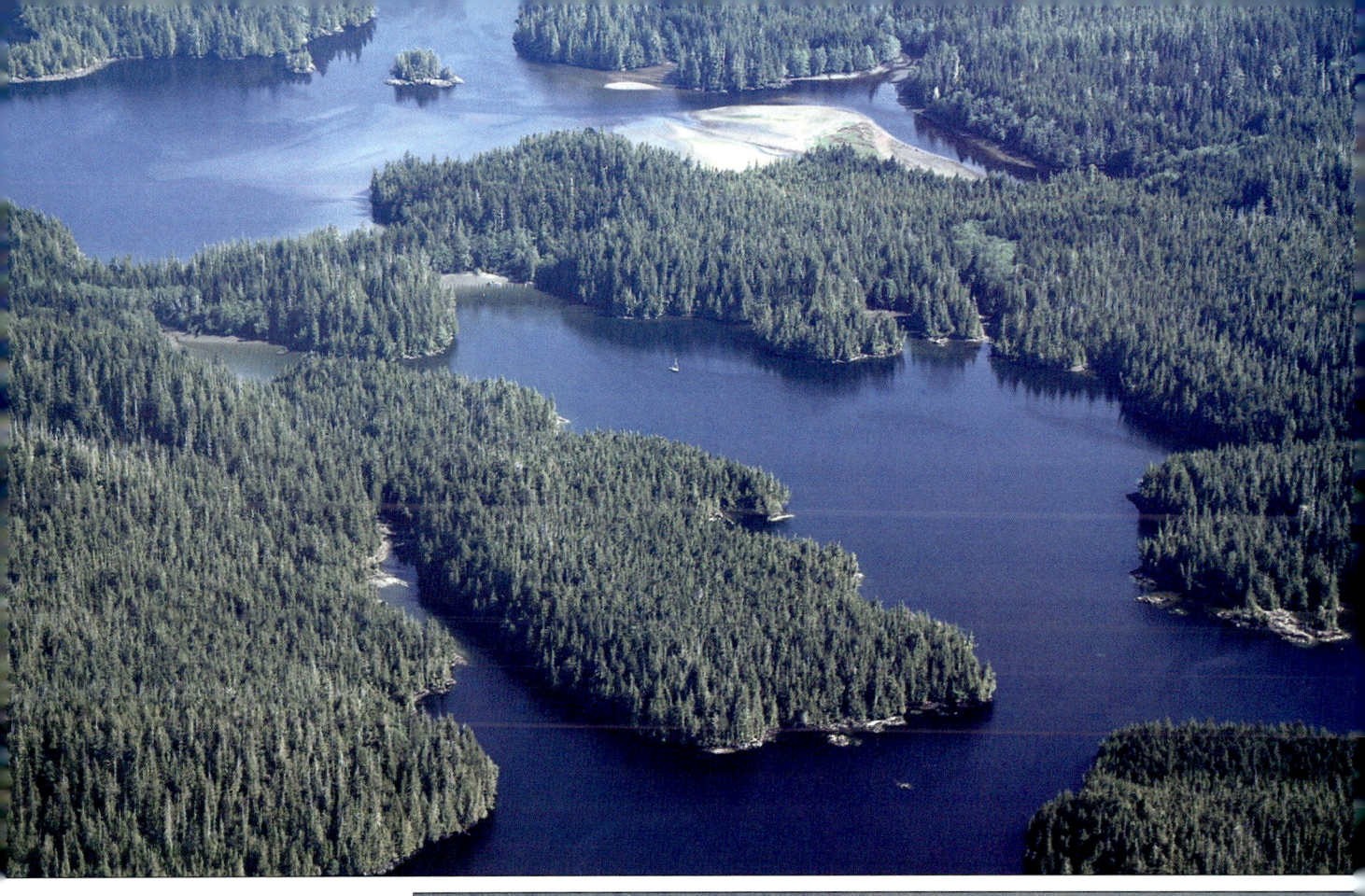

*Opposite, top: Egg Island is a weather reporting station, lighthouse and major navigation aid.*
*Above and right: Takush Harbour. It is a popular anchorage and easily accessible near the entrance to Smith Sound.*

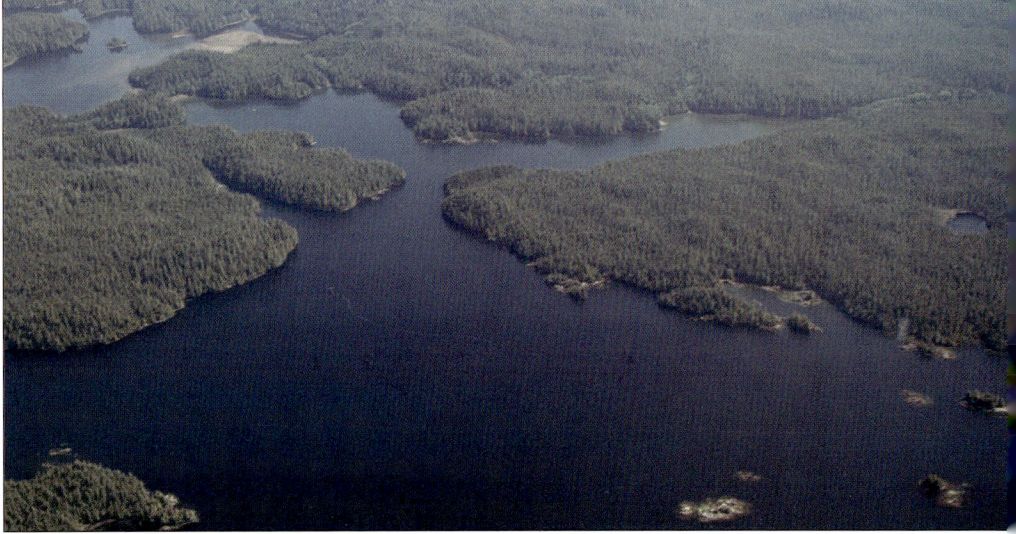

shelter en route past Smith Sound. Among anchorages it is generally the preferred one in the area. It is about 2.5 miles from Egg Island. When passing Smith Sound in either direction temporary anchorage could be taken overnight in mild weathern in the lee of Egg Island.

Entering Smith Sound **Leroy Cove** offers sheltered anchorage for one or two boats. It lies to the west of Leroy Island just south of the lower tip of Indian Island. Make sure you set your anchor well. Both Leroy Cove and Jones Cove are reported to have uncertain seabed holding.

## Takush Harbour   chart 3931

Opening off Browning Channel, Takush Harbour is a quiet scenic anchorage with cosy nooks and basins where calm conditions generally prevail. The harbour lies just beyond Indian Island. After passing Wakas Point and Bloxham

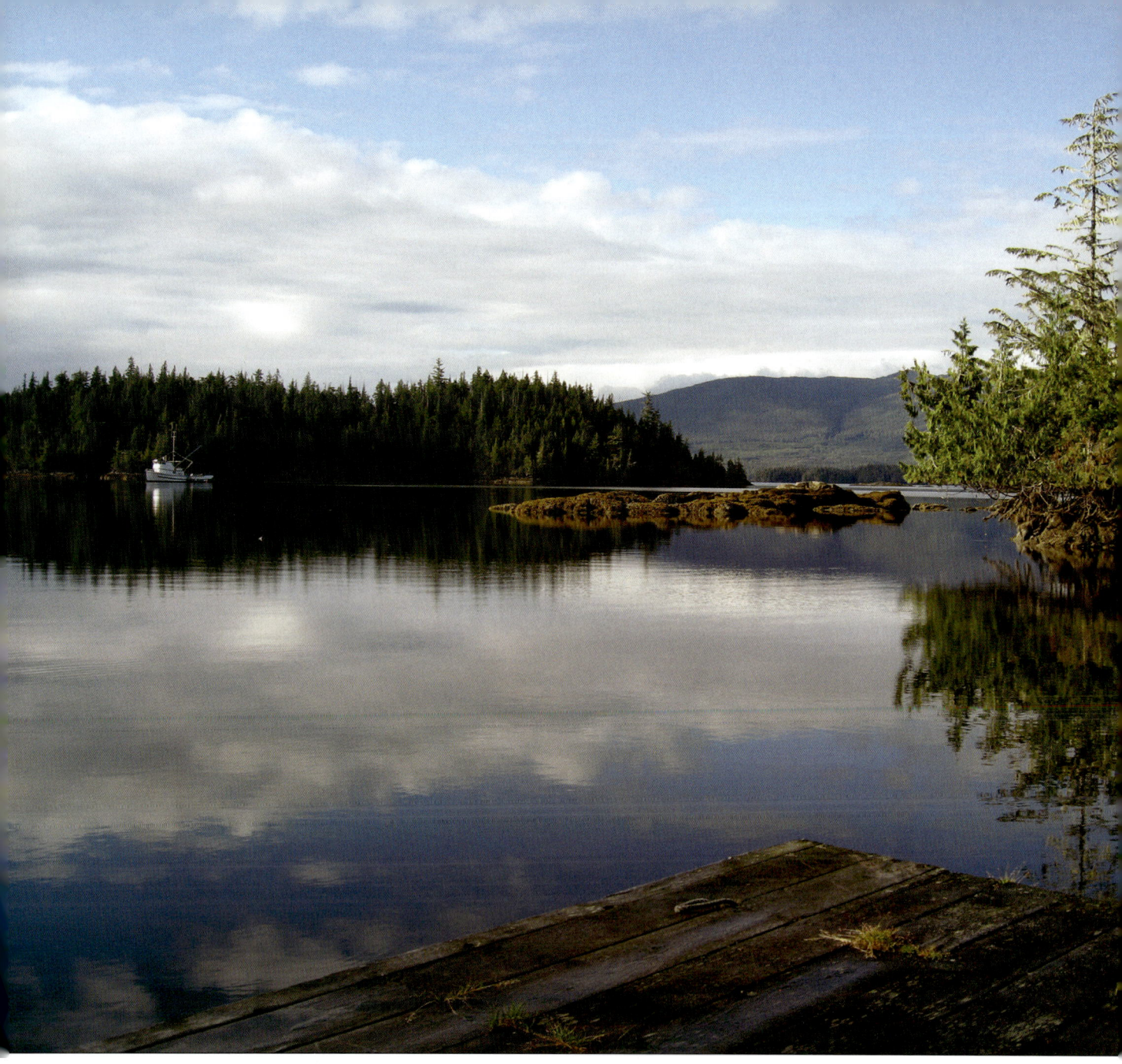

Point enter **Anchor Bight** through the narrow pass between Gnarled Islets and Anchor Islets. A shoal extends to the east of Anchor Islet. A good spot to drop anchor is just beyond Ship Rock on the south shore and in line with Abrupt Point on Indian Island. Takush Harbour has other suitable places to anchor as well as many nooks to explore including **Fly Basin**, which is protected by reefs and submerged rocks. Be mindful of these when you are entering to drop the hook.

### Millbrook Cove  chart 3934

On the opposite shore of Smith Sound, opening off Blackney Channel Millbrook Cove offers an easier and more expansive entrance to the anchorage than the entrance to Takush Harbour. This is the anchorage of choice for most mariners stopping in Smith Sound. Shelter can be reached from Blackney Channel, to the east of Shield Island and west of Millbrook Rocks in the entrance. Give the shoal off Shield Island a wide berth as you pass. Rocks and reefs are scattered along the west side of the cove entrance. Drop the hook in 7.3 metres at the head of the cove or in about 3 metres at the opening on the west side, about half way in. Millbrook Cove was the site of an old cannery.

There were many canneries in the area in the early days. All that remains of some of them today are pilings and remnants of buildings where those that have been abandoned once stood, and the odd one, mostly in Rivers Inlet, that has been turned into a fishing lodge.

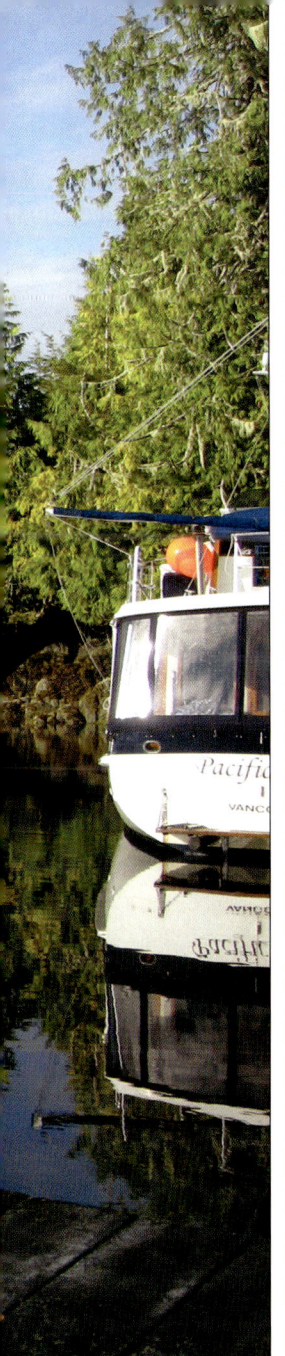

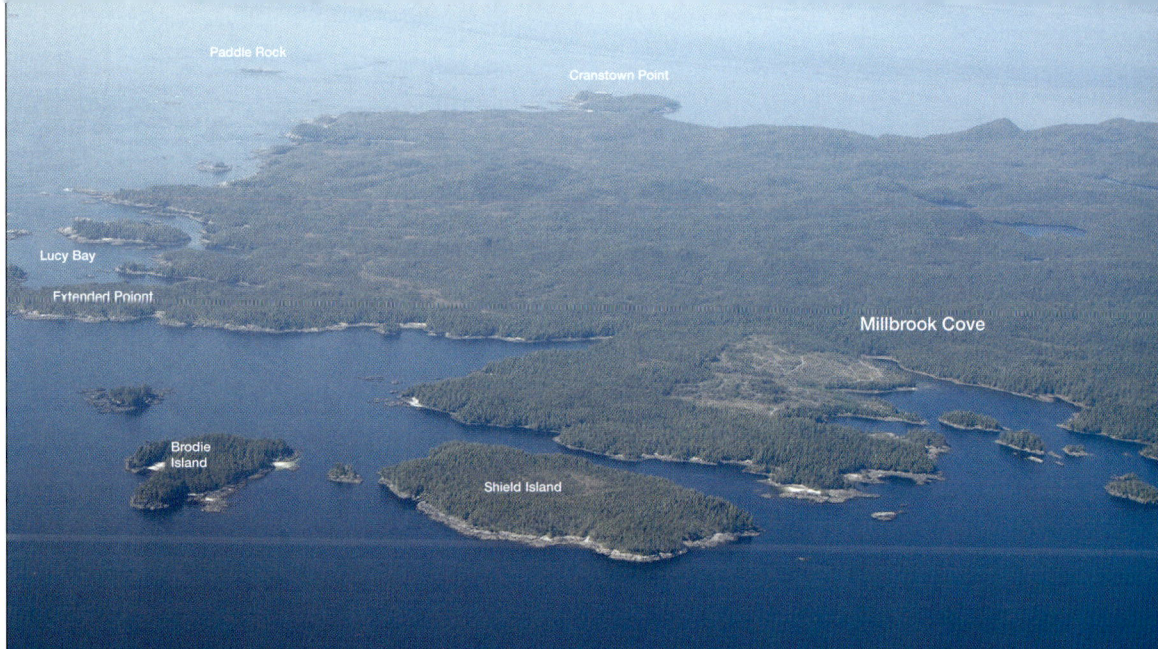

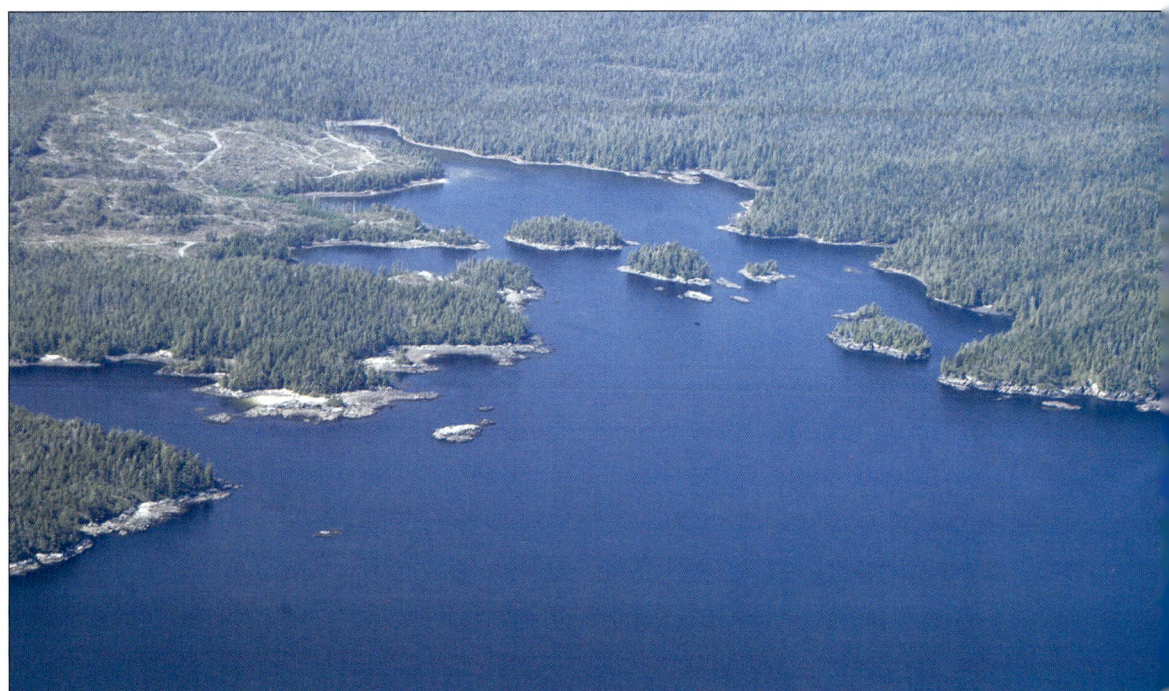

Farther inside Smith Sound, at the entrance to Smith Inlet, **McBride Bay** offers temporary sheltered anchorage. This bay is exposed to winds from the north, so find a suitable spot to drop the hook in the lee of the drying reef on the west side of the bay or in the lee of Oblong Island.

**Margaret Bay**, between Boswell Inlet and Smith Inlet, was once the site of a store and post office that served the local canneries and probably homesteaders, loggers and fishermen for many years. As you enter Margaret Bay beware

*Opposite: Vessels anchored at Takush Harbour. This sheltered harbour with several coves is conveniently located off the south shore of Browning Channel in Smith Sound near the entrance to Smith Inlet. Photograph courtesy of Noreen Rudd and David Hoar.*

*Above: Millbrooke Cove, on the opposite shore of Smith Sound from Takush Harbour. It is a large anchorage with sheltered nooks.*

*The view of Millbrook Cove at top includes Shield Island and Brodie Island in the foreground and Extended Point, Lucy Bay and Kelp Head to Cranstown Point beyond. Dugout Rocks and Paddle Rock can be seen to the left of Cranstown Point at the top of the photograph.*

244

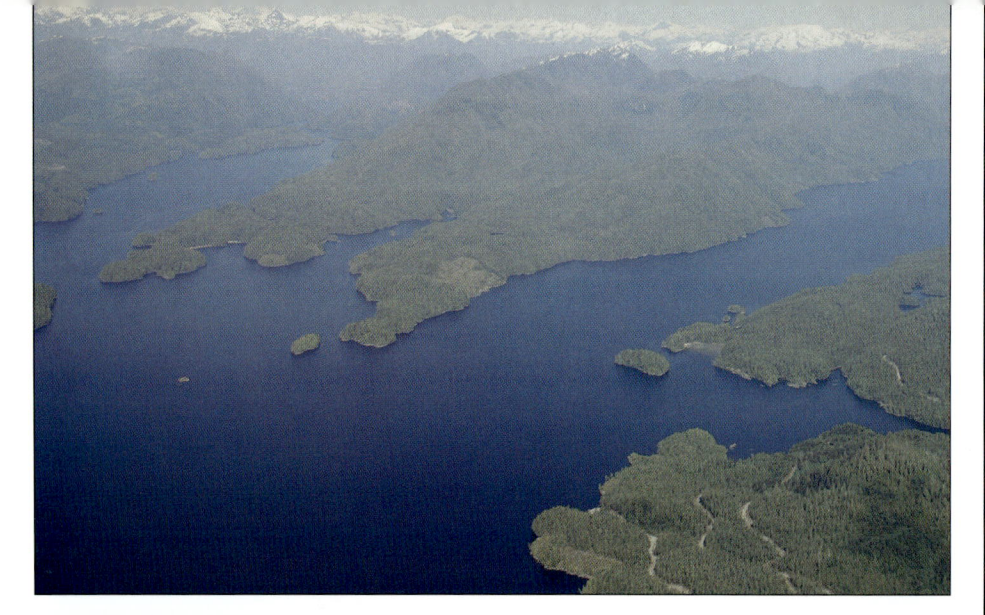

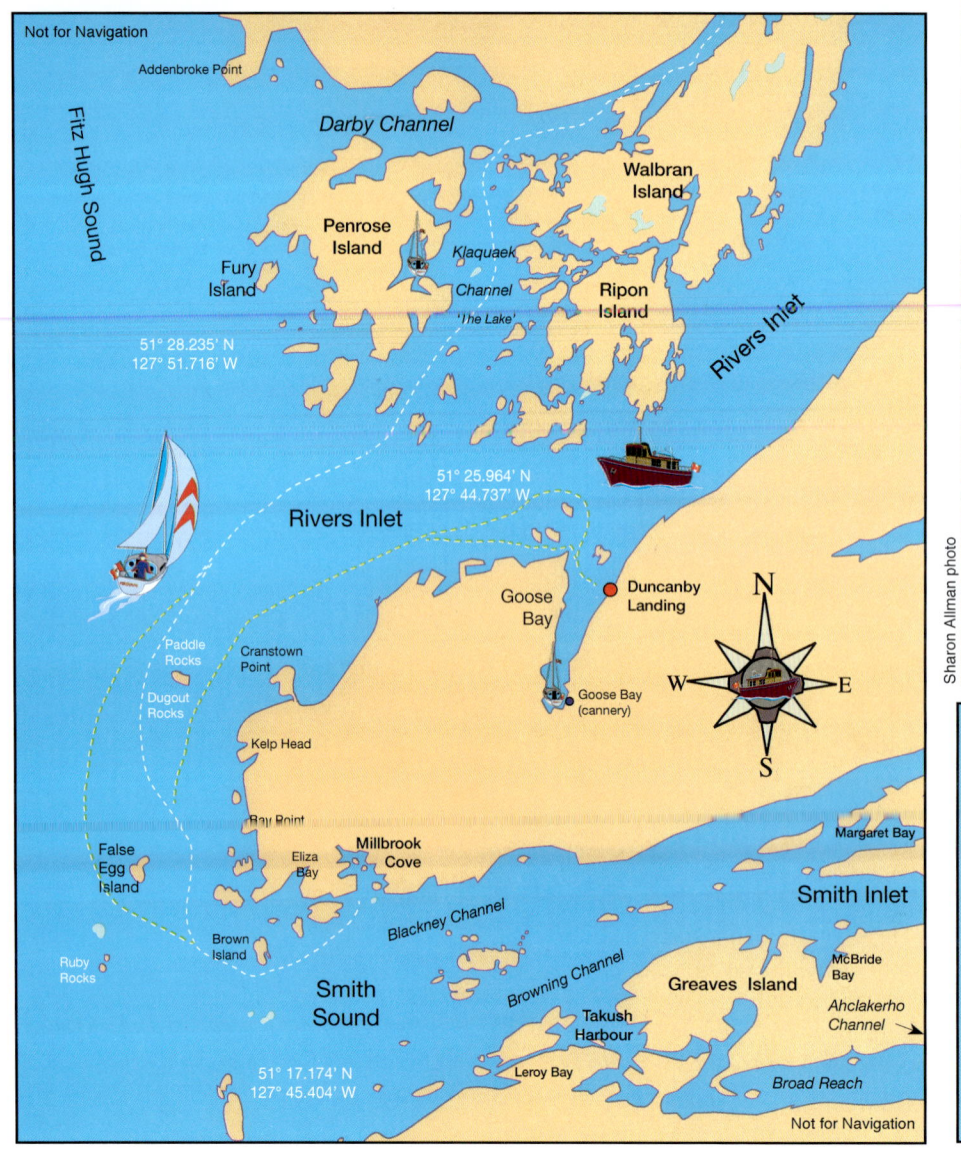

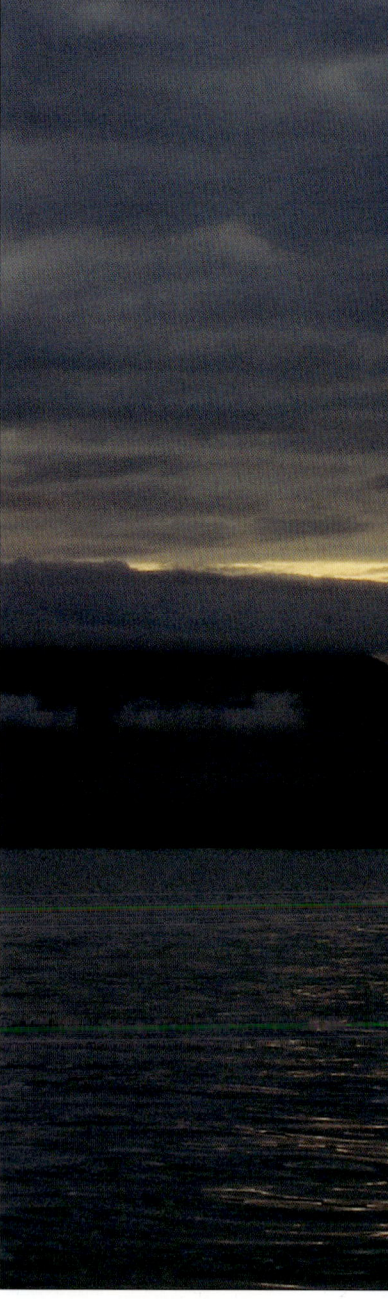

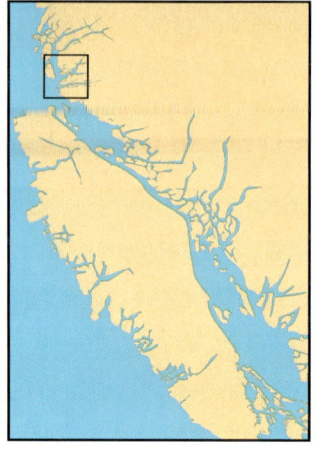

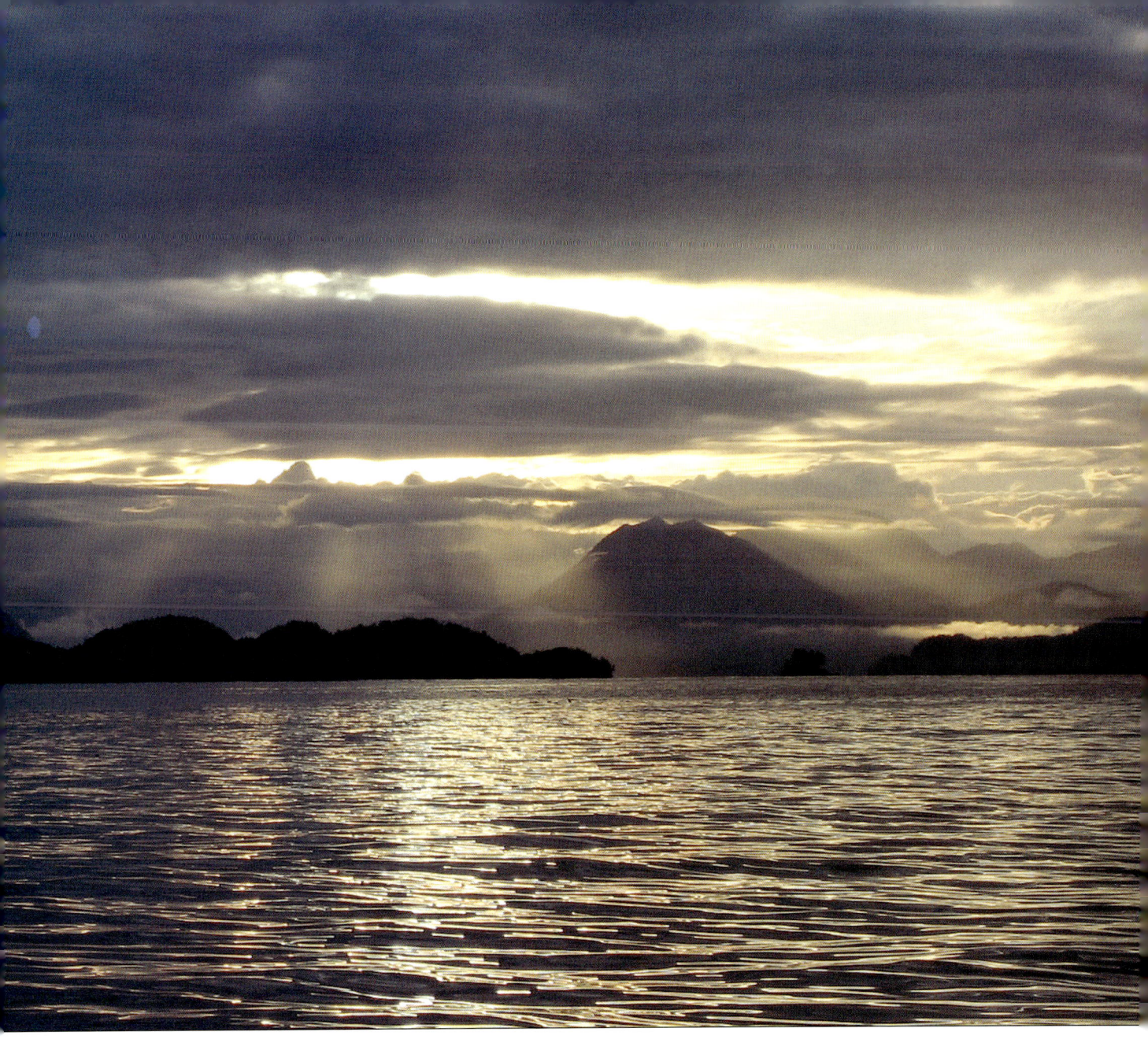

of Camosun Rock and some rocky shallows off Chambers Island in the middle of the bay. At the head of the bay there are remnants of a cannery. It was built in 1916 for Western Packers and later sold to the Canadian Fishing Company who operated it until 1945. It later became a camp for the gillnetter fleet but was eventually closed in 1959. In Rivers Inlet, Good Hope Cannery has a longer history. It was built in 1895, and was turned into a fishing lodge in the 1950s.

If you are an explorer by nature you may want to poke about Ahclakerho Channel and the east end of Greaves Island to Naysash Inlet near the head of Smith Inlet (see diagram page 238). To reach the channel that washes the south shore of Greaves Island you would have to cruise east along the north shore of the island and don't expect to return by way of the south shore as the passage connecting Ahclakerho Channel with Takush Harbour is simply not navigable by anything much larger than a canoe. Captain Vancouver explored these waters in 1792, but he was on a mission. Charting the coast kept him and his crews very busy, leaving little time to take leisurely strolls on the beach or lie daydreaming in an anchorage.

*Opposite: Smith Inlet with Margaret Bay and McBride Bay just beyond the entrance to Takush Harbour.*
*Above: Sunrise over Smith Sound.*

## Goose Bay, Rivers Inlet  charts 3934, 3931

If the weather is calm, or you feel confident in following

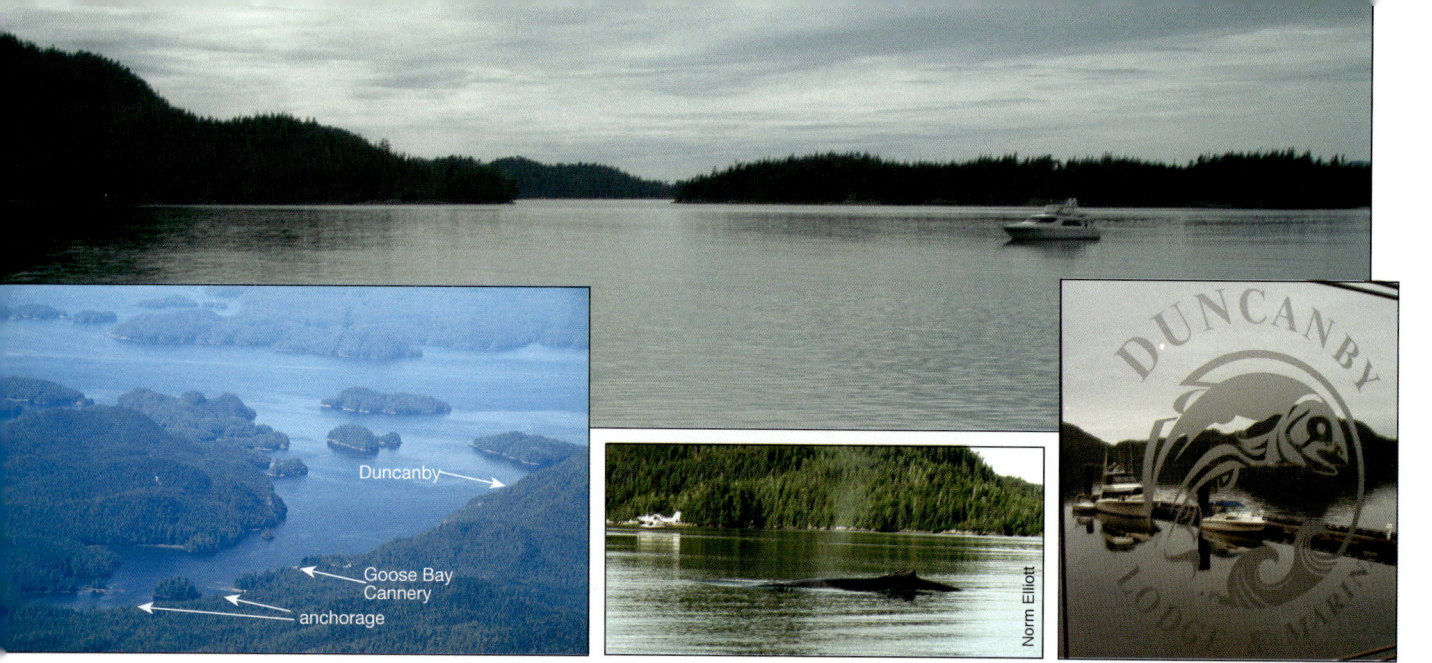

close to the shoreline from Smith Sound to Rivers Inlet, you can wend your way around the outside of Brown Island then pass between False Egg and Tie Islands to continue to the west of Spur Rocks and Cranstown Island. Beware of the reef to the southwest of Cranstown. Pass Open Bight and head into the entrance of Rivers Inlet. If you want to pass to the west of False Egg Island and Spur Rocks use Irving Passage. Once southwest of Egg Island take a bearing on the visible island at Dugout Rocks and follow a curving route to avoid the rocks that lie off Kelp Head. If you choose to enter Rivers Inlet wide of Paddle Rocks give them a good amount of clearance as you enter the south end of Fitz Hugh Sound. Follow your chart carefully making reference to your GPS as a secondary source for accurate navigation.

Cruising to Rivers Inlet from Cape Caution follow South Passage, pass west (or east in calm conditions) of Egg Island then round Paddle Rock and head for Sharbau Island. East of this island is an easy entrance to Goose Bay and Duncanby Landing. There is good water among the islands at the west entrance to Goose Bay (see chart 3934). Alternatively, continue on the outside the islands and enter west of Bull and Cow Islands. The lodge at Duncanby is almost in the lee of Cow Island. It is a popular fly-in fishing destination, favoured also among transient mariners. Moorage is available for visiting boats and the restaurant offers fine cuisine and sunset views over Rivers Inlet.

Fishing activity in Goose Bay began in the early 1900s. The old cannery was abandoned in 2002 after various tenants occupied it since its closure in the 1970s. Since its abandonment much work has been done to clean up the site as part of a restoration project to eliminate environmental contaminants. It has a fine new dock and overnight visitors are encouraged to stay for a fee. There is good, shallow anchorage nearby in the lee of a small island. Mind the shallows as you navigate the head of Goose Bay.

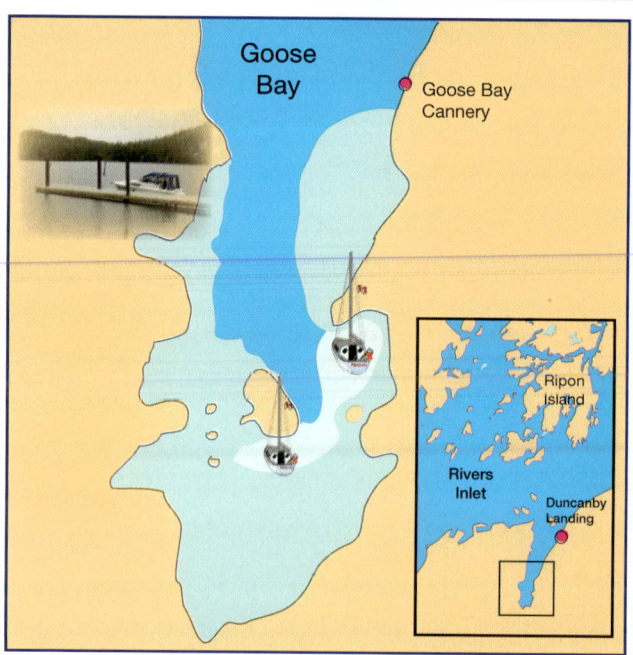

## Duncanby Landing Lodge and Marina
### Rivers Inlet
**Phone 1-877-846-6548**

admin@duncanbylodgemarina.com   www.duncanbylodgemarina.com

This is a fishing lodge with overnight moorage available. Power at the docks has 50 and 30 amp supply. The marina offers fuel, water, showers and laundry facilities. Guests can sign up for fishing excursions and there are fishing supplies and equipment available for sale at the lodge. Fish cleaning and vacuum sealing of guests' catches is offered. The marina has wireless internet access.

There is a spacious restaurant that serves breakfast, lunch and dinner. A store on site offers snacks and supplies, including ice, bait, books and other items.

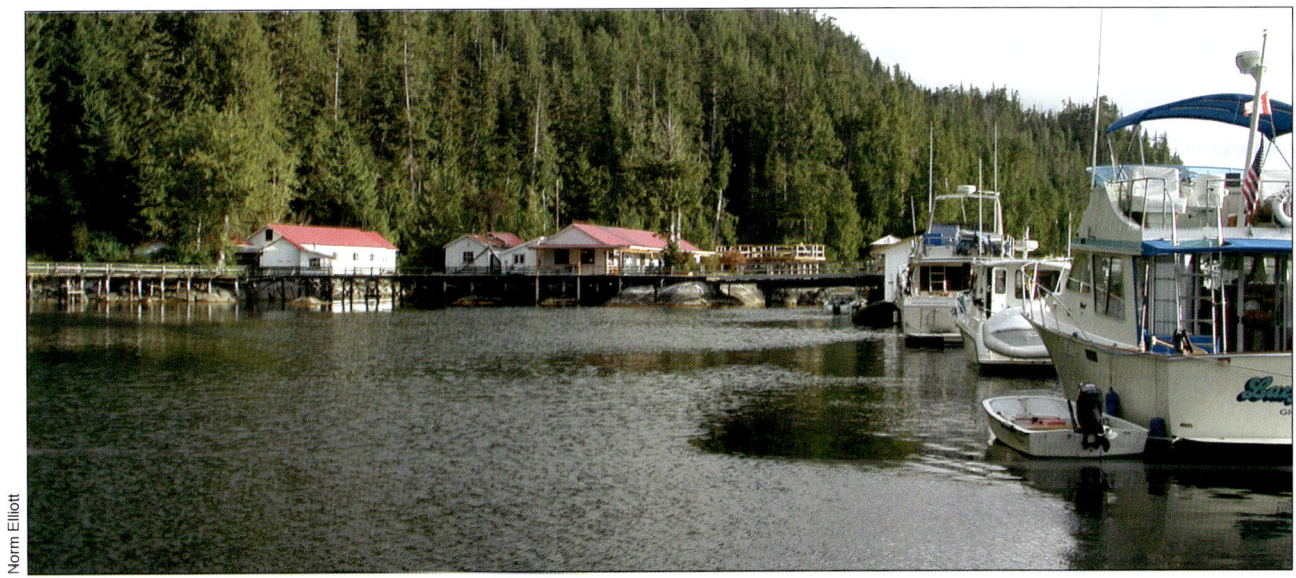

*Above: Duncanby Landing is a popular sport fishing lodge with docks and facilities for transient overnight guests.*

*Right: Old cannery buildings at Goose Bay. They are being renovated with the help of moorage fees collected at a new guest dock. Anchorage can be taken in the lee of the island seen in the photograph below, that also shows remnants of the wreck of the Haroc, an old fish collector vessel.*

*Opposite: Outlook from Duncanby Landing in Goose Bay, Rivers Inlet. Inset photographs show Goose Bay, a Minke whale making an appearance near the marina and boats at the dock, looking through a window of the restaurant.*

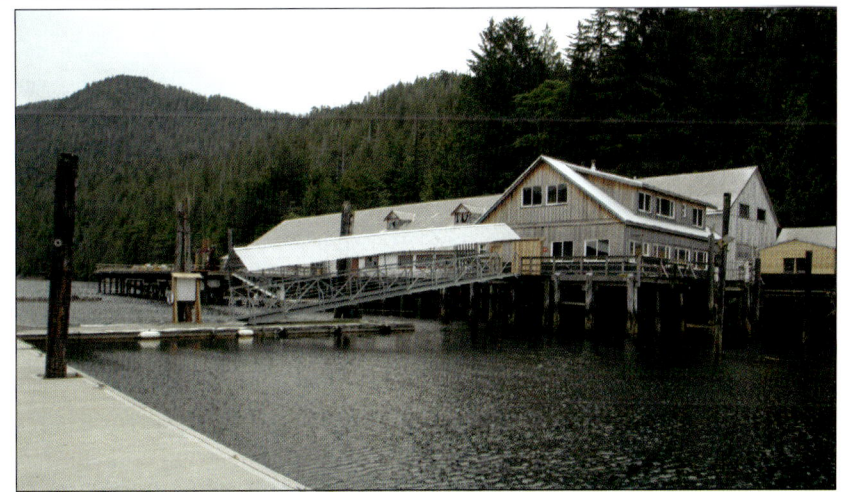

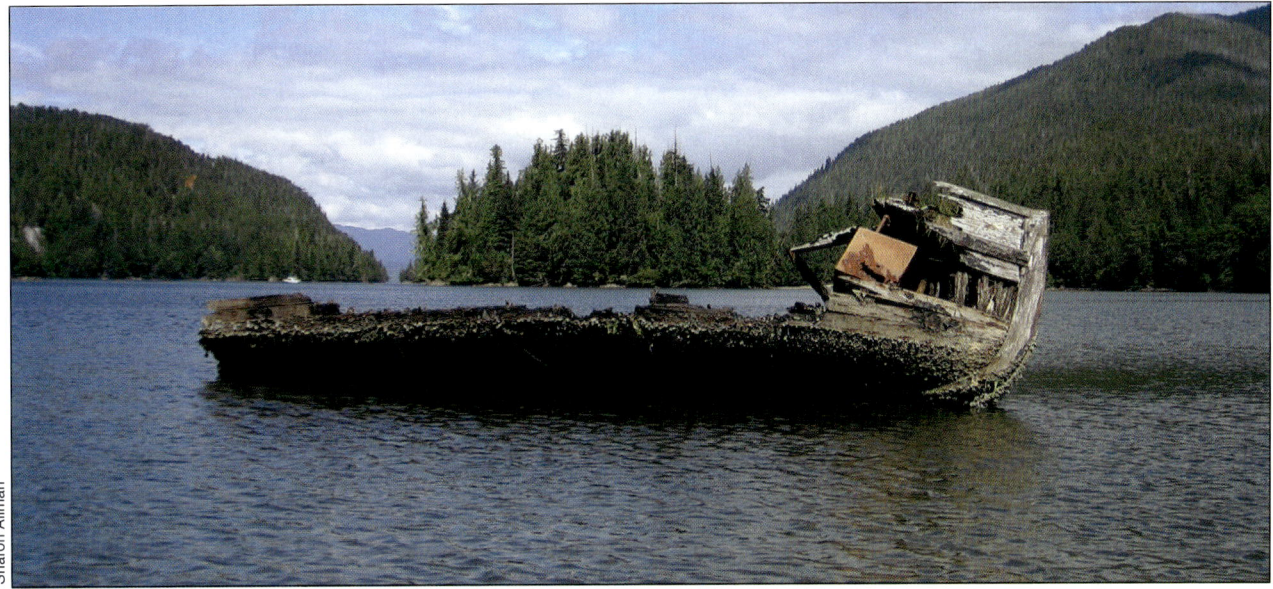

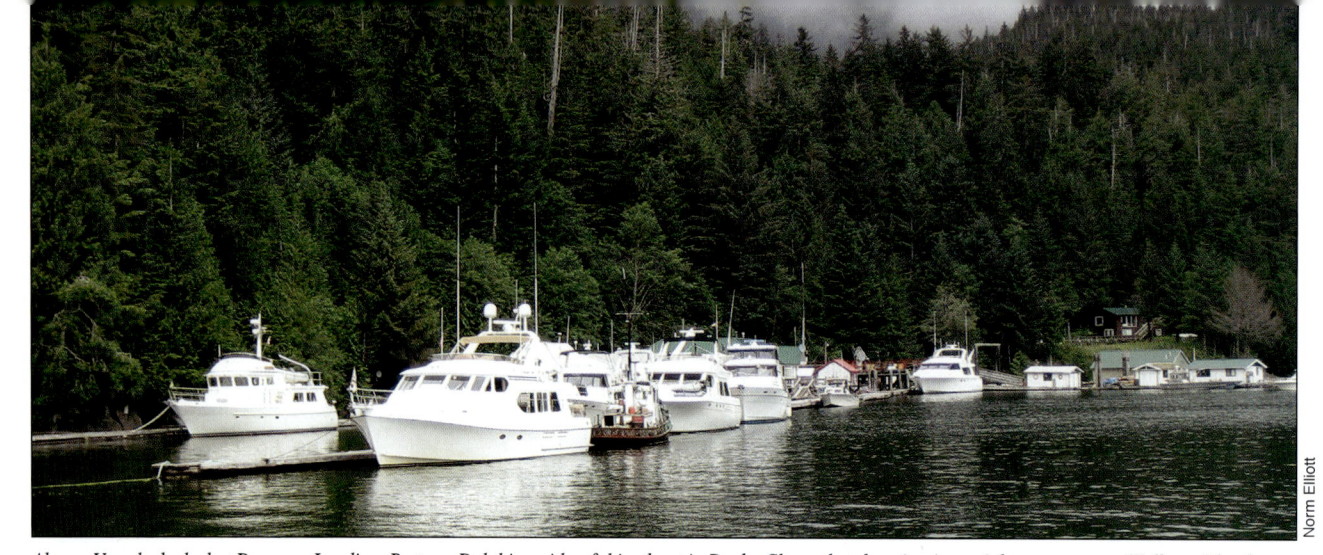

*Above: Vessels docked at Dawsons Landing. Bottom: Dolphins with a fishing boat in Darby Channel and navigating a tight waterway on Walbran Island.*

Another structure not far from Goose Bay is Good Hope Cannery. This was one of the first canneries on the central coast. Today it is a thriving fishing lodge and not a suitable overnight stop for mariners. It is a busy place in summer and there is little time on the management's busy schedule to cater to any needs of passing boaters. We have been advised from time to time that overnight stays by visitors is possible subject to available space.

Wadhams is another lodge, belonging to the same owners as Good Hope, and it too does not cater to transient marine traffic. It is located at the site of the former largest cannery in Rivers Inlet.

The cannery was founded in 1897 by E.A. Wadhams and run by the BC Packers company until 1942. When I first saw it in the 1970s there were still significant buildings at the site, on land and on pilings. Today nothing is left of the old cannery, but new cottages and lodgings have replaced the derelict buildings and it has become a pristine waterfront.

## The Lake, Rivers Inlet  charts 3934, 3932

To the north of Goose Bay, across Rivers Inlet entrance, is a group of islands and islets that include the larger Penrose, Ripon and Walbran Islands. Klaquaek Channel that divides the islands is known locally as 'The Lake'. This waterway and its myriad small islands and passages was for many years the playground of the late George Ardley and guests at his Rivers Lodge in Sleepy Bay. George took me on an exciting ride in his runabout once, to show me the narrow passages leading to Geetla Inlet, coves such as Sunshine Bay and the intricacies of Magee Channel.

George Ardley was known locally as Hurricane Ardley. He got the name because of his many trips to and from Port Hardy in practically any kind of weather. He operated several power boats over the years and one day he arrived home at his fishing lodge after a quick trip to pick up supplies at Port Hardy. Wife Pat, greeting him at the dock asked in horror what had happened on the trip. Surprised by her strained greeting, George came down off the bridge to see the cause for her concern. The windows in the main cabin were all but gone and the supplies were strewn about the cabin, awash from having taken heavy seas that blew out the glass and saturated the interior. It is gratifying to know that even a small powerboat can take a lot more than we expect in conditions such as those that occur off Cape Caution.

For the adventurous, there are a few possible anchor-

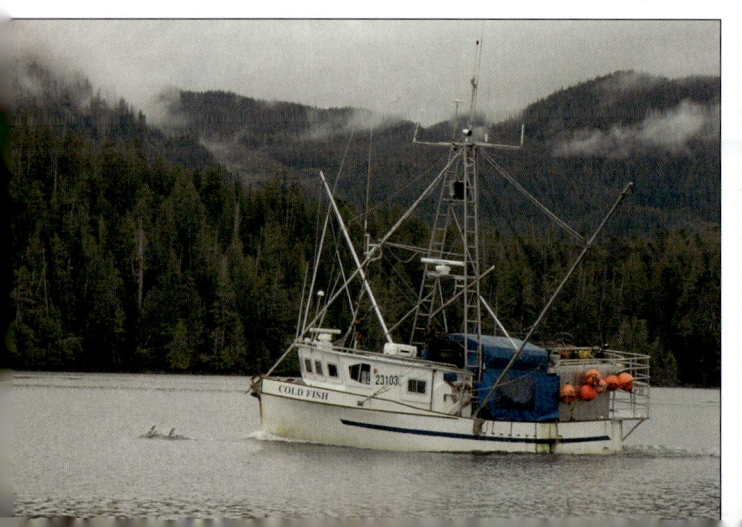

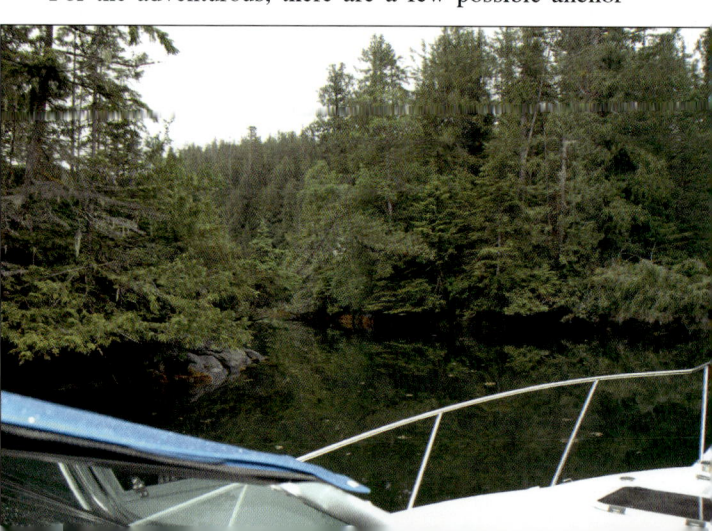

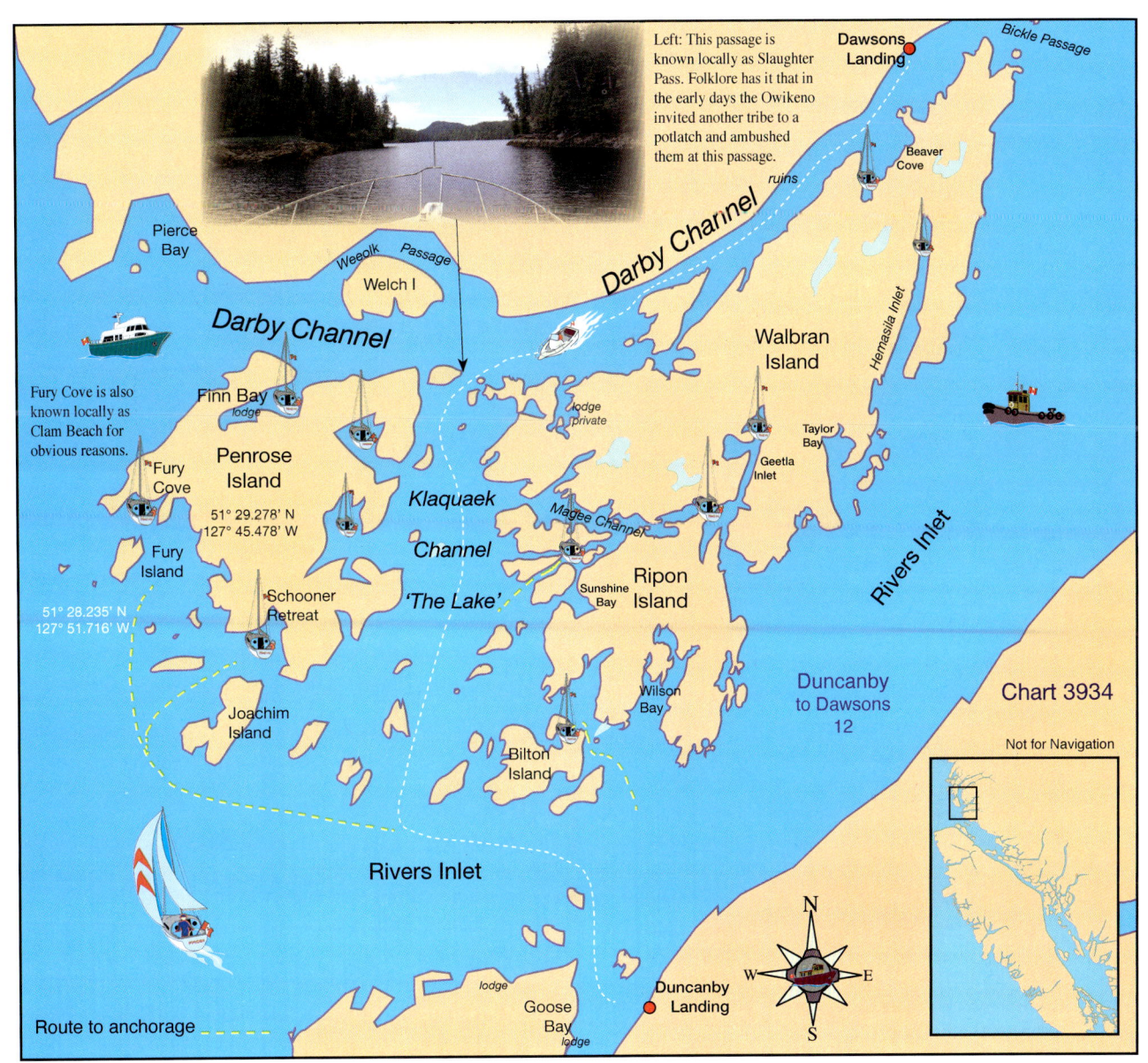

Left: This passage is known locally as Slaughter Pass. Folklore has it that in the early days the Owikeno invited another tribe to a potlatch and ambushed them at this passage.

ages on the east side of Walbran Island. A couple are located inside **Geetla Inlet** and another at the head of **Hemasila Inlet**. Both of these inlets require very careful navigation and avoidance of reefs and rocks. One of the anchorages in Geetla Inlet is in a cove at the east end of Magee Channel near its intersection with Geetla Inlet. The other is at the head of Geetla Inlet. Mind the rocks at the entrance. Anchor also in the north side of **Bilton Island** in a cove formed by the small islet adjacent to it.

It is a pleasant cruise up the narrow Darby Channel to **Dawsons Landing**. Here supplies and fuel are available, as well as a place to stay at a dock overnight. The store at Dawsons has a large inventory of groceries and supplies and other conveneinces for mariners. Anchorage may be taken at the head of **Beaver Cove** nearby.

## Dawsons Landing
**Dawsons Landing BC V0N 1M0**
**Phone 604-629-9897**

*dawsonslanding@dawsonslanding.ca   www.dawsonslanding.ca*
The dock at Dawsons Landing has seen the coming and going of all forms of vessels for many decades. It is a well-known fuel stop with gas and diesel as well as stove oil available. Overnight mooring guests will find washrooms, showers and laundry at the marina.
The store has fishing licences and tackle as well as block and cube ice, groceries, books, charts and some marine supplies. It is also a post office and a scheduled air service stop connecting to Port Hardy.
Owners are Rob and Nola Bachen. Rob's family has owned Dawsons Landing for many decades.

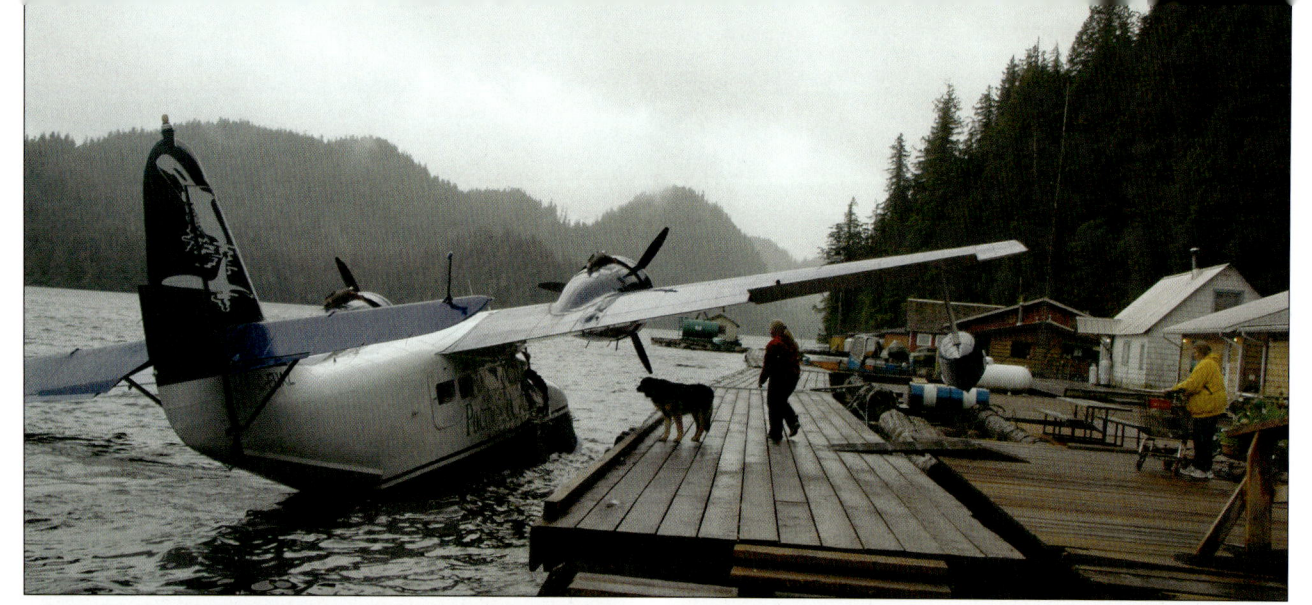

Beyond Dawsons Landing, the short Bickle Passage between Walbran Island and Edna Mathews Island returns the cruise into Rivers Inlet and just across the way is Good Hope and Wadhams, former cannery sites. These two facilities have been operating as recreational fishing lodges for many years since the closure of their canning facilities. New structures and some of the old canning buildings remain, in refurbished condition, to accommodate guests.

There is a public dock at the head of Rivers Inlet, but it is poor for overnight shelter. There are few choices and it is best to find moorage or anchorage at Dawsons, Duncanby or the anchorages described earlier. A short distance beyond Edna Mathews Island is Sandell Bay, site of a former hospital, long since abandoned and left to the encroachment of the forest. There are a few shallow areas near the head of this bay but anchoring should be temporary. Anchor in fair weather. Watch for southerly winds.

Moses Inlet, opening off Rivers Inlet is a long waterway with deep water and little if any shelter (diagram opposite). Hardy Inlet is also deep and inhospitable. Nelson Narrows off Inrig Bay, farther up Moses Inlet, is deep enough for easy passage.

The mouths of **Kilbella River**, Chuckwalla River and Wannock River offer some temporary anchorage. A native village is located on the Wannock River at the head of the inlet. Besides promising catches of big salmon, Rivers Inlet offers the possibility of viewing wildlife, including killer whales, eagles and grizzlies. Check for fishing restrictions.

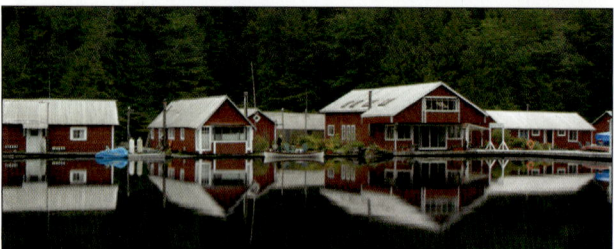

*Above: A rustic lodge on Walbran Island and an aerial view of Dawsons Landing. Top: A Pacific Coastal Airlines Goose arrives at Dawsons Landing.*

## Penrose Island  chart 3934

Anchorage is available at **Finn Bay** at the north end of Penrose Island and in the lee of **Fury Island** on the west and southwest side. Finn Bay is easy to reach at the entrance to Darby Channel. It is a large bay with a wide entrance and sheltered anchorage to the south of the islet at its head.

The **Schooner Retreat** group of islands, which includes Fury Island, offers shelter in **Exposed Anchorage, Frigate Bay** and **Secure Anchorage**. Use good ground tackle in these anchorages for secure holding in the event of strong winds. Our favourite anchorage is in Fury Bay.

To reach **Fury Island's** anchorage approach the south west side of Penrose Island and enter the passage northwest of Stunted Islets and Folly Islet then pass east of Cleve Island. To the south of Exposed Anchorage is Rocky Bay, Secure Anchorage and Frigate Bay. These can be reached by way of **Safe Entrance** between Ironside Island and Joachim Island. There are reefs in the entire group that demand careful, slow navigation to reach sheltered moorage.

Once safely anchored in one of the above basins explore the sandy beaches, nooks and crannies, in your dinghy or runabout. Remember, there is good fishing and crabbing in the area, hence the number of busy fishing lodges in Rivers Inlet. The area is also suitable for clear water visibility scuba diving. Use heavy neoprene diving suits, preferably dry,

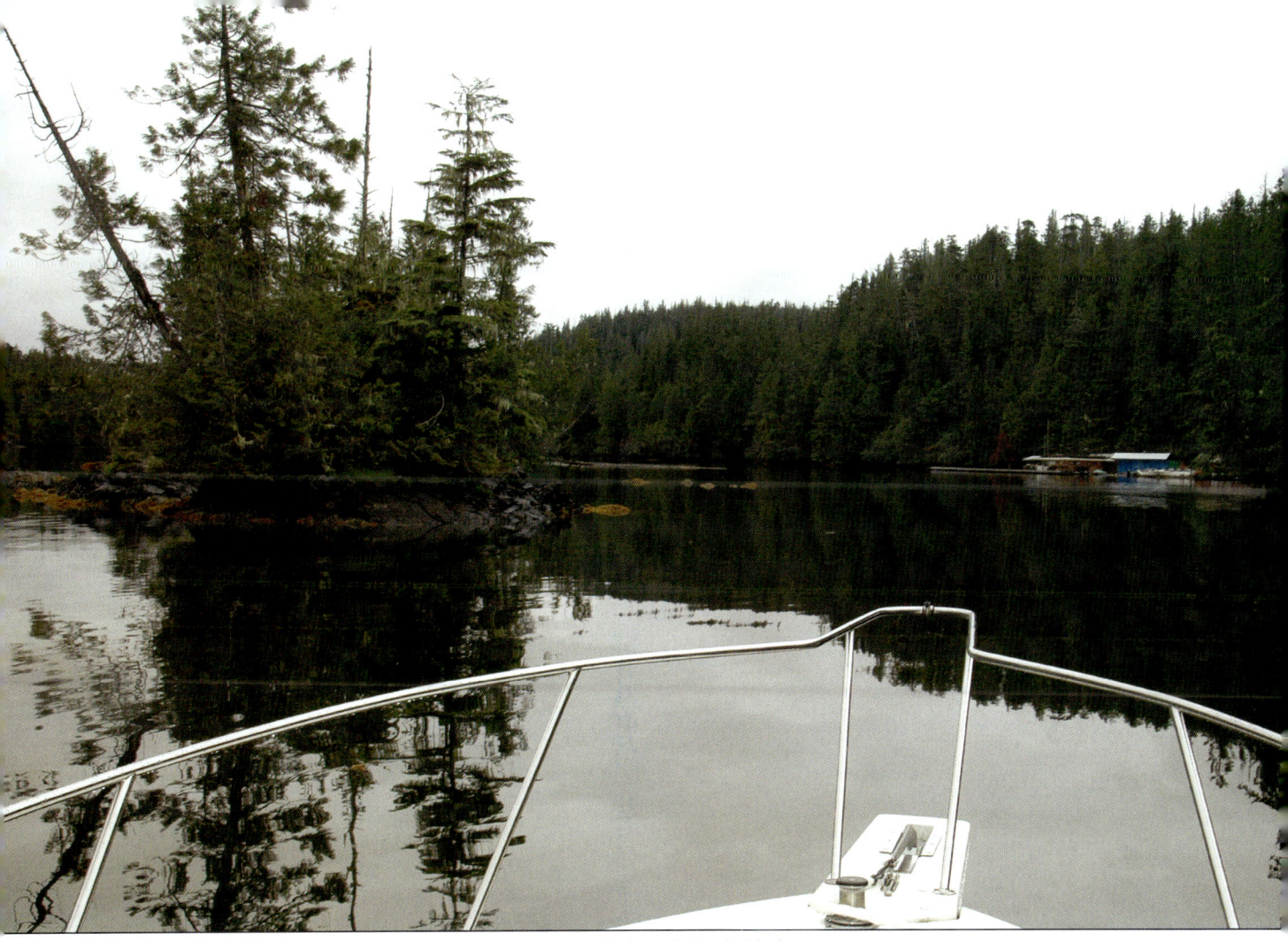

*Above: Sheltered anchorage in Finn Bay can be taken in the lee of the small islet at the head of the bay.*

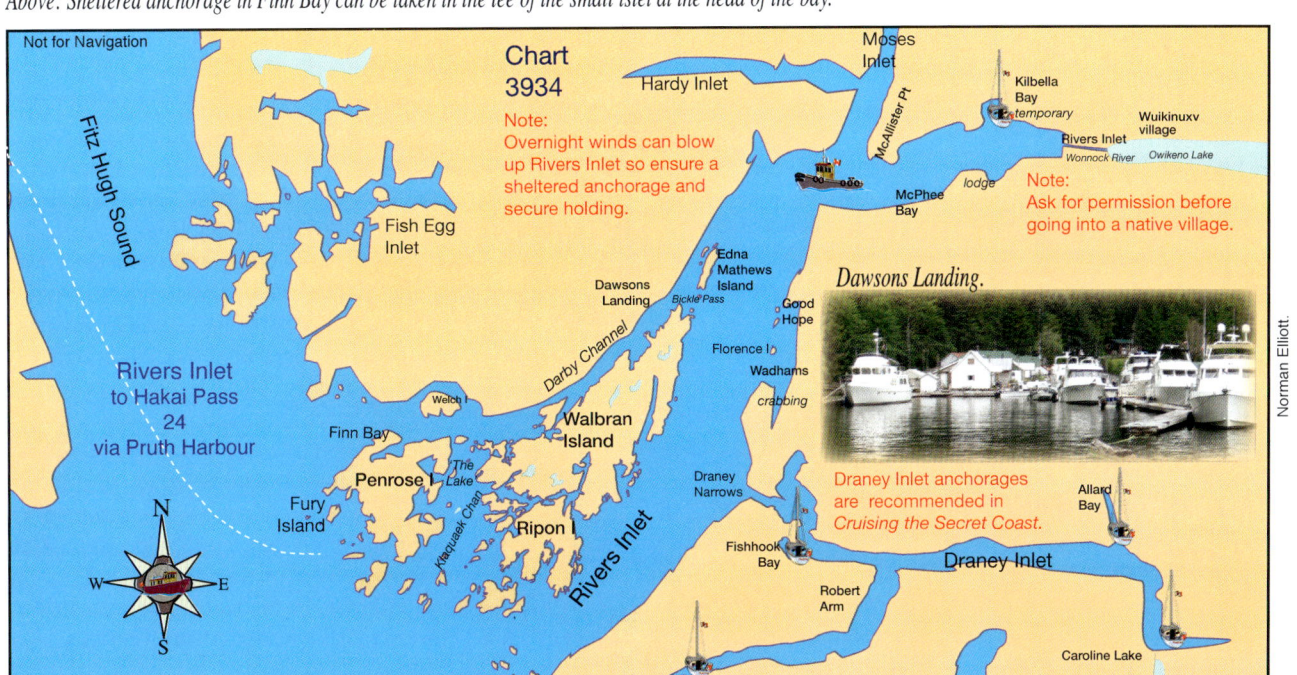

**Chart 3934**

Note: Overnight winds can blow up Rivers Inlet so ensure a sheltered anchorage and secure holding.

Note: Ask for permission before going into a native village.

*Dawsons Landing.*

Draney Inlet anchorages are recommended in *Cruising the Secret Coast*.

Norman Elliott.

251

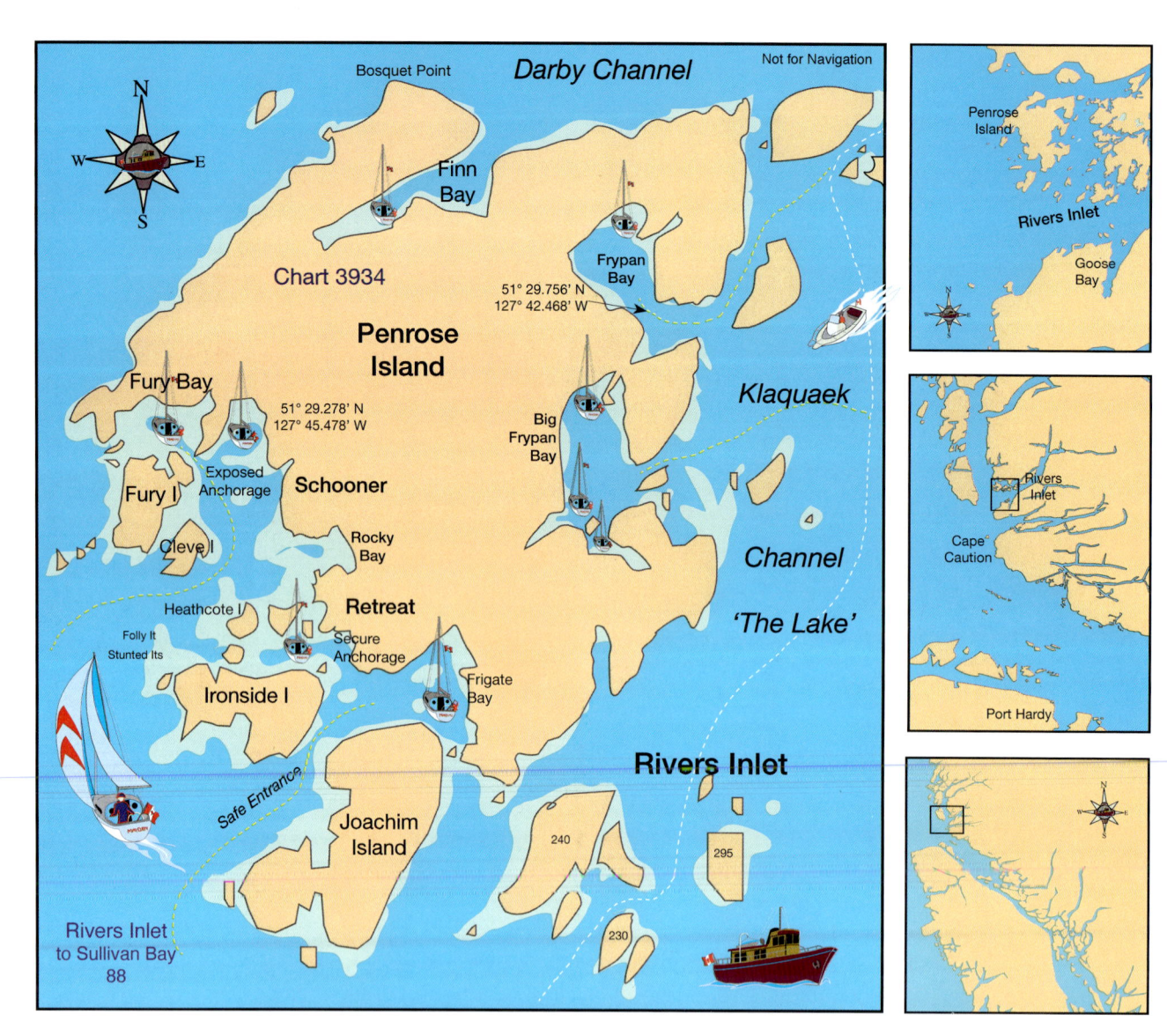

because the water temperatures are very cold. It is equally important to be well protected against cold when kayaking, another popular activity in the area.

Penrose Island is an undeveloped marine park. In addition to its anchorages at Finn Bay on the north end and Schooner Retreat at the south, it has sheltered nooks off 'The Lake' in **Frypan Bay** and **Big Frypan Bay**.

The south and west of Penrose Island are exposed to the open weather of the Pacific Ocean. When winds are blowing from the south west, in particular, care should be taken when planning any excursions. Note that after stormy weather large swells continue a while before abating, so be careful in kayaks and other small craft.

Mariners are advised against harvesting bivalves as the entire area is subject to red tides. Use of holding tanks is appreciated by the local Oweekeno First Nations who use the area around Penrose Island as a shellfish harvesting site.

Rivers Inlet was named for George Pitt, first Baron Rivers of Strathfieldsaye. When Captain Vancouver gave it the name he called it Rivers Channel, which, like numerous other inlets so named during his Voyage of Discovery, was changed later to reflect the true nature of the waterway. Vancouver's ship *Discovery* was lying in Safety Cove with her consort *Chatham* on the east shore of Calvert Island at the time of the exploration of Rivers Inlet. During an extensive examination of the coast by small boat out of Safety Cove, the expedition's men covered a lot of shoreline extending as far north as Burke Channel. It was Whidbey and Puget who explored Rivers Inlet. Safety Cove was also named by Vancouver, although Calvert Island was named a few years prior to Vancouver's visit, by Captain Charles Duncan, an earlier explorer on the coast, in his sloop *Princess Royal*. Duncan is also believed to have named Milbanke Sound and Chatham Sound.

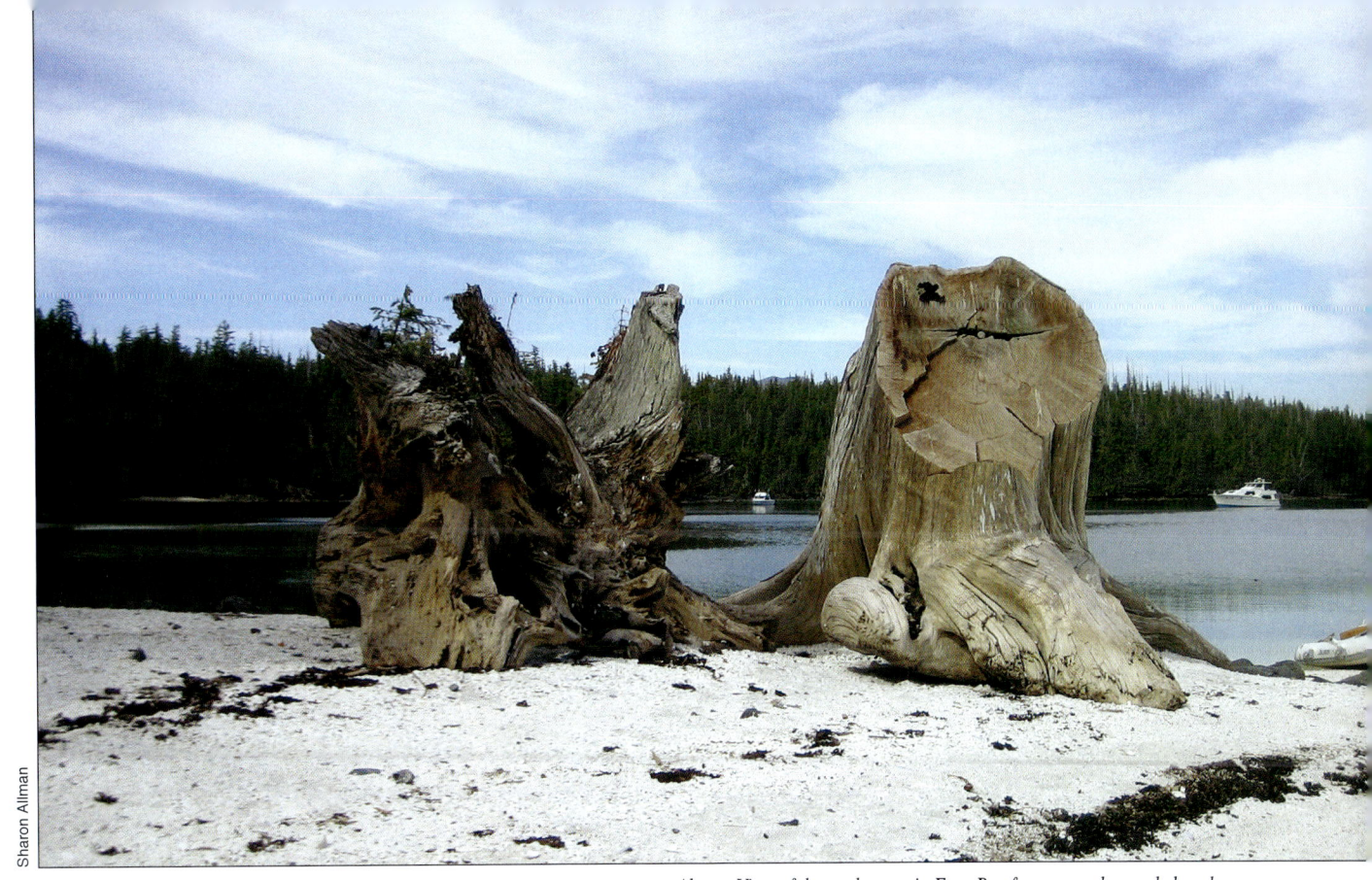

Some historians differ about the name of Duncan's ship. Walbran refers to it as *Princess Royal* while Marshall/Mitchell refer to it as *Prince of Wales*. It appears that the *Princess Royal* and *Prince of Wales* sailed out of England together under command of Duncan and James Colnett respectively. After accomplishing his mission in the Pacific Northwest, Duncan handed over the *Princess Royal* to Captain William Hudson and took command of the *Prince of Wales* to return to England. Duncan's mission had been to capitalize on the burgeoning fur trade.

## Draney Inlet   chart 3931

Draney Narrows has a tidal current of up to 10 knots. Use the Prince Rupert tidal reference plus 25 minutes. Once inside look for spectacular vistas and sheltered anchorage. These can be found primarily in **Fishhook Bay**, Allard Bay Caroline Falls or Robert Arm (diagram page 251).

## Fitz Hugh Sound   charts 3934, 3935, 3936

As you make your way out of Darby Channel from Rivers Inlet into Fitz Hugh Sound you will pass Addenbroke Point and its adjacent Swan Rock. Just north of Rivers Inlet **Philip Inlet** offers some shallow anchorage in about 30 feet. Continue to Blair Island and Addenbroke Island and find temporary anchorage in **Fifer Bay** (diagram page 254). Using Convoy Passage enter **Fish Egg Inlet** or continue

*Above: View of the anchorage in Fury Bay from a nearby sandy beach.*
*Below: Going ashore on Penrose Island while lying at anchor in Fury Bay.*

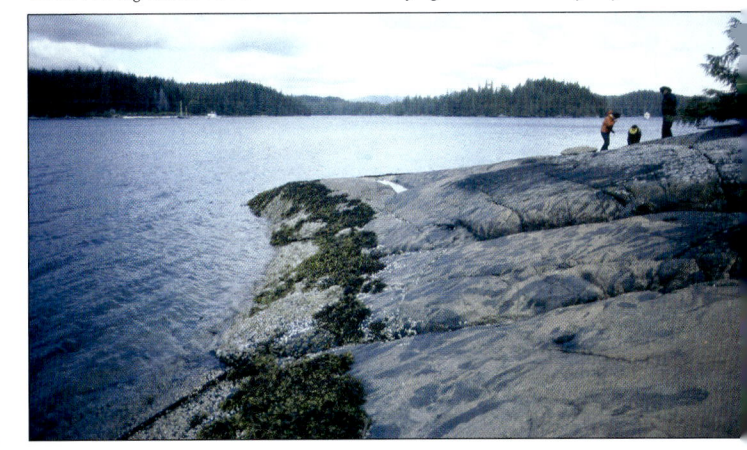

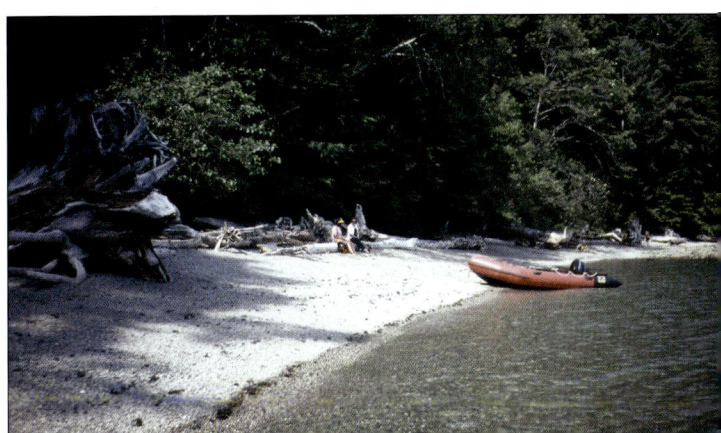

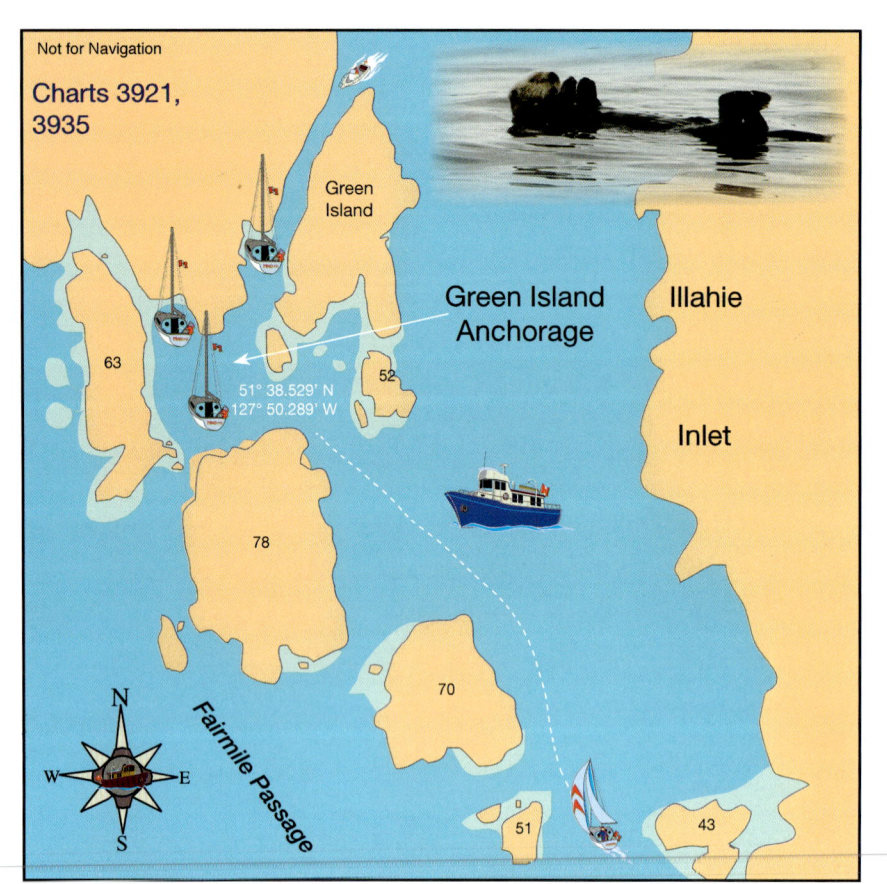

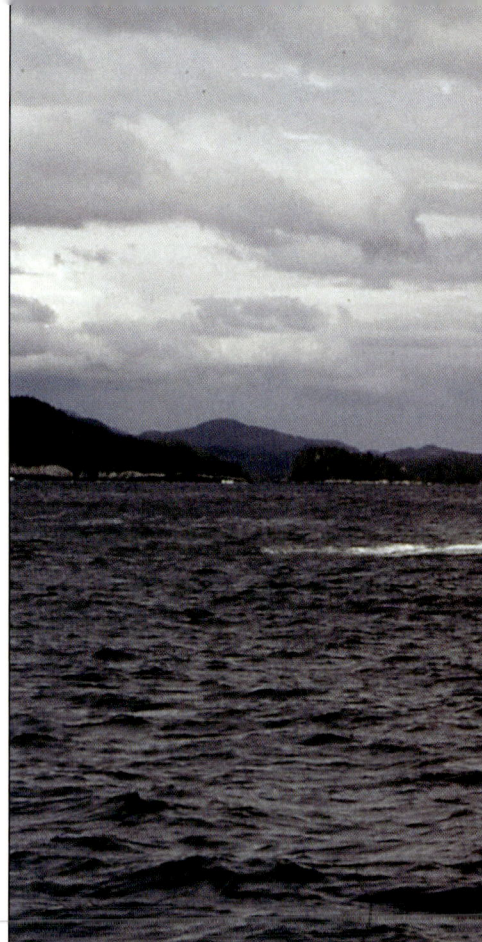

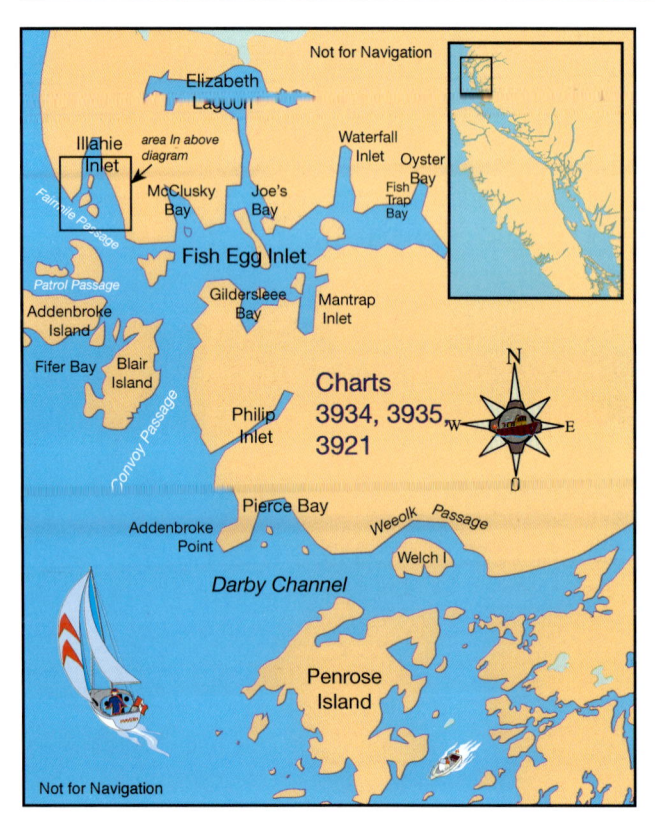

by way of Fairmile Passage to **Illahie Inlet**. **Green Island** anchorage lies in the lee of Green Island near the entrance to Illahie Inlet. The first time I visited Fish Egg Inlet, like Drany Inlet off Rivers Inlet, it had not yet been charted.

We ventured in a short way, watching the depth sounder with great attention and the waters ahead for shallows or reefs. We anchored in **Gildersleeve Bay**. The water had been calm and the bay tranquil. The inlet would be surveyed within a few years of that visit and today it is a popular place for the few who have time to explore and enjoy its many features. Poke around **Mantrap Inlet** and **Joe's Bay** for possible good overnight anchorage. Joe's Bay is at the entrance to Elizabeth Lagoon.

Deeper in Fish Egg Inlet are Waterfall Inlet, Fish Trap Bay and Oyster Bay, all of which bear exploring. A small boat may be preferred for these, as there are some winding, narrow passages strewn with islands, islets and rocks.

## Hakai Pass (Hakai Recreational Area)

Cross Fitz Hugh Sound to Hakai Pass or continue along the mainland shore where you will find delightful anchorages along the way in the vicinity of Hakai Pass.

On the Calvert Island side of Fitz Hugh Sound there are many interesting anchorages and waterways. We have avoided **Safety Cove** because it is deep with a steep drop-

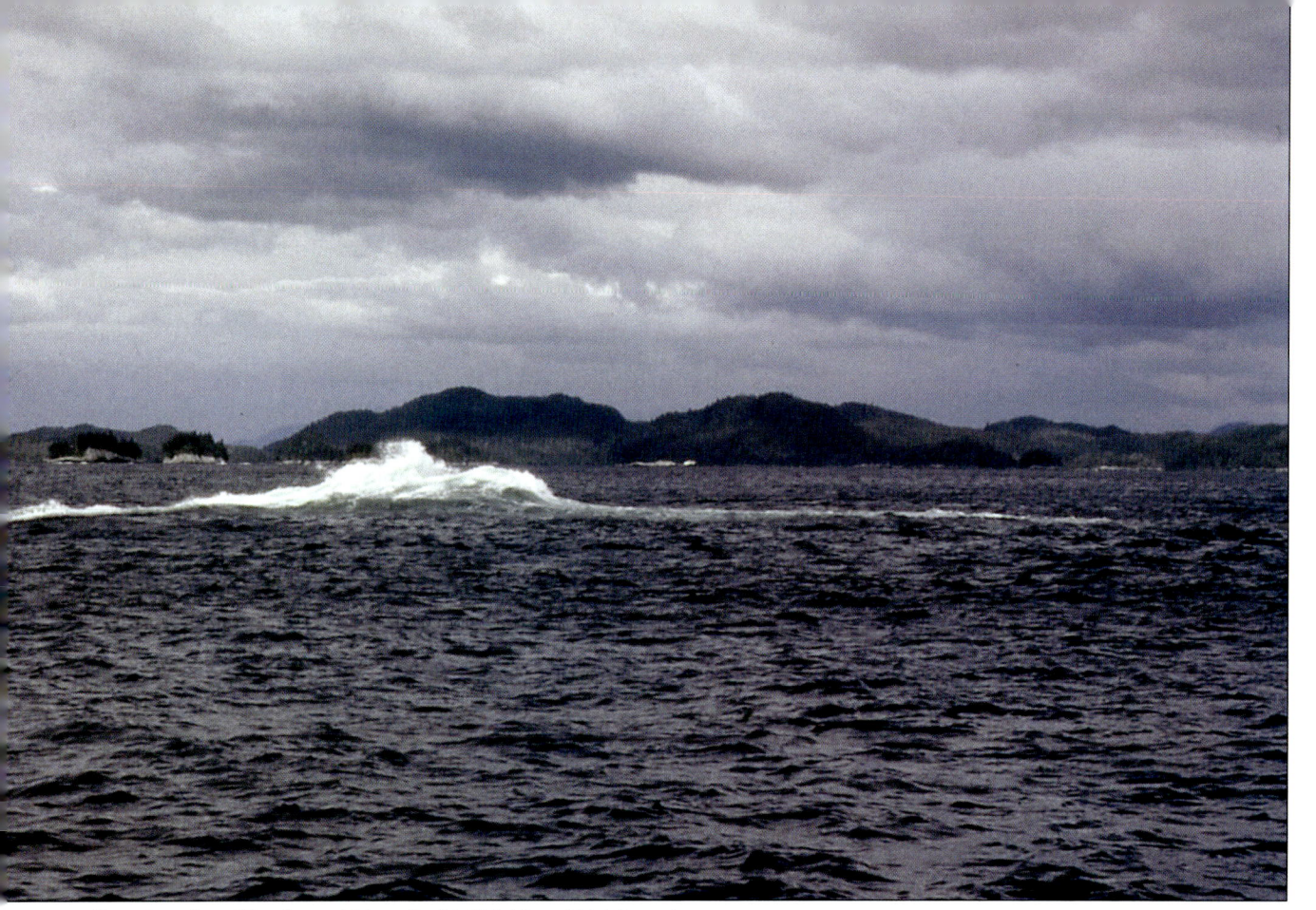

*Above: A gentle swell breaks over Mainguy Rock in Hakai Pass. This is located just into the pass when entering from Pruth Harbour.*

off from shore, and is a fairly exposed anchorage. Captain Vancouver anchored there while exploring the area.

Move up to Kwakshua Channel separating Calvert Island from Hecate Island. This channel leads to **Pruth Bay** and Keith Anchorage and gives access to the outer waters of Hakai Pass. A former lodge and fishing resort landing is located at the very head of Pruth Bay. Today the property is occupied by the Hakai Beach Institute, a privately owned family foundation. There is a trail that leads from the landing to a beautiful sandy beach on the west side of the island.

The head of Kwakshua Channel is a good place to find anchorage. A small cove opens off Pruth Bay that provides fairly good anchorage. Nearby **Keith Anchorage** is also quite good but more exposed than Pruth Bay. Opposite Keith Anchorage a channel leads to Hakai Pass.

There is a beautiful bay off Hakai Pass at **Adams Harbour.** We have walked the beach in this bay and kayaked around the adjacent rocks and islets in calm conditions while anchored near the northern entrance to the harbour.

At the northeastern tip of Hecate Island the popular **Goldstream Harbour** is a protected place in the lee of Hat Island. Anchor deep inside the harbour for the most protection from wind and seas.

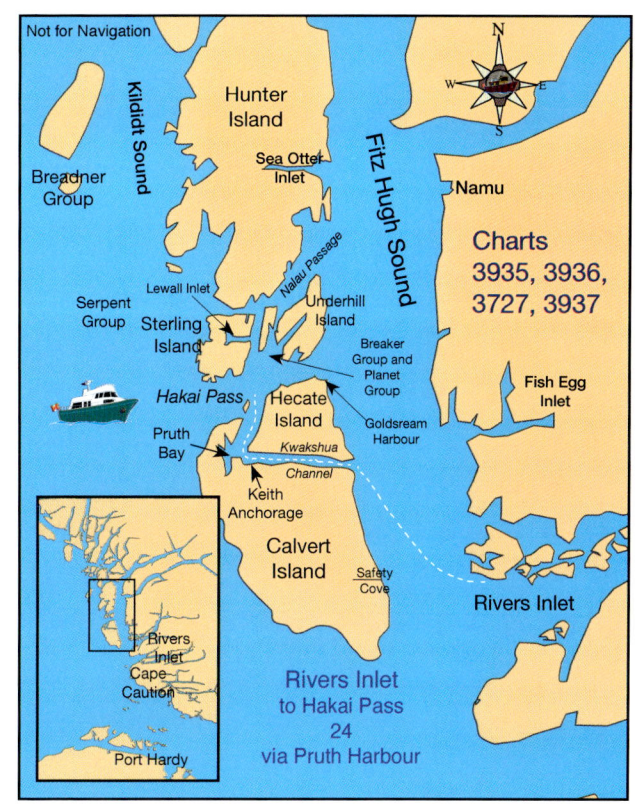

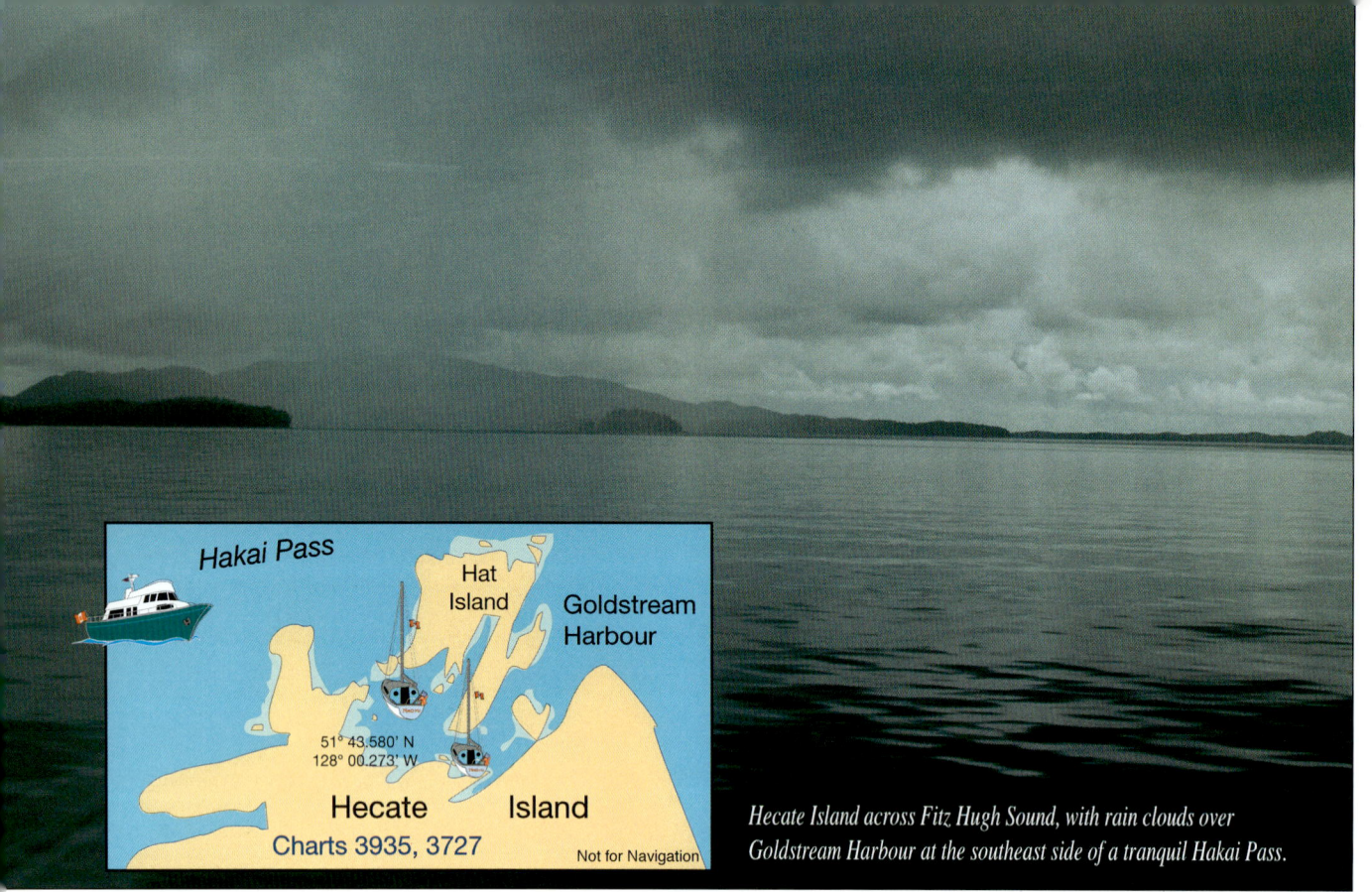

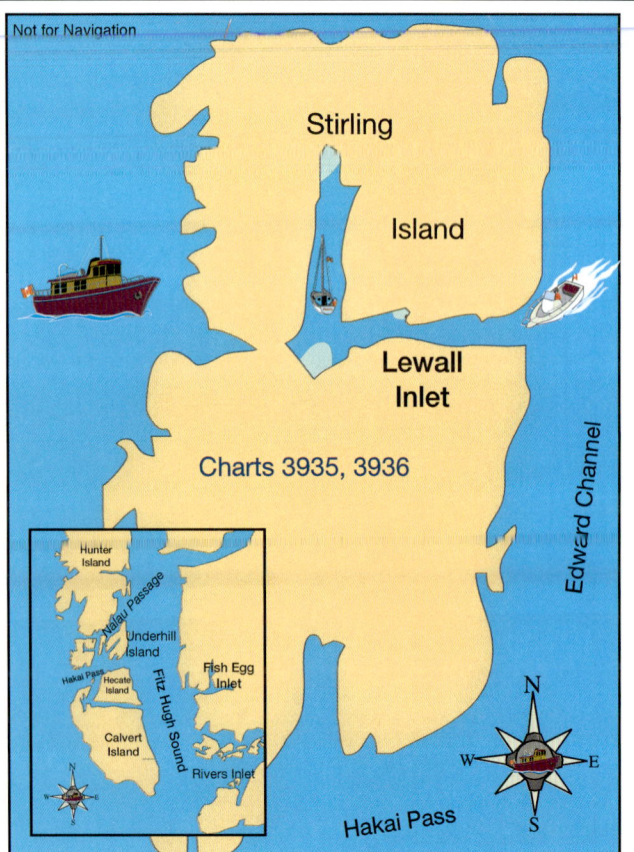

*Hecate Island across Fitz Hugh Sound, with rain clouds over Goldstream Harbour at the southeast side of a tranquil Hakai Pass.*

A tranquil anchorage not to be missed is at **Lewall Inlet**. This opens off Edward Channel on Stirling Island on the north side of Hakai Pass. It can be reached beyond the Breaker Group and the Planet Group (page 255), carefully wending your way through the islets and rocks between Stirling Island and Underhill Island. Lewall Inlet can be reached also from the north east of Underhill Island by way of Nalau Passage, a route we use when leaving the anchorage to head across Fitz Hugh Sound for Namu and Ocean Falls.

If you are continuing north along Fitz Hugh Sound or crossing over to Namu but want to linger a while longer in the vicinity of Hunter Island you will find that Sea Otter Inlet, opening into the east shore of Hunter Island, is a good all weather anchorage (diagram page 255).

There are other anchorages in this area, both inside Hakai Pass and on the outside. Those outside the pass are found in the Kildidt Sound area and include the Breadner Group and the Kittyhawk Group. In this archipelago there are anchorages well known among the relatively few who make them a regular destination. They are found in the proximity of Spider Anchorage and, along with many others, are comprehensively covered in the guide *Cruising the Secret Coast* by Jennifer and James Hamilton. The guide includes remote passages and anchorages to the south and north.

To continue to anchorages and marinas beyond these destinations please consult this author's guides ***Anchorages and Marine Parks*** and ***Docks and Destinations.***

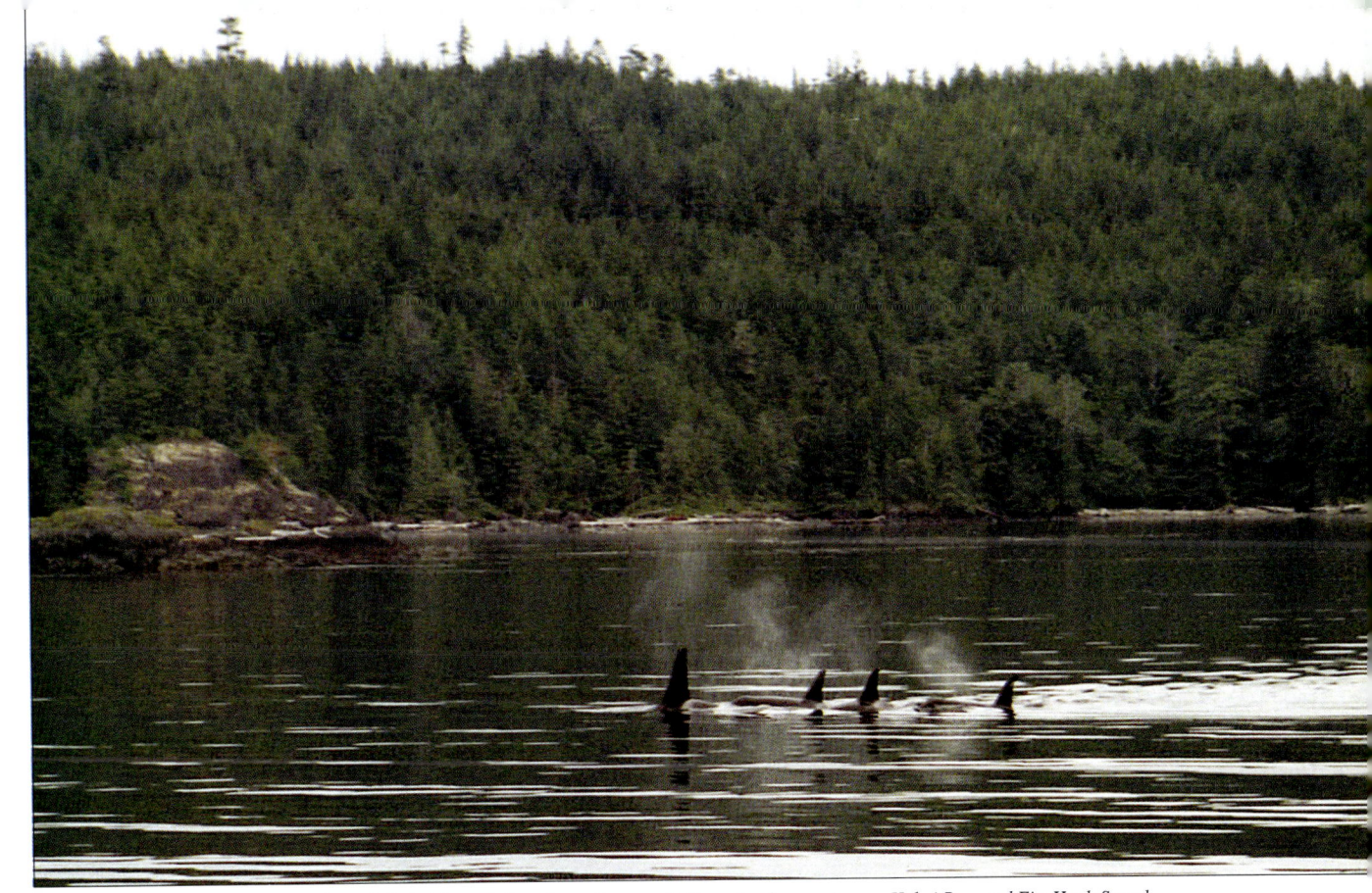

*Above: A pod of killer whales going through Hakai Pass. Below: Late afternoon light as clouds move in over Hakai Pass and Fitz Hugh Sound.*

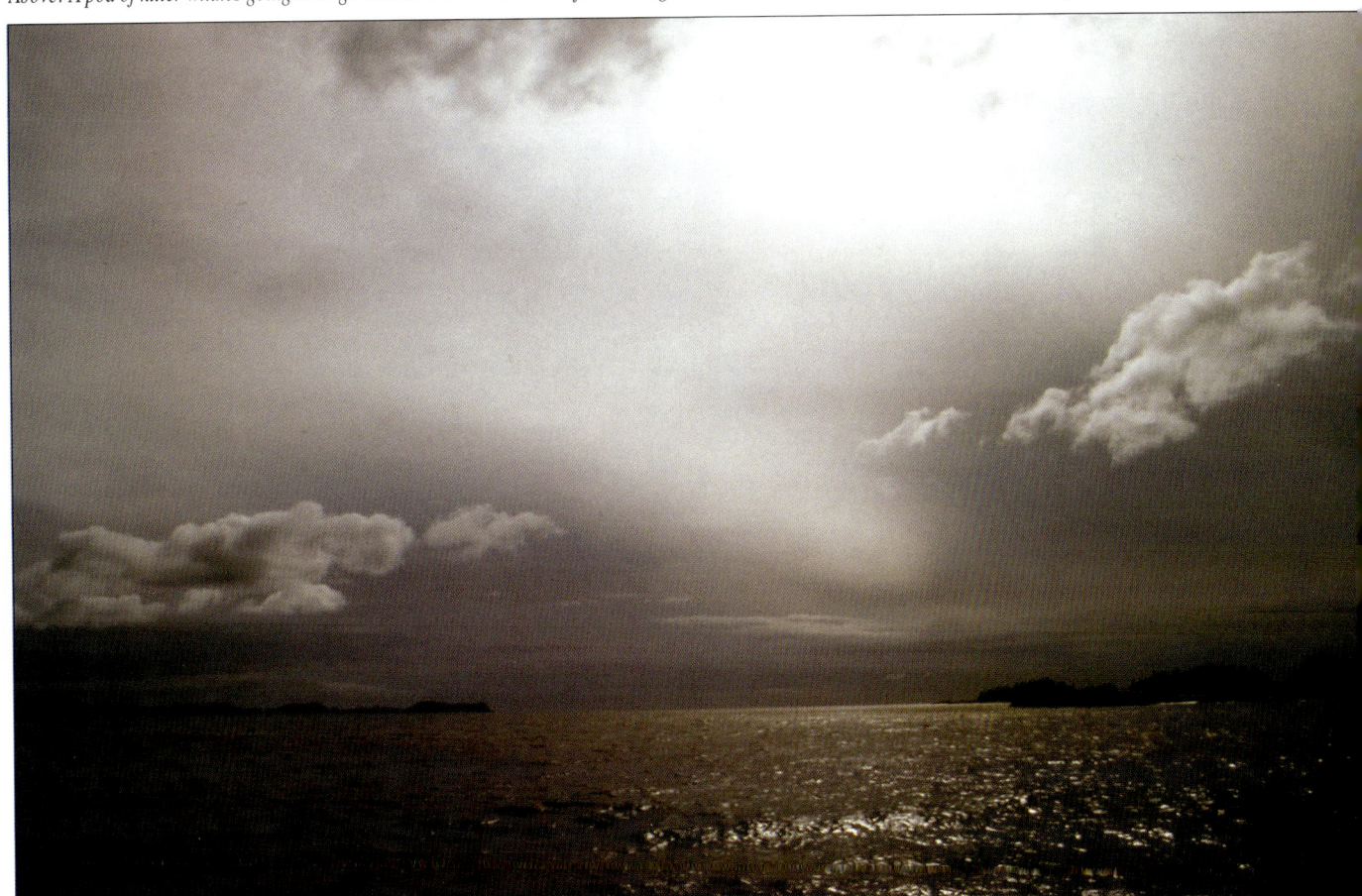

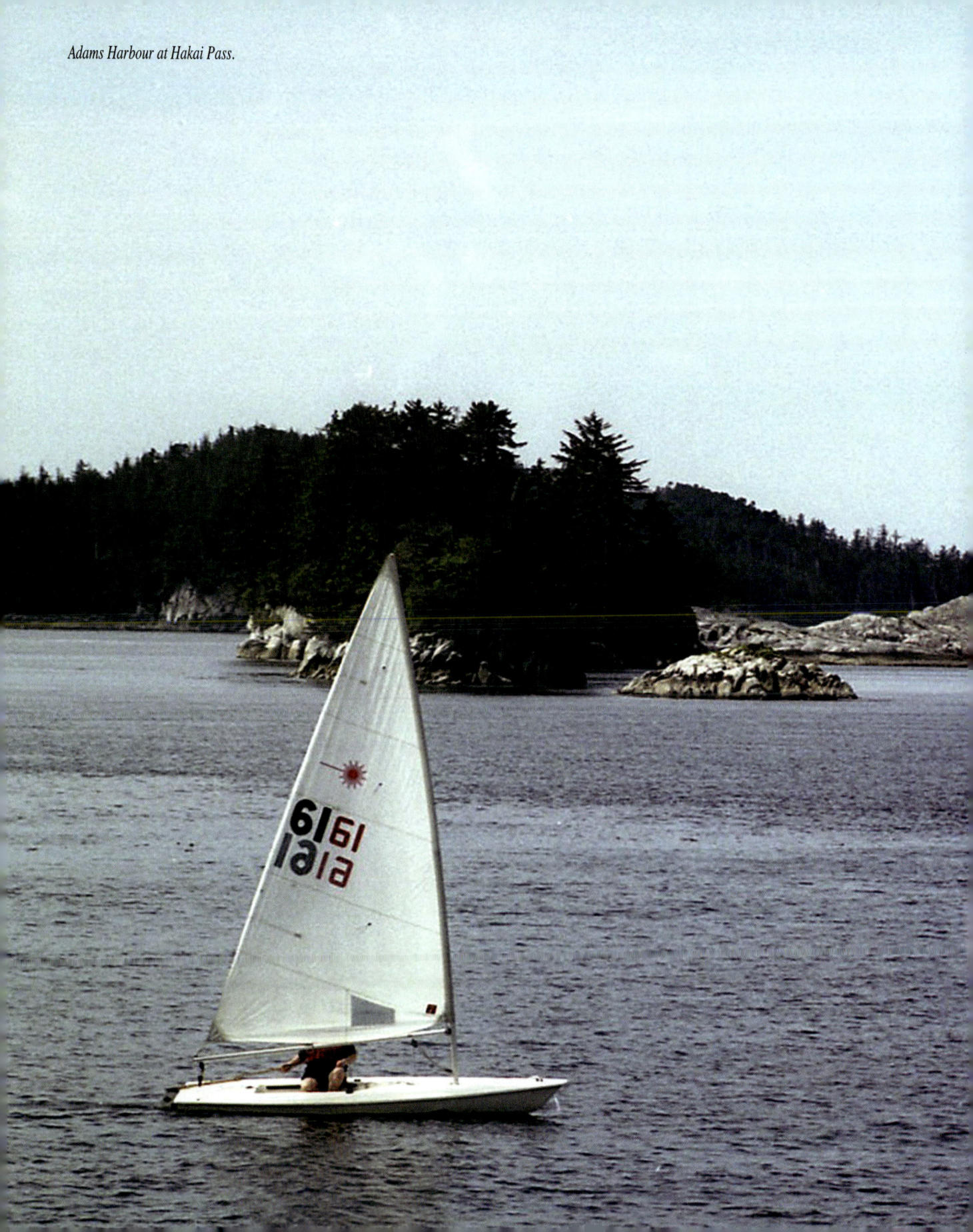

*Adams Harbour at Hakai Pass.*

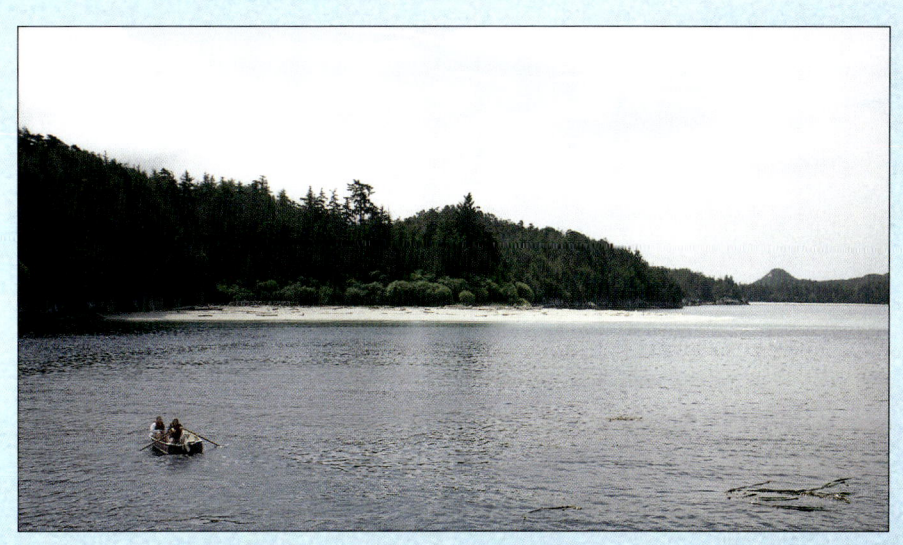

*Above and bottom right: Boating fun in Adams Harbour and adjacent waterways at Hakai Pass.*

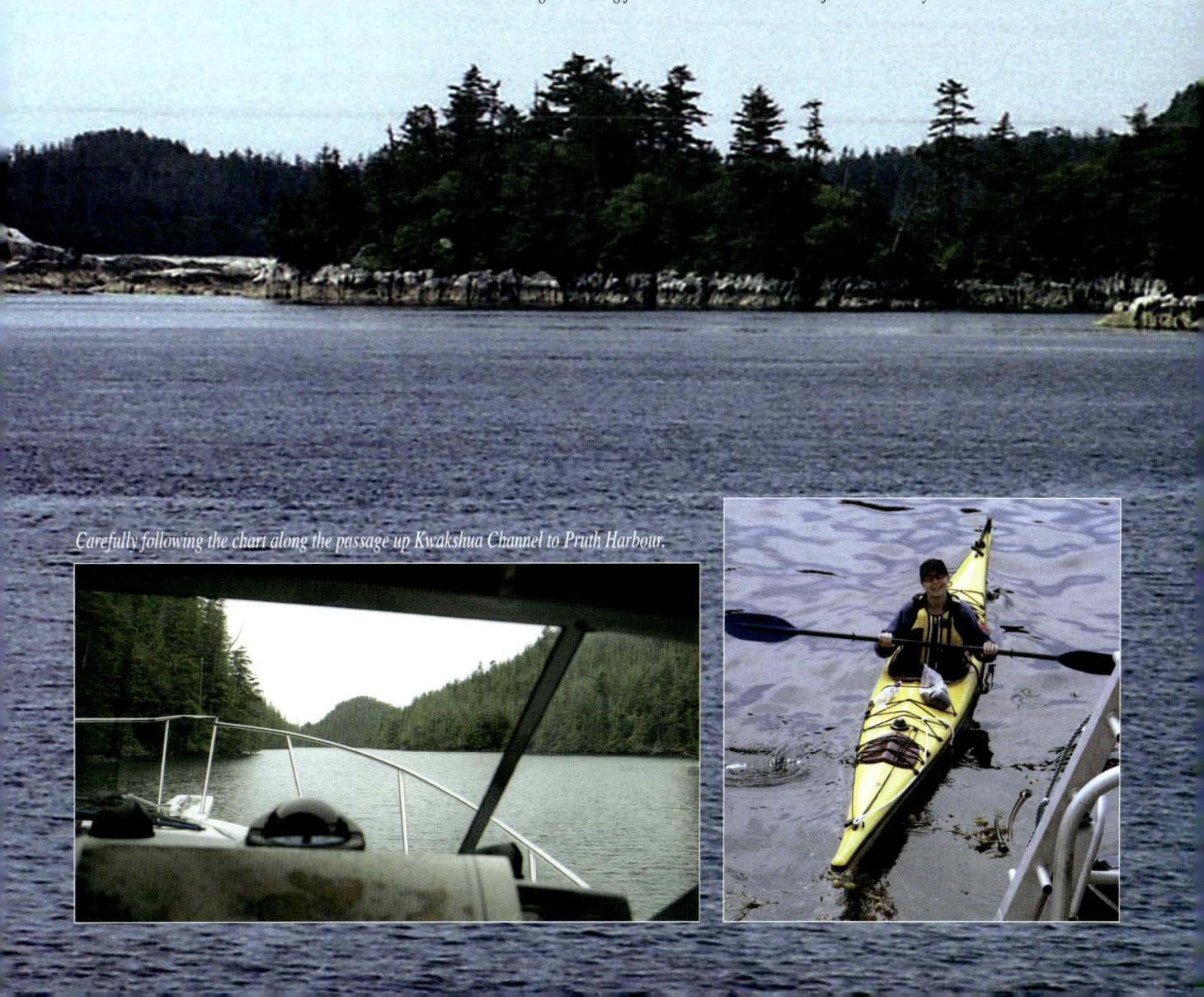

*Carefully following the chart along the passage up Kwakshua Channel to Pruth Harbour.*

# INDEX

*This index provides primary and some secondary reference to names of anchorages, marinas, passages, islands and features of the coast deemed to be notable. Most are found as headings, titles, subtitles and in bold typeface. Some appear only on the diagrams and/or in plain reference in the text. They may appear also elsewhere in the guide, not indexed, in a less notable reference.*

## A

Actaeon Sound  173, 182
Actress Passage  182
Adams Harbour  255
Ahclakerho Channel  245
Alert Bay  202, 213
Alert Bay public docks  217
Alexandra Passage  239
Allard Bay  253
Allison Harbour  192
Allison Sound  199
Anchorage Bight  241
Anchorage Cove  146
Anchor Islands  198
Anchor Islet  242
Angular Island  121
Apple Islet  106
Arran Rapids  23
Arrow Pass  116
Atchison Island  65

## B

Baker Island  86
Barber Passage  23
Baresides Bay  58
Baronet Passage  88
Baron Reef  88
Bauza Cove  211
Bear Cove  232
Beaver Cove Van I  203
Beaver Cove Rivers  249
Beaver Harbour  227
Beaver Inlet  42
Belleisle Sound  146

Bell Rocks  88
Bend Island  75
Benjamin Group  120
Bere Point  224
Bermingham Island  148
Berry Cove  150
Berry Island  104
Bessborough Bay  44
Beware Cove  95
Beware Passage  91, 94
Bickley Bay  35
Big Bay  22
Big Frypan Bay  251
Billygoat Bay  56
Billy Procter  130
Bilton Island  249
Blackfish Sound  203
Blackney Channel  242
Blackney Passage  89
Blenkinsop Bay  47
Blind Channel  40
Blind Channel Resort  38
Block Island  31
Blunden Harbour  190
Blunden Bay  238
Boat Bay  60, 88, 202
Bockett Islets  65
Bond Lagoon  183
Bond Sound  78
Bones Bay  68
Bonwick Island  86, 118
Booker Lagoon  124
Bootleg Bay  117
Boughey Bay  62
Bowers Islands  67
Bradley Lagoon  190
Bramham Island  195
Broughton Lagoon  151
Broughton Lake  154
Broughton Strait  203
Brown's Bay  49
Brown's Bay Marina  49
Browning Pass  239
Bughouse Bay  175
Burdwood Group  134
Burial Cove  65
Burly Bay  172
Bush Islets  202
Butress Island  195

## C

Call Inlet  65

Calm Channel  26
Cameleon Harbour  31
Campbell River  49
Canoe Passage  98
Cape Caution  237
Care Island  94
Care Rock  94
Carey Group  98, 100
Carriden Bay  167
Carrie Bay  117
Carter Passage  156, 185
Cattle Islands  227, 232
Caution Cove  95
Cecil Island  151
Chained Islands  49
Chancellor Channel  42
Charles Bay  37
Charlotte Bay  196, 200
Chatham Channel  65, 67
Chatham Point  49
Chief Nollis Bay  199
Christie Passage  239
Clapp Passage  77
Claydon Bay  164
Clio Channel  68, 88
Clock Rock  89
Cockatrice Bay  189
Compton Island  91
Cook Island  95
Cooper Reach  42
Cordero Channel  37
Cordero Islets  37, 39
Cordero Lodge  37
Cormorant Island  213
Cougar Inlet  195
Cramer Pass  134
Crawford Anchorage  37, 39
Crease Island  86, 97, 104
Creasy Bay  183
Crib Island  121
Cullen Harbour  123
Current Passage  54
Cutter Cove  69
Cypress Harbour  150

## D

Darby Channel  249
Dawson's Landing  249
Davis Bay  173
Deep Harbour  124
Deloraine Islands  192
Dent Island Resort  29

Dent Rapids  22
Devil's Hole  22
Dickson Island  125, 187
Discovery Passage  49
Dorman Island  70
Double Bay  106, 108
Douglas Bay  44, 46
Draney Inlet  253
Drury Inlet  173, 180
Duck Cove  114
Duncanby Lndng Marina  246
Dunsany Passage  167
Dusky Cove  118

## E

Earl Ledge  56
East Bay  203
East Cracroft Island  75
East Eden  118, 120
East Thurlow Island  39
Echo Bay  77, 126
Ecological Park  216
Eden Island  86, 120
Edith Cove  42, 43
Edna Mathews Island  250
Egg Island  238, 246
Eliot Passage  89, 98
Ellis Bay  200
Embley Lagoon  165, 167
Erasmus Island  37, 39
Exposed Anchorage  250

## F

Fanny Island  55
Farewell Harbour  105
Farquharson Island  70
Fifer Bay  253
Finn Bay  250
Fish Egg Inlet  253
Fishhook Bay  253
Fish Trap Bay  254
Fitz Hugh Sound  253
Florence Lake  31
Fly Basin  242
Fort Rupert  227
Forward Bay  60, 202
Forward Harbour  44
Fox Rock  150
Frazer Bay  42
Frederick Arm  35
Frederick Bay  196
Freshwater Bay  106

Freshwater Cove  185
Frigate Bay  250
Frypan Bay  252
Fury Island  250

# G

Gator Gardens  216
Geetla Inlet  249
George Point  122
Gildersleeve Bay  254
Gilford Island Village  116
Glendale Cove  114
Gnarled Islets  242
Goat Island  97, 104
Gods Pocket  233, 239
Goldstream Harbour  255
Goletas Channel  239
Good Hope Cannery  246
Goose Bay  245
Granite Bay  51
Grappler Sound  164
Grebe Cove  117
Greene Point Rapids  42
Green Island  254
Greenway Sound  154
Griffiths Islet  39
Growler Cove  88, 202
Gunner Point  47
Gwa-yas-dums  116
Gwa'yi  146

# H

Haddington Island  213, 219
Hadley Bay  67
Hakai Pass  254
Hand Bay  183
Handfield Bay  31
Hanson Island  108
Harbledown Island  86, 97
HardyBay  232
Hardy Inlet  250
Harriet Point  198
Havannah Channel  60, 202
Hayle Bay  148
Health Bay  116
Helen Bay  173
Helmcken Island  54
Hemasila Inlet  249
Hemming Bay  32
Henrietta Island  114
Heydon Bay  43
Hooper Island  178

Hopetown Passage  167
Hornet Passage  136
Hoy Bay  164
Hudson island  118
Hull Island  62
Humpback Bay  54

# I

Illahie Inlet  254
Indian Channel  97
Indian Islands  65
Insect Island  122
Irving Passage  246

# J

Jackson Bay  47
Jamieson Island  91
Jennis Bay  180
Jennis Bay Marina  180
Jesse Island  58
Jimmy Judd Island  23
Joe Cove  118, 120
Johnstone Strait  49
Jones Cove  239
Jumble Island  89

# K

Kamano Island  94
Kanish Bay  49
Karlukwees  92
Keith Anchorage  255
Kelsey Bay  54
Kenneth Passage  164, 167
Kilbella River  250
King Bay  196
Kingcome Inlet  145
Kinnaird Island  167
Klaoitsis  88
Klaquaek Channel  248
Knight Inlet  89, 113
Knox Bay  53
Kuldekduma Island  211
Kumlah Island  77, 78
Kwatsi Bay  78
Kwatsi Bay Marina  79

# L

Lady Boot Cove  118
Lagoon Cove  70
Laura Bay  148
Laura Cove  148
Leche Islet  173

Leroy Cove  241
Lewall Inlet  256
Lewis Cove  189
Lewis Rocks  189
Little Nimmo Bay  172
Long Island  124
Loughborough Inlet  42

# M

Macgowan Bay  173, 180
Mackenzie Sound  164
Magee Channel  248
Malcolm Island  223
Mamaliliculla  98
Maple Cove  114
Margaret Bay  243
Marsh Bay  190, 192
Mars Island  86, 118
Martin Islets  77
Mary Island  48
Masterman Islands  227
Matilpi  61, 65
McBride Bay  42
McBride Bay, Seymour  243
McEwan Rock  239
McIntosh Bay  137
McLeod Bay  47
Meade Bay  117
Mereworth Sound  199
Mermaid Bay  29
Midsummer Island  89, 114
Miles Inlet  192
Millar Group  190
Millbrook Cove  242
Millbrook Rocks  242
Miller Bay  150, 151
Milly Island  58
Mink Island  39
Minstrel Island  68
Mist Islet  61
Misty Passage  122
Mitchell Bay  224
Monday Anchorage  121
Monk's Wall  96
Moore Bay  139
Moore Rock  190
Morgan's Landing  28
Morris Islet  173
Mound Island  106
Mount Ick  154
Muirhead Islands  173
Murray Labyrinth  192

# N

Nakwakto Rapids  194
Napier Bay  185
Naysash Inlet  245
Negro Rock  68
Nepah Lagoon  164, 167
New Vancouver  103
Nickoll Passage  77
Nimmo Bay  164, 172
Nixon Rock  51
Nodales Channel  31
Nugent Sound  198

# O

O'Brien Bay  137
Old Passage  122
Open Cove  60
Otter Cove  51, 53
Oyster Bay  254

# P

Pack Creek  199
Parson Bay  106
Parson Island  88
Pearse Islands  108, 211
Pearse Passage  211
Pearse Peninsula  148
Peel Rocks  35
Peet Bay  199
Penphrase Passage  148
Penrose Island  250
Perley Island  70
Philip Inlet  253
Phillips Arm  35, 42
Piddell Bay  31
Pierre's Bay  134
Pierre's Echo Bay  128
Plumper Islands  108, 203
Polkinghorne Islands  125
Port Elizabeth  114
Port Hardy  231
Port Harvey Resort  62
Port McNeill  218
Port McNeill Boat Hbr  218
Port McNeill Fuel/Marina  218
Port Neville  58
Potts Bay  89, 114
Potts Lagoon  90
Pruth Bay  255
Pulteney Point  227
Punt Rock  106

## Q

Quarterdeck Marina  232
Queen Charlotte Strait  202

## R

Race Passage  54
Raleigh Passage  134, 148
Range Island  60
Raynor Group  184
Restless Bay  173, 175
Retreat Pass  117
Richards Channel  184
Richmond Bay  173
Ridge Islets  117
Ripple Rock  49
Ripple Shoal  55
Rivers Inlet  245
Roaringhole Rapids  165
Robbers Nob  58
Robson Bight  60, 203
Rock Bay  53
Rocky Islets  32
Rough Bay  227
Round Island  227

## S

Safety Cove  254
Sail Island  114
Sambo Point  68
Sandell Bay  250
Sarah Islets  104
Sargeaunt Passage  77
Scarlett Point  239
Schooner Channel  192, 194
Schooner Retreat  250
Scott Cove  134
Seabreeze Island  114
Seagate wharf  231
Secure Anchorage  250
Seymour Inlet  194
Shawl Bay  134, 139
Shawl Bay Marina  143
Shelter Bay  192
Shewell Island  77
Shield Island  242
Ship Rock  242
Shoal Bay  34
Shoal Bay Lodge  34
Shoal Harbour  125
Sidney Bay  42
Simoom Sound  137
Simpson Island  153
Sir Edmund Bay  150
Sir Edmund Head  150
Siwiti Rock  190
Skeene Bay  182
Skull Cove  192
Slate Point  106
Slingsby Channel  194
Small Inlet  51
Smith Sound  239
Soderman Cove  65
Sointula Harbour  223
Sonora Island  29
Sophia Islands  91, 202
Spiller Passage  118
Spout Islet  106, 108
Spring Passage  89, 117
Spur Rocks  246
Stackhouse Island  150
Steamboat Bay  172
Steep Islet  118
Storm Islands  239
Strachan Bay  199
Stuart Island  22
Stuart Island Dock  27
Stuart Narrows  175
Stubbs Island  108, 211
Sullivan Bay  161
Sullivan Bay Resort  159
Sunday Harbour  121
Sunderland Channel  44, 47
Sunshine Bay  249
Sutherland Bay  173
Sutlej Channel  136, 184
Swanson Island  86

## T

Takush Harbour  241
Tallac Bay  37, 39
Tancred Bay  173
Telegraph Cove  205
Telegraph Cove Marina  206
Telegraph Cove Resorts  206
The 'Mainland'  125
The Blowhole  70
The Lake  248, 251
Thief Island  139
Thief Rocks  139
Thompson Sound  78
Thurston Bay  31
Thurston Marine Park  31
Topaze Harbour  42, 47
Tracey Harbour  185
Tracey Island  118
Treadwell Bay  194
Tribune Channel  77
Trivett Island  148
Trivett Rock  148
Tsibass Lagoon  182
Tully Island  31
Tuna Point  47, 56
Turnbull Cove  164
Turn Island  53
Turnour Point  95
Turret Rock  195

## U

U'mista Cultural Centre  217

## V

Vere Cove  55
Village Cove  196, 199
Village Group  100
Village Island  86, 97
Viner Sound  137
Viscount Island  77

## W

Waddington Bay  117
Wadhams  246
Wahkana Bay  78
Waiatt Bay  51
Walbran Island  249
Walkem Islands  53
Wannock River  250
Warren Islands  65
Waterfall Inlet  254
Watson Cove  79, 85
Watson Island  164
Wawatle Bay  196, 200
Wedge Island  89
Welde Rock  173
Wellbore Channel  41, 44
Wells Passage  184, 237
Westerman Bay  196, 199
Weynton Passage  211
Whirlpool Rapids  42, 44
Whitebeach Passage  91, 97
Woods Lagoon  198
Woods Point  151

## Y

Yorke Island  55
Yucultas  22
Yuki Bay  165

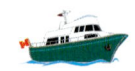

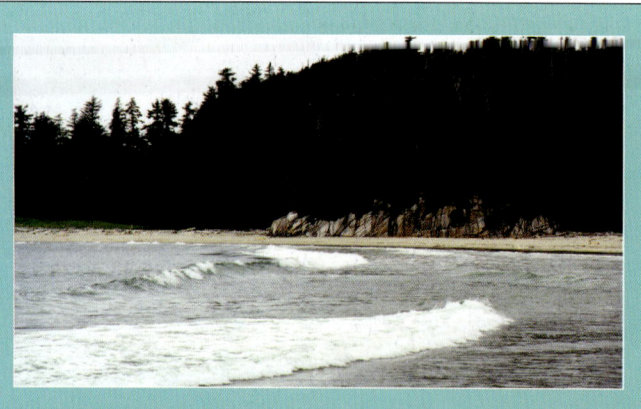

---

Use of metric in this guide:
Metric has been used extensively in the guide in keeping with Canadian hydrographic charts. Therefore depths are in metres.
Distances are approximate, and have been shown in nautical miles. Canadian English has been used for the spelling of metres and kilometres.

# Bibliography and recommended marine books on the areas covered in this guide

**A Guide to the Western Seashore**. Rick M. Harbo. Hancock House, Surrey, BC. 1988.
**Accidental Airline.** Howard White and Jim Spilsbury. Harbour Publishing.
**Anchorages and Marine Parks**. Peter Vassilopoulos. Pacific Marine Publishing. Marineguides.com. Guide to anchorages and marine parks in British Columbia and the San Juan Islands. 2008.
**Best Anchorages of the Inside Passage.** Anne Vipond and William Kelly. Ocean Cruise Guides. 2006.
**British Columbia Coast Names**. Captain John T. Walbran, Douglas and McIntyre
**Canadian Tide and Current Tables.** Pacific Coast all volumes. Ottawa-Department of Fisheries and Oceans. Annual.
**Charlies Charts North to Alaska.** Charles E. Wood. Margo Wood. PO Box 352. Seal Beach, CA. 90740.
**Coastal Villages.** Liv Kennedy. Harbour Publishing.
**Cruising Beyond Desolation Sound**. John Chappel.
**Cruising the Secret Coast.** Jennifer and James Hamilton. Weatherly Press. Bellevue Washington. 2008.
**Desolation Sound and the Discovery Islands**. Bill Wolferstan.
**Docks and Destinations.** Peter Vassilopoulos, Pacific Marine Publishing. Marineguides.com. Guide to marinas in British Columbia and Puget Sound in Washington State. GPS coordinates included. 2011.
**Dreamspeaker Cruising Guides**. Laurence and Anne Yeadon-Jones. Harbour Publishing.
**Encyclopedia of Raincoast Place Names.** Andrew Scott. Harbour Publishing. 2009.
**Exploring the Inside Passage to Alaska**. A Cruising Guide. Don Douglas. Fine Edge Productions. Bishop, California.1995.
**Exploring the South Coast of British Columbia.** 2nd edition by Don Douglass and Réanne Hemingway-Douglas. FineEdge.com, 1999.
**Exploring Puget Sound and British Columbia Olympia to Queen Charlotte Sound.** Stephen Hilson. Evergreen Pacific Publishing. Revised 1996.
**Following the Curve of Time.** Cathy Converse. Touchwood Editions. 2008.
**Full Moon, Flood Tide.** Billy Proctor and Yvonne Maximchuk. Harbour Publishing, 2003.
**Grizzlies in Their Backyard.** Beth Day. Heritage House, 1994.
**Heart of the Raincoast**. Billy Proctor and Alexandra Morton. Horsdal and Shubart, 1998.
**High Boats**. Pat Wastell Norris. Harbour Publishing.
**Journeys Through the Inside Passage**. Joe Upton
**Local Knowledge**. Kevin Monahan. Fine Edge. Anacortes, WA.
**Marine Weather Hazards Manual**. A guide to local forecasts and conditions. Vancouver. Environment Canada. 1990.
**Naturally Salty**. Marianne Scott. TouchWood Editions, 2003.
**Navigating the Coast**. J.W. Langlois.
**North to Alaska**. Hugo Anderson. Anderson Publishing Co. 1993.
**Oceanography of the British Columbia Coast**. Richard E. Thomson. Ottawa. Dept of Fisheries and Aquatic Sciences. 1981.
**Sailing Directions. British Columbia Coast (North Portion and South Portion)**. Ottawa. Dept of Fisheries and Oceans.
**Sailing with Vancouver**. Sam McKinney. Touchwood Editions.
**Secret Coastline I and II**. Andrew Scott. Heritage Group.
**Sea Kayaking Vancouver Island**. Gary Backlund and Paul Grey. Harbour Publishing. 2003
**Seven Knot Summers**. Beth Hill. Horsdal and Shubart, 1994.
**Sointula**. Paula Wild. Harbour Publishing.
**Spilsbury's Coast.** Howard White and Jim Spilsbury. Harbour Publishing.
**The Inlet**. Helen Piddington. Harbour Publishing.
**Time and Tide: A History of Telegraph Cove (Raincoast Chronicles 16)**. Pat Wastell Norris. Harbour Publishing.
**Totem Poles and Tea**. Hughina Harold. Heritage House, 1996.
**The Curve of Time**. M. Wylie Blanchet. Whitecap Books.
**Two Wolves at the Dawn of Time**. Judith Williams.
**Upcoast Summers**. Beth Hill. Horsdal and Shubart, 1985.
**Waggoner**. Fine Edge Publishing. Seattle. Annual cruising guide to the Washington ad BC coast.
**Weatherly Waypoint Guides**. Robert Hale. Volume 3: Includes Desolation Sound to Port Hardy.
**Woodsmen of the West**. M. Allerdale Grainger. 1908.
**Whistle Up the Inlet.** Gerald Rushton.

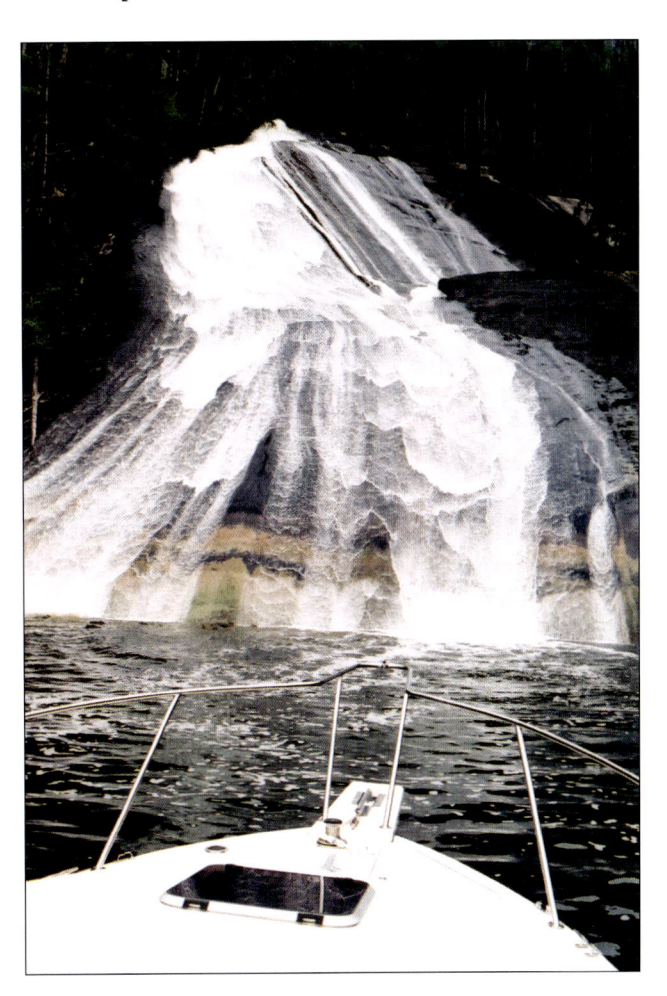

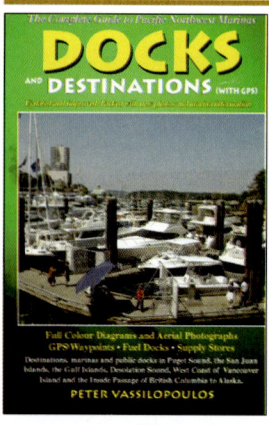

## Docks and Destinations
ISBN 0-919317-43-7    2010
With GPS. (Eighth edition)
Colour pages included.
This is a complete guide to marinas on the coast of British Columbia and Puget Sound, Washington State. It covers the inside passage in geographical sequence to Ketchikan, Alaska from the San Juan Islands. The west coast of Vancouver Island is included from north to south ending in Olympia, Puget Sound. The book is filled with many aerial and ambient photographs and descriptive diagrams with pertinent information on marina services and facilities. GPS Waypoints are included for all entries in this popular marine guide.

Author Peter Vassilopoulos has travelled extensively throughout the entire area during more than 35 years of boating in the Pacific Northwest, and provides up-to-date information on where to go, what to look for and why to visit the destinations included.

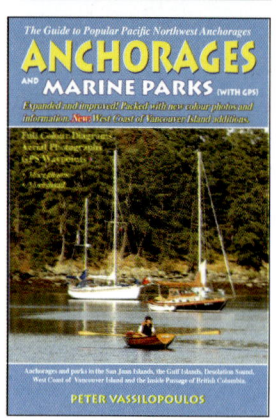

## Anchorages and Marine Parks
ISBN 978- 0-919317-44-4    2008.
A companion to Docks and Destinations, this book is a complete coastal guide to marine parks and anchorages. It covers the area from the San Juan Islands to Ketchikan following the coast in geographical sequence from south to north, returning down the west coast of Vancouver Island in a north to south progression. The guide is loaded with aerial and ambient photographs and numerous diagrams clearly depicting location of anchorages and parks.

Bind your books. The best way to keep them is to have them spiral bound at an office supply or print shop.

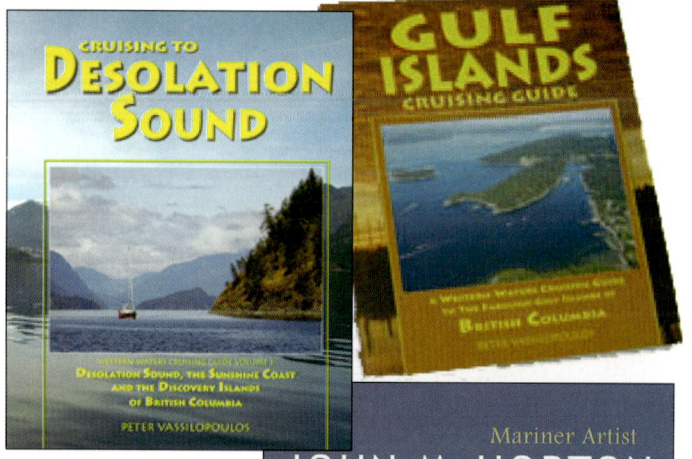

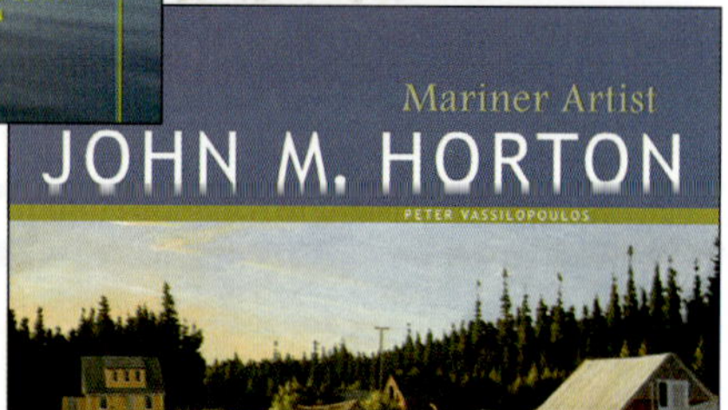

## Cruising to Desolation Sound
ISBN 978-0-919317-45-1
Peter Vassilopoulos    2009.
This well-illustrated, comprehensive cruising guide takes the user to Desolation Sound by way of Indian Arm, Howe Sound and the Sunshine Coast. It also features the fabulous Princess Louisa Inlet and the Discovery Islands.

## Gulf Islands Cruising Guide
ISBN 0919317-38-3
Peter Vassilopoulos    2006
The most popular cruising destination in the Pacific Northwest is fully covered in this guide to the Gulf Islands. It includes anchorages, towns and villages, marinas and public docks with hundreds of photographs and diagrams.

## Mariner Artist John M Horton
ISBN 978-1-894974-34-9
Peter Vassilopoulos    2007
Published by Heritage House, this magnificent coffee-table book features large page images of this marine artist known for his significant, historic works.

*Hundreds of aerial and ambient photographs are featured in all of Peter Vassilopoulos' marine guides.*

Enquiries to
**Pacific Marine Publishing**
boating@dccnet.com
**Phone
604-943-4198**

You are welcome to email the author at *boating@dccnet.com* to discuss questions or your cruising travel plans on the BC coast.